7 X 1/10 ✓ 2/10

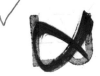

2X 12/04 ✓ 6/05

FEB 27 2003

Screaming to be Heard

Hormone Connections Women Suspect and Doctors *Still* Ignore

Screaming to be Heard

Hormone Connections Women Suspect and Doctors *Still* Ignore

Completely Revised and Expanded

ELIZABETH LEE VLIET, M.D.

M. Evans and Company, Inc.
New York

M. Evans and Company, Inc.
216 East 49th Street
New York, NY 10017

Cartoons and the original artwork for diagrams used in this book are by Gordon Vliet.

Library of Congress Cataloging-in-Publication Data

Vliet, Elizabeth Lee, 1946–
    Screaming to be heard : hormonal connections women suspect . . . and doctors ignore /
Elizabeth Lee Vliet. — 1st ed.
        p.   cm.
    Includes bibliographical references and index.
    ISBN 0-87131-914-4
    1. Women—Health and hygiene.   I. Title.
RA778.V55   1995
613'.04244—dc20   94-49419
                                                                        CIP

Design and type formatting by by Bernard Schleifer

Manufactured in the United States of America

.9   8   7   6   5   4

This book is dedicated to:

• The courage and persistence of my women patients—and their partners—who listened to their inner voice of knowing, and who pursued answers to their health questions in spite of medical teachings that often seemed to contradict women's wisdom and insights. As I have listened, you have taught me; your wisdom and experiences will now benefit others as your words are given a voice in this book.

• My mother, Virginia Lee Hutcheson Davis, and her mother, Nellie Butler Hutcheson, women of strength and faith in the face of adversity, women of intellect and wisdom, women who taught me to stand firm for what I believed in, women who taught me to listen well to the voice of wisdom.

• My husband, Gordon Cheesman Vliet, a quiet strength and soulmate, who has shared this journey of helping others and blessed my life richly. He was among the first who encouraged and nurtured me in my pursuit of a medical career as well as the exploration of new avenues for healing.

• Our Creator, who has given us this incredible blessing of life, who sustains us through adversities, and who has provided guidance, insights, and strength to carry out my life's work.

ACKNOWLEDGMENTS

I would like to once again give my deep appreciation to all of those teachers and encouragers I acknowledged in the First Edition of *Screaming to Be Heard*. Thank you for your role in helping me grow and develop as a physician and author.

As the years have passed, there are additional special people without whose efforts and support I would not be able to sustain our mission to gain attention for the overlooked hormone connections and provide help to the hundreds of women we see in each of the *HER Place* centers.

Kathryn A. Kresnik, who saw the enormous need for this work in women's health and has invested time and energy above and beyond our initial agreements. Without her dedication, persistence, calm presence, and commitment, we would not have been able to build the successful women's center in Texas or sustain the outreach efforts with my speaking and writing.

James Talmadge Boyd, M.D., FACOG, a caring and capable gynecologist who has long seen the need for more individualized approaches to women's health and hormonal needs. Since joining our group, he has shown that it is the *person* of the physician that makes a women's health specialist, not the *gender*. I have continued to learn from his experience and expertise, and he has added much to our practice, in both the art and science of medicine.

Carolyn Margraf, M.S., R.N., C.S., Clinical Specialist, and Donna Gilson, R.N., M.S.N., C.M.T/Clinical Specialist—both are extraordinarily gifted healers and advocates for women. Their dedication to the highest standards in the healing arts from many traditions, and their courage in the face of their own health challenges and life struggles have been an inspiration to me and to our staff and patients. Their spiritual and physical presence are gifts that enrich all of us at *HER Place*.

To Gordon Vliet, Linda Snyder, Samia Yasmin, Brandi McCoy, and Susan Anderson, my grateful appreciation for your efforts to keep the offices running well, to be responsive to the needs of our patients while supporting me in my writing responsibilities. And to Victoria Hahn, once again, the computer wizard who helped solve the technical difficulties so the book project could proceed.

Our business advisors, Tony Rickert (and his assistant, Debbie White) and David Cohen, have provided indispensible guidance, support, and encouragement through challenging times, helping us to grow responsibly.

My publisher, George C. de Kay, who has continued to be committed to seeing that my work and message reach a broader audience of women.

My editors, Betty Anne Crawford, who understood the importance of the message, and shaped and guided me as a beginning author with the First Edition; and PJ Dempsey, who helped hone and focus the Revised Edition while keeping the qualities that have touched responsive chords for readers. Both are women who understood why this book was so important and took a personal interest in seeing it done well.

And I also thank you, each of the women and men, who have given me the great priviledge of your trust as you came for consults and guidance on your heath problems. I have been awed by the courage you have shown in the face of your adversities, and your persistence in seeking answers. As I have listened to your insights, you have also taught me much that goes beyond the textbooks of medicine. Your experiences and words woven throughout this book are your legacy passed on to touch and help others. This book is your voice, too.

Contents

1: Screaming to Be Heard! Listening to Women's Voices   1

Challenges and Controversies in Women's Health: Issues That Affect YOU • The Invisible Woman in Health Research • Medical Problems That Hit Women Harder • Behind the Headlines: Alarming Facts You Still Don't Hear • Shocking Facts in Women's Health • Impediments to Improved Health Care for Women • Why Women Aren't Heard: Stereotypes and Negative Labels • Women's Traditional Healing Wisdom: Devalued and Ignored • Setting the Stage for Change

2: Hormones: A Guide to Your Body Cycles   24

What Is a Hormone? • Brain–Body Hormonal Communication Pathways • The Menstrual Cycle RHYTHM of Changes Through Our Lives • What Happens When Estrogen Declines: Hormone Changes Through the Decades • The Thyroid: The "Great Imitator"—Problems Often Missed in Women

3: Hormones and the Brain   54

The Brain: Master Conductor of Our Body's Orchestra • New Understandings of the Brain's Chemical Messengers • It's Not All in Your Imagination! The Biology of Mood Changes • Insights on Depressive and Anxiety Symptoms versus Psychiatric Disorders • Estrogen Effects on Serotonin and Other Mood Regulators • The Brain's Alarm Center: Hormone Triggers of "Anxiety," "Racing Heart," and "Flutters" • Progesterone Effects on the Brain • Progesterone Effects on Growth Hormone Production • Testosterone and the Brain • Future Directions

4: Hormones of Pregnancy and Stress: Progesterone and Cortisol

Progesterone's Discovery • Natural Body Cycles and Progesterone's Roles • Progesterone and Progestins: Understanding the Important Differences • Progesterone Effects on Sleep • Progesterone Effects on Pain Regulation • Progesterone Interaction with Oher Hormones: Insulin and Cortisol • Progesterone Effects on Muscle and Connective Tissue • Progesterone Effects on Metabolism • Laboratory Tests • Current Issues Concerning Progesterone • Cortisol and Stress: Interactions with Our Ovary Hormones

5: The Big Question: Has Anybody Seen My Estrogen?

...And Will Someone Help Me Look for It? What about Blood Tests for Hormones? • The Three Types of Estrogen for Human Females • What Do We Mean by Natural or Synthetic? • Sources and Components of Various Estrogen Products • New Research on Estrogen and a Woman's Body • Different Estrogens, Different Effects • Effective Evalution of Hormone Levels to Assess Therapy • Beyond Bones: Estrogen Effects on Skin, Hair, Eyes, and Other Fun Facts

6: Testosterone amd DHEA: The Forgotten *Women's* Hormones:

Myths About "The Male Hormones" for Women • Women's Sexuality: An Overlooked Concern in Health Care • Women's Bodies Do Make Testosterone • Synthetic versus Natural Micronized Testosterone • My Response to the Myths about "Male Hormones" for Women • DHEA: Promises and Pitfalls • Finding What's Right for You: Options Available • The Role of Hormone Testing: Blood versus Saliva • Keeping Your Sexual Vitality As You Age • Resources to Help You Rekindle the Sexual Fires

7: The Persnickety P's: PMS, PCOS, Premature Menopause, Perimenopause, and Postpartum Depression

Is It PMS, PCOS, or Perimenopause? • Just What Is PMS? • Common Sympton Clusters in PMS • What Are Some of the Causes of PMS? • Is It the Blues, the Blahs, or Major Depression? • Stress: Vicious Cycle Effects on Hormones, Anxiety, and Depression • How Are All of These Phenomena Related? • How Can I Tell What My Problem Is? Getting Checked Out • Options for Feeling Better • Summary: Heading into the Future

My Hormones? • What Exactly is Incontinence, or "Leaky Bladder"?
• Help Ahead: Hormonal Balance, Biofeedback, Exercise, and Other
Options • One Woman's Experience • Summary

The Use of "Doctors" in the Title

When I use the word *doctors* in the title of my book, I am *not* referring just to physicians, or medical doctors. Indeed, it is doctorate-level professionals in many fields who, as teachers and researchers, have ignored the biological gender differences that are the focus of this book. In the original meaning, doctor meant "teacher" or "great teacher." Historically, the first "doctor" degree was doctor of philosophy (Ph.D.), not doctor of medicine (M.D.). Philosophy is derived from Greek words meaning "love of wisdom." Individuals who loved learning and gaining wisdom enough to continue their studies for an advanced degree were then awarded the doctor of philosophy. The new "doctors" typically then became "teachers" of others. Today we have a variety of doctorate-level degrees in diverse fields: the branch of medicine known as osteopathy (D.O.), education (Ed.D.), social work (D.S.W.), science (Sc.D.), Ministry/Theology (D.Min.), and others.

An example came up a while ago illustrating ways in which doctorate-level professionals in diverse fields have failed to consider the crucial biological differences in women's health. At the annual meeting of the Society of Menstrual Cycle Research at which my paper on "Hormonal Relationships in Perimenopausal Mood Changes" was presented, many of the Ph.D.s, Ed.D.s, and doctorate-level nurses (all of whom were women) seemed to discount the *biological* hormonal connections. One presenter in another session said: "Forget all this stuff about serotonin and estrogen; we all know that mood problems at menopause are caused by life stresses. The medical industry is just trying to medicalize everything." Think about the ramifications of this comment. Does seeking good science to explain how women's bodies function mean we have "medicalized" it, or just that we are trying to get answers we all want and need?

Which is more stigmatizing: to think that suddenly, when you reach menopause, you can't cope with life stress and become depressed or anxious because you suddenly lost the coping abilities you have had all along, or to explore whether hormonal changes may be adversely affecting how you feel and altering your usual coping strategies? Collectively, our culture accepted the disempowering view that women are weaker and anxious or neurotic. Why should it be difficult to acknowledge or accept the idea that changes in body chemistry might detract from our usual psychological strengths and coping abilities? It seems to me that it is actually more empowering to recognize the role our biology plays in how we feel emotionally, spiritually, and physically and then use this understanding to explore choices and options so that we may feel our best.

The presenter I just described was a woman, speaking to an audience of all women professionals. We can't blame only men for these attitudes. Perhaps I am even more disappointed when women aren't any more sensitive to other women's needs than male physicians. Clearly, medical doctors are not the only ones who fail to see the integrated picture of women's health in its totality. In my view, doctors in many fields ignore crucial biological links in women's health. How can we truly have gender-based biology and medical approaches if we do not use reliable methods of measuring women's hormone levels? This is a major reason that we still don't have answers to the crucial questions women consumers have been raising about their health for decades. In my view, all of this must change if "women's health" is to truly meet women's needs for the twenty-first century and beyond.

A Special Note to Physicians

Although we were taught "about" hormones in medical school and residency, we were not taught about the hormonal connections I am raising. My comments are meant not to be an indictment of medicine but to stimulate a broader view of the integration needed in women's health research and clinical care and in physician education. I also hope to help you see women patients with new insights about important *overlooked* hormonal connections, and to hear what women have been trying to tell us. We have much we can learn and share with our profession to improve the way women's health services are conceptualized and delivered. Our patients can teach us a great deal, if we just stop to listen to the wisdom of their voices of experience.

ELIZABETH LEE VLIET, M.D.
Founder, HER Place:
Health Enhancement Renewal for Women, Inc.
Tucson, Arizona, and Dallas–Ft. Worth, Texas

Introduction to the Revised Edition: Reflections and Comments

It has been an amazing journey for me over the past five years since *Screaming to Be Heard* was first published. Thousands of women have heard my talks around the country and come up to me afterward to share experiences similar to those in the first edition of my book. Letters from women here and abroad have described poignant and painful journeys through the health care maze, trying to find answers that make sense and help them feel better. Women have called our offices, identifying with the descriptions I wrote in *Screaming to Be Heard,* saying "Hello, I am chapter 10, or I am chapter 7 . . . " Patients coming for consults in Tucson and Dallas–Ft. Worth have written detailed summaries of their arduous efforts to regain their health. And in all, the stories remain the same as I first described years ago: Women aren't being listened to, their insights are discounted, their theories written off, their requests for appropriate blood tests ignored or made fun of, and their requests for consideration of hormone issues still being dismissed by such inane statements as "You're too young for menopause (or perimenopause)" or "It's just stress, dear, you need to see a therapist." I recently received a four-page fax from a women sharing her experiences in health care settings over the last twenty-five years—she began her fax with "eeeeeeEEEEEkkkkkKKK—that's my 25 year scream trying to be heard and get these problems addressed!"

This woman expresses the consumer perspective I hear daily in my offices, letters about my book, responses to my former radio show, women's feedback at talks I have done across the country over the last twenty years, and even on the phone when clerks (male and female) ask me what kind of doctor I am—as soon as I mention hormones, I get unsolicited comments about *their* hormone questions and experiences. A recent example occurred when I called to arrange a ride to the airport, commenting that the driver might have to wait a few minutes while I finished a talk. The woman asked what I was talking about, and when I told her the topic, she said, "I've had ten children and I sure know about what those hormones can do! I should come to that talk."

Do I speak for all women? No. Some women are truly blessed to have an easy transition from reproductive years to menopausal years. But even these women still need encouragement to practice the positive lifestyle habits that will keep them healthy and aging gracefully and well. In my writings and clinical work, I speak for those who *don't* have this easy transition. I speak both as a physician and a consumer, one who has been a patient many times. I speak for those who have been disenfranchised by the way medicine is practiced for women in this country. I speak for those who have had their problems overpsychologized without having even a basic workup of ovarian function. I speak for those who have difficulty getting help from our fragmented, male-physiology-based model of western medicine. And I speak for the husbands and partners of these women, many of whom have broken down in tears watching the women they love not get the help they need. My mission in health care is to speak for those who have shared their voices and their struggles with me in these many settings.

If you are one of the women who has a difficult time with hormonal changes and problems, my book is for you. This book is about these *overlooked and ignored hormonal connections;* what we *do* know about hormonal effects on brain-body systems and how these hormonal effects interact with the endocrine, immune, metabolic, cardiovascular, respiratory, musculoskeletal, reproductive, urinary, and nervous systems. In writing about all these hormonal connections, am I saying all women at menopause need or should take supplemental hormones? NO. I do think, however, that *all* women deserve balanced information, proper evaluation, compassionate assistance in making an individual risk assessment, assistance in sorting out their priorities and values for their health, and help in making decisions suited to their needs at a given time. I also think women deserve the same approach to individualizing amounts and types of hormones as we give to men with cardiovascular medications—as is standard practice for almost all other medications we use today.

Although I may sometimes sound critical of my fellow physicians, they don't carry all the blame for the issues I am raising. There is plenty of blame to go around—from the media hype, television news "health" sound bites, to headlines and articles written to increase sales rather than be accurate, to companies (alternative and conventional) focused on pushing their products, to insurance carriers that deny services tailored to women, to the FDA's use of outdated information for estrogen package inserts, based on Premarin rather than newer information on the natural human estradiol or the safer transdermal estradiol patches. We need constructive changes in all of these areas. As you read *Screaming to Be Heard,* consider what I have to say not as criticism, but as ideas for change, for growth, for finding ways to create a true partnership between patient, physician, allied health professionals, hospitals, insurance carriers, pharmaceutical companies, and health products suppliers.

To those of you readers who are professionals working with women's health programs and services around the country, remember that you are in a position to make a difference for today's women and those who will follow. You are with organizations, big and small, that have the power to bring balance and reason back to women's health, to bring back the heart and soul of the healing arts through your consumer education and services, and with your influence in the insurance industry and your development of physician education programs.

My vision for the twenty-first century is that we will celebrate the science we have available, disseminate it more effectively, and take advantage of ways to apply it in new approaches for our care of women. My dream is that we will listen to and value the insights, wisdom and experiences of our women as patients and create effective partnerships as we work together to help women achieve optimal health now that we have the opportunity to live so much longer. I hope this next millennium will bring these needed changes in how we approach women's health to help prevent the tragic consequences that have happened in the past to so many women and their families when these hormone connections are ignored. Let's make "power surges" have a new meaning . . . a health care relationship *powered* by respect for women's marvelous beings, by understanding of women's unique and wonderful biology, and by collaboration in shared partnership so that we are all *surging forward* with zest.

ELIZABETH LEE VLIET, M.D.
Tucson, Arizona

Introduction

Women are *still* not being listened to, not just in doctors' offices, but everywhere. Women's wisdom is ignored. Women's body knowledge is dismissed as "neurotic," "hypochondriacal," "hysterical." Women suffer in silence, alone with their fears: "Am I crazy? I know something is different about my body, but the doctors keep saying there's nothing wrong."

It's not just *male* physicians who don't listen or who discount women's ideas about what may be wrong. We physicians have all been taught by the same flawed system of education that does not fully listen to women's voices, does not adequately address women's body differences or value women's insights and experiences. Women physicians have also been taught the same negative stereotypes of women patients that male doctors have been taught. I will never forget a woman family physician I was considering asking to join my medical practice. She said, quite disdainfully, "I don't want to just work with women patients; they're so neurotic and complain all the time." I was shocked by her comments. Even with the advances in life and career options and opportunities for women, there is still a vast undercurrent of stigma women face when they enter the health care system as patients. This stigma permeates all levels, from doctors to nurses to insurance claims case managers who see women as "overutilizers of services." Actually, I think the primary reason that women utilize medical services more often than men is due to their body awareness, their being astute consumers, their willingness to dig for answers that make sense. Unfortunately, the fact is that their questions and problems often go unresolved since our medical approaches are based on male physiology and function.

Another key factor women face in getting good health care is their conditioned passivity. Women have been socialized to accept without question what an authority figure, in this case the physician, tells them. In spite of several decades of emphasis on teaching women to be more assertive, to ask questions, to seek second opinions, I still see this passivity by women unquestioningly accepting explanations and approaches with both traditional Western-trained physicians and with alternative or complementary medicine practitioners. Standing up for yourself and asking questions is not bitchy or aggressive; it just makes good sense when your health is at stake. Yet women who speak up are more likely to be labeled negatively by health professionals than are men who ask the same questions. At the same time, men and women who are more involved in their health care, who ask questions, who seek more information and alternatives, actually have better outcomes when illness strikes.

Women *are* able to make a difference when we ask questions and demand appropriate attention to our gender differences in health needs. Menopause is a good example of the success we achieve when we speak out. At first, just a few women spoke out, then more joined in as these realizations hit. What were whispers became louder as more women were talking, finding that others had similar experiences. Gail Sheehy published *The Silent Passage* in 1991, bringing menopause, the "M word," out of the closet, enabling us to more openly share experiences. The massive pioneering U.S. study of women's health needs, the landmark Women's Health Initiative, was launched about the same time. Since then, Women's Health has become a major *hot topic,* finally gaining the national attention it needed—BUT, and it is a big BUT—it often becomes even more frustrating when you are trying to find help amid the confusing, often conflicting information and media hype about menopause and other women's health topics.

For the woman approaching menopause, fears mount: "Am I getting Alzheimer's?" "Will I get breast cancer?" "What to do?" "Do I take hormones?" "What are the alternatives?" "What's natural, what's not?" "Where do I find answers that make sense?" Our questions still get blank stares from physicians. We are bombarded with media hype. We feel deluged with information. We feel confused. Silence again. Our voices become quiet. We discover that once more there are no set answers to our questions and concerns, and often not much interest or time on the part of physicians to explore these issues. Instead, doctors say, "There, there, dearie, it's just menopause. Everyone goes through it. Why are you so upset? You can take hormones or you can live with it." Feminists say "Doctors make too much of hormones. Menopause is just a natural transition. Just eat right, take herbs, exercise, and you'll be fine."

Meanwhile, your sleepless nights continue, your energy seems to have suddenly disappeared, fatigue becomes overpowering and you feel like you are slogging through quicksand to get through your day. Your memory seems less sharp and familiar words seem to have evaporated from your brain cells; joints ache, muscles hurt, eyes are dry, contacts don't seem to work anymore; the work demands pile up; family needs have to be met; tempers flare; crying spells hit out of the blue for no reason; and sex drive? What's that? Also totally gone, zip, zero. You say, "I don't feel like me anymore. Whose body is this, anyway?"

Then you want to scream when your doctor says "You can't be in menopause; you're too young. It's just stress. Take it easy. Take a vacation. Take Prozac. Don't get so wrought up. [Men are "concerned"; women are "wrought up."] See a therapist. You just need to get a grip on things." Then another betrayal: Women leaders who have previously spoken out for women's issues trivialize menopause or use their own easy transition as a marker of how other women should handle it. Accusations are stated or implied: If you have symptoms and problems with menopause, you are either afraid to face the reality of aging, or you are less of a woman, somehow not "doing it" right (sounds a lot like the macho ideas men have labored under). One feminist activist was heard to describe her own menopause this way: "I think it lasted about an hour. I don't see what all the fuss is about." While I am glad she had such an easy time, not every woman is so lucky. Menopause is *not* another "should" that we have to *do right* or we have failed.

Once again, we are led to doubt ourselves and our perceptions of reality. The voices of inner knowing scream inside our heads: "Wait a minute. I used to handle stress in life just fine. Why *now,* when I have everything going for me, does it seem to get me down? I don't have reasons to cry like this. I *know* there is something changing with my hormones, but I'm told there's no connection. I'm told I'm *fine,* but I am not. It is real. I *know* it. Will *someone* just listen to me?"

Is it any wonder, then, that we feel disenfranchised, devalued, and discounted by the medical professionals and turn to alternative therapies for help?   Women are angry. Women are becoming increasingly proactive. They turn to alternative practitioners, herbalists, pharmacists, massage therapists, and a host of others, hoping for compassion and answers. But are we getting *all* the care we may need from these nonmedical options? Many times the answer is no. Each group of practitioners has its own set of biases, blinders, and "pieces" of the puzzle, but very few are really putting all the pieces together into a coherent and cohesive whole.

As a physician who has been listening to women's voices and experiences for many years, I have felt a deepening disquiet as my work continues. I have found, over and over again that many health problems women have go unrecognized, overlooked, or ignored because their wisdom and knowledge are not being heard and heeded. I feel a scream growing inside my own mind: "She's describing it so thor-

oughly. Why haven't her other doctors listened to what she is saying?" My inner voice crying out was barely audible to me at first. I
had to grow in wisdom and experience as a woman physician and
be better able to trust *my own intuition*. I could not depend on the
limitations and rigidity of my specialty training in internal medicine
and psychiatry that had ignored the entire ovarian endocrine system
and the ways it affected basic brain-body function beyond reproduction. Day in and day out, women continued to tell me stories of
hormonal connections they experienced that were not being listened
to or addressed. Their stories needed a strong voice. My own inner
voice became louder and more insistent, until it, too, became a voice
that must be heard. This book is that voice. It is intended to give you
the specialized "hormone health" information you need to be able
to ask intelligent questions and seek new medical options. I hope to
open doors you might never have found using the traditional "cookbook approaches" using the Premarin-Provera recipe for all women.

What led me to branch out from internal medicine and psychiatry to begin working with the hormonal aspects of women's health
that are usually addressed by gynecologists? During my residency
days and early days of practice, physicians would refer women to me
for "psychogenic" problems such as PMS, anxiety, stress-related illness, sexual concerns, or depression. I would see the person, expect-
ing to help with those issues. But patient after patient, a pattern
emerged and I often found myself saying to the woman and her
physician, "The problems you are describing have a clear pattern
related to your menstrual cycle, and I don't think you have a major
depression [or whatever happened to be in question]. I do not find
a psychiatric disorder; I think you are experiencing hormonal
changes that are affecting your moods." I thought the referring
physician would be glad to have the information. The woman typically was relieved that she now had some answers that made sense
to her. What I discovered, however, was that most commonly her
physician didn't listen to me, either. I struggled for many years to get
other physicians to understand and accept that hormonal shifts can
effect brain chemistry and trigger changes in mood, anxiety, pain,
headaches . . . you name it.

Finally, I decided I had had enough of this battle. I knew the
women were right, and I could relate what they told me directly to
the normal physiology of a woman's body rhythms and hormone
shifts. I undertook a more systematic study of endocrinology and
reproductive hormones, searched the international medical literature and read hundreds of articles, attended many continuing medical education programs on menopause and gynecology, joined the
Menopause and Climacteric Medicine societies, subscribed to journals I couldn't find in my own medical library, and began to inte-

grate whatever I could find with the knowledge I had already gained from internal medicine and psychiatry. Much of the scientific work I could locate came from the international menopause journals and research done in Europe, Australia, and Canada over many years, in addition to the pioneering work in this country by Dr. Robert Greenblatt, Dr. Edward Klaiber, and Dr. Phillip Sarrel.

I learned more and more about the differences in the various types of hormones and saw how well these differences fit with what women were describing to me. I was finding the pieces of the puzzle that had been overlooked and these pieces were fitting beautifully with other pieces of the puzzle that were discovered at Johns Hopkins, where extraordinary neuroscience research was happening during my residency. It was exciting and rewarding for me at both the personal and the professional levels. The improvement women described as a result of fine-tuning of their hormonal balance further validated my belief that I was heading in the right direction. Obviously, not every woman needed hormones, but those who did clearly benefited from the changes we made together to address these issues.

I began speaking around the country, doing what I could to educate women and groups of physicians. Women still had so many questions and they kept asking me, "Is there a book on this anywhere? Is there something I can read about what you are saying? It makes so much *sense.*" I gave the usual references, but the bottom line was that there was no book that addressed the *integration* of all these hormonal issues *with* other traditional women's health concerns. So, I had to write this book. I could not ignore the "screams" any longer.

Screaming to Be Heard is an outgrowth of more than twenty years of clinical work and outcomes research that measured ovarian and other hormones at specific times in women's menstrual cycles using reliable and standardized methods. I also carefully tracked women's menstrual symptom calendars, their own descriptions of how they ate and exercised, what medications they took and how they felt emotionally from day to day. I used objective rating scales for mood, pain, headache, and anxiety problems so that we could together see the "before and after" changes. I included reliable tests of bone density as early as 1985, and measures of cholesterol and cortisol and thyroid and glucose so that I could see what other factors were affected by the changes in the ovary hormones. As my patients and I worked to figure out their individual puzzle pieces for a whole picture, I also began to see ways that we as physicians could take a more *integrated* approach to the multiplicity of factors affecting women's health: from the biological to the spiritual.

The model I have developed over the years has been useful, practical, results-oriented, as well as cost-effective, since we often eliminated many other medications women had been taking. Another important aspect is that the approaches I use could be taught to others in the programs I gave for physicians, nurses, psychologists, physical therapists, and as well as women themselves. Best of all, the women themselves described feeling better overall, often could stop other medications, and their improvements with the hormone interventions validated their own insights. *Screaming to Be Heard* has become a tapestry woven of women's experiences. The voices of wisdom of women patients, family members, friends, and colleagues have taught me much. The voice of my own experiences through several ordeals as a patient has been a great teacher, if a painful one. The voices of women who have not been heard yet, as well as the voices of our ancestors whose writings gave us the legacy of *their* wisdom, pain, joys, struggles, and achievements in the face of adversity . . . all have contributed to this complex and beautiful tapestry. I hope you will add your own voice to the tapestry as you read these pages.

My Experiences as a Patient

I have had my own adversities. I was a patient who was not listened to until I lost the function of my left leg, bladder, and bowel and had reached a point requiring emergency back surgery for a fully ruptured disk compressing my spinal cord. I know firsthand the pain, suffering, fear, self-doubt (*"I must be crazy. NO. I'm NOT!"*), the helplessness of not being listened to or believed, the frustrations of wanting to be well and not being able to make progress. I was a physician; I was also the patient. And when the patient is female, the old stereotypes and patterns of relating take precedence over her professional status as physician.

As the patient, I *knew* something crucial had happened. I had followed directions and stayed in bed for a month; yet, I wasn't getting better. In fact, my ability to stand up for more than three or four minutes was getting progressively worse. I had problems with bladder control that were really worrisome. My brain felt like it was in a fog; I couldn't even think clearly enough to focus on my medical reading. I began to berate myself, lying there telling myself that I must be lazy or something; that I really should be using this time to catch up on reading my medical journals. I would start to read, and I couldn't focus on the pages. Several years later, while at Johns Hopkins, I found out that I had not been imagining this "foggy brain" feeling. It was real, and a side effect of the Valium that had been prescribed four times a day for muscle relaxation. There was something *terribly wrong* with my body, but my doctors were telling me there was *nothing wrong*. I thought I *was* going crazy!

"*Nothing wrong?* Nothing? What do you *mean?* I collapse when I try to stand. I can't go to the bathroom. What *is* this? How could it be something in my mind? I just don't understand." I went back for a checkup. The neurologist thought I "might" have a worsening herniation of the disk and sent me to his partner, a neurosurgeon. This doctor did not even recheck neurological function. He just patted me on the shoulder saying, "Now, you're just fine. You're just too anxious. All you have is a back strain, and it will be fine if you just get out of bed and go on about your business. It's time for you to get back to work." I felt chastised for avoiding my work responsibilities. So, having been raised in the southern tradition of responding like a dutiful little girl to an older male authority figure (even though at the time this happened, I was an adult woman, a physician through medical school and internship), I went back to work at the hospital.

I lasted half a day before my legs collapsed once again and I couldn't stand. I was getting really frightened by this time, although I tried not to show it. "Remember, Lee, physicians don't cry. If you cry, they'll just think you're anxious and neurotic," I said to myself. My internal medicine doctor said he thought I should be admitted to the hospital for a week of traction to see if that would help. So I did that. As the week went on, I could barely walk well enough to go to the bathroom; once I got there, I had trouble urinating, and I became unable to have a bowel movement. Thinking I was constipated from inactivity, my physician ordered regular daily doses of Metamucil as a stool softener. But the problem wasn't constipation; it was nerve damage to the bowel from spinal cord compression. My abdomen was blowing up like a balloon from the Metamucil because I couldn't have a bowel movement on my own. It was awful. I must have looked like a snake that had swallowed a pig. When I first wrote this in 1994, I could see the humor in the mental image that flitted across my mind. In 1979, when I was going through it, I was terrified, and it was not at all funny. But I still did what I was told, like the proverbial "good girl." I didn't know what else to do, and no one seemed to be listening. My confusion and fear were compounded by the fact that I was reminded I was the patient, not the doctor, and to follow directions.

Finally, after lying there a week in the hospital and getting worse, I called my medical school and asked one of my former professors for a psychiatric consultation. He was concerned and sympathetic but astutely said, "Lee, I'll be happy to see you professionally, but I don't really think you have a psychiatric disorder. I think you should get a second opinion from a back surgeon." Two days later, Dr. Henry Wilde, from Houston, Texas, came to Williamsburg for a business meeting with my husband, who mentioned that I was in the hospital with unexplained back problems that weren't getting better. When Henry, an orthopedic surgeon who specialized in back surgery, came to my hospital room, I felt a sense of relief. I just knew he would take me seriously. He listened to my description of what had happened, did a thorough neurological examination, and said, "Lee, you don't have a muscle strain, you have a centrally herniated lumbar disk with compression of the end of the spinal cord. You have lost function in your leg, bladder, and bowel because of the nerve compression over such a long time. You need surgery, and you need it *now* in order for to have any chance of the neurological function coming back."

Needless to say, I felt an overwhelming sense of relief at finally having confirmation that something *was* wrong, what it was, and what needed to be done. Dr. Wilde listened, did a thorough examination, and gave me a diagnosis that explained all that I had been experiencing. It made sense. What I was experiencing was real. I wasn't imagining this. I certainly wasn't at all eager to go through major surgery, but I felt a tremendous weight lifted from my shoulders because I now knew what was wrong. I can deal with *known* problems a lot better than with all the uncertainty that only intensifies my fear. Understandably, I did not want to go back to the neurosurgeon who had failed to properly diagnose my problem. Two days later, I was in Houston having the surgery I had needed all along.

Thanks to Dr. Wilde's visit and, I believe, God's hand in all this, I had surgery in time. In addition to the technical skill of his surgery, Henry also gave me a vitamin and exercise regimen that helped the healing process, and helped me regain my strength. The nerve function returned, the pain gradually lessened as I diligently swam my mile a day and did my walking program. Several months later I was able to go on with my specialty training. Dr. Henry Wilde has now retired from his very successful career, but his legacy of listening and using integrated approaches lives on every single day of my life. His legacy is passed on to many others in the work I do with individual patients, in my writing and in my teaching. Dr. Wilde's intervention was one of those life-transforming moments, and I am profoundly grateful to him for listening when I was in such pain. I want to continue to share that gift with others. But for many of my patients over the years, the outcomes have not been as positive. They have told me of lost years of productive careers due to hormonally triggered health problems that weren't addressed. Some have had their families broken apart when their spouse didn't realize that hormonal problems were the trigger of behaviors that just seemed "difficult and witchy." Some women had even experienced irreversible damage—heart failure, spinal deformity from incapacitating bone loss, dementia—because they did not have proper attention to the hormone issues they had been describing. I hope the next millennium will bring changes in how we approach women's health to help prevent such tragic consequences for so many women and their families.

Richard Bach said *"Every problem has a gift for you in its hands."*[1] For me the *problems* were certainly clear at the time. The *gifts* have emerged in many ways since 1979. One of the most meaningful gifts from my herniated disk problems has been the gift of hearing patients more clearly and trusting that if I listen carefully, they will tell me what I need to know to help them. Another *gift* from my own surgical experience was that I learned very early in my medical career just how crucial exercise, vitamins, healthy food, and a positive mindset are to enhancing the healing process.

"Won't *someone* please listen to me? I *know* I am right. *Something* is wrong. It's *not* all in my head!" These are the silent and the spoken, sometimes whispered, screams. It is time for women to be heard. It is also time for men to be heard because these problems have an impact on them as well. As Helen, a business executive in her fifties, said to me:

> I think women are getting short-changed in all this lack of information about hormones and how they can affect our minds and our well-being; and it affects interpersonal relationships, business relationships, and I think a lot of us are suffering."

So for all of you who have not been listened to or answered and for the men in your lives, this book is your voice. It is also a guide for those of you who have not yet heard your inner cry or who have heard it and not found avenues of help. Most women have incredible *body wisdom*. They are attuned to their body rhythms and sensations in a positive way; indeed, in my opinion, this is one of women's gifts that enhances our survival. Women commonly are keen observers of their bodies, seem to have an *intuitive sense* about body changes and what might be wrong, and ask intelligent, well-thought-out questions of us physicians. All of this adds up to what I call "body wisdom." In working with male patients, I find very few who have this body wisdom. Most men have been taught not to pay attention to their bodies and to "gut through" the pain. For men, this "no pain, no gain" attitude often works to the detriment of their health, leading them to delay seeking medical attention for problems that could be serious, or even fatal.

For women's body wisdom to be useful, however, we health professionals must *listen* to it, learn from it, respect it, and incorporate it into our approaches for healing. Listening to patients, under-

---

1. *Illusions: The Adventures of a Reluctant Messiah*

standing the person as a whole being is where the art and science of medicine began thousands of years ago. Fundamentally, we must come back to this basic foundation of the interaction between the healer and the person coming for help in the healing process. This is the *soul* of the healing arts to which we must return if we are to truly reform health care.

Listen to the words of Sir Francis Peabody *in 1926:*

> *The application of the principles of science to the diagnosis and treatment of disease is only one limited aspect of medical practice. The practice of medicine in its broadest sense includes the whole relationship with the physician and the patient. It is an art, based to an increasing extent on the medical sciences, but comprising much that still remains outside the realm of science.*

I have tried my best to practice this blend of art and science, and to focus on the integrated needs of the whole person with my patients over the years. Even when I cannot personally provide all the services for a given person, I can at least do my best to see that they are identified and suggestions given on how best to find someone to help. Isn't this what we are all asking for from our health care in the new millennium? At another time, in his wisdom, Dr. Peabody said to the graduating class at Harvard Medical School in 1931: *"The secret of the care of the patient lies in caring for the patient."* His comments are as relevant today as they were in 1931, and his words should be indelibly etched in the minds of all who would call themselves "physician."

Robert T. Manning, M.D., the founding dean of my medical school and an important role model for me as I observed him to be one of the true practitioners of the art and science of medicine, reiterated to us over and over: *"Listen to your patients, and they will tell you what is wrong."* Over and over, each day I am in medicine, the truth of this voice rings out. Dr. Manning's legacy of wisdom, commitment to patients as people, and dedication to teaching lives on in all of us who were his students.

Remember, no book can take the place of your personal physician in determining your individual health program. No one authority has all the answers for every woman. But my promise to you is that I will tell you what I *know* I know—from medical research, from listening to women's experiences and descriptions, from clinical study of women's hormone levels at the time of the cycle they have the symptoms they describe, from psychological and cross-cultural research findings, and from my own experience as a patient who has been through much of what this book addresses. I will also tell you honestly what I don't know or what isn't yet known from scientific research. My commitment to you, the reader, is the same commitment I have always given my patients: I will do my best to be honest with you, to give you the best information I am able to find, and to *admit* I don't know, and to help identify resources for you to get your questions answered. I don't expect you to find the answers to *all* your questions in this one book, but I do hope that you will find answers that you have *not found* addressed in other books.

My commitment to you is that *I have not made any recommendations or any interpretations* from the medical literature in this book *that I would not use myself for my own health needs* or recommend to my own family to consider with their physicians. I also have *no* financial interest in any products that I describe in my books or talks. I am not trying to sell you any products. I am only providing information for you to choose to use or not as you see fit. My book cannot address the needs of all women, but it does aim to help those of you who have had or may experience these hormone-related problems.

Let's turn now to the voices of women who must be heard, and *heeded,* for us to better meet the intricate health needs for women of all ages. I hope you will find encouragement to trust your perceptions and body wisdom as you read these pages. I hope you will find answers that have eluded you before to guide you as you work to enhance all levels of your health.

ELIZABETH LEE VLIET, M.D.
Tucson, Arizona
January 1995

x x x /

CHAPTER 1

Screaming to Be Heard! Listening to Women's Voices

With all the recent apparent public attention to the crucial health needs of women, are things *really* changing for the average woman patient headed to her doctor's office seeking help? I would honestly have to say that at this point, *not a lot has changed for the average woman in this country.* In the words of one young woman who recently came to see me for migraine headaches and mood changes before her menstrual period:

> *What bothers me is that I am thirty-six years old and with all the medical doctors I have seen, only one psychologist (a nonmedical person, who was also a woman), who saw me for four sessions for depression recognized that I may have a hormonal imbalance. It surprises me and makes me angry that I have possibly had this problem for twenty-three years. I always told my physicians my headaches happened right before my period, but they dismissed my ideas. Where is the physician who will listen to my observations about my body?*

And this is not unusual. I hear this same story every day from women of all ages, from all parts of the country. There simply is not the information and awareness of *just how different* male and female bodies really are. The medical establishment is so dominated by men's thinking and male physiology that women's different hormonal makeup and health needs are rarely even in the conscious awareness of physicians, much less adequately addressed even by caring physicians. A medical publication in late 1999 illustrates this issue: A woman urologist wrote a review article on interstitial cystitis for publication in a women's health medical journal. In spite of multiple well-known effects of estrogen on all aspects of bladder function, there was *not one* word mentioning potential adverse effects in this disorder due to declining estrogen. Yet, look at the

profound list of estrogen effects I outline in chapter 12 on the bladder and you will see there are many ways that declining estradiol in
the years leading up to menopause could potentially play a role in
the development of Interstitial Cystitis. We have a long way to go.
After seminars I have given on women's health, I have had male
physicians come to up me and say, "What you are saying makes so
much sense. Why hasn't anyone talked about these connections
before? Why hasn't this been in the medical literature? It certainly
fits with *what my patients tell me*, but I have not known how to put
it all together."

The sad part is that women will guide us in being effective physicians *if we will listen to what they say and think about what is happening to them*. For the woman quoted above, her migraines did
indeed have a major hormonal trigger each month. With treatment
to address that hormonal trigger, her recurring premenstrual
migraines have been eliminated. She is still susceptible to weather
and food triggers for her migraines, but she described feeling an
enormous sense of relief that a significant dimension of her migraine
problem has been resolved by stabilizing the hormonal changes, a
factor she herself had been asking about for many years.

Challenges and Controversies in Women's Health:
Issues That Affect YOU

In 1989, the United States General Accounting Office (GAO) audit
revealed that less than 3 percent of the National Institutes of Health
(NIH) budget had been spent on total women's health issues, less than
2 percent on obstetrical and gynecological health concerns, and less
than 0.5 percent on basic research in the area of breast cancer. Have
we made any progress in the years since the GAO first realized women
were ignored in most research studies? Yes. Are we where we need to
be so women will get the gender-specific health care they need and
deserve? No. In fact, we are still a long way away from this goal.

First, let's review some areas of progress:

1. Federal mandates to include women as subjects in all NIH-funded
   clinical research trials
2. Launching of the NIH Women's Health Initiative
3. Establishment of the Office of Women's Health at the NIH
4. Publication of the results of the Postmenopausal Estrogen and
   Progestin Intervention (PEPI) trials, the first major U.S. longitudinal
   double-blind, placebo-controlled study of menopausal hormone
   therapy regimens. Although this study used only *one* type of estrogen (native to horses), it did compare synthetic and natural prog-

esterone for the first time in the United States.

5. Discovery of genes linked to hereditary breast-ovarian cancers
6. Discovery of the new estrogen receptor beta
7. Discovery of new causes and treatments for osteoporosis
8. Development of selective estrogen receptor modulator drugs
9. Decline of 6 percent in breast cancer deaths in this country, a trend first noted in this country between 1991 and 1995
10. Passage of more rigid regulatory requirements to improve quality in mammography settings around the United States
11. Improved recognition of the multiple health consequences for women victims of domestic violence and childhood abuse; with increased shelters and support networks for battered women
12. Improved access to prenatal care nationwide—today more than 80 percent of women are getting prenatal care in the first trimester
13. Decline in infant mortality rates, and finally, a beginning decrease in teen pregnancy rates
14. More openness to inclusion of complementary medicine approaches from traditional healing practices of many cultures
15. More physicians willing to discuss hormone therapy options and alternatives with their patients; there is a *little* less of the "cookbook" approach with Premarin or PremPro for everyone; more physicians are using the bio-identical (sometimes called "natural") hormone products that are on the market, both commercial FDA-approved ones such as Estrace, Vivelle, Climara, and Alora, as well as ones compounded by specialty pharmacies
16. More extensive use by physicians of the serum (blood) hormone tests that are the gold standard for reliable hormone levels in menopause and perimenopause research, particularly in the international menopause field
17. FDA approval of two new natural progesterone commercial products (Prometrium, Crinone) that are typically covered by health insurance prescription plans (whereas the compounded prescriptions generally were not covered by such plans)
18. Improved protection from HMO abuses of patients in a few states that have passed patient protection bills (Texas legislators were the first to be so progressive in passing a law that allowed patients to sue their health plan for adverse outcomes that occurred due to denial of care, although this bill passed without Gov. Bush's support.)
19. Formation of new consumer groups for women's health
20. Establishment of new medical journals devoted to women's health
21. Increase in newspaper and magazine articles and television and radio programs on women's health topics, regardless of their accuracy, depth, or focus
22. Increase in hospital-sponsored women's health programs that address health concerns beyond birthing and childcare

23. Increased numbers of women taking charge of their health and not settling for answers that don't make sense, seeking new opinions and changing physicians when needed

24. Most importantly, women doing what we have always done: networking with each other, starting self-help support groups, nurturing each other, and making efforts to ask questions and to learn more about our individual and collective needs

However, we still have a long way to go. Much more work has to be done by all of us with an interest in women's health and a commitment to sound, responsible approaches. Fundamental and basic hormonal effects must be addressed to better understand crucial needs in health care for women. For example, it is well known clinically that the menstrual cycle is an important factor affecting drug metabolism and interactions; yet, few systematic studies have been done to determine exactly how best to adjust medication dosages according to the menstrual cycle. These clinical observations of menstrual cycle hormonal effects on medication and disease severity and frequency have been observed in areas as diverse as herpes outbreaks, epileptic seizure activity, allergies, migraine headaches, yeast infections, bipolar affective disorder, and depression. But we *still* have not studied HOW hormonal changes affect these cyclic changes in various disease flare-ups.

Drs. Buchwald and Garrity, authors of a 1994 study of similar clinical patterns in chronic fatigue syndrome (CFS), fibromyalgia syndrome (FMS), and multiple chemical sensitivities (MCS) looked at many characteristics of these clinical problems more common in women. They did correctly identify these disorders as being much more common in women in their forties. Yet, there was *not one* word in the study about, or any methods used to assess, possible *ovarian hormonal factors* contributing to these diseases. Interestingly enough, both researchers were women, so we can't just sit back and say men don't listen. It seems incredible to me that in the era of "gender-based medicine," not even women physicians were addressing such an obvious potential trigger factor as the ovarian hormones. The blind spots are overwhelming, and health care professionals must remove the blinders when conducting women's health studies.

The relationship of premenopausal hormone changes to a variety of disorders seen more commonly in women, such as depression, fibromyalgia, and migraines, have also not been adequately addressed. I have included a chapter on each of these important subjects because each one affects women *much* more frequently than men. The fluctuations and declines in hormone levels are normal physical changes that may have a significant impact on pre*menstrual* and pre*menopausal* sleep and mood changes.

Mood changes in the years before menopause (from about age

thirty to age fifty) have traditionally been *assumed* to be primarily the result of life stresses and psychological transitions, but almost nothing has been done in systematic research to study hormonal effects on the brain as a factor causing these problems. We live in a culture that hasn't even been fully convinced that women *have* a brain, much less that it is connected to the body. If you think I am being too harsh, just look at the cartoons, ads, and body images used to sell products and present health information and notice how many headless bodies there are and how many jokes are printed daily about "brainless" or "nutty" women. We must remember, the brain *is* connected to the body, and hormones are one of the most potent chemical messenger systems affecting the brain and all its functions, including, of course, mood, sleep, and memory. In particular, both estrogen and progesterone have profound effects on the serotonin, norepinephrine, dopamine, and endorphin receptor systems that are involved in mood regulation; yet, almost no clinical research has integrated these findings to identify effective treatment regimens for premenopausal women. Because this crucial information is so woefully neglected in women's health, it is a major focus of this book.

The Invisible Woman in Health Research

In the past, women have been excluded from health and medical research studies for a variety of reasons, *including the presence of the very hormonal changes that need to be studied.* Here are some of the complex factors that have contributed to the problem:

- The hormonal cycling and complexity of women's physiology were considered "background noise" that complicated study design.
- The male body has been considered the "norm." What was learned about men was assumed to apply equally well to women.
- Research done on males without hormonal cycling was deemed to be more reliable. The bias against excluding women in research studies had even extended to a preference for male laboratory rats.
- Men dominated the research-funding committees, medical school, and university research settings, and they determined where the dollars went and for what types of studies.
- Most disorders that were known to be more common in women, such as migraines, FMS, MCS, et cetera, were assumed to be primarily psychological in origin and not as important to study as the "real" diseases more common in men.
- Women in general, until the past two decades, have been almost invisible, apart from their reproductive functions, in our culture as a whole.

Women's invisibility in health and medical research also extends far beyond what I have just described. For example:

> The Baltimore Longitudinal Study of Aging was started in 1958 but **excluded women until 1978.** The last major report was published in 1984 and was titled *Normal Human Aging,* and this report contained *no data on women.* It appears that, even though women generally live longer, in this research, women weren't even considered "human"!

Medical Problems That Hit Women Harder

Bernadine Healy, M.D., the first woman to be appointed director of the NIH, said,

> It is now time for a **general awakening.** Women have unique medical problems. They have greater morbidity [medical term for suffering, disability] than men and are affected by more chronic debilitating illness. Although women live longer than men—i.e., as much as seven years on average—the quality of life of those years is exceptionally burdened by cancer, particularly of the lung, breast, and colon, by heart disease and stroke, osteoporosis, depression and social isolation, Alzheimer's disease and general frailty. These conditions, which tend to afflict women in the last third of their lives, are not the inevitable ravages of age but are in many cases highly preventable and eminently treatable. We must awaken fully to these facts and address the diseases of women as different from the diseases of men but of equal importance.

To illustrate Dr. Healy's point about the quality-of-life concerns for elderly women, osteoporosis alone is a major factor in the increased cost of health care and the rising need for nursing-home care for elderly women. It is striking that **over 75 percent of nursing home residents over sixty-five are female.** The even more tragic aspect of this statistic is that women in this age group who end up so debilitated that they are forced to be in nursing homes are suffering from diseases that are largely *preventable* through early education about risk factors and emphasis on healthy lifestyle changes.

What contributes to women not getting the information and education they need on these potentially preventable later-life diseases? One factor is clear: The media imbalance in focusing predominately on breast cancer has significantly distorted the *real* health issues that affect you as you grow older and adversely affect your quality of life: The disabling and potentially deadly conditions of osteoporosis and heart disease.

Osteoporosis

Osteoporosis has become a national health epidemic, with $8 to $10 billion spent annually on health care for osteoporotic-related fractures and subsequent long-term disability. And these figures do not include the dollar and human cost of pain and suffering or the devastating effects on quality of life. A hip fracture is definitely not easily resolved by a "total hip replacement," as a popular magazine solution would have you believe. After a hip fracture, nearly one in five women die from complications within three months, and 50 percent *never* walk independently again. Pretty scary, I think. I am concerned that women do not get an accurate picture of the consequences of bone loss and osteoporosis complications, especially since greater emphasis on preventive approaches to osteoporosis in the twenties, thirties and forties, could dramatically reduce the frailty and debilitation seen in older women.

The issues of older women and bone loss represent only the tip of the iceberg of the potential osteoporosis *epidemic* in this country. We aren't even really addressing the millions of young women who are starving themselves to be thin to reach some "magazine ideal" for their bodies. In the process, they are losing bone at the very time in their lives (teens, twenties, and thirties) when they should be building bone toward peak bone density. These women do not even *arrive* at menopause with optimal bone density. Often, however, they appear healthy on the outside and don't even know that "silent termites" are eroding their bone from the inside. We think these young women look "great," "healthy," "vibrant" because they are thin. The "thin look" is what we have been conditioned to think is normal. But women need about 20 to 25 percent body fat in order to have normal menstruation, fertility, bone growth, hair and nail growth, and other measures of good health. I assure you, the models you see in most of the magazines have less than the 20 percent healthy body fat level. Have *you* had your body composition checked recently?

Alcoholism

Alcohol is another area of challenge in women's health. Alcohol abuse and alcoholism hit women *harder* than men in all dimensions: physically, on the body and brain; psychologically; financially; and sociologically. I include it as another one of the risks you don't hear much about relative to other topics in the popular press. A 1990 study in the *New England Journal of Medicine,* by a team of Italian and American researchers, revealed that women had smaller quantities of the protective enzyme alcohol dehydrogenase, which breaks down alcohol in the stomach, and that as a result women absorb about 30 percent more alcohol into their bloodstream than do men. The researchers also made another startling discovery: Alcoholic men have about half as much alcohol dehydrogenase as healthy males do, but alcoholic women show almost *no* enzyme activity. The researchers concluded that alcoholic women appear to lose all gastric protection in the absorption of alcohol; this is one of several reasons alcohol hits women harder and sooner than men.

Tobacco

I hear from women around the country who are terrified of breast cancer. I understand this fear. Did you know, however, that cigarette smoking represents one of the *worst* threats to women's health? In 1991 alone, 51,000 women died of lung cancer, and 191,000 new lung cancer cases were diagnosed in women. In 1965, there were 14,000 tobacco-related deaths in women; in 1995, there were about 240,000 tobacco-related deaths in women, almost SIX times the number of breast cancer deaths.

Tobacco use is a hidden epidemic that is killing women. In 1986, lung cancer became the leading cancer death in women, exceeding breast cancer, and remains the leading cause of cancer death in 1999 (American Cancer Society 1999 estimates: 68,000 to 43,300). The dramatic rise in lung cancer in women is directly attributable to the rise in smoking among women since World War II. But 90 percent of women still think their leading cause of cancer death is breast cancer. Other disease risks associated with smoking include heart disease, early menopause, osteoporosis, emphysema, infertility, miscarriages, low-birth-weight babies, and possibly ovarian and breast cancer. Adolescent and young adult women are beginning to smoke in alarming numbers. Those of you who are mothers, take note of this: The fastest-growing group of smokers in the United States are girls under age *eleven*.

Why don't you know this? The bottom line is money. All the women's magazines except *Good Housekeeping* and *Ms.* (which accepts no advertising at all) in the United States are heavily supported by advertising from the tobacco companies. Women's magazines, whose bottom lines would be jeopardized by offending their large advertisers, have not been running stories on the health consequences of cigarette smoking. A study published in the *Journal of the American Medical Association* objectively documented the correlation that had been long suspected: The *greater* the percentage of advertising revenue from tobacco companies, the *less likely* a magazine was to publish any information on the health effects of tobacco use. Go back and look at your typical women's magazines. How many articles about lung cancer in women do you find? How many full-page color ads do you see showing pretty, smiling, *thin* young women smoking?

Cigarette smoking has been shown to cause earlier menopause and bone loss both in female smokers and in *nonsmoking* women whose spouses are smokers; yet, the number of women smokers is increasing, not decreasing. **Fewer women than men quit smoking. Reason? Women value their appearance more highly than their health, thinking, "If I quit smoking, I'll gain weight."**

The bottom line is that tobacco companies sell glamor, glitz, thinness, and an image of good health in advertisements that specifically target young women to buy a product that will enslave and potentially kill them. Just as we were outraged over the inadequate research and funding for breast cancer, we must raise our voices against this larger threat to the health of the next generation of women, our collective daughters. Cigarette smoking has been found to impair fertility, although the components of cigarette smoke that are toxic to ovarian follicles are unknown. Cigarette smoking has also been implicated as a factor that increases the risk of breast cancer, perhaps by increasing cell mutations. If this turns out to be as important a link as many physicians and researchers suspect, women will have been sold literally a **lethal** bill of goods. Yes, "you've come a long way, baby." But is more *disease* what you intended or wanted? Smoking-related costs and deaths affect us all, whether we smoke or not, whether we have daughters or not. We must all have the courage to speak out to stop the glamorization of cigarette smoking and help our young people, especially vulnerable adolescent girls, make the choice not to start smoking.

Eating Disorders

Eating disorders are other behind-the-scenes problems that affect women in enormous numbers, but rarely generate the same degree of media interest as topics like breast cancer. The cultural "thinness mania" began with Twiggy in the 1960s, continued with the 1993 "waif" look, and is still present in 1999 with the character Ally McBeal and a host of other popular stars. Idealizing extreme thinness in the "star" culture has created a female obsession with weight, dieting, and being thin no matter what the price to one's health. The ads bombard us constantly with headlines and images: Change your body. Change your self. Fix your flaws. Blast those jig-gly hips and thighs. Get that tummy FLAT. Have a "tummy tuck" (major surgery and painful recovery, but they don't mention *that* in the ads). Become new and sexy, more attractive and exciting to your man: Spray, powder, paint, nip, and tuck your body until you reach PERFECTION. No matter the cost.

The idealized female body shown in our magazines is thin, bony, slouched, lean, and usually devoid of the normal female curves. These images have been a major factor in the creation of a multibillion-dollar diet industry in the United States, largely aimed at YOU—the women. These ads and images play on our cultural obsession with thinness to ensure continued sales of products. It is an entrepreneur's dream: Sell the same products over and over to the same group of people. The reason it tends to be the same group of people is that 95 percent of people who go on repeated quick-weight-loss diets end up regaining the weight they lost, and usually an additional five or ten pounds. Chronic "yo-yo" dieting has a major adverse effect on your health; going on and off diets stresses the heart, brain, bones, and other organs. Excessive thinness is associated with increased cancer risk, early menopause, osteoporosis, ulcers, anemia, and emphysema. There has been little research done on the connection between underweight and illness. The preliminary evidence suggests that it is actually healthier to be a little overweight than to be chronically dieting, going on and off fasts and other quick-fix approaches. Chronic dieting can be lethal. With the increased participation in women's athletics at all levels, perhaps the image of the active, exer-cising, *healthy* female will prevail.

Behind the Headlines: Alarming Facts You Still Don't Hear

Prevention of osteoporosis is a compelling reason for prescribing estrogen to postmenopausal women; yet, many of these women are reluctant to take estrogen because of the distorted picture in the media about the risk of breast and uterine cancer. In an article enti-tled "Endometrial Cancer From Estrogen Replacement Therapy (ERT): An Unfounded Fear," distinguished menopause researcher Dr. R. Don Gambrell reported that the absolute risk of endometrial (uterine) cancer is quite small, occurring in one in every thousand women over age fifty each year. This type of cancer is easily detected, very treatable, and less aggressive in women using hormones than in women who are not on hormone therapy. Dr. Gambrell also stated that *estrogen itself is not carcinogenic*. In patients diagnosed with endometrial cancer while on estrogen therapy, the five-year survival rate is 95 percent, a significantly *better* survival rate than that of women diagnosed with endometrial cancer who are *not* on estrogen therapy. Many specialists think that the type of cancer that occurs in women who don't take hormones is a more aggressive form of cancer than in those who do take hormones. You don't see this information in the magazine and newspaper articles. It disturbs me, both as a physician and as a consumer, that the available information is not more balanced and current.

Breast cancer is another example. Women who are *on* estrogen at the time of diagnosis actually have been found to have less aggressive forms of breast cancer, better treatment outcomes, and longer survival times. But you don't hear about that data either. Estrogen has never been shown to *cause* breast cancer, yet this is the impression that the majority of women have from reading the popular press articles. Yet another example occurred the week of January 24, 2000. A study published in *JAMA* reported that women using the combined estrogen-progestin combination had a higher risk of breast cancer than women using estrogen alone. But in my view, one of the most crucial points of all was omitted from national media reports. This point was that Premarin and medroxyprogesterone acetate (MPA or Provera, a synthetic progestin) were the hormone products used by the women in this study, and both of these products are "unnatural" hormones for the human female body, with very different effects from those produced by our own ovary hormones. It seems such an obvious point, and even the study authors failed to mention this in their conclusions as a limitation of the study. I will talk more in chapter 14 about these critical issues with regard to *what* information you get about breast cancer and *how* this information is presented. The same types of incomplete or incorrect information are perpetuated in article after article.

Shocking Facts in Women's Health

Fact You Are Not Told:

Heart disease is an equal-opportunity killer. It is the number one cause of death in women over forty—yet it is generally assumed to be a disease of *men*. Prior to the Nurse's Health Study, women had been *excluded* from every major study of heart disease prevention, diagnosis, and treatment.

Fact You Are Not Told:

Women who are seen in the Emergency Room for chest pain and palpitations are far more commonly given a diagnosis of "anxiety" and sent home with a prescription for a tranquilizer rather than having a full evaluation for heart disease. Young women may die when true heart disease is missed. See cases I describe in chapter 13. Men with similar symptoms are more likely to be kept overnight to rule out a heart attack.

Fact You Are Not Told:

Between the ages of forty to sixty-five, almost 500,000 women die each year from cardiovascular disorders, versus 60,000 deaths annually from *all reproductive cancers*: breast, uterine, cervix, ovarian, and vaginal. But women and their physicians often don't think to start screening for heart disease risk factors in women in their forties.

Fact You Are Not Told:

A 1991 study published in the *New England Journal of Medicine* provided further evidence of sex bias in the management of coronary artery disease: Women were significantly less likely to have prescribed coronary angiography, angioplasty, or bypass surgery when admitted with a diagnosis of myocardial infarction, angina, chronic ischemic heart disease, or chest pain. Men are routinely offered these options. In 1999, **44 percent of women—but only 27 percent of men—who have a heart attack *die* within a year,** because men are treated more aggressively earlier.

Fact You Are Not Told:

Postmenopause estrogen therapy (ET) dramatically reduces (more than 50 percent in recent studies) risk of heart disease and osteoporosis, yet *less than 15 percent* of postmenopausal women take estrogen, in part because of an exaggerated fear of breast cancer in media reports, and lack of adequate information and screening for individual health risks.

Fact You Are Not Told:

Despite the fact that a *natural human form of estradiol has been FDA-approved in the United States since 1976,* women in this country are usually given only one recipe for hormone therapy [I call it the "cookbook approach" with Premarin and Provera or PremPro]. Rarely are other options offered to women, even if they have adverse reactions and unwanted side effects with the standard therapies.

Fact You Are Not Told:

The United States is 20 years behind Europe in our options for natural hormone therapies for menopause. In other developed nations, many different forms of native human estradiol, progesterone, and testosterone are routinely prescribed.

How many of these facts and health risks did you already know? I suspect not many, since these don't often make the headlines. The more you look at coverage of women's health, the more you see the imbalance in focus on topics that are more likely to have an emotional "hook" that gets you to *buy* the magazine. The distortion in risk has an impact on choices women make in lifestyle changes as well as other interventions to reduce disease risk.

My intent is not to make this a political book. I raise these issues for three primary reasons: (1) to help you see the undercurrents that enhance or distort the health information you receive, (2) to paint an overall picture for you to critically evaluate, and (3) to emphasize the importance of YOU being active in getting information YOU need to make YOUR OWN decisions. When you become an informed consumer working with your physician to individually assess your various health risk factors, you can select the options that best meet your *individual* needs. What are some of these challenges that still lie ahead during the new millennium? What are some of the impediments to greater improvement in the delivery of health services tailored to the unique needs of women? The following are a few that I see and ones I hear from women consumers.

Impediments to Improved Health Care for Women

- **Cultural stereotypes of women as hypochondriacal, stressed, neurotic, anxious, or depressed.** These stereotypes prevent physicians from looking carefully at underlying causes of symptoms. Such symptoms may have many different causes: from psychological ones such as a history of sexual abuse or domestic violence to physiological ones such as premature decline in ovarian hormones.

- **Restrictive HMOs and "managed" (rationed) care plans.** These plans abysmally fail to see the importance and cost-effectiveness of properly assessing women's body chemistry, including hormone levels. In our practice, we encounter daily examples of such short-sighted thinking: health plans that would rather pay $100–200 every month for Prozac or Zoloft or Celexa, but say "it's too expensive" to check hormone levels and find out that what a woman may need could be thyroid or ovary hormone options that might cost $20 a month.

- **Focus on use of "magic bullets" for menopause, PMS, and peri-menopause, including soy supplements, progesterone and "wild yam" creams, OTC forms of DHEA, and melatonin.** All of these have potentially harmful effects for women who are already having thyroid or ovarian hormone imbalances. See chapter 16 for critical information on ovarian effects of soy products. Consumers do not usually get this information from their health professionals because most physicians are so overwhelmed with just keeping up with the basics of medical therapies that they are unable to keep up with all the newest supplements. And even doctors get mixed information. As an example, in the summer of 1999, the U.S. medical journal *Menopause* ran two-page color ads for a red clover isoflavone supplement called Promensil. This happened the same month the international journal *Climacteric* published the first two placebo-controlled, prospective, randomized, double-blind studies showing that Promensil had *no effect* greater than placebo on *any* of the menopausal symptoms measured, including objective measures of estrogen effect. That same month, I received my copy of *Menopause Management* (a U.S. journal sent to doctors all over the country), and this journal went a step further in promoting soy products—they actually shrink-wrapped with the issue an advertisement and a sample soy protein drink package. Personally and professionally, I found this offensive in view of the very mixed results on soy's effectiveness and its known potential problems for women with thyroid disorders and early ovarian decline. I was pleased to see that the international editors of *Climacteric* took a higher road than the U.S. journals: They wrote a position statement that the international menopause journal would not accept advertising for any health product that had not been proved to be effective on the problems for which it was advertised.

- **A spate of books with conflicting, out-of-date, or just plain inaccurate information about female hormones and the options available to restore a healthy balance.** Books in this category that are designed to sell the authors' various products end up having the tragic result of leaving consumers more confused.

- **Continued dominance of a "cookbook" approach to hormone therapy using one form of estrogen (derived from pregnant mares' urine) dominating more than 85 percent of all ERT for decades, whether women feel well on it or not.** This reliance on the oldest product occurs in spite of options available in the United States since 1976 using hormones *identical* to those the human ovary makes. Using one product in the same dose for every woman doesn't make sense to thinking consumers. They know that we don't approach any other areas of health care that way. Can you imagine giving every patient with an infection the same antibiotic? Do you think that all diabetics are prescribed the same dose and type of insulin? Are all men with heart disease given the same type of medicine? Of course not. So women reject such a one-size-fits-all approach. Study after study on hormone use in the United States has shown that about two-thirds of women who start hormone therapy discontinue it on their own within a year; over a third of women given a prescription never have it filled and usually don't tell their physicians. One of the primary reasons for this is that women are individuals and require individualized hormone therapy—a concept that makes intuitive sense to women, who then decide not to use the standard "recipe."

  Why does this "cookbook" approach to hormone therapy exist? Because gynecologists, family physicians, and internal medicine physicians have not been adequately trained in the finer nuances of individualizing and fine-tuning hormone therapy. There was little emphasis on this in either medical school or specialty training. Many physicians get their primary information from drug manufacturers. The company with the largest market share has also the largest budget for advertising and marketing, and obviously focuses its educational efforts only on its product rather than the many options now available from competitors. In addition, with the limits imposed by HMOs and other forms of managed care, physicians don't feel they have enough time to spend with women to explore options and answer hormone-related questions.

- **A lack of comparative research on the different effects of the various types of estrogens and progestins.** As a result, women are often told by their physicians, "we don't know enough about natural hormones." Most of the hormone studies done in this country are financed by grants from the makers of the conjugated horse-derived estrogen product.

- **The continuing focus on fear to sell products.** The fear of breast cancer is used as a tactic to sell new and expensive medications called "designer estrogens" as well as soy supplements and Chinese herbs with unknown components. Instead of educating women with balanced articles, we are inundated with fear tactics, leading many women to develop a terror of estrogen.

- **The limits of modern medicine in being unable to heal many patients—the majority of whom are women—who suffer from *chronic* debilitating disorders.** There is a marked female predominance in many of the common, chronic disorders that rob sufferers of quality of life, work productivity, social involvement, and money both in direct dollars spent on health care and indirect dollars from lost productivity or work time. Disorders such as arthritis, migraines, fibromyalgia, depression, anxiety, dementia, asthma, diabetes, allergies, chemical sensitivities, environmental illness, incontinence, osteoporosis, autoimmune disorders, thyroid disease, and others affect women in numbers far greater than men.

- **A dichotomy between physicians' thinking and approaches oriented to *treating disease* versus consumers, particularly midlife women, focusing on healthy "natural" approaches for *staying well*.** Women are identifying that there is a hormone connection to the symptoms and illnesses they are experiencing, but they are getting turned off by the doctors who are discounting what they are saying . . . this leads them to turn to alternative sources for information and treatment (some reputable, others not—and it is hard to differentiate between the two). Many consumers have become so disenfranchised by traditional medicine that they are questioning everything a physician says and are wary of all prescription medications—but will try anything "natural" or over-the-counter, thinking it must be safe and have no side effects because it comes from a health food store. Yet we need to remember that there can be harm from "harmless" therapies—such as taking a supplement *thinking* it will preserve bone, only to find out a few years later that it did not and osteoporosis has developed. I have seen some of my patients who have experienced such frustration with the way traditional medical settings and physicians have functioned become so enamored with complementary or herbal medicine that they attribute all of their benefits to the alternative approaches and nothing to the traditional medical treatments they are receiving at the same time.

Why Women Aren't Heard: Stereotypes and Negative Labels

Additional problems include the media's substantial role in perpetuating other stereotypes that adversely effect women. Think of the many negative labels applied to women: *anxious, overworried about their health, complainers, difficult patients, crocks, neurotic, emo-*

tionally-starved, empty-nesters, ditherers, bitchy. As a culture, we laugh at the cartoons about PMS, and we do not take seriously the women who struggle with the problematic symptoms of PMS that can at times be severe enough to adversely affect work, family, and social relationships. Feminists complain that physicians try to make PMS a psychiatric disorder. Women who *have* PMS complain that physicians aren't listening. Many physicians who have worked extensively with PMS patients are frustrated that the culture trivializes and discounts the very real physical and psychological symptoms of PMS to such a degree that even physician advocates don't get listened to when we try to speak up on behalf of our patients.

Women with breast cancer have been treated as *breasts* rather than persons. One woman wrote an eloquent piece about her experience in a cancer center, describing her depersonalized treatment as feeling like "a piece of baggage on an airline baggage carousel," going from one physician to another. When women *do* speak up about their health care desires and needs, they tell me over and over they are then labeled "difficult, demanding" by both nurses (still mostly female) and doctors (still mostly male). How is a woman to figure out what to do? My personal advice is for her to be a well-informed, knowledgeable, articulate "squeaky wheel" armed with thought-out questions, organized symptoms, and a brief history.

Older women in this country aren't valued for their experience and wisdom as we see in countries of Europe and Asia. So if menopausal women aren't valued as being very important, then perhaps it isn't "worth" taking the time to work out an individualized approach. Older, menopausal women are also viewed as *complainers,* so they are often just given the standard approach and sent home.

To illustrate my points, here is an exercise I would like you to do now, as you are reading this:

TASK: Quickly write down the first three words that come immediately to mind with the phrase "An older man is _____." Just spontaneously fill in the blank with whatever words pop into mind. What did you come up with? Now do the same thing with this phrase: "An older woman is _____."

Do you see any pattern to your responses? When I ask these two questions in my seminars, the words that most frequently come to mind in the audience for describing older men are "distinguished," "successful," "powerful," "attractive." I rarely hear a negative word used to characterize older *men.* The common audience responses for the statement about older women are words like "dowdy," "old," "tired," "fat," "alone," "invisible," "poor," "over the hill," "unattractive." These stereotypes of older women are so deeply ingrained in our minds that we don't even consciously realize how *differently* we view aging men and women. We can't help but feel these images and incorporate them into our sense of self. The cumulative impact for women, adds up to an even lower sense of self-worth as we grow older, since we have been part of the culture far too long to easily shrug off such belittling messages. We need to know such stereotypes are alive and thriving in our culture in order to understand why our questions and concerns are frequently overlooked or ignored.

Women's Traditional Healing Wisdom: Devalued and Ignored

"Healing wisdom" is women's *intuitive sense* about body changes and what might be the cause. Women have been living with body changes since adolescence and recognize when their body is out of sync, and they often have ideas about why. They want to be affirmed and informed and involved. Without research specifically taking into account women's body chemistry, however, physicians are hampered in suggesting what changes to make or how to make them. If scientific advances were able to put a man on the moon *in 1969,* why haven't we been able to determine whether we can give a woman half an aspirin a day to help prevent strokes or whether medication should be adjusted according to the menstrual cycle?

I have been making medication adjustments based on the menstrual cycle phase for my patients for about fifteen years, but this is not an approach I was taught in medical school or found in the medical literature. I learned it by *listening* to my patients, and by observing cyclical patterns to their experiences. Women's body wisdom knows the hormonal rhythms; women's mind wisdom knows there are connections to these hormonal shifts. It is a magnificent symphony each month, but sometimes one section may be out of tune with the rest, creating discord and disharmony. Women know this, *feel* it, observe it, ask good questions about it. This is another aspect of what I mean by women's body wisdom. Why have health professionals not done a better job of paying attention to and heeding what our female patients have been telling us for decades?

One answer may be that our scales and formats of evaluation are a result of research based on males and male body physiology and the assumption that those findings would apply equally well to female patients. Of course, this assumption of similarity ignores a fairly obvious fact: Women's body chemistry and hormonal cycles are markedly different from men's. Symptoms female patients report may not fit in any one column or they may cut across several columns. I keep reading about diseases that are 60 percent, 70 percent, or 80 percent female predominant, followed by comments such as, "We don't know *why* there are these gender differences." There is rarely ever mention of studying the most obvious factor that differentiates males and females: the *hormones* that make women *female*! Why have we overlooked or ignored researching something so obvious? It certainly isn't because *women* are unwilling to accept a hormonal connection. We already know it is there. Women would like to know more about what it is and what to *do* about it.

This book is about these **overlooked and ignored hormonal connections;** what we *do* know about hormonal effects on brain-body systems and how these hormonal effects interact with the endocrine, immune, metabolic, cardiovascular, respiratory, musculoskeletal, reproductive, urinary, and nervous systems. Every cell of our bodies participates in the flow of our menstrual rhythm. Changes occur in almost all body functions and secretions as the levels of female hormones rise and fall every month. These changes have been measured and objectively documented in *many* factors as the following *partial* list illustrates.

Menstrual Cycle Measurable Body Changes

- body temperature
- blood glucose regulation
- breast size, texture, skin/nipple color
- energy levels and sleep patterns
- neurotransmitter production
- thyroid and adrenal hormone production
- red and white blood cell counts
- fluid balance
- skin color, texture, permeability
- respiration functions: CO_2, O_2
- blood pH
- memory and concentration
- citric acid (Vitamin C) content of mucus
- brain wave (EEG) patterns
- heart rate and rhythm
- balance, fine motor coordination
- ESR ("sed rate") measure of inflammation
- pupil size and reactivity
- platelet counts
- basal metabolism rate
- estrogen levels in blood and urinary metabolites
- progesterone levels in blood and urinary metabolites
- levels of brain hormones
- bile pigments (to digest fat)
- blood levels of adrenaline
- body weight
- GSR (galvanic skin resistance)
- pulmonary (lungs) vital capacity
- blood protein levels and amounts
- vaginal mucus characteristics
- vaginal cytology (cell types)
- visual, auditory, olfactory acuity
- serum bicarbonate
- pain threshold
- feeling state and behavior
- Concentrations of vitamins A, C, E, and B group
- cervix changes: size, color, position
- urine volume, pH, specific gravity

© Elizabeth Lee Vliet, M.D., 1995, revised 2000

Does this list begin to give you an idea of just how *profound* the relationships are in every part of our body to the changing hormone levels each month? It seems to me there is a wealth of opportunity to study these and learn ways of working *with* women's natural body cycles for optimal health and well-being.

Setting the Stage for Change

The Women's Health Initiative (WHI), launched by Dr. Bernadine Healy and the NIH in the early 1990s, was long overdue and much welcomed by physicians, health professionals, and researchers in many fields, as well as by patients. The landmark decade-long study focused on the effects of hormone treatment on breast cancer risk, the role of diet in contributing to cancer, the effects of taking or not taking hormones on weight gain after menopause, and the effectiveness of estrogen in preventing bone fractures and in modifying heart disease risk factors. The WHI study results are due to be reported in 2005. Other major studies of medications are being implemented to specifically include women and to address public outcry over the lack of such information, but even these studies aren't optimal. Only one type of estrogen, derived from horses and not natural to a woman's body, has been used in most of these studies, and this product doesn't even deliver adequate levels of the native *human* estrogen, *17-beta estradiol*. As a result of using only this "foreign" estrogen, even the WHI results won't provide all the answers we had hoped to find about the overall benefits of 17-beta estradiol. We still have a long way to go. We need to keep the pressure on. It helps that women's interest groups have taken up the banner and are raising the public consciousness and politicians' awareness.

We as women also need to challenge medical schools to see that they are in a primary position to elevate awareness of gender concerns in the new generation of physicians. I am a strong advocate of having continuing medical education (CME) programs better designed to address the male-female differences in disease recognition and treatment. I have designed a number of CME programs with this integrated approach.

Pharmaceutical companies must demonstrate their involvement in increasing the knowledge of male-female body/mind differences through research and support of educational programs for all health professionals as well as consumers. It is very aggravating to me that some of the same groups who criticize physicians and "those bad drug companies" for such jointly sponsored programs are often the same people who have a vested interest in *their own* products: vitamins, herbs, over-the-counter hormone creams, evaluation kits, self-improvement tapes—you name it.

Women have sometimes asked why I agreed to be on national speaker's programs that have educational grants from pharmaceutical companies. Although I resigned my position on all of the pharmaceutical-sponsored speakers' bureaus as of 1998-99 to maintain complete independence from potential commercial sponsors, this is why I participated in the past:

- I would convey the message I knew to be sound, based on insights taught by my patients and my clinical experience, based on basic principles of normal physiology and current science, *regardless of who was providing financial support.* If a company or organization did not agree with my position and my clinical program content, then they didn't invite me as a speaker. I have continued to be alarmed by the fact that women are not told about available options such as FDA-approved products of natural hormones. If there are products on the market deemed safe by the FDA, and they are ones I would use myself or recommend for my family and patients, wouldn't you want me to also be telling *you* about such options?

- I want to advance the knowledge base in women's health issues by speaking to as many groups of both consumers and practitioners as possible, and I believe it is part of the social responsibility of for-profit companies to invest some of their profits back into the educational process. Educational grants from large companies are one way to accomplish these goals.

I don't have many illusions about what has motivated the current surge of interest in women's health when many of us have been "screaming to be heard" for many, many years. Women's collective *economic* clout is finally too great to ignore any longer. Collectively, we women have in our hands about 500 *billion* health care dollars. Two out of every three health care dollars are spent by women. With $500 billion in our pockets, we ought to be more demanding, more assertive about getting our needs met. Our economic potential gets the attention of businesses in all sectors.

Even women's health has become a hot topic, getting more attention in magazines because it sells. Have you noticed how many new women's health newsletters have popped up in the last few years? Many of these contain the same information recycled in a new design. There is very little that I have read in any of these "new" newsletters that is truly *cutting-edge* information for women. You are buying magazines and books because you are hungry for the information and answers. I am glad to see *more* such articles, newsletters, and shows on these topics. I also want to see information available that is sound and up to date, not just perpetuating old myths and old polarizations. I say to all of you: Be aware of underlying motives that may bias the selection of information presented, and evaluate carefully what you hear in the news, in magazines, in health education programs, in conversations with friends, or wherever. Follow the "money trail"—if the author or speaker is trying to get you to buy products on which they make commissions, then you need to be more skeptical of the claims being made. If something sounds like a miracle cure, it is probably too good to be true. Remember, each of us is an individual with different needs. No one approach works for everyone, and no one authority has all the answers for everyone.

Setting the stage for, and implementing, change will continue to be our task in the interest of future generations of women. We can work to see that pressures are intensified in the search for answers by encouraging research and educational activities, and by helping to develop sources of funds to create more health care options and choices for all of us. We must become "activated" patients, in a *partnership* with our health professionals, to improve communication, increase awareness of the special needs of women's bodies, and further enhance awareness of gender differences and gender concerns as they impact prevention and health care. We can, and should, "vote with our feet" by changing physicians and other health professionals when we feel we are not being listened to adequately.

Another resource is the increasing number of women in the health professions in all fields. We must be the ones to lead this agenda into the twenty-first century. We can be, and should be, in the forefront of the women's health agenda efforts. Health **costs** can be reduced and health **care** improved by attention to the significant differences between the needs and body chemistry of men and women. You will find in this book some often unrecognized connections, and issues, that are crucial to our understanding of how women's bodies work. You have known or suspected some of these hormonal connections because you live them. Some will seem so obvious you will wonder why they haven't been addressed before. Some will make you cry; some will make you angry. "I *knew* it was real," women say in my office. "At least I don't feel like I'm crazy. There's something going on that now makes sense." "Finally, someone is telling it like it is and putting it together." For example, I have drawn a number of diagrams throughout the book to show hormonal connections that seem *basic* to me. I have never seen these connections laid out like this before. I continue to be astounded by the apparent blind spots about the role of female hormones in so many different body-brain functions.

I have provided a lot of medical information in the chapters ahead. Use this information to become a powerful advocate for your own health and well-being. Write me with your comments, your feedback, your experiences in health care settings, and your ideas or suggestions for how we can all work together to reach our goals to improve the delivery of women's health care: for ourselves, for our collective daughters' and granddaughters' generations. Because of my daily patient appointments and my writing and speaking schedules, I won't be able to respond personally to your letters. I can assure you, however, that your voice WILL be heard, taken seriously, and I will incorporate your letters and comments into future programs, courses, services, and research in women's health. Each of you reading this can make a difference. Let's work together to make the slogan "You've come a long way, baby" mean something HEALTHY!

Chapter 2

Hormones:
A Guide to Your
Body Cycles

HORMONES. Whenever I mention the word *hormones*, women have almost instantaneously an intense reaction, either very positive or very negative, not much in-between:

"I don't want strange chemicals in my body."

"Being on estrogen has given me my life back."

"All doctors ever do is prescribe hormone pills."

"Why didn't anyone tell me about natural hormones before . . . I feel so much better now!"

"Those are drugs. I don't take drugs; I want to take natural herbs."

"I know it's my hormones out of whack that's making me feel so bad, but my doctors won't listen. Why won't anybody give me hormones?"

"I felt like being on hormones has lifted the fogginess off my brain and I have more energy now."

This polarization of opinions crops up everywhere these days. Betty Friedan, in a speech at Omega Institute in 1994, called hormones, specifically estrogen therapy, a *hoax* perpetrated on women by the medical industry. The same year, Dr. Trudy Bush of Johns Hopkins said in several publications that the majority of women after menopause would benefit from estrogen therapy. Both speakers are women, yet 180 degrees apart in their views.

Why such emotional intensity and polarization over hormones? Why is this? What are these things called *hormones*? What do they do? Why are they important? How do we tell when a woman (or a man, for that matter) needs hormones? This chapter will help clarify these questions. In later chapters, we will look more closely at factors I think contribute to the polarity in views and the intense emotionalism on these issues. I will also provide you with the latest research and clinical information that helps to show often unrecognized hormonal connections affecting many conditions that occur more commonly in women.

What Is a Hormone?

A hormone is "a product of a living cell that circulates in body fluids or sap (in plants) and produces a specific effect on the activity of cells remote from its point of origin; or a synthetic substance that acts like a hormone" (*Webster's Collegiate Dictionary 10th edition*). I think of hormones as "chemical communicators" or "connectors" that carry messages to and from all organs of the body and serve to connect one organ's function with another organ's function to keep the body balanced and functioning optimally. Without our hormones to keep the connections and messages flowing smoothly and our organs functioning in a balanced and integrated manner, we would die. It's that simple. The secretion and interaction of hormones throughout our bodies every day is a highly complex and ongoing process.

For many years, as I have explained these complex processes to patients and students, I have used the visual analogy of a "key in a lock" to describe the way brain chemicals fit at special receptor sites in the brain and body and the way hormones bind at their specific receptor sites to trigger their action on the target cells. Each hormone, neurotransmitter, neuropeptide, or other chemical messenger is a unique molecular "key," and each has a "lock" (receptor site) into which it fits (see diagram). Similar keys may fit in a lock, but not be able to turn it. This is a simplistic model, and the hormone-receptor interaction is really more complex than this, but it helps visualize the basic principle to think of it this way.

The receptor sites may be located on cell surfaces (membrane receptors) or inside cells (cytoplasm or nucleus receptors). Each hormone provides a specific set of directions or messages to the target cells to enable the cells to perform certain functions. The cells of the body are like manufacturing plants, making the many chemicals the body needs to function. Hormones have a variety of functions, some similar to those of assembly-line supervisors directing the manufacturing processes, and some similar to those of team facilitators acting as catalysts for chemical processes to occur in the cell. Hormone actions may be extraordinarily rapid if they trigger immediate chemical release via effects on membrane receptors. Hormones act more slowly when they act at the cell nucleus receptors to influence the DNA and direct the manufacture of specific enzymes and proteins. The shape and molecular structure of each hormone fits exactly into the proper receptor site; changes in the molecule shape or makeup produce different notches on the molecule "key." This means that a different shape may not work, or work as well, at that receptor. This effect of changes in the molecule is evident from the way in which the various types of estrogen molecules produce different results at the estrogen receptors throughout the brain and body. We also see this difference in response with many other hormones and their synthetic "look-alikes." If the hormone molecules don't bind just the right way and "click into the lock", it's like a key getting stuck in a lock. The door doesn't open easily (or sometimes at all); the cell doesn't function properly, and you may experience the body effects of missing that particular hormone.

As a specific example of the importance of molecule shape and makeup, consider the primary human estrogen, 17-beta estradiol, and the primary horse estrogens, called equilins, components of Premarin. All of these types of estrogen have four connecting rings as the basic shape of the molecule. But the equilins have some important differences in the makeup of the rings, which makes them slightly different keys. Consequently, these estrogens don't fit exactly the same way at the estrogen receptor. The equilin estrogens sometimes keep the human estradiol key from fitting into the lock (receptor), which means the *effects* can be different from those of the natural human 17-beta estradiol. Horse-derived equilin estrogens attach more strongly, and longer, to our bodies' estrogen receptors than does our own human estrogen. The *process* for the body to *metabolize* equilins also takes much longer because the equilin metabolites are not normal ones for the human body to process, and we don't have the enzymes needed to break them down. All this because of a few changes in one ring! The body is quite amazing in its ability to recognize its exact molecular keys.

The human female produces three types of estrogen that I will describe more in later chapters so I just want to name them here: *estrone* (E1) made in the ovary, liver, and fat tissue; *17-beta estradiol* (E2) the premenopausal estrogen made in the ovary; and the weaker *estriol* (E3) produced by the placenta during pregnancy. Premarin contains small amounts of two of these human estrogens (estradiol and estrone), but much higher amounts of the equilin estrogens unique to the horse. All that is needed to activate the human body's estrogen receptors is the 17-beta estradiol, but the remaining equilin hormones still have to be processed by the liver for excretion in the urine. Equilin isn't necessarily "bad," especially for the horse, but it

Diagram 2.1—Hormones and Receptors:
A Look at How They Work

Each hormone has its own receptor site "lock" at target cells throughout the body. The body's own hormone molecular "key" fits into its receptor to trigger hormone effects. Molecules with different shapes may also occupy the "lock" for that hormone, but may or may not trigger the hormonal action in the way your body's molecules do. These different-shaped molecules (examples: equilin, genistein, SERMS) may actually block the body's own hormones from working properly.

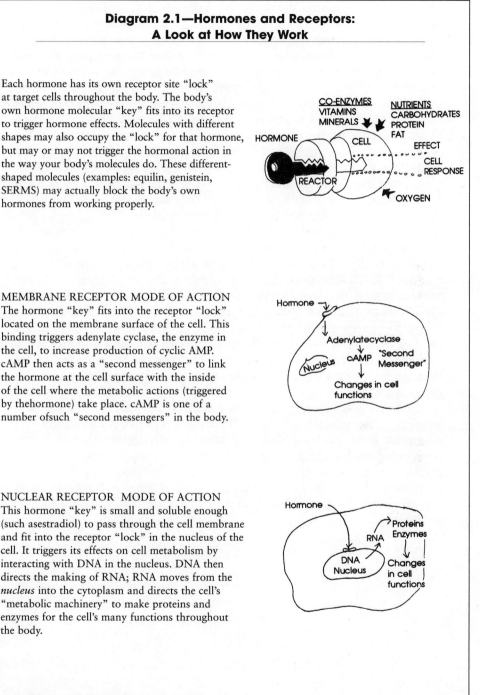

MEMBRANE RECEPTOR MODE OF ACTION
The hormone "key" fits into the receptor "lock" located on the membrane surface of the cell. This binding triggers adenylate cyclase, the enzyme in the cell, to increase production of cyclic AMP. cAMP then acts as a "second messenger" to link the hormone at the cell surface with the inside of the cell where the metabolic actions (triggered by thehormone) take place. cAMP is one of a number ofsuch "second messengers" in the body.

NUCLEAR RECEPTOR MODE OF ACTION
This hormone "key" is small and soluble enough (such asestradiol) to pass through the cell membrane and fit into the receptor "lock" in the nucleus of the cell. It triggers its effects on cell metabolism by interacting with DNA in the nucleus. DNA then directs the making of RNA; RNA moves from the *nucleus* into the cytoplasm and directs the cell's "metabolic machinery" to make proteins and enzymes for the cell's many functions throughout the body.

does place an unusual extra demand on the human body that isn't needed for our bodies to have estrogen's beneficial effects. For many women this appears to be one of the reasons that they still have symptoms of estrogen loss, even when taking the accepted dose of conjugated equine estrogen (Premarin). The horse estrogen keys are not opening the receptor locks quite as well, or perhaps the horse's mixed estrogens aren't providing quite enough of the human form (17-beta estradiol) that woman may need. This may be why the dose is often increased, but that then means even more equilins for the body to have to process, and this contributes to the bloating and breast enlargement women describe. I will talk more about the many effects of some of these differences in the chapters ahead, but I wanted you to begin to realize the crucial importance of the *fit* of hormone molecules into their receptor sites throughout the body.

Hormones are very potent molecules, and it usually takes miniscule amounts, sometimes as little as a *billionth* of a gram (nanogram), to exert their effects on cells of the target organs. Estradiol, for example, is measured in picograms, one *trillionth* of a gram. After initiating actions at the target organs, hormones are broken down and "inactivated" by the target cells themselves or carried by the blood to the liver to be metabolized. The metabolized hormones are used again by the body's synthesis processes to make new hormone molecules, or the metabolic breakdown products are excreted in the urine (tests can measure hormone breakdown substances in urine or feces).

Some of the major hormones, where they are produced, and what they do, are described in the diagrams and charts below. As you read them, think about the brain as the orchestra conductor who provides direction to the various "instruments" (hormones) to produce the "symphony" of our body rhythms and functions. Hormones affect the brain, and the brain affects hormone production and interactions. The brain and the body *really are* intimately connected.

Diagram 2.2—The Endocrine System:
A Look at Key Hormones And What They Do

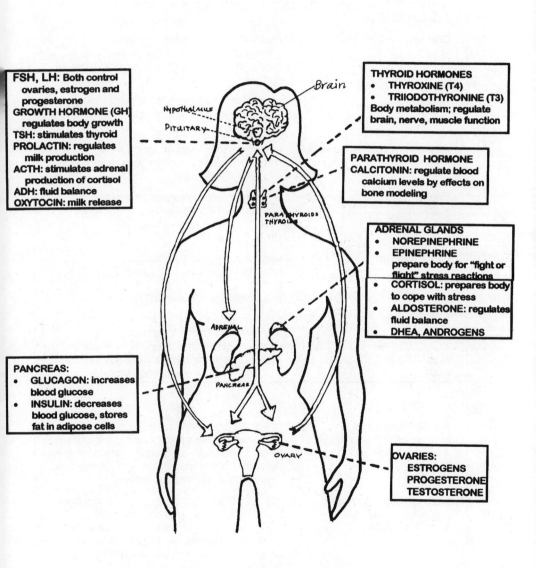

FSH, LH: Both control ovaries, estrogen and progesterone
GROWTH HORMONE (GH) regulates body growth
TSH: stimulates thyroid
PROLACTIN: regulates milk production
ACTH: stimulates adrenal production of cortisol
ADH: fluid balance
OXYTOCIN: milk release

THYROID HORMONES
• **THYROXINE (T4)**
• **TRIIODOTHYRONINE (T3)**
Body metabolism; regulate brain, nerve, muscle function

PARATHYROID HORMONE
CALCITONIN: regulate blood calcium levels by effects on bone modeling

ADRENAL GLANDS
• **NOREPINEPHRINE**
• **EPINEPHRINE**
prepare body for "fight or flight" stress reactions
• **CORTISOL:** prepares body to cope with stress
• **ALDOSTERONE:** regulates fluid balance
• **DHEA, ANDROGENS**

PANCREAS:
• **GLUCAGON:** increases blood glucose
• **INSULIN:** decreases blood glucose, stores fat in adipose cells

OVARIES:
ESTROGENS
PROGESTERONE
TESTOSTERONE

Brain

HYPOTHALMUS
PITUITARY

PARATHYROIDS
THYROID

ADRENAL

PANCREAS

OVARY

CLASSES OF HORMONES AND WHAT THEY DO

Primary Actions

I. STEROIDS

Cortisol . . . . many metabolic actions, anti-inflammatory actions, produced in higher amounts during stress and may suppress normal immune function

Aldosterone . . . . regulates fluid balance by stimulating kidney to retain sodium and water, excretes potassium

Androgens (DHEA, others) . . . enhance sex drive, produce mild male features in women (e.g., facial hair, male body shape)

Estrogens (three) . . . . produces female secondary sex characteristics; key role:
• ESTRADIOL
• ESTRONE
• ESTRIOL
menstruation, pregnancy; 400 other functions

Progesterone . . . . helps maintain pregnancy, many metabolic effects, high levels give sedative, analgesic effects at brain may produce depressed mood

Testosterone . . . . produces male secondary sex patterns; triggers sex drive and arousal in both males and females, many metabolic effects (bone and muscle growth, etc.)

II. AMINES

Thyroid hormones:
• THYROXINE (T4)
• TRIIODOTHYRONINE (T3)

stimulate body metabolism by increasing cell energy release; increasing heart rate, heat production, and brain activity. Helps normal regulation and growth of nervous, and musculoskeletal systems

"Adrenaline" hormones:
• NOREPINEPHRINE (NE)
• EPINEPHRINE (EPI)

"fight or flight" (stress) hormones, prepare body by increasing heart rate; act on brain to lift mood (or in excess, cause anxiety), increase alertness; dilate arteries to key organs to provide more oxygen, glucose, and nutrients

© Elizabeth Lee Vliet, M.D., 1995, revised 2000

III. PEPTIDES AND PROTEINS

Insulin . . . . *lowers* blood sugar (moves glucose into cells), stimulates fat storage and protein synthesis

Glucagon . . . . *raises* blood glucose (glycogen breakdown and glucose release from liver, gluconeogenesis)

Somatostatin . . . . mild effect to raise blood glucose

Parathyroid (PTH) . . . . major role: increase blood calcium levels by stimulating bone breakdown, calcium release

Calcitonin . . . . involved in regulating blood calcium levels by inhibiting bone breakdown, calcium release

Thymosin (thymus gland) . . . . major role in development of immune system

ACTH . . . . adrenocorticotropin hormone; stimulates part of the adrenal gland to make cortisol

FSH . . . . stimulates ovaries, activates and promotes follicle growth to produce estrogen

LH . . . . triggers ovulation, formation of the corpus luteum, secretion of progesterone, estrogen

Growth Hormone (GH) . . . . oversees entire process of normal body growth

TSH . . . . stimulates the thyroid gland to release T3, T4

Prolactin . . . . stimulates breast enlargement during pregnancy and milk production after delivery

Anti-Diuretic Hormone (ADH) . . . prevents dehydration by stimulating kidneys to increase reabsorption and retain water

Oxytocin . . . . stimulates uterine contractions during labor, helps trigger milk release after delivery

Melatonin (pineal gland) . . . . regulation of sleep cycles, body rhythms

Brain-Body Hormonal Communication Pathways

The brain and body are interconnected by an incredible array of chemical and electrical circuits, each one interacting with and affecting others. The brain has a multitude of ways to direct the orchestra of the body to respond to what the brain perceives, from inside the body physically, from inside the mind's thoughts and feelings, or from outside the body. In women's bodies, the entire process is even more complex, with the menstrual cycle rhythm of changes causing the brain-body systems to continuously adapt to the changing hormonal environment. Unlike the male body, which maintains a fairly steady production (*tonic* pattern) of testosterone all month, the female body has a *cyclic* pattern of ovarian hormone rise and fall.

The major underlying influence of these crucial female hormonal rhythms has never been fully appreciated for the diverse effects on all parts of the female body, not just reproduction. The diagram that follows shows some of the ways that these stimuli (stressors) of all kinds require the body processes to change and adapt. Hormonal change is another one of those stimuli that trigger the body systems to constantly change and adapt. When the body systems are overstressed, a variety of things may occur: we call these changes *symptoms* if they feel unpleasant to us, or we call them *phenomena* if they are just normal and don't bother us. These changes themselves may then become additional "stressors" on the body and contribute to more overload and possible illness. The interconnections and the ways in which hormonal production may in turn be altered by stress on the body are often overlooked when women seek medical care. Keep in mind that Mother Nature's protective plan is to prevent pregnancy when animals or humans are stressed or sick. It shouldn't be a surprise to learn that prolonged stress can suppress the ovaries and cause decreases in hormone production. The two-way nature of these pathways is a critical connection throughout all facets of women's health that is so often overlooked.

Diagram 2.3—STRESS EFFECTS

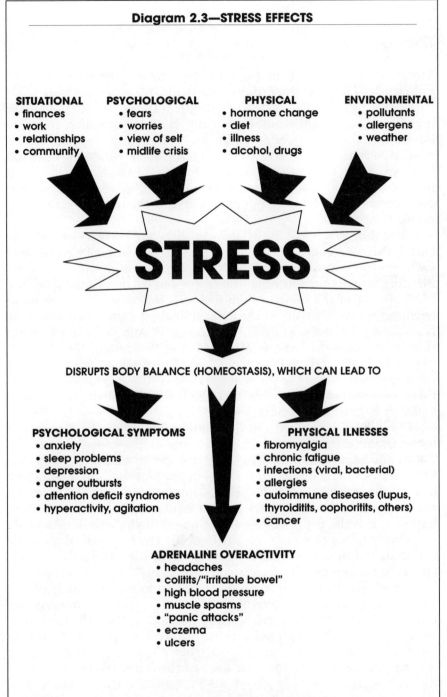

SITUATIONAL
- finances
- work
- relationships
- community

PSYCHOLOGICAL
- fears
- worries
- view of self
- midlife crisis

PHYSICAL
- hormone change
- diet
- illness
- alcohol, drugs

ENVIRONMENTAL
- pollutants
- allergens
- weather

STRESS

DISRUPTS BODY BALANCE (HOMEOSTASIS), WHICH CAN LEAD TO

PSYCHOLOGICAL SYMPTOMS
- anxiety
- sleep problems
- depression
- anger outbursts
- attention deficit syndromes
- hyperactivity, agitation

PHYSICAL ILNESSES
- fibromyalgia
- chronic fatigue
- infections (viral, bacterial)
- allergies
- autoimmune diseases (lupus, thyroiditits, oophoritits, others)
- cancer

ADRENALINE OVERACTIVITY
- headaches
- colitits/"irritable bowel"
- high blood pressure
- muscle spasms
- "panic attacks"
- eczema
- ulcers

Medical Content © Elizabeth Lee Vliet M.D., 1985, rev. 1995, 1999

The Menstrual Cycle RHYTHM of Changes Through Our Lives

Most women learn about menstruation initially from mothers or girlfriends. The first scientific explanation we receive about what happens is often in health class, about the sixth or seventh grade. We then live it each month and don't really think about which hormone is doing what at any given time. In case you've forgotten your health education material, I'd like to give you a quick rundown on what happens in the normal menstrual cycle. My description is based on the average cycle length of twenty-eight days, but keep in mind that cycle variations in length from twenty-five to thirty-five days may be perfectly normal.

We arbitrarily mark the cycle by labeling the first day of bleeding Day 1 (M). We could define any day as Day 1, but it helps to have such a clear-cut marker as bleeding to use as a starting point. Bleeding is really the finishing of the previous cycle with the shedding of the lining of the uterus (womb) that is not needed if there is no fertilized egg to nourish. As the uterine lining is being shed, the body is preparing for the next cycle. The follicle ("little sac") in the ovary that will become the egg is already being "recruited" by the hormonal changes directed by the brain. Progesterone and estrogen both dropped sharply in the waning days of the previous cycle, and these two hormones are now at their lowest point of the cycle as bleeding begins (Day 1 of next cycle).

From Day 1 onward until ovulation, estradiol (E2), and to a lesser extent estrone (E1), levels are rising as the growth of several follicles is being stimulated by FSH (follicle stimulating hormone). Once estrogen reaches a certain level in the bloodstream, all but one of the follicles shrink and die. That dominant follicle remains as the one destined to be the egg released at ovulation. For the entire first half of the cycle, progesterone levels remain extremely low, usually less than 1 nanogram per milliliter (ng/ml). The first half of the cycle is dominated by estrogen and is called either the *"Follicular* phase" (refers to the egg development in the ovary) or *"Proliferative* phase" (refers to the process of growth of the endometrial lining of the uterus). Estradiol levels average about 200 pg/ml (picograms per milliliter) across the first two weeks of the cycle, with the low point being Day 1 and the high point being OVULATION, usually about Day 14. Peak estradiol levels at the ovulatory phase are in the range of 350 to 500 pg/ml. The first few days of the cycle, (Days 1–3) estradiol levels are optimally about 80–90 pg/ml, until the decline in estrogen with premenopausal years when estradiol typically drops to less than about 40 pg/ml during Days 1–3 of the cycle.

Thus, keep in mind that in the first two weeks each cycle until ovulation occurs, estrogen levels are *high*, and progesterone levels are *low* (in fact, there's very little progesterone at all present for these first two weeks of each month). Days 1–14 are typically the phase of the cycle during which women experience a sense of well-being, optimal energy level, normal sleep, and an "up" mood; that is, they feel good. Estrogen has an activating effect on brain centers and contributes to enhanced energy and mood as well as clarity of thinking, sharper memory, and ability to concentrate. In chapter 3, I will show you some of the many ways estrogen acts on the brain that are similar to the actions of present *antidepressant* medications.

FSH is the brain hormone that stimulates the growth of the follicle that contains the egg. FSH begins to rise in the cycle when the brain senses the drop in estrogen at menses, and then FSH stimulates the ovary to produce the next follicle. FSH and LH (luteinizing hormone) are the two primary brain hormones that govern the egg maturation and release for the menstrual cycle. I won't focus as much on FSH and LH because I want you to have more of an overview about the estrogen and progesterone patterns and effects in the normal cycle. In the perimenopausal years, as estradiol production from the ovary *declines,* the brain produces *more* FSH and LH, trying to stimulate the ovary to produce more hormones. So you will see high levels of FSH and LH prior to and after menopause because estradiol levels are then low (usually less than 30 pg/ml).

In the first ten days of each new cycle, rising estradiol levels stimulate the release of LH from the brain. When estradiol reaches its peak level (about 400–500 pg/ml) at mid-cycle, LH triggers the follicle to be released as an egg, called ovulation. Some women can feel ovulation as a brief, sharp pain in the area of the ovary (called "mittelschmerz"); other women do not feel any physical sensations at ovulation. The rapid drop in estradiol as the egg is released may trigger onset of a migraine in some women. It may also contribute to brief disruption in sleep; and for some women, it may trigger brief mood swings as the brain chemicals are changing in response to the drop in circulating estrogen. I will talk more about these important connections in upcoming chapters.

The egg develops into the *corpus luteum* (from Latin for "yellow body," due to its yellowish appearance). This half of the cycle is called the *luteal phase* (if referring to the ovary changes) or *secretory phase* (if referring to the further thickening of the uterine lining to prepare for fertilization and implantation of the egg). This phase of the cycle is dominated by the hormone progesterone, produced by the corpus luteum. Progesterone is the "pro-*gestation*" hormone and its primary role is to prepare a woman's body to sustain and nourish a pregnancy. It is the *dominant* hormone of the second half of the cycle, with blood levels higher than the level of estrogen. Circulating levels of progesterone reach a peak between 10–25 nanograms per milliliter by about Days 20 to 22, the midpoint of the second half of the cycle (or about the third week from last Day 1 of bleeding). If the egg is fertilized, progesterone levels stay high until the placenta takes over producing the progesterone for pregnancy. If there is no fertilization of the egg, the corpus luteum begins to disintegrate and no longer makes progesterone so the progesterone level drops sharply, triggering the onset of bleeding. Estrogen also drops at this time of the cycle, and the falling estradiol level can be a trigger for migraines, restless sleep, anxiety symptoms, palpitations and pain flares. It is the decrease in progesterone that causes bleeding to occur. Shedding the uterine lining is part of the process of preparing the body to begin a new cycle. Falling progesterone levels may further add to insomnia and anxiety triggered by the falling estradiol.

Estrogen (estradiol) levels also rise again from ovulation until about Day 20, reaching the peak for the second half of the cycle at the same time progesterone is peaking. The optimal level of estradiol in the luteal phase of a healthy cycle is somewhat less than in the follicular phase of the cycle. Average peak luteal phase estradiol levels are about 200–300 pg/ml. I find that women we see have worsening premenstrual symptoms when luteal phase estradiol levels fall below about 160–170 pg/ml.

Since progesterone prepares the body for pregnancy, it makes sense that some of the changes you notice—water retention, increased appetite, breast enlargement—are triggered by the metabolic effects of progesterone, since these are necessary changes to help the body provide for a growing fetus. Hormones, such as insulin, that control blood glucose levels are affected by progesterone, and this contributes to some of the "sweet cravings" women describe in the premenstrual week. Tufts University researchers show a 12 percent increase in appetite and metabolic rate under the influence of progesterone. You're not imagining it, you *do* notice feelings of hunger more in this half of the cycle for very real, physiological reasons based on the higher levels of progesterone at this phase of the cycle. Progesterone makes you want to eat more so your body could sustain a pregnancy.

Another effect of progesterone is to slow down the movement of food through the gastrointestinal (GI) tract by decreasing the muscular waves (peristalsis) that move material through the entire digestive system. As a result, you hold more contents in the intestine when progesterone is high, so this is one reason you feel full or bloated at this phase of the cycle. Our low-fiber diet is another lifestyle factor that intensifies the natural constipating effects of progesterone. In Stone Age cultures, humans may have eaten 100 grams of fiber a day or more. Thus there was an evolutionary advantage for survival of the species to have progesterone effects in women slow down the gastrointestinal tract, enabling more nutrients to be absorbed from the food into the blood stream. With a high-fiber diet (which causes "rapid transit" through the GI tract) and in times when food was scarce, the hormonal effect of progesterone further helped a woman's body retain nutrients to sustain a pregnancy. In the typical American high-fat diet, women may get only 10 grams of fiber a day. Slowing down the gastrointestinal tract when you're eating a low-fiber diet has some very unpleasant side effects, among them *constipation*. Women in the progesterone-dominant luteal phase (or when taking progesterone or progestins for HRT) frequently describe feeling constipated, bloated, headachy, irritable, and lethargic from fluid retention.

Progesterone and its metabolites have a tranquilizing effect on the brain, much like our current antianxiety medications. For some women, progesterone has *such* a calming effect that it acts more like a sedative. For some women, the "slowing down" effect of progesterone feels "wonderful," "soothing," "relaxed," "more centered." For other women these progesterone effects feel like "depression," fatigue, tiredness, or lethargy. These women say, "I don't have any get up and go." "I withdraw." "I can't get out of bed." "I don't have any energy." You can see how a hormone having a calming, tranquilizing effect is an evolutionary advantage in the early stages of pregnancy: being calmer or "slowed down" would facilitate diminished activity at a time when the egg is being implanted, thereby helping prevent expulsion from the uterus. This facilitates early development of the embryo. In pregnancy, progesterone levels decrease sharply at the sixth to eighth week and do not rise again until about the thirty-fourth week of gestation to prepare the body for delivery. If you have been pregnant, think about how you felt the last six weeks of pregnancy (when progesterone rises very high) compared with the middle months of pregnancy, when estrogen levels are quite high. You can then see some of the physical and psychological differences between estrogen and progesterone.

The hormonal ebb and flow, which occurs in this cyclical manner, has widespread effects on the brain-body processes, as well as on our psyche. When you understand the specific effects and roles of each of the primary female hormones, you can see how beautifully orchestrated the female endocrine system is for its role in bringing new life into being and keeping the species alive. These hormonal actions make sense from an evolutionary standpoint for the tasks they govern in the body. The problem today is that in our culture, food is no longer scarce; for most people, it is overly available. We don't eat as much fiber in fruits, whole grains, and vegetables; we have too much sugar, caffeine, and alcohol easily at hand. We're not getting pregnant as often, and we are trying to do multiple tasks, with a marked increase in overall stress levels. Consequently, some of the natural hormonal metabolic effects are now experienced as *negative, unwanted* physical-psychological "symptoms" because of our unnatural lifestyles and diet. I think this is one of a number of reasons that we see so many more women experiencing PMS in today's culture compared to women at the turn of the century when diets had lower overall fat, sugar, salt, alcohol, and caffeine intake and a far higher intake of fruits, whole grains, and vegetables.

All these underlying physiological changes then have a bearing on how we respond to the external world and the impact of external stresses on our brain-body pathways. Please don't think that I'm saying we are at the mercy of our hormones. If we understand what is happening, we can learn to "go with the flow" in positive ways, rather than making things worse with poor lifestyle choices. What I am concerned about is that we need to better understand the differences and the physiological changes women experience. We desperately need more gender-specific research on these issues so that we can learn to constructively manage our very complicated lives when living in a body that is much more complex than the male body. I don't think that the hormonal cycles mean that we should do anything less than whatever it is we would like to do with our lives. However, in order to really understand what is happening, we need to know about the hormonal cycles, and we need better medical and health research that will help our therapeutic approaches take into account the unique and natural needs of the female body.

It is important to understand how these hormone messengers are carried in the bloodstream throughout the body. Sex steroid hormones are carried in the bloodstream three ways: bound to two different carrier proteins (sex-hormone–binding globulin (SHBG) and albumin) and in the free form, not bound to carrier protein. Thyroid hormones are carried by thyroid-binding globulin (TBG). Cortisol is carried by corticosteroid binding globulin (CBG). The free amount of all of these hormones is a much smaller percentage than the total circulating hormone.

It was previously thought that only the *free* form was biologically active, but newer research has shown that *both* the free portion and the portions *weakly bound* to albumin are biologically active, at least for the sex steroid hormones. It is less clear whether this is also true for thyroid hormones and cortisol. Serum (blood) assays for ovarian hormones, thyroid, and cortisol include all of these circulating forms: total, weakly bound, and free. The serum assay provides a complete picture of the steroid hormones available to act at tissues of the body. When needed, the "free" fraction of a given hormone can also be measured in the serum.

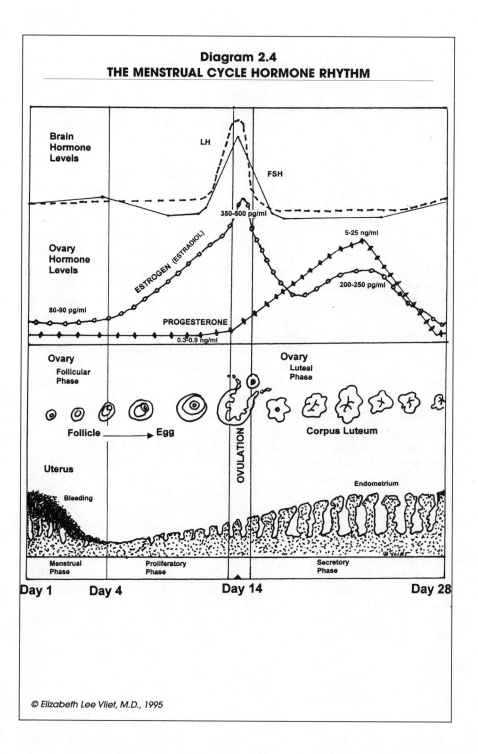

Diagram 2.4
THE MENSTRUAL CYCLE HORMONE RHYTHM

© Elizabeth Lee Vliet, M.D., 1995

There has been a great deal of current consumer marketing effort aimed at use of saliva measures of ovarian and other hormones. The makers of the saliva test kits claim that a measurement of the free hormone in saliva gives a more reliable result than the combined fractions measured in serum. These claims have not been borne out in menopause research settings showing saliva hormone testing is a reliable tool for use in assessing adequacy of clinical response and therapeutic effect. In fact, as further research has clarified the complexity of estrogen action at receptor sites and the ability of some tissues to actively utilize both protein bound and free forms of these hormones, it appears to be even more important to use the serum assays that reflect bound and free fractions. Saliva hormone tests only show the small part in the free fraction, and the amount of the free fraction that is excreted into the saliva from serum.

Urine hormone assays are measuring only the metabolic breakdown products of the various forms of the hormones, not the active forms. The urinary hormone tests are the most *indirect* (and therefore less useful) measures of circulating levels of the active forms of the ovarian hormones. Compared to the serum assays, the saliva and urinary hormone tests are much less clinically useful in making treatment decisions regarding ovarian hormone therapy because we really need to know more than just the free fraction in order to have a complete picture of what is happening in your body. Serum measures remain the worldwide gold standard in research settings addressing crucial issues in women's health and certainly are the measure that should be used in making assessments of hormone effects on complex problems.

Many factors affect the amount of hormone that is "free" at any given time. I have shown some of these in the chart that follows. Other factors include medications that are highly protein bound. Such medications compete for the carrier proteins and displace more of a given hormone into the free form, possibly producing symptoms of hormone excess. Or the converse may happen. Some medications will push more of the hormone into the bound and inactive form, leaving less in the free, active fraction. A good example of this problem is the effect of birth control pills on thyroid hormones. BCPs cause more of the thyroid hormones to bind to TBG, moving out of the free and active fraction. This is one way that women on BCPs sometimes develop symptoms of hypothyroidism even thought their TSH and total hormones appear normal on the blood tests.

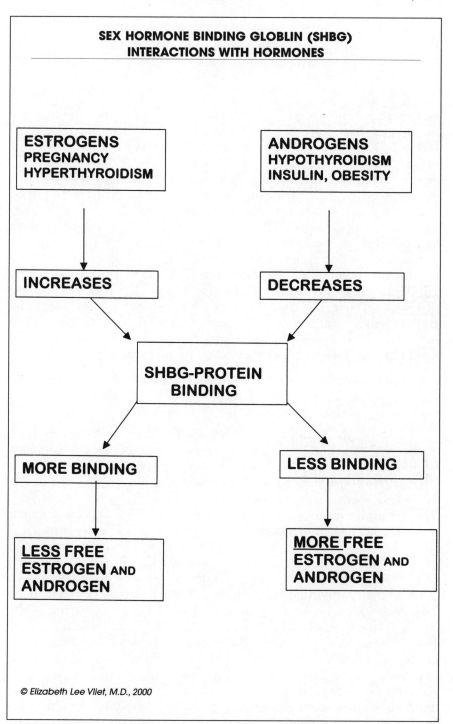

**SEX HORMONE BINDING GLOBLIN (SHBG)
INTERACTIONS WITH HORMONES**

ESTROGENS
PREGNANCY
HYPERTHYROIDISM

ANDROGENS
HYPOTHYROIDISM
INSULIN, OBESITY

INCREASES

DECREASES

**SHBG-PROTEIN
BINDING**

MORE BINDING

LESS BINDING

**LESS FREE
ESTROGEN AND
ANDROGEN**

**MORE FREE
ESTROGEN AND
ANDROGEN**

What Happens When Estrogen Declines: Hormone Changes Through the Decades

At birth, a newborn girl's ovaries contain about 500,000 follicles, and these are the source of her future eggs. By puberty, the number of follicles has decreased to 300,000, and by age thirty-eight to forty, the average woman has only 5,000 to 10,000 follicles remaining. Several follicles are "recruited" each cycle, but only one egg will be released at each ovulation. The follicles and maturing eggs produce estradiol; when the ovaries run out of follicles (and therefore out of eggs), they also run out of the supply of estradiol, our body's most active form of estrogen. The brain senses the decrease in estradiol, and produces more FSH and LH to try to stimulate the ovaries to produce more hormones. This effort is to no avail because there are no more follicles to develop into hormone-producing eggs. Fundamentally, when our follicle supply is depleted, this is the end of a woman's *reproductive* stage, and we no longer menstruate. The end of menses is **menopause.** The journey from puberty to menopause has many developmental stages along the way. Here are some of the highlights of those stages as they relate to hormone cycles.

Early Puberty and Adolescence

Girls in the United States typically enter puberty anytime between about nine and fourteen years of age. Breast development begins to appear first, followed by the appearance of pubic hair. Menstruation usually doesn't occur until the breasts are well developed and a critical body weight of about 110 pounds is reached. This generally follows soon after the girl's adolescent growth spurt, at about age eleven or twelve. The average age at the onset of menstruation is about eleven and a half to thirteen, although it may take several years for the menstrual cycle to stabilize into a regular pattern. During these years, a young woman's ovaries are beginning to develop their individual cycle rhythm. It can be a time of erratic periods, feelings of uncertainty about what's happening to the body, mood shifts, new physical sensations, and unpredictable menstrual flows. Some young women experience only mild cramps, or no cramps at all, with bleeding; while others have severe and sustained cramping. Some can tell physically when ovulation occurs; others have no awareness of it. Fertility (the ability to conceive and bear children) occurs when ovulation begins. The problem for many adolescent girls is that since ovulation may be erratic in the first year or two of menstruation, it may be difficult to know when they are fertile. This is one reason girls in this age group are surprised when they accidentally become pregnant. It is important for girls who are sexually active at this time to use some form of contraception.

Throughout history many cultures have had ceremonies (rites of passage) for young girls to mark this transition into womanhood. In our culture, this has not been a usual practice, and many young girls are embarrassed by the onset of menstruation. In our culture there is a lot of negative language about menstruation: "on the rag," "the curse." Such demeaning terms don't help young girls feel proud about becoming a woman. Having meaningful ceremonies marking this as a special dimension of being a woman could serve to provide positive images and role models for girls today as they become young women.

Reproductive Years: The Twenties and Thirties

During her twenties and early thirties, a woman's menstrual cycle tends to be fairly regular, unless altered by lifestyle (e.g., extreme dieting, cigarette smoking, strenuous athletic activity, alcohol or drug abuse) or the presence of endocrine or other medical disorders. Polycystic ovary syndrome (PCOS) is an example of an endocrine metabolic disorder that disrupts normal ovary cycles in this age group and often causes infertility. Fertility usually peaks by age twenty-five, and the body is at its physiological optimal point for childbearing during the early and mid-twenties. That does not mean that women cannot become pregnant at a later age; it simply means that in the decade of her twenties, a woman's circulatory, respiratory, and digestive systems are at their peak to meet the physiological demands of pregnancy with the least stress on the mother's system.

Hormone production during the twenties and early thirties is more predictable than during either puberty or perimenopause and typically follows the pattern I outlined: estrogen levels high in the first half, and progesterone dominating the second half of each cycle, and testosterone fairly constant throughout the cycle. By the mid-thirties, the menstrual flow may begin changing, at first imperceptibly, and by the late thirties more noticeably, as flow may become lighter and shorter, and cycle length may become either longer or shorter. By the later thirties, women often begin to notice more pronounced premenstrual mood, energy, and appetite changes, which are described as the premenstrual syndrome (PMS) for short. For some women, there is no PMS at all; others experience a minor degree of discomfort; still others have more bothersome symptoms lasting a week or more; and for a small percentage of women, PMS may be severely disruptive of work, family, and social relationships.

I describe these changes and some of their causes in chapter 7. As estradiol begins to decline, this is also a time we may see worsening migraines, fibromyalgia, bladder problems, vulvodynia, and other annoying changes.

Pre- and "Peri"-menopausal: The Forties

Between the ages of approximately thirty-five and fifty women enter the phase called the "climacteric" or premenopausal years when the ovaries' production of estradiol and progesterone begin declining as the woman's follicles are diminishing. This is a transition phase from our optimal reproductive hormone levels that make us fertile to the lower levels that still produce menstrual periods but don't necessarily maintain "optimal" metabolic function throughout the body. This is the time that so many women begin having "vague" symptoms as I have been discussing throughout this book. Depending on your lifestyle habits and your genetic makeup, the climacteric may start in the early thirties or may not begin until the mid- or late forties.

During the climacteric or premenopausal years, hormonal levels begin to decline, the amount of estrone rises relative to decreasing estradiol, cycles become more erratic, there are more cycles when you don't ovulate, and there is more fluctuation in the actual amounts of estrogen and progesterone produced. In cycles when you do ovulate, you will have higher levels of progesterone, and those cycles are usually ones when you have much more PMS: feeling bloated, headachy, irritable, tearful, and just generally awful. In cycles when you do not ovulate, there isn't much progesterone, so you sail through and don't notice these PMS-type changes.

As estrogen declines, there are many body functions that are affected: sleep, memory, mood, energy level, immune system, body fat distribution, circulatory system, digestive tract, bone metabolism, skin changes (such as increased acne), sexual function, bladder function, and many others that I will be addressing in more detail throughout this book. These changes are gradual and take place over several years; they do not all occur at a single point in time and suddenly you wake up and say "that's it, it's menopause." The final menstrual period happens at a definite (albeit unpredictable) point, but the hormone changes have been leading up to it for a decade or more. These changes in the balance of estradiol, testosterone, DHEA, and progesterone cause a wide variety of physical and psychological experiences. For example, intermittent palpitations around menses and premenstrual migraines may begin to occur for the first time or may suddenly get worse if you have had problems with either one in earlier years.

Another frequent early indicator of declining estradiol, characteristically occurring in the early to mid-forties is changes in sleep patterns. Are you waking up multiple times during the night? I found that for a while I was waking up, looking at the clock, then going back to sleep; an hour later I'd wake up, look at the clock, and go back to sleep. Disrupted sleep is one of the earliest hallmark changes affecting the brain as estradiol levels decline. Mood swings, episodic tearfulness for no reason, irritability, angry outbursts, and brief spells of feeling depressed prior to your period may also occur as a result of estradiol drops that trigger changes in the mood-regulating chemical messengers in the brain.

Another effect of decreased estradiol is the rise in total cholesterol production, decreased HDL, and increased LDL cholesterol that can lead to heart disease. Decreased estradiol also causes loss of bone that can result in osteoporosis. I've had a lot of women in their late thirties and forties who were told categorically, without any further evaluation, that they were too young to be having any menopausal symptoms, yet their estradiol levels were already far too low. This is the time that we need to be checking these various health measures so that we can take preventive steps for the future. If you are having premature ovarian decline at age forty, thirty-nine, or even younger, you need to know that, so you can take the necessary steps that will help reduce your risk of heart disease and bone loss in the next five to ten years . . . as well as reduce or eliminate the annoying symptoms that negatively affect your quality of life at this time.

Menopausal Years: The Fifties

The onset of menopause is defined as one year from the "last menstrual period." Ovarian function has been declining for several years, and now the levels are so low that menstrual periods cease. The decline in ovarian hormones is sufficient to end the cycling pattern of our reproductive years and produce the steady, low levels of a noncycling hormone pattern characteristic of the postreproductive years.

Menopause is a rather unique situation because it's the only thing I know of in the medical world that is officially recognized *twelve months after it has happened*. It is a little hard to plan for it or to take proactive steps to decrease health risks if you don't define it until twelve months after it has happened. Most of the time women won't even know when their last menstrual period will be until months have gone by.

At menopause, the ovaries do not cycle any longer, and the overall hormonal production has decreased considerably. After menopause women lose almost all of their estradiol production, and no longer make

progesterone. We also lose anywhere from 50–60 percent of our testosterone production. The female ovary produces testosterone and DHEA,
so as estradiol is lost after menopause, we begin seeing the "unmasking"
of the testosterone that is present. That's when you notice some changes
in skin and facial hair, along with changes in body fat. The "pear" shape
female (gynecoid) fat pattern around the hips and buttocks suddenly
begins moving up toward the middle of the body to become the "apple"
shape (android) more typical of men. Then you wonder, "Gee, what
happened to my waistline?" I show this change in the following diagram. These are some of the testosterone effects that begin the body
changes that are characteristic of the male body pattern. During these
years, the enzyme lipoprotein lipase starts to decrease in the lower body
fat tissue and increase in the upper body fat, which further adds to the
pattern of increasing body fat around the waist, chest and shoulders,
hips and thighs. We see a rise in blood pressure and cholesterol in
women that is similar to the pattern in men as the testosterone effects
become more pronounced relative to estradiol declines.

As women **lose the biologically active estradiol,** we begin to see
one of the gender *differences* become a gender *similarity*: the incidence of cardiovascular disease (CVD) increases dramatically for
women. Regardless of age at menopause (whether it's a *natural*
menopause at age forty-five or a *surgical* menopause at age forty), the
rate of CVD increases. It is based on *menopausal hormone levels,* not
just your *chronological age.* It is important to know a woman's
endocrine status in order to more completely assess her risk of CVD.
You cannot go by age alone, since women experience declining
estradiol levels at a variety of numerical ages. This loss of estradiol
sends your cholesterol profile into a really negative spin.

Postmenopause: The Sixties, Seventies and Beyond

Let me share with you a different perspective on menopause and
the years that follow. I think we've heard many conflicting points
about menopause. In our culture it has often been treated with a sense
of taboo as well as fear and apprehension. Part of that has to do with
the fact that at the turn of the century the average age of death for
women in this country was forty-eight; the average age of menopause
was fifty-one. Which means that as recently as 1900, most women did
not live very long after menopause and ovarian decline. Five hundred
years ago women died on average by age thirty-five.

When we read about the wise women of Native American cultures,
Asian cultures, and the Celtic and other traditions, the wise, elder
women were typically those *over thirty,* past the age of childbearing in
those times. Yet you and I are reading that same material in the con-

text of an *unparalleled increase in longevity* in the human population. It has only been in the last two to three generations that we have had large numbers of men and women living long enough for us to see some of the brain-body effects of declining ovary hormones for women and declining testicular hormones for men. When I talk about menopause and women's health needs, I am discussing it from the perspective that we now have an extraordinary length of time—perhaps thirty to fifty years—to live beyond menopause. For many of us, that means we have the potential to live *at least half* of it after the ovaries have stopped producing the normal quantity of biologically active estradiol and testosterone. Loss of these crucial hormones has an enormous impact on every dimension of our body's function, literally from head (hair, itchy scalp, and brain function) to foot (joint pain, heel pain), and most everything in-between (skin, teeth, muscles, joints, bones, heart, intestinal tract, immune function, blood pressure, bladder function, and sex drive). You need to be empowered with up-to-date, accurate information to help guide you in your choices for optimal health as you grow older. We now have an incredible wealth of information from outstanding scientific research to show the far-reaching effects on a woman's body after we lose our optimal estradiol—whether we are twenty or thrity or forty or fifty when that happens. Well-done studies from around the world show that giving estrogen after menopause decreases by 40 to 60 percent the risk of heart attacks, stoke, Alzheimer's disease, osteoporosis, incontinence, and colon cancer. Loss of estrogen has the potential to rob us of energy, sex drive, sleep, muscle strength, balance, memory, concentration, and general zest, as I will explain further throughout this book.

I recently saw an eighty-nine-year-old lady who is very active, very sharp mentally, and who enjoys traveling all over the world. She was having trouble with incontinence and wanted to see if estrogen would help. I gave her a script for Estrace 0.5 mg. The pharmacist for her insurance company refused to fill the prescription, saying she was too old for estrogen! When she said she needed it to help incontinence so she could enjoy her activities and travel, he said the insurance company allowed only Detrol for this. Of course Detrol has unpleasant side effects and none of the other benefits of estradiol, but that didn't seem to matter to the insurance company. I encouraged this woman to go ahead and pay the $25 for Estrace and see how she felt on it. Then she could appeal the insurance company decision later if she thought it had helped. Her daughter reported later that within twenty-four hours of starting Estrace twice a day, the urinary incontinence had significantly improved. After three or four months, the urinary incontinence was very insignificant; she no longer had to wear any kind of protective padding and was feeling great, had more energy, and was so busy traveling she forgot to come in for her follow-up appointment.

Diagram 2.5—WOMEN'S MIDLIFE BODY SHAPE CHANGES

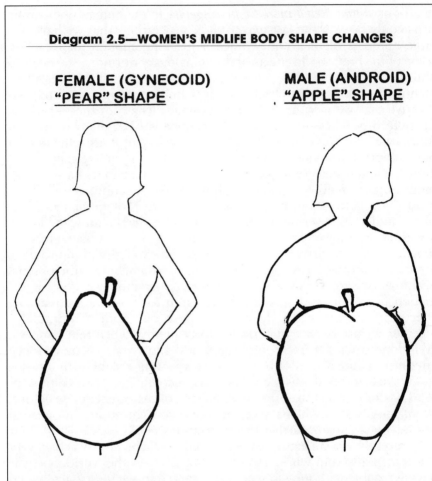

**FEMALE (GYNECOID)
"PEAR" SHAPE**

**MALE (ANDROID)
"APPLE" SHAPE**

Characteristic of women prior to menopause, when estradiol (E2) greater than estrone (E1), and normal female level androgens.

Characteristic of women after menopause (if *not* on hormone Rx); E1 greater than E2. Associated with higher risk of heart disease, hypertension, diabetes, insulin resistance. Also seen in women with PCOS due to higher androgens, lower E2, higher than normal E1.

© Elizabeth Lee Vliet, M.D., 1995, revised 2000

My message to you is straightforward: **Menopause is not a disease,** it is a natural transition in our lives if we live long enough. We now have the opportunity to go through this transition and *live an extended period beyond.* That was not the case for our great grandmothers and their ancestors. Primates such as monkeys, chimpanzees, and gorillas die at the end of their reproductive years, and do not then show postmenopausal changes seen in human females. I think the most critical point for women to understand is that we need to learn what we must know about maintaining our long-term health and reducing our long-term individual disease risks so we can live these additional thirty or forty years with the best possible quality of life and good health. Don't focus on just *treating* or *"getting through"* symptoms now. Look at your big picture and make decisions based on what is needed for your overall vitality and health for many years to come.

The Thyroid: The "Great Imitator"— Problems More Often Missed in Women

Thyroid disease has sometimes been called "the great imitator" because both *hyper*thyroid and *hypo*thyroid diseases produce myriad symptoms that can be confused with many different illnesses. *Hyper*thyroid syndromes produce an excess of thyroid hormones, whether you have a disorder such as Graves' Disease, or are simply taking too much thyroid medication. *Hypo*thyroid disorders involve too little thyroid hormone production, or interference with normal hormone action, such as Hashimoto's thyroiditis. Thyroid disorders of all types are far more common in women, as much as *eight to twenty times* the frequency found in men. The incidence of thyroid disorders increases with age in both sexes, but there is a more dramatic increase in women from the mid-forties and on into the seventies. There are a variety of laboratory tests that can identify these problems. What often happens for women is that only the total thyroid hormones themselves are checked without looking also at the brain hormone TSH (thyroid stimulating hormone) that is a much more sensitive indicator of excessive, or declining, thyroid function. Or, if TSH is checked, thyroid antibodies and free hormones are not, and this means early phase thyroiditis (with normal TSH) is missed.

One facet of thyroid disease not generally recognized is its tendency to cause disturbances in mood and in menstrual cycles. Menstrual irregularity, infertility, worsening PMS, atypical depression, new onset depression later in life, postpartum depression, anxiety syndromes, fibromyalgia, excessive fatigue—all of these may be caused or aggravated by thyroid disorders and are "red flags" to me that may indicate an underlying thyroid problem. Yet, all too commonly, women with these syndromes and symptoms are given a psychiatric label, referred to a therapist for "stress management," and are not evaluated medically any further than a cursory exam and basic blood chemistries. Studies of patients admitted to psychiatric hospitals have repeatedly shown a high incidence of previously unrecognized thyroid disorders that were thought to be the causative factor in the mood disorder. Women at midlife in particular need careful evaluation of thyroid function as part of their medical check-ups, and this needs to include more sensitive tests than just the standard profile.

A comment I hear frequently is "you couldn't have thyroid problems because your TSH (thyroid stimulating hormone) is normal." When the cluster of symptoms I described above are present in women, I think it is important to go a step further in evaluating the thyroid. I have a series of several hundred patients, all but *two* are *women,* who had a normal TSH and turned out to have significantly elevated thyroid antibodies, indicating an autoimmune thyroiditis disorder. This also meant they needed thyroid medication in order to feel normal. This type of oversight is particularly common with a type of thyroid disease called thyroiditis, which is about *twenty-five times* more common in females than males. There are several different types of thyroiditis, but in general this is an inflammation of the thyroid gland that can result in production of antibodies to the gland tissue (microsomal antibodies) or antibodies to the thyroid hormone itself (thyroglobulin antibodies). These antibodies act like "blocking agents" to keep the gland and its hormones from working properly, and the patient begins to experience the clinical symptoms of declining thyroid gland function. For some period of time (actual length may vary greatly from person to person), there is a gradual or abrupt elevation in the thyroid antibodies *before* there is a compensating rise in TSH produced by the brain in response to the failing gland. This means a woman may experience the symptoms of disease *months to years* before TSH goes up. The prevailing "dogma" among endocrinologists and thyroid specialists is that you don't test for thyroid antibodies if the TSH is normal, even if the patient has classic symptoms of hypothyroidism. That's where we often run into trouble and fail to diagnose thyroiditis. All too often, and particularly with women, the clinical problems are present and the antibodies are elevated even when TSH is normal. Adding low-dose thyroid medication can be dramatic for these women, and has even helped some of my infertile patients become pregnant!

I do *not* advocate using thyroid hormone if *all* of the laboratory studies are completely normal, *including* thyroid antibodies. There are potential serious adverse effects of taking thyroid when you don't actually need it, and these problems are worse for women: heart rhythm disturbances and bone loss are the two most important. The problem I have found is that too often women are told their thyroid is normal *without having the complete thyroid tests done*. Of course, what most people, and many physicians, don't realize is that (1) a "normal range" on a laboratory report is just that: a *range*. A given person may require higher or lower levels to feel well and to function optimally. I think we must look at the lab results along with the clinical picture described by the patient. After all, we are supposed to be treating people, not lab values. (2) It is also possible that one or more lab measures may still fall in the normal range and yet other, more subtle measures, may be abnormal. Hashimoto's Thyroiditis may often occur with *normal* total T4 and T3 but markedly elevated antibodies and very low free T4 and/or free T3. We have to listen to the woman and her descriptions with an open mind and with trust in what she says and knows about her body. Several cases from my practice will illustrate this point very clearly.

Arla was thirty-two when I first saw her. Her last child (of two) had been born five years earlier. Over the past three years, she had been experiencing marked loss of energy, decreased concentration at work, premenstrual mood swings, and severe chocolate cravings. She described feeling "so tired I can hardly make it through the day, that just isn't like me. My memory isn't as sharp as usual, I get dark circles under my eyes all the time, I can't lose weight no matter how much I exercise. I just feel so loggy all the time. I thought there might be a thyroid problem, but my family doctor said my thyroid hormones were normal. What's wrong with me?"

Her routine lab studies were normal, and there was nothing particularly unusual on her physical exam except for the moderate degree of obesity. Her standard thyroid profile was normal for the T3, T4 hormones and her TSH was 2.21 (normal range is 0.3 to 5.0 and the standard teaching is that no thyroid treatment should be given until the TSH reaches about 7 or 8). The striking *abnormality* was the thyroid antibody result: her antithyroglobulin antibody was 370 when the normal range is 0.00 to 0.30 units/ml. She had a level of 1,660 on a later check of her antithyroglobulin antibody, even though her *TSH was still normal* at that time also. The antibody to the thyroglobulin was acting like a "blocking agent" keeping the thyroid hormone from being able to attach to the receptor sites and work properly, even though the thyroid gland was making enough of the hormone. She was certainly relieved to know what had been causing her diverse symptoms. I started her on Synthroid, initially at a small dose of only 0.025 mg. She felt better fairly soon but had to have several more dose adjustments before she reached the optimal amount of medication. A year later, she described feeling "back to my old self"!

Another woman, a twenty-year-old college student, illustrates the potential for marked effects on brain phenomena when the thyroid function is diminished. Her father asked if I would do a consult for her because they had not been able to find help for her severe PMS. She had not been doing well in school although previously had been an excellent student. When I saw her, she described having a lot of difficulty keeping her concentration focused to be able to study, her memory was much worse than normal, and she had a deterioration in her grades even though she was studying more than usual. She talked about feeling embarrassed by severe anger outbursts before her period, "I'd be so irritable I thought I would explode, and then I would cry over little things and couldn't stop." Her family described her as usually very energetic and vivacious, but over the past year, she said she could barely make it through the day and often cut class to take naps in the afternoon because she was so tired. She had gained about twenty pounds over the past year and had not previously had a weight problem. There was no evidence of a major depression. Her primary doctor had told her that all her tests, including the thyroid hormones, were normal—**TSH was not done.** The physician suggested she see a counselor to help her cope with the stress of being away from home at college. When I interviewed her with her parents, I did not find any indication that she had problems adjusting to the school setting. I did, however, find out an interesting point in the family history: the patient's mother had thyroid disease and had been on thyroid medication for many years, as had her maternal grandmother.

Shellie had a complete evaluation that came back normal *except* for the thyroid antibodies and TSH. Her antithyroglobulin antibody was 6,000 IU/L (the normal range this time was 0 to 100 IU/L), the antimicrosomal antibody was 475 (same normal range of 0–100). Her TSH was 7, a level that many doctors simply "watch" for six months and recheck. But since we had the critical information about the marked abnormalities of the antibodies, I thought it was important to begin thyroid medication right away. Clearly she was significantly hypothyroid, even though the T3 and T4 were normal. A thyroid scan showed a diffusely enlarged gland typical of thyroiditis. The high antibody levels were preventing the thyroid hormones from working properly at critical body pathways, especially the brain. She was started on thyroid medication and gradually increased to the right amount for her. The brain symptoms have resolved, and her PMS is no longer a major problem. She is gradually losing weight with exercise and a healthy meal plan combined with her thyroid medication.

Both of these women show how important it is to pay attention to changes like this in brain function when the person has previously

not had such difficulties. The brain is often the first organ to show the effects of subtle changes in either thyroid or ovarian hormone function because the brain is so exquisitely dependent upon normal balance for optimal function. When I talk with physicians about these issues, I emphasize that the overall "pattern" is what helps determine the tests to do. We are treating *patients,* not lab values. Since space is limited in this book, you may want to read *Living Well with Hypothyroidism,* by Mary Shomon, or *The Thyroid Solution* by Dr. Arem, for excellent and much more in-depth discussions on getting help for thyroid problems. I also have explained more about the thyroid connection in PMS and fibromyalgia in upcoming chapters.

COMMON SYMPTOMS OF HYPOTHYROIDISM

- severe fatigue, loss of energy, feeling "sluggish"
- weight gain, difficulty losing weight
- depressed mood, usually not as severe as major depression, but may be mistaken for primary depression
- menstrual irregularities, difficulty becoming pregnant/infertility
- low body temperature*
- PMS symptoms, with pre-menstrual mood changes common
- dry, scaly, itchy skin and scalp
- dry, brittle hair and nails
- losing hair (alopecia)
- hoarseness
- chronic constipation
- puffiness of face, lower legs, and feet
- slowed heart rate, unusually low blood pressure
- diminished reflexes

- difficulty tolerating cold environments, climate ("can't get warm")
- sleeping much more than normal
- tingling in wrists/hands, mimicking "carpal tunnel syndrome"
- clotting problems
- multiple joint aches (arthralgias)
- achy muscles (myalgias), leg cramps, muscle weakness
- diminished or lost sexual desire (libido)
- decreased memory, concentration (also brain effect of low thyroid may be misdiagnosed as dementia in an older person)
- Worsening allergies
- ABNORMAL LAB TESTS: high TSH, low thyroid hormones, high total cholesterol, lower than normal HDL, possibly elevated liver enzymes

---

*keep in mind, many of these changes including low basal body temperature may also occur in other conditions, particularly when estradiol and testosterone loss occurs. You can't go by symptoms or basal body temperature alone—you must have the proper hormone levels fully checked to determine *which* problem you have.

© Elizabeth Lee Vliet, M.D., 1995, revised 2000

Chapter 3

Hormones and the Brain

The Brain: Master Conductor of Our Body's Orchestra

What is the brain? To look at it, not much. To live with? Ah, that's another story entirely. Although it is out of sight and we often take it for granted, the brain is truly the organ that defines each of us as an individual, unique person and personality. With it, we perceive the world, we laugh, we cry, we scream, we talk, we joke, we learn, we relate to others. It governs our eating, sleeping, breathing, heartbeat, immune function, water balance, hormone output, and our sex drive, sexual fantasies, and sexual function. The heart may beat with a mechanical pump, and we still survive. If the brain dies, which it will in the absence of oxygen for more than just a few minutes, we lose all dimensions of who we are as an individual; indeed, perhaps our very soul is lost. The brain is a powerhouse organ, more creative and adaptable than the world's fastest computer, yet soft enough to crush with your fingers without the protection of its bony case (the skull) and tough fibrous sac (dura mater) inside the skull. It is often compared to a computer, but that analogy hardly does it justice. If a computer is faced with a new command or task or is given incorrect directions, it simply shuts down; overloaded, it quits. Our brain, however, responds rapidly with new solutions; almost without even realizing it, we adapt and change to meet the new tasks or directions. The brain is able to remember and to forget; your computer can only remember. The computer operates only in an either-or, on-off, "binary" mode. Our brain appreciates infinite "shades of gray" along a continuum of choices and options. In many ways, it is far too complex for me to find a good metaphor or analogy for its function.

When talking about fears of disease in my seminars, I have commented on the way in which many magazine articles lump women together by calling breast cancer our greatest fear. It isn't for me. My greatest health concern would be developing a disease that destroys my brain, since it is the organ that makes ME who I am. I could work and be ME without my breast. I could no longer work, and I could no longer *exist as ME* without my brain. It has only been in the last decade or so that we have truly come to appreciate just how completely the brain defines our total being.

As I mentioned in chapter 2, *the brain is the master conductor of the "orchestra" made up of all the "instruments" of our body.* Without the conducting, coordinating functions of our brain, there would be no "music" from our existence; all our body parts would be chaotically playing individual notes and pieces of tunes, like the discordant notes we hear as an orchestra is warming up, with all the musicians playing individual parts of songs and scales. Not the sort of music you attend a symphony to hear. But when the conductor appears on stage and brings the orchestra to life as an entity, the symphonic music begins. As we listen to the orchestra, we often forget how crucial the conductor's role is or how many different individual instruments are being guided into playing together to create the drama and beauty of the music. The essence of the brain (and of woman) lies not in the parts, but in the *connections between the parts* that create the totality of the whole.

To give you an adequate appreciation of the many functions of the brain and its complex structure would require an enormous textbook. I would like to give you an overview of the major areas of the brain and some of the broad areas of function that are orchestrated by these key areas. This information is based on current understandings of the brain; keep in mind, however, that neuroscience research is an exploding area of new knowledge, increasing almost daily, so there will be more that we know about this marvelous organ in years to come. The brain diagram below will help you understand where these areas are and will serve as a reference point for the discussion of the hormone connections that follows.

The brain rests inside the bony protective cover of the skull, with a number of openings in the base of the skull through which pass the nerves and spinal cord. The spinal cord carries bundles of nerve tracts from the head down the back to the lower body. The *cortex* mediates thinking functions and is divided into two halves, the left and right *cerebral hemispheres,* which have different specialization of functions. The *left* hemisphere specializes in verbal, analytical, and sequential (or linear) information processing; the *right* hemisphere specializes in visual-spatial, nonverbal, intuitive (or nonlinear), and Gestalt information processing. Both hemispheres are further divided into areas called *lobes,* named for the overlying skull bones: *frontal, temporal, parietal,* and *occipital.* The cortex is the part of the brain that makes us uniquely human, since it governs speech, reading, and

Diagram 3.1—The Human Brain, Side View of Major Areas

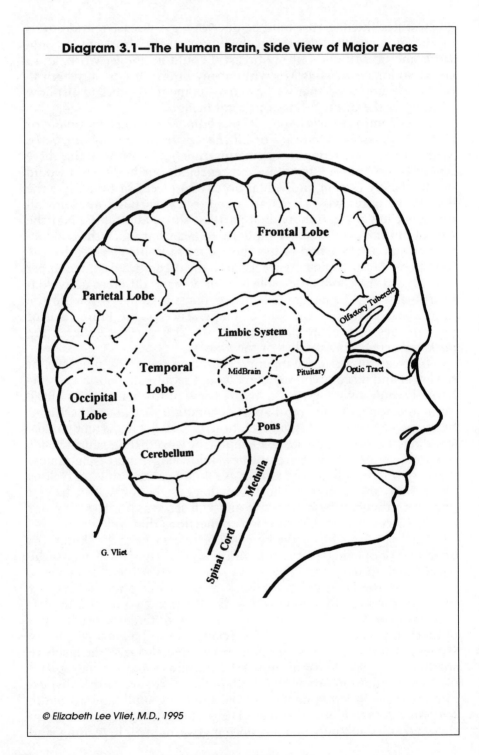

G. Vliet

writing of language. There is overlap among many of the brain areas to a significant degree, both structurally and functionally, which gives us an enormous capacity for adaptability.

At the interior center of the brain, lying below the cortex, is the area of structures collectively called the *limbic* system. This collection of structures is the primary center integrating emotion, memory, pain, sleep, appetite, sex, and basic functions vital to life. The *brainstem* group of structures (lying below the cortex) regulates the "vegetative" functions that keep us alive, such as breathing, blood pressure, and heart rate. The *cerebellum* lies somewhat above the brainstem but below the cortex and is the primary center regulating movement, balance, and motor coordination. Bundles of nerve fibers leaving the cortex, limbic system, brainstem, and cerebellum come together to form the *spinal cord* that extends to the base of the vertebral column in the lower back area. Chart 4.1 summarizes these major functions; you may find it helpful to refer to it as I discuss the chemistry of mood and hormonal effects on various brain functions.

New Understandings of the Brain's Chemical Messengers

How do all these areas of the brain communicate with each other? We talk about "nerves," which are fibers. But how do messages get from one nerve cell to another? I have found it helpful to think about the brain as an enormous three-dimensional network of many different "communication centers" that turn on and off rapidly, send out bursts of electrical impulses, and then communicate further by releasing chemical messenger molecules called *neurotransmitters*. The visual image that pops into my mind is the large flashing network of fibers in the TV commercial for a worldwide communications company. There are billions of nerve fibers, all with hundreds of potential connections to other nerve fibers. To try to comprehend all this complexity can be overwhelming to most of us.

The basic process of communication between nerve cells, or neurons, and other body cells is both electrical and chemical. The electrical impulse travels along the neuron to the end of the cell called the *synapse,* or junction point, where it fires off the release of the chemical messenger molecules that have been made in the cell and stored in little sacs called *storage vesicles*. The chemicals are released to travel across the space between cells, called the *synaptic cleft*. The messenger molecules fit into a receptor site, and this "unlocks" the next nerve cell to allow the message to be processed and acted upon. This is often illustrated as a neuron connecting with only one other

BRAIN AREAS AND THEIR KEY FUNCTIONS

BRAIN AREA	FUNCTIONS
FRONTAL Lobe	• integrates thinking, feeling, creative imagining, decision making • oversees "social appropriateness" of behavior, insight-judgment abilities • has role in expression of personality • helps control body movements
TEMPORAL Lobes	• process auditory information, • control language (usually left hemisphere) and memory, • help modulate emotions
PARIETAL Lobes	• receive information about body sensations ("somatosensory area") • modulate spatial orientation ability
OCCIPITAL Lobe	• receives and processes visual information
BRAINSTEM: Midbrain, Pons, and Medullas:	• regulates "survival functions" such as: respiration, heart rate, blood pressure • receives information via multiple connections (brain and spinal cord)
LIMBIC SYSTEM: Amygdala, Hippocampus, Mammillary Bodies, Fornix, Basal Ganglia (BG), Thalamus, Hypothalamus, Pituitary, and Cingulate Gyrus	• memory processing • mood-emotion regulation • attention, alertness, focus • human "drives": appetite, thirst, sex, aggression, sleep-wake cycles • governs "starting and stopping" behavior • hormone regulation (especially hypothalamus, and pituitary) • has role in modulating *chronic* pain, acute pain paths bypass limbic area • integrates sensory information and role in movement (basal ganglia)
CEREBELLUM	• integrates and coordinates movement (with cortex), balance, coordination
SPINAL CORD	• carries nerve tracts and chemical messengers back and forth between brain and body; • origin of nerve tracts to body areas

© Elizabeth Lee Vliet, M.D., 1995

Diagram 3.2
ANDROGEN AND ESTROGEN RECEPTORS IN THE BRAIN

ANDROGEN RECEPTORS IN THE BRAIN

Cortex

Thalamus

Preoptic Region

Hippocampus

Pituitary

Amygdala

Brain Stem

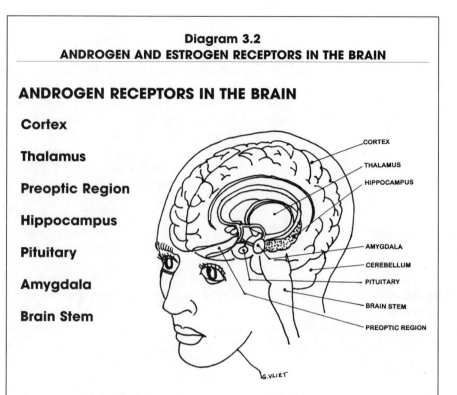

ESTROGEN RECEPTORS IN THE BRAIN:

Hippocampus (memory)

Pituitary

Amygdala (well-being, sexuality)

Cerebellum (balance, coordination)

Brain Stem: olive (synchronizes movements)

Cortex (higher cognitive functions)

neuron, but in reality, each neuron has perhaps hundreds of connections with other cells. What I have described is a *greatly simplified* version of a very complex, multidimensional, continuous process occurring every second of every day we are alive. It is awesome to consider the incredible intricacies of the body.

There has been an exponential growth in our understanding of the actual modes of communication between the brain and body since Dr. Candace Pert and Dr. Solomon Snyder first discovered the opiate receptor in the brain in 1973. This opiate receptor is the site where drugs such as morphine, heroin, and their derivatives plug into brain cells to produce their pain-relieving action. It seemed logical to these researchers that the brain would not be equipped with a special "lock" (receptor site) if it did not also produce a "key." In 1975, they found the natural "key" for this "lock" in the discovery of the endorphin and enkephalin neuropeptides, the pain-killing molecules produced in the brain and body. Since that time, researchers have identified many more "molecular messengers" that provide the "courier information service" between the brain and various body sites. These biochemical information substances produced in the body have been grouped into various categories, including *neurotransmitters, neuropeptides, hormones, growth factors,* and *lymphokines.* They all have powerful effects on multiple aspects of body function, including mood and emotion. You can think of these informational molecules as "biochemical words" or messages used by the brain to "talk" directly to body cells and organs and by the body to "talk back" to the brain. These molecules link the brain and immune system, the endocrine and immune systems, the brain and the endocrine system, the brain and the gut, the brain and the heart, and so on throughout all the possible connections between brain centers and body organs.

Some of the most important chemical messengers I will be describing with regard to hormone influences on mood and physical symptoms are: serotonin (5-HT), norepinephrine (NE), dopamine (DA), acetylcholine (ACh), and gamma aminobutyric acid (GABA). These molecules function to convey and modulate information going back and forth between the brain and the body. They provide an important link between emotional and physical health. This link is not surprising in view of the critical role of emotions in regulating behavior that ultimately affects our very survival. These information-carrying substances are made in the brain and body from "building blocks" called *amino acids* found in the food we eat. The body's metabolic processes to make the neurotransmitters require the presence of various vitamins and minerals as catalysts and cofactors for the synthesizing enzymes to work properly. Perhaps you are beginning to see why a healthy, balanced diet is so crucial to your good health and optimal function.

We are just beginning to discover the incredible diversity of roles and functions the neurotransmitters have. Serotonin research, for example, has given us extraordinary new insights about the biological basis of many behavior problems we previously thought were caused by psychological conflicts—everything from compulsive shoplifting to gambling, from compulsive sexual behaviors to hand-washing and hair-pulling (*trichotillomania*) behaviors. Overeating is mediated by serotonin imbalances, and so are pain and sleep patterns. Anxiety syndromes may be set off by changes in serotonin function, as well as by excessive production of norepinephrine. Mania results from excessive levels of norepinephrine and dopamine, while depression occurs when both of these and serotonin are either produced in inadequate amounts or the receptor sites are not functioning properly.

Major depression is a *biological* disorder occurring as a direct result of marked changes in these chemical messengers and an alteration in the receptor numbers and sensitivity—it is not a "character" problem or lack of willpower. Attention deficit disorders are also affected by the balance between serotonin and norepinephrine and affected by decline in estradiol and testosterone as women grow older. Abnormalities in dopamine production and function are thought to be the primary disturbances causing Schizophrenia and Parkinson's Disease. Loss of acetylcholine, accentuated by loss of estradiol, is the primary deficiency leading to Alzheimer's dementia. Irritable bowel syndrome and fibromyalgia are two of many so-called "vague" medical problems aggravated, if not caused by, serotonin and norepinephrine imbalances along with the loss of estradiol. As you can see, these deceptively simple molecules have a profound impact on many aspects of our health.

SUMMARY OF THE ROLES OF
TWO KEY NEUROTRANSMITTERS

♦ *Increased* Serotonin (ST, or 5HT)
- diminishes **anxiety**
- lessens **pain**
- improves **sleep**
- diminishes **depression**
- decreases **obsessions**

♦ *Increased* Norepinephrine (NE)
- diminishes **depression**
- worsens **anxiety**
- intensifies **pain**
- causes **restless, fragmented sleep**
- triggers **palpitations**

© Elizabeth Lee Vliet, M.D., 1995

Another fascinating connection that has been overlooked and under-appreciated in women's health is the existence of specific estradiol, progesterone, and testosterone receptor sites in key areas throughout the brain and body. These hormone receptor sites are found throughout the body's organs and tissues, far beyond reproductive organ sites you would expect to respond to circulating ovarian hormones. In the brain, the estrogen receptors in particular are heavily concentrated in the cortex and in the limbic system areas. As I described, the limbic system is the major center for regulating **mood, memory, sleep, sex drive, appetite,** and **pain.** There are multiple connections between the limbic system and all the other parts of the brain and spinal cord, which carries messages to all parts of the body. The rise and fall of estrogen alters serotonin, which affects pathways in the limbic system, which then produces changes in mood, sleep, memory, pain, appetite, and many other mind-body functions. Changes in hormone levels, in turn, affect the *amount* of neurotransmitters produced as well as the *sensitivity* of neurotransmitter receptors to the chemical messengers. No wonder changing hormone levels at puberty, in pregnancy, after delivery, and at menopause can produce such a wide variety of physical and emotional changes.

We have only begun to scratch the surface of appreciating how widespread these connections are. You may have been told that mood changes aren't due to your hormones, but there is a great deal of science to explain the hormone connection. What you experience with menstrual mood changes is **very real and has profound hormonal connections**. Contrary to popular opinion, the brain and the body really are connected. It is not all in your head in the "imaginary" sense; it *is* "in your head" in the real physical changes that take place regularly between the hormone messengers and the brain's own mood-altering messenger molecules.

It's Not All in Your Imagination! The Biology of Mood Changes

It has long been observed in worldwide studies that both depressive syndromes and anxiety disorders are two to three times more common in women than in men. I think it is important to explore links between women's hormone cycles and our expanded knowledge about mood-regulating mechanisms in humans. The *cause* of mood changes that occur around and during the menopausal transition or with the menstrual cycle luteal phase has been hotly debated in scientific journals and the lay media for a long time. There is a lot of intense emotion on both sides of the debate: Is it hormonal change?

Is it the combination of life stresses? Consider this example from a nationally syndicated column by Jane Brody, published in September 1994. The headline in my newspaper was "Menopause Doesn't Have to Be Depressing." The article began this way:

> In her newly published memoir, Barbara Bush reveals that in the mid-1970s she was overcome by depression so severe that she feared she might purposely end her life by crashing her car. The former first lady attributed her emotional distress to the hormonal changes of menopause compounded by the stress of her husband's job as director of the Central Intelligence Agency. By linking her depression to menopause, Bush perpetuates a centuries-old belief that the hormonal swings that accompany this life stage can touch off what had long been called involutional melancholia (involutional is a term referring to the body's changes at menopause).

Ms. Brody then goes on to say that "studies show there is no particular link between depression and menopause; if anything, it is far more common among younger women than in those from 45–55 when most women enter menopause."

But in reality, we do not have adequate studies that have addressed this issue. None of the studies Ms. Brody referred to measured hormone levels, a fairly critical factor, if you are trying to see whether there's a link between hormones and depressive symptoms! Most of these studies did not even determine whether a woman was still menstruating or whether she had undergone a hysterectomy. Many have based menopausal status on age alone, which you will find as you read further is not at all accurate in identifying which women are actually menopausal by *endocrinological measures*.

Under Barbara Bush's picture is this quote (in large type and bold letters), which I think reflects even worse stereotypes of women and certainly is not based on well-done studies:

> Barbara Bush had led a traditional family life with her major role being raising children. As her children left home, the loss of this role may have made her more vulnerable to depression at that time. When women are not in the work force, depression may be more common at menopause, reflecting the woman's stage of life, not necessarily her hormones. (Myrna M. Weissman, Ph.D, as quoted in the nationally syndicated column by Jane Brody, September 27, 1994)

How does this quote make you feel? Is Dr. Weissman perpetuating the old stereotype that women "can't cope" with life-stage changes and become depressed? I think this attitude perpetuates an appalling stigma, one that unfortunately continues today in the new millennium. I also think it is rather arrogant to suggest that women who are "in the work force" somehow cope better with menopause *because* they work. Any woman who is a full-time homemaker will tell you she has a full-time job, even if she isn't paid for her labor.

Moreover, Dr. Weissman's view *still* hasn't been confirmed by sound research. Dr. Philip Sarrel of Yale has found the opposite: Women in the work force describe *more severe* symptoms of menopausal distress than women who do not work outside the home, perhaps related to the higher levels of stress experienced by women who are juggling multiple roles of home and career. Such stresses can further *decrease* ovarian hormone levels. Dr. Sarrel reported his research findings at the inaugural meeting of the North American Menopause Society in the fall of 1989, but most doctors still don't take this seriously. Dr. Sarrel said,

> *Most important in impairing a woman's capacity to function [at her optimal ability] in the workplace are symptoms due to hormone deficiency: sleep disturbance, hot flashes, anxiety attacks, depression, and altered [i.e., decreased] short-term memory. In approximately 67 percent of women who work outside of the home, and approximately 50 percent of homemakers, menopausal symptoms [such as above] have a moderate to severe effect on the ability to do work.*

These observations have been borne out as we evaluate more women now going through the "perimenopausal" phase.

We are not facing our "mother's" menopause. Women today lead much more complex lives and want a higher level of cognitive performance and energy level than our mothers commonly had. Women today experience greater demands than ever before—at work, at home, taking care of the extended family, taking care of home repairs—just look around Home Depot on a Saturday! More and more women are tackling multiple roles and jobs that used to be "men's work" but then still have to carry out the traditional female roles as well. This is not to complain, it is to acknowledge that our lives are much more complex. The old pats on the back or standard treatments will not do and are not acceptable now. Our society demands we operate at a constant high-performance level; we also expect this of ourselves and find it devastating when we can't.

As one woman so eloquently said it, "I survived the depression era, I raised six kids, my parents died when I was in my twenties. When I was 32, my husband was killed. I have had lots of stress in my life. Why did everyone say it's 'stress' causing my sleep problems and irritability when I went through menopause? Relative to what I had already lived through, menopause was *not* a stressful time, but I certainly had a lot of bothersome symptoms." Many women I see tell me that they feel *validated* in their own perceptions when I find low hormone levels contributing to their unpleasant symptoms.

Perhaps the hormonal changes, along with life stresses, were factors that aggravated Mrs. Bush's symptoms around the time of her menopause. In addition to overlooking the reality of hormone effects on brain function, I do not think any of us should *assume* that Barbara Bush became depressed because her role as a mother had changed. This statement is made as if it were an established fact, but Dr. Weissman's quote was not based on a confirmed causal connection. So, once again, a stereotype is perpetuated and possible physical factors are discounted. I think there are at least two possible *endocrine* causes for Mrs. Bush's depression: her thyroid condition, a condition which has been recognized for 100 years or more to cause depression; and the changing ovarian hormone levels around the time of menopause that affect brain chemicals regulating mood. Instead of such an "either-or" mentality evident in the Brody article, why not approach these issues with a "both-and" mindset and look at all the interrelating factors that make women unique and contribute to the observed higher frequency of depressive symptoms and disorders in women?

If we look at the patterns of major depression, we have known for more than fifty years that there are several *common predisposing factors* (this is true worldwide):

- prior depressive episodes
- family history of depression
- **female gender**
- **postpartum state**
- severe, prolonged, or unanticipated stress

Two of the five factors that have been known for ages as predisposing factors to the medical (biological) illness of depression are directly related to being female: female gender, and the postpartum state. Since these patterns of female dominance have been noted in primitive and industrialized cultures, there must be some biological reasons for this. Why do we continue to stigmatize and blame women as being "weak" and "not coping well" because they have a higher frequency of depression? I find it hard to fathom why researchers and physicians haven't made, or paid attention to, these hormonal connections long before now. Perhaps they don't want to see them. Perhaps that's a product of the concern expressed by many feminists that if we acknowledge the hormonal influences, we may lose some of the gains women have made to move into new occupational fields. I understand such fears. We have all suffered long enough from the stereotype of the bitchy, cranky, moody woman.

But on the other hand, if we *don't* acknowledge possible hormonal factors, we cannot develop the most effective therapies to help women who *do* have these problems. Such women will continue to suffer from lack of recognition or from overuse of other medication or surgery that may have more side effects or higher costs. I believe these are crucial issues that must be addressed.

A good example of profound hormone change is seen in the postpartum phase. A woman's hormonal levels drop over a hundred-fold in the twenty-four to thirty-six hours after delivery. That's a major adjustment for both the brain chemistry and the chemical messengers that regulate sleep and mood. Then add to that the fact that there is now an infant who's keeping you up much of the night, so you're not sleeping very well. Sleep deprivation is also known to cause biological depression. But a woman who becomes significantly depressed following her baby's birth is still more likely to be told she has *psychological* conflicts about being a mother. The biological factors are overlooked. There are social and cultural factors involved, and these have been studied exhaustively. But I think we have not paid enough attention to the obvious hormonal changes, especially postpartum, that have to do with the biology of being female and may profoundly disrupt mood-regulating chemical messengers in the brain. In Europe, and in my own practice, there are good reports of the positive response to estradiol therapy after delivery in women who have a postpartum depression due to hormonal decreases. Dr. John Studd from England has published studies of successful use of transdermal 17-beta estradiol patches to treat postpartum depression. Many of these women then did not need antidepressant medication. If the postpartum depression is severe, some women benefit from the combination of estradiol and a serotonin-augmenting antidepressant. We need to be more open-minded to *individualization* of the best options for a given woman.

I have long been struck by the repetitive, commonly occurring pattern of mood changes and physical symptoms and their relation to the normal changes in estrogen and progesterone levels throughout the menstrual cycle. Most women who have menstrual periods (or ovarian cycles if they have had a hysterectomy) have *some* physical or emotional cues that tell them that their periods are about to begin. Women also experience changes that signal the beginning of the midlife transition, or *climacteric*. In my medical practice, I have found a significant percentage of patients who have luteal-phase PMS symptoms severe enough to interfere with optimal function at home, at work, and in relationships. These women would like to at least have someone check their hormone levels and offer some constructive, well-thought-out options to help them feel better on these days. I don't think that is too much to ask of a health system that can now achieve successful organ transplants, develop Viagra to enhance men's erections, clone sheep, and other wonders.

Even when women have had a hysterectomy, many who still have their ovaries can describe quite well the body-brain markers of the residual ovary cycle. They tell me they have breast tenderness, bloating, food cravings, constipation, and other markers, just like they used to the week before their menses began. Or they will describe a few days of restless, fragmented sleep, emotional changes, crying easily, loss of energy, feeling mentally "foggy," or having anxiety attacks and palpitations like they did the first few days of bleeding (when estradiol is at its lowest point of the cycle). Yet they are often told they "couldn't possibly" have PMS. I think many physicians forget the ovaries still cycle and produce these changes. Another cause of these changes is the fact that ovaries decline *sooner* after hysterectomy due to interruption in ovarian blood flow when arteries are tied off in order to remove the uterus. Many women, and doctors, don't know this.

It has been my hypothesis from years of observing patients, listening to the ways women describe their experiences, and studying the extensive science of hormone effects on brain function, that there is an unrecognized and unaddressed connection between declining estrogen levels in women and the pattern of female dominance in depression and anxiety disorders. Consider these observations (based on women who still have regular menstrual cycles):

- PMS symptoms commonly become worse in the late thirties and early forties.
- The late thirties to early forties represent the peak age range of *new onset* depression and anxiety syndromes in women, but not in men.
- The late thirties to mid-forties is the time frame for onset of *erratic* and *declining* ovarian hormone production, creating the potential for adverse effects on brain neurotransmitters to destabilize mood-regulating mechanisms.
- By the time menses have stopped at menopause, hormone levels are "even" at a new *lower* level, and no longer cycle, making mood swings less likely.
- Researchers, however, have focused only on the time of *menopause* in trying to correlate hormone changes and depression.
- In most studies of depression around *menopause*, hormone levels are not measured.

I think a key factor in the connection between hormones and mood effects is the **degree of fluctuation**, or **rate of change**, in hormone levels. In all the studies I have reviewed, this crucial factor has *not* been addressed. I have studied this connection by measuring hormone levels at times in the menstrual cycle when women describe their most distressing mood symptoms, and at times in the cycle when estradiol is at its lowest point and its highest point. Then I "connect the dots" to see the pattern that emerges as I show the symptom clusters side by side with the actual hormone results. It has been striking to find that approximately 85 percent or more of these women in their mid thirties and early forties who described "worsening PMS" had *below normal* estradiol levels at these points during their menstrual cycle.

The prematurely low estradiol levels were *even more likely* to be present in women who had experienced a surgical procedure that affected blood flow to the ovaries, such as *tubal ligation* or *hysterectomy* (even when the ovaries were left in place). According to the currently accepted age-based definitions, these women were *too young* in most cases to be considered pre- or perimenopausal. When I measured the hormone levels, however, I confirmed that they indeed had reached the *endocrinological* stage of perimenopause. I offered these women treatment with low-dose estrogen supplementation to optimize their estrogen levels instead of using antidepressants. I have been astonished at the results. Women who fit this profile described a consistent pattern of improved mood, diminished irritability, improved sleep, improved libido, improved energy level, and diminished mood swings prior to their periods, after starting on a low dose of natural human estradiol. Only a few of these women required the addition of antidepressants once hormone levels were returned to the usual optimal levels for a menstruating woman. (See menstrual cycle diagram in chapter 2 for desirable ranges.)

A variety of studies in recent years has demonstrated that neuro-receptors respond to circulating hormones of all kinds, including the sex hormones estradiol, progesterone, and testosterone. Researchers have shown that hormones can increase or decrease the release of neurotransmitters. Hormones have both presynaptic and postsynaptic nerve cell actions, as well as indirect influences that modify the function of neurons. Both the brain (central) and the body (peripheral) nervous systems have cells with receptor sites sensitive to 17-beta estradiol, progesterone, and testosterone. The brain clearly responds to the withdrawal and absence of these ovarian hormones. There are a wide variety of physical phenomena and psychological effects of decrease or withdrawal of the ovarian hormones, and I discuss these connections in the next sections, as well as in chapters 4–7. But first, I think it is important to clarify some descriptions of terms you will see in various articles, which may be one of the reasons there is so much confusion about hormone effects on mood.

Insights on Depressive and Anxiety Symptoms versus Psychiatric Disorders

As you read the upcoming sections, it is important to keep in mind the difference between (1) experiencing *symptoms* on an episodic or cyclic basis with your menstrual periods and (2) having sustained physical and emotional changes that would be severe enough to be considered a *disorder* or an illness. Many women have mild to moderate symptoms or experience mood, sleep, and energy-level changes around the time of hormonal changes or in conjunction with situations that are stressful. When I talk about this cyclic type of pattern, I am not referring to the *illness* of major depression, which indicates a more severe, debilitating degree of depression. The same is true with anxiety. The term *anxiety* may be used in many different ways, so it is important to know how it is being used in a given context. Some people use it to mean a *mood*: "I'm in an anxious mood now," or "I'm feeling anxious." Others use it to mean a *characteristic or trait* of a person—"He's always been anxious and uptight." It may mean a brief *symptom*: "I had an attack of anxiety over my bounced check." It may be used to mean a *sustained pattern* of physical and emotional changes that we call generalized anxiety disorder. In these chapters on hormone connections, I am generally referring to fairly short-lived, episodic anxiety *symptoms* that occur in relation to *changes* in physiological variables such as levels of glucose, thyroid hormone, estrogen, testosterone, and progesterone.

As a global observation, I have not found the hormone shifts of the menstrual cycle to be a *primary cause* of the psychiatric syndrome generalized anxiety disorder, since this illness typically is present on an almost daily basis. On the other hand, I *do* commonly see women who have panic attacks only around the menstrual-cycle phase of dropping estrogen and progesterone levels. I think this pattern of menstrually-related panic attacks is different from the psychiatric syndrome we call panic disorder. The cluster of symptoms (I sometimes use the nonmedical, descriptive word *phenomena* instead of *symptoms*) is often the same because the same brain-body pathways are involved. In my view, the *pattern* of a particular symptom cluster provides the most important clues to contributing causes. I certainly am *not* saying that all women who experience premenstrual depressed moods or feelings of anxiety are suffering from a psychiatric disorder. Quite the contrary. I think *far* too many women are given a psychiatric diagnosis and psychotropic medication, without the realization that the "symptoms" are occurring around the menstrual period and *may be triggered by hormonal changes.*

Estrogen Effects on Serotonin and Other Mood Regulators

There still have not yet been good systematic, prospective studies of the effect of rate of change in estrogen levels on the frequency and severity of mood symptoms in perimenopausal women. We have known for a long time, however, that estrogen does affect many brain-mediated phenomena. Experimental data indicate that the sex hormones (estradiol, testosterone, progesterone) are the *most potent* body-generated chemical signals affecting nerve cell activities in the brain. All three major sex hormones alter the electrical and chemical features of cells in the central nervous system (CNS), especially in the hypothalamus and limbic system—areas that regulate key functions like sleep, mood, memory, pain, sex drive, appetite, weight, temperature, and thirst. Changes in levels of estrogen and progesterone have been shown to influence multiple brain-chemical messengers: dopamine, norepinephrine, acetylcholine, and serotonin, all of which are powerful modulators of mood.

Dr. Malcolm Whitehead and his associates did an excellent study that showed marked improvement in memory, anxiety, and irritability in menopausal women taking estrogen, compared with menopausal women not taking estrogen. This information isn't exactly hot off the presses; it was published in the British medical literature *in 1977*. So we've had this kind of information in the medical literature for a long time; it has just been ignored. Women tell me every day that they have been told *categorically* by their doctors: "Hormones don't affect mood. Your memory changes aren't due to hormones. It's just stress. See a therapist and learn to relax."

Since the 1950s at least, a number of clinical reports have indicated that estrogen supplementation helps alleviate mood swings and depression as well as the physical symptoms such as hot flashes, headaches, insomnia, and memory disturbance associated with the midlife phase. Most have been dismissed because they were not double-blind, placebo-controlled studies. Instead of ignoring these important findings, researchers should have been using those early studies as guides for well-designed double-blind studies. With the development of the first modern psychotropic drugs in 1954, however, the brain effects of all kinds of hormonal influences have been forgotten and overlooked as the focus shifted to using antidepressants, antianxiety agents, neuroleptics, and sedatives. With exciting new information from neuroscience research in the past decade, and with the use of more refined diagnostic criteria rating scales to systematically assess mood characteristics, there is increasing measurable evidence that mood symptoms and physical reactions described by perimenopausal women *are* related to their hormone changes and may respond to supplemental estrogen even before menses stop.

Dr. Sarrel of Yale said in 1989 at the NAMS meeting that "estrogen addition over a six-month period appeared to relieve sleep disturbance most significantly, and resulted in a marked improvement in *all* categories of perimenopausal symptoms in 40 percent of women." He went on to say that it was "of concern that women don't realize how much their quality of life may be improved with proper estrogen therapy and that *only 15 percent* of *all* menopausal women received hormone therapy at all. Many women simply do not seek medical help, even though hormonal therapy may be a benefit to them." Bruce McEwen, Ph.D., at Rockefeller University, has done extensive basic science research on brain-hormone connections and has found that estradiol, testosterone, and progesterone affect the brain directly, acting at specific hormone receptors unique for each hormone. These receptors are concentrated in areas of the brain that are highly hormone-sensitive and dense with receptor sites: the hypothalamus, limbic system, cortex, prefrontal regions and others. Current research indicates that progesterone and testosterone brain receptors in women must *first be "primed" by estrogen in order to work properly*.

Dr. McEwen and other scientists have shown that hormone effects on the brain can be *gradual and long lasting,* that is, on the order of hours, days, or even weeks in some cases; or may be *rapid onset and shorter duration of effect*. The rapid hormone effects typically occur at the cell membrane receptor, while the longer-lasting effects occur at the cell nucleus receptor. All of these observations have many profound implications for an *interactive* model of thinking about the role of women's ovarian hormone cycles producing psychological phenomena such as mood changes. The brain mechanisms and pathways already exist. We need to put the pieces of the puzzle together to see the complete picture. The problem is that women's health has some pieces left in the "box" of gynecology, and some pieces left in the "box" belonging to psychiatry, and they don't get put together by separate specialists working on different body parts.

Acting at their specific receptor sites, hormones influence the production, release, and breakdown of the mood-regulating neurotransmitters. Antidepressants and antianxiety medications are also given to influence these same neurotransmitters to lift or stabilize moods. The ability of these medications to work optimally appear to be affected by circulating hormones, especially estradiol and progesterone. Dr. Kendall and coworkers found that the presence of estrogen increased the binding of the antidepressant drug imipramine (Tofranil) to serotonin-2 receptors involved in mood. In animals, this imipramine-receptor-binding effect was *abolished if the ovaries were not present* and was *reestablished by giving estrogen.* Many case reports describe similar changes in antidepressant response based on a woman's phase in her menstrual cycle.

Early in my career, as I listened to women describe side effects with antidepressants, I found that I frequently needed to make dosage adjustments depending on menstrual cycle phase. Women often needed *higher* doses in the *progesterone-dominated* luteal phase and *lower* doses in the *estrogen-dominated* follicular phase. I never saw anything about this in the medical literature until 1993, but my patients taught me what they needed and I usually gave different doses depending on phase of menstrual cycle. This fits with what we know about estradiol having its own *antidepressant* effects on the brain centers, so less additional medication is needed when estradiol levels are high. Progesterone, on the other hand, has more of a "dampening-down," a sedative, or (for some women) a depressant effect on mood-regulating neurotransmitters. Progesterone also decreases receptor binding of both estradiol and testosterone. Thus, when progesterone levels are high in the second half of the cycle, it is reasonable that more antidepressant medication may be necessary.

Ovarian hormones also have been found to have effects on several other mood-altering neuropeptides: endorphins ("morphine within" pain-reducing chemicals), oxytocin, vasopressin, and prolactin, which are involved in modulating memory, motor coordination, and a variety of behaviors. Studies have demonstrated a decrease in some serotonin measures (either plasma-free tryptophan or platelet serotonin) in the menopausal and perimenopausal years that correlates with the age of peak suicide rate for women (a comparable peak has not been seen in men). Recent studies have found that brain levels of 5-hydroxyindoleacetic acid (5-HIAA), a serotonin breakdown product, are low in patients who attempted or completed suicide. If 5-HIAA is low, it indicates that brain serotonin levels are also low. Decreases in serotonin production and increases in serotonin breakdown are seen in (1) the human aging process, (2) as an effect of *declining estrogen in women*, and (3) as an effect of prolonged stress, chronic alcohol overuse, and cigarette smoking. Numerous worldwide studies over the past two decades have shown that *reduced* serotonin levels are a primary cause of depressed mood, increased irritability, increased generalized anxiety, increased pain sensitivity, eating disorders, obsessive-compulsive disorders and disruption of normal sleep cycles.

If you then add the factor that declining estrogen *also decreases serotonin,* the symptoms of PMS, postpartum, perimenopause, and menopause make even more sense *physiologically.* Many factors affect serotonin balance, but the loss of estrogen may be a key gender difference that contributes to a greater susceptibility to depression and suicide in women. Along this line, investigators from several countries have a greater incidence of psychological symptoms (irritability, mood swings, etc.) in women aged forty to forty nine, when estrogen is decreasing most rapidly, compared with both younger and older women. You aren't a hypochondriac. Your body *is* changing. Much later, after all the "ups and downs" of hormone change, women reach a new balance point with overall lower hormone levels, less estradiol, and more estrone. But while the changes are occurring, some women tell me they feel like they are on an emotional roller coaster. Most of us don't like to feel so out of control, and these feelings are compounded when doctors do not explain what is happening to us.

Such mood changes, which are clearly cyclic and related to the menstrual cycle, often respond better to **natural human 17-beta estradiol** than to antidepressant or antianxiety medication because the addition of estradiol actually normalizes the body chemicals that are out of balance. A number of clinical studies that monitored psychological measures along with physical changes in perimenopausal and early menopausal women have found that giving estrogen does result in marked improvement in women's sense of well-being, energy, clarity of thinking, short-term memory, and quality of sleep. At the same time, women report marked decreases in hot flashes, vaginal dryness, and other typical physical symptoms. I have certainly seen these kinds of dramatic improvements in the women I have treated for these problems over the past twenty years. In addition to the open clinical studies, such as the work I have been doing, recently published randomized double-blind placebo-controlled studies have also shown that estrogen therapy effectively improves general well-being, reduces the frequency of hot flashes, and objectively improves the quality of sleep as defined by increases in length of rapid-eye-movement (REM) sleep and total sleep time.

Changes in endorphins have also been shown to play a role in premenstrual and postpartum mood disorders, particularly the anxious-agitated depressive subtypes. Estrogen has an effect on levels of endorphins: High levels of endorphins occur in the late stage of pregnancy when estrogen levels are at their peak. At delivery, when the sharp drop in both estrogen and progesterone happens, there is a rapid decline in endorphin levels. The withdrawal of endorphins produces effects similar to withdrawal from heroin or morphine: irritability, tearfulness, anxiety, stomach upset, diarrhea, and sweating. I think it is reasonable to think that declining levels of estrogen associated with either postpartum, perimenopause, or menopause can cause reductions in endorphin levels and thereby play a *contributing,* if not a *causative,* role in the onset of the anxiety, depressive, and pain symptoms described by women in these phases.

To summarize: Estradiol has multiple effects on the brain that collectively act in ways similar to antidepressants, memory enhancers, and nerve growth factors. Overall, these pharmacologic effects of estrogen on the nervous system fit well with current theories of antidepressant actions and the action of potent nervous-system-regulating molecules. It has always made sense to me that changes in any aspects of body chemistry, especially changes in such potent chemical messengers as hormones and neurotransmitters, might first be evidenced by changes in brain-mediated phenomena such as irritability, depression, anxiety, and sleep. These are symptoms women notice first, *earlier* in the climacteric, I think because the brain is so exquisitely sensitive to small changes in its biochemical balance and to alterations in the interactions of the various neurotransmitter systems. It is not an either-or split between psychological and biological. Both have to be seen as operating *together* in an *integrated* manner. There is much more to come in our understanding of this key female hormone, but it is clear that estrogen plays a major role in maintaining our sense of well-being, vitality, and zest.

ESTRADIOL EFFECTS ON THE BRAIN

- enhances CNS availability of norepinephrine and dopamine
- increases production and/or prolongs action of serotonin
- regulates sleep centers
- regulates body temperature, vasomotor tone
- improves pain tolerance, (raises pain threshold)
- inhibits the monoamine oxidase (MAO) enzymes that break down serotonin, dopamine, and NE (prolongs mood-lifting action of these chemical messengers)
- increases production of the enzyme needed to make acetylcholine, a crucial memory-enhancing neurotransmitter
- prolongs neuronal responses to excitatory amino acids in the cerebral cortex, cerebellum, hippocampus, hypothalamus, midbrain, and pons
- acts directly on glutamate receptor binding and inactivation
- enhances attention and concentration mechanisms
- increases sensory perception for fine touch, olfactory, and visual stimuli
- increases dendrite connections between nerve cells in memory centers
- has effects that alter seizure threshold, dependent upon type of seizure

©Elizabeth Lee Vliet, M.D., 1995, revised 2000

The Brain's Alarm Center: Hormone Triggers of "Anxiety," "Racing Heart," and "Flutters"

You hit age thirty-nine, have been in good health, maybe you exercise three or four times a week, and wham! All of a sudden you start having horrendous palpitations and pounding sensations as if your heart were going to literally jump out of your chest. Maybe you start feeling anxious; your stomach is a little upset; your skin is clammy. "What's going on? This can't be me? I'm healthy, and I never had these problems before. What is happening? I must be having a panic attack. Maybe I'm having a heart attack. No, that can't be; I'm too young. What is this? I'd better see the doctor." So you see your family doctor, who checks you over and says you're fine, but you need to relax more and reduce your stress. With a deep sigh of relief, you leave and go on about your daily routine. Then, a few weeks later, it happens again. *What is this?*

If you have been checked out and do not have heart disease or thyroid problems or another medical condition that can trigger such episodes, it may be due to ovarian hormone changes. Have you noticed *where* in the menstrual cycle these palpitations or panicky episodes occur? You might find it helpful to keep track of this pattern. If your physical symptoms (heart flutters, heart racing or pounding, feeling queasy or nauseous, sweating, feeling anxious for no apparent reason) come right *after ovulation*, a day or so *before your period starts*, or the first *two or three days of bleeding*, you may be experiencing one of the brain effects of dropping estrogen levels. I can hear you saying to yourself as you read this, "How does estrogen affect the brain to cause heart symptoms?" Well, by some of those chemical messenger molecules I was just talking about. A drop in blood levels of estrogen affects the brain in several ways. Take a look at the following sequence of events:

Decreased estradiol (ovary) ———> Decreased estradiol (at the brain) ————> decreased brain endorphins ———-> burst of brain adrenaline (increased norepinephrine—NE) ———-> brain-body responses to the *stimulation* from norepinephrine: *increased heart rate, palpitations, rise in blood pressure,* being awakened suddenly from sleep, dilation of body blood vessels triggering the "hot flash," sweating, "butterflies" in the stomach, diarrhea, headaches.

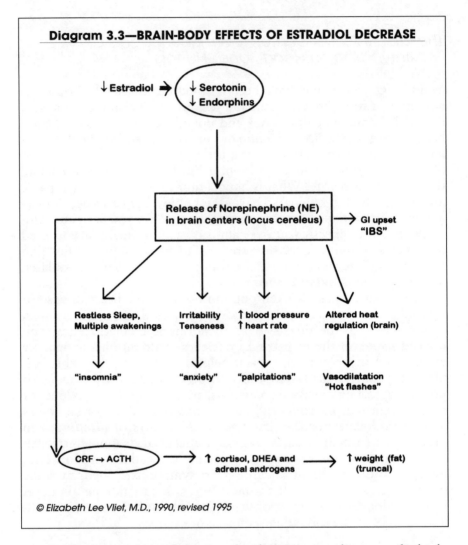

Diagram 3.3—BRAIN-BODY EFFECTS OF ESTRADIOL DECREASE

↓ Estradiol ➡ (↓ Serotonin ↓ Endorphins)

Release of Norepinephrine (NE) in brain centers (locus cereleus) ➝ GI upset "IBS"

Restless Sleep, Multiple awakenings

Irritability Tenseness

↑ blood pressure ↑ heart rate

Altered heat regulation (brain)

"insomnia"

"anxiety"

"palpitations"

Vasodilatation "Hot flashes"

CRF → ACTH ➝ ↑ cortisol, DHEA and adrenal androgens ➝ ↑ weight (fat) (truncal)

© Elizabeth Lee Vliet, M.D., 1990, revised 1995

So there you are, a whole cascade of events spreading over the body from a direct hormone-triggered release of brain chemicals. Remember that endorphins are the body's natural painkillers and mood regulators, so you see how *psychological* (brain) symptoms can be related to the *physical* hormonal drop. This is such a common occurrence, many women don't even notice it until the hormone drops become greater during perimenopause. As estrogen production declines, a fall in estrogen before menses triggers a much more pronounced physical response. Most doctors have *not* been taught these hormone-brain-body connections, so they don't realize these are *clues* to hormone shifts for women. Women tell me they know "its a physical, chemical kind of thing," and they are correct.

In fact it wasn't until the late 1970s that doctors accepted scientific proof that women's hot flashes were a real physical phenomenon. They had been assumed to be psychological and a figment of the woman's imagination. The surging hormones prior to menopause trigger pulses of LH and drops in estradiol that fire off norepinephrine (NE) in the limbic system, and this burst of NE disrupts the normal function of the heat-regulating center in the hypothalamus. The thermoregulatory center then sends its chemical messengers to the arteries, dilating them to allow excess heat to dissipate. The dilation is accompanied by sweating, body temperature begins to drop, and you feel a chilly sensation sweeping over you. If it happens at night, this whole sequence wakes you up each time it happens, and you are often soaked in sweat.

When estrogen is dropping, it triggers a decrease in serotonin. Since serotonin helps maintain sleep and decrease anxiety, a drop in serotonin *adds* to the episodes of awakenings at night, and aggravates the adrenaline-induced feelings of irritability, tension, palpitations, and chest discomfort. It is important to have palpitations and chest discomfort evaluated and the possibility of heart disease ruled out. It is *also* important that we look at changing hormone levels as contributing factors and not immediately jump to the conclusion that it's just psychological stress.

Situational and psychological stress obviously makes all this worse by further suppressing ovarian function along with its many other effects on the body. I will discuss the stress-induced connections in greater detail in upcoming chapters. A lot of the mood swings women experience are not due *only* to external stresses; mood swings also result from the *interaction* of external stresses and our internal body hormonal changes. These are also stressors requiring the body to change and adapt. So, when you experience heart flutters and palpitations, keep in mind that it's not all in your imagination or just due to anxiety, it can also be your hormones changing.

Progesterone Effects on the Brain

With all the headlines talking about progesterone as a "wonder hormone" to prevent osteoporosis and solve all of women's problems, I think it's time to clarify what we know about this hormone. I will elaborate on this further in chapter 4 and just focus on brain effects here. Some of the promoters of the natural "wild yam" progesterone cream have got it backward as to which hormone does what in the female body—but then most of these promoters are men, who don't live with our body experiences every month.

Many women have told me over the years that they become

depressed when they take progesterone or use the "wild yam"–progesterone creams. This is to be expected due to progesterone's effects on the brain, since several metabolic breakdown products of the natural human progesterone molecule are *very potent* depressants of brain (CNS) function. One of the metabolites of progesterone (3-alpha-OH-DHP) has been found to be about *eight times* more potent as a CNS depressant producing antianxiety, sedative effects than the most potent barbiturate known today, methohexital. Studies looking at the anticonvulsant actions of 3-alpha-OH-DHP have found it to be more potent than clonazepam (Klonopin), a high-potency benzodiazepine used for epilepsy and panic disorder. Depressed mood occurring with progesterone is similar to the depressant effects some women have when taking Klonopin or Valium.

The neuroendocrine studies that have identified these progesterone metabolic products and their effects at brain receptors go back several decades, but much of this literature has not made its way into general clinical settings, particularly in the fields of psychiatry and gynecology. The progesterone metabolites above actually attach to GABA receptors, the same ones that bind the benzodiazepine drugs (Klonopin, Valium, Xanax, Ativan, and others in this group of medications). At higher levels, progesterone actually acts very much like these antianxiety medications by attaching to the GABA receptor sites and causing release of the inhibitory neurotransmitter GABA, just like Klonopin, Valium, and the others in this group of medicines do. Inhibitory action at the GABA receptor complex causes *decreased* anxiety, a *decrease* in seizures, *increased* sedation, *delay* in word recall and verbal responses, and potential *increase* in depression. The depressant effects seem to occur at higher doses than are needed for antianxiety effects, again similar to the type of effects we see with benzodiazepines. The depressant effects of progesterone are now thought to primarily occur from one of its metabolites, 3-alpha, 5-alpha-THP or allopregnanolone. Levels of allopregnanolone have been shown to correlate well with circulating levels of progesterone in the bloodstream.

An interesting observation in several studies is that progesterone given to *either* men *or* women produces effects like Valium (and others in the benzodiazepines) on such measurable variables as heart rate, blood pressure, respiratory rate, and the electrocardiogram patterns. It also causes quite pronounced daytime sleepiness for many, male or female. The flip side of this effect is that progesterone produces *withdrawal* effects similar to other medications that act at the GABA receptor, such as benzodiazepines and barbiturates. This effect has been shown in men and women. This withdrawal syndrome includes increased anxiety, restlessness, insomnia, tearfulness, among other effects.

The binding of progesterone metabolites to the GABA receptor complex appears to be one of the primary reasons that high doses of progesterone help decrease anxiety in some women with severe PMS. The doses typically used for PMS treatment may run anywhere from 400–1600 mg a day and produce blood levels actually higher than the levels of progesterone seen in the third trimester of pregnancy. Such high doses are actually providing a *pharmacologic* effect on the brain, similar to benzodiazepine medicines, rather than a *physiologic* one mimicking the levels and functions of a normal menstrual cycle. At these higher doses, the anxiety-relieving metabolites of progesterone are found to be depressogenic, much like what happens to some people when taking higher doses of Valium or Ativan over a period of time. The brain actions are essentially the same, so in susceptible women, using progesterone may initially relieve anxiety, but then over time, it can make depressed, dysphoric moods worse. There is clearly a lot of additional information we need about the varied brain effects of progesterone before any responsible physician should suggest that women buy over-the-counter progesterone creams to use on a daily basis.

Progesterone has some other rather interesting effects on the brain. It has been found to act as an antiestrogen (similar to Tamoxifen) to reduce estrogen binding at brain receptors and to also decrease testosterone effects by several mechanisms, including a down-regulation or "dampening" of estradiol and testosterone receptor activity in the brain, so that it offsets some of the usual mood-*lifting* effects of both estradiol and testosterone. Progesterone also increases the flow of calcium ions into nerve cells, *decreasing* the release of important chemical messengers (neurotransmitters) that boost mood. This is yet another way that progesterone and its metabolic breakdown products may trigger depressed mood, especially if a woman has a history of depression.

If you started using one of the progesterone creams and are wondering what happened to your sex drive, it turns out that progesterone also competes with testosterone for uptake from the blood into the brain and decreases the conversion of testosterone into its most active form. In fact, progesterone is sometimes described as one of the most potent naturally occurring antagonists of androgens. Progesterone competes with testosterone and other androgens at the receptor sites in androgen-dependent tissues and prevents these target tissues from overly responding to the androgens present in women. This reduction in the amount of active testosterone at the brain has the result of further decreasing sexual interest (libido), particularly if estrogen levels are also low. In addition, both estradiol and testosterone have mood-elevating effects, so when progesterone diminishes the binding of estradiol and testosterone at brain receptors, it's not surprising that you may notice your mood is grumpy, irritable, tearful, and depressed.

Women who experience PMS, and those who have FMS that is worse in the second half of the menstrual cycle typically say that their mood and pain become progressively worse from right after ovulation through the first few days of bleeding, which tracks with the time that progesterone rises in the second half of the menstrual cycle. Irritable, depressed mood and increased pain is especially common if estradiol levels are lower than normal at the same time that progesterone is rising. While some women find the "calming" effects of progesterone pleasant, other women really are uncomfortable and "out-of-sorts" with the depression-producing effects of progesterone. The irritable dysphoric mood effects of progesterone and progestins have also been widely observed in menopausal women on HRT, who report feeling very well on the estrogen-only phase of hormones but then become lethargic, bloated, irritable, "PMSy," depressed, and miserable during the days when progesterone or progestin is added.

If you have begun using a wild yam or progesterone cream and experience weight gain; an increase in FMS or bladder-vulvar pain; or a decrease in energy, sex drive, or mood, you may feel better by stopping the progesterone product. Have your hormone levels checked by a reliable method (not just saliva tests) to see what hormones may actually be low, and what you may need supplemented to restore your body to optimal levels. We once again come back to the importance of a healthy balance of the ovarian hormones Mother Nature provided us. There's no quick fix, no magic bullet, and rarely is anything going to give us 100 percent positive effects, without the possibility for some offsetting negatives.

Progesterone Effects on Growth Hormone Production

Studies of progesterone have also shown that it *decreases* the brain's production of human growth hormone, GH. This is a desirable effect in late pregnancy to help the baby not grow too large to be born, but it is an undesirable effect in non pregnant women, especially those with FMS who need GH effects for normal muscle repair. This effect of progesterone was also demonstrated to occur in *non-pregnant* women in excellent medical studies from several centers (Frantz, 1965; Mintz, 1968; Tyson, 1969; Yen, 1967), published in the 1960s. Suppression of growth hormone by progesterone was shown to occur if the amount of progesterone given resulted in blood levels similar to late pregnancy. So what is the daily dose of progesterone that it takes to do that? Bhatia and colleagues at the Medical College of Wisconsin addressed this question in a 1972 study. They found that a daily oral dose of 300–400 mg of progesterone given to healthy nonpregnant women caused a significant blunting of GH concentrations in *all* patients, as well as produced the unwanted effect of significant rises in insulin levels and an exaggerated (abnormal) response of insulin to oral glucose. The rising levels of insulin also caused further decrease in GH release. The hypothesis was that progesterone decreased plasma levels of GH by a suppressant effect on the central nervous system, rather than by direct action on the pituitary cells that synthesize it.

Another critical point regarding progesterone effects on growth hormone is the *duration* of higher progesterone levels. Women in the Bhatia study were only given progesterone for slightly *less than one week,* but I routinely see patients that have been using it for *months to years*. The cumulative negative effects can be severe. Similar suppressive effects on GH secretion were also found for the synthetic progestin, medroxyprogesterone acetate (Provera and other brands) by Simon (1967), Lawrence (1970), and Malarkey (1971). The broad suppressive effects of progesterone (and progestins derived from it) on pituitary gonadotropin, ACTH, and GH release suggest that progesterone produced by the placenta is one of the major ways the pregnant body shifts its endocrine "manager" from pituitary control to control by the placenta as the baby grows. Such a shift helps to ensure that the mother's body will change appropriately to nourish the growing baby.

I think it is important to point out that the *decrease in GH* from progesterone was demonstrated with doses of progesterone *lower* than amounts being recommended today by some practitioners for PMS treatment and relief of menopause symptoms. Typical doses of progesterone used for PMS are often suggested as 400 mg to 1600 mg a day. And keep in mind, that this study used oral doses. If you use a non oral delivery, such as cream or suppository, the dose is supposed to be *decreased* to about 10 percent of the oral dose due to better absorption of the non-oral forms. This means that a 100 mg dose for oral use should be decreased to 10 mg per gram of cream, since the cream bypasses the liver when it is absorbed directly into the bloodstream through the skin. Yet, I have frequently had patients come in to my office using progesterone creams that are marked on the container *100 mg/gm*, about ten times the recommended amount. No wonder they feel so bad!

In addition to incorrect dosages for *prescription* creams, many of the currently available over-the-counter "wild yam" and progesterone cream products deliver amounts of progesterone in excess of those in the Bhatia study. While this is not a complete list, some examples of progesterone-containing creams with greater than 400 mg/oz are Angel Care, DermaGest, EssPro7, Fair Lady, Fem Crème, FemGest, GreenPastures, Progestacare, ProGest, Today's Man, YamCon (Pro) Extra (reference: PIC Analysis, Aeron Laboratories).

Based on my analysis of decades of medical literature summarizing the adverse metabolic consequences I describe, my medical opinion is that the concentration of progesterone in these products is far in excess of what is safe or reasonable for daily use. The extensive data on adverse effects of progesterone on major metabolic functions of the body, including growth hormone production, seems to be ignored by those who are advocating the regular daily use of supplemental progesterone in body creams and other forms, particularly since over-the-counter ones vary so greatly in the amount of progesterone added. If you are using an over-the-counter progesterone or wild yam product, please talk with your doctor and have the important lab tests I discuss in upcoming chapters.

Testosterone and the Brain

In chapter 6, you will read how testosterone is crucial for normal sex drive in women, since it activates the brain "sexual circuits" in both women and men. For now, I just want to emphasize that it is another hormone produced by the ovary that helps to improve a woman's sense of well-being, energy level, and stimulates normal bone growth and muscle development. We know that a certain level of estradiol (estrogen) must be present in our brain areas in order for testosterone to function properly. It is now thought that the brain testosterone receptor is *created* by the presence of estradiol. Without enough estrogen to "prime the pump" so to speak, testosterone produced by the ovary cannot attach properly in brain centers to stimulate sexual arousal for women. So your level of estradiol also plays a role in how well your body's testosterone can work. When I have explained this biology to women and their partners, it has helped improve many hurts in relationships where the partner thought she was no longer attracted to him.

As another illustration of the connection between estradiol and testosterone, we have seen in women who have had breast cancer and cannot take estrogen, that providing supplemental testosterone may only *partially* improve their sexual desire and ability to have an orgasm. The important role of "estrogen-priming" for optimal testosterone response may explain these clinical observations. Other studies have demonstrated a mood-lifting or antidepressant effect of testosterone, which many women in my center also describe after testosterone therapy is added to their program. It is rewarding to me to hear my patients describe how they feel after taking natural testosterone, when they have typically experienced low testosterone levels for quite a long time: "GOSH, I FEEL LIKE MY OLD SELF AGAIN. I have my energy back. I'M INTERESTED IN SEX AGAIN. I have my get-up-and-go feelings." Using natural testosterone at doses designed for women, it is uncommon that I see unwanted side effects. I will describe in chapter 6 the different types of testosterone available and how I use blood levels and women's descriptions to find the right amount for a given person.

Future Directions

For centuries, medical observation has written about the connection between reproductive hormones and changes in mood and behavior, but these observations have been largely dismissed due to problems in methods, lack of "adequate" biological evidence, and lack of the necessary interdisciplinary studies. Recent developments in the study of the endocrine system and brain function have certainly shed light on the ways that changes in hormones through the menstrual cycle may contribute to perimenopausal mood *disorders* and *symptoms*. Mood disorders and milder mood-change symptoms are a significant source of distress to many women in the perimenopausal years; yet, they often fall between the cracks in our fragmented health care system.

The model I have developed for HER Place: *Health Enhancement and Renewal for Women* Centers in Tucson and Dallas–Ft. Worth are examples of the integrated approach we crucially need for women's health care services, as well as educational and research paradigms. Now we need to view hormonal effects on mood from a similarly integrated perspective. We need to focus on the internal biological factors, such as hormones, that interact with external events to increase the likelihood of *exaggerated* or *abnormal responses* to *normal* hormonal changes. Areas of future research need to also include evaluation of the

- Possibility that different types of estrogens, progestins, and testosterone, as well as different doses, have very different effects on the brain, especially mood, sleep, and pain pathways;
- Mood effects of estrogen and progesterone in women who have never had previous depression;
- Effect of different hormone preparations in women who have a history of hormone-related depressions;
- Effects of different types of estrogens, testosterone, and progestins in various subtypes of depressed patients (unipolar, bipolar, those with normal estradiol levels, those with proven low estradiol levels, etc.);

- Differential effects of brief and ongoing estrogen use along with how it is taken;
- Prospective evaluation of estrogen and testosterone roles as an augmentation approach as traditional antidepressant medications;
- Evaluation of the role that stress plays in suppressing ovarian function;
- The effects of hormone interactions with other medications.

These are clearly critical areas affecting women. Why are these issues not being addressed? I think one factor is economic. There is more money to be made in the current proliferation in development and use of antidepressants rather than natural hormones, many of which have been around so long they have gone off patent. Once medications are off patent, the companies that developed them no longer make much money on them, and other companies begin to compete with generics. So the race is always to find new medications, new supplements, new products that will bring profit to the company that creates them.

But using antidepressants or over-the-counter supplements to reduce symptoms is like putting a Band-Aid on a wound that needs stitches—it may give some relief but doesn't get at the underlying cause of the problem. Getting at the underlying hormone imbalance and finding the right "recipe" for a given person takes time and detective work. Time is expensive in today's health care environment. It is easier—and takes less time—to write a prescription for an antidepressant than to check hormone levels properly, listen to the woman's concerns, answer her questions, address her fears about hormones, and fine-tune a hormone prescription to achieve optimal hormonal balance. Many times, doctors can't or don't want to spend the time it takes, and many consumers aren't willing to pay for the extra time or put up with the initial difficulties encountered trying to find the right combination. So there really isn't any one "cause" or "fault" in all this; there are many factors. Only when women themselves have reliable information and become assertive about getting their needs met, will we have more individualized approaches widely used.

But if you really think about how valuable your health is, taking the approach I have outlined, is *less* expensive (in time and money) in the long run because you are addressing the underlying causes, and you are restoring body balance with natural hormones that your body has always made. If this is addressed really well, you will likely need far fewer other medications, hospitalizations, or surgeries to "fix" problems. Think about these points as you read the chapters ahead, in which I will give you many more specific examples and actual case stories from women themselves who have taken this journey. Remember, menopause is not a Prozac or Zoloft or Paxil deficiency. It is the loss of hormones that have overseen our body function for most of our lives. Don't let anyone make you take the easy way out. Educate yourself—and ask to try approaches that feel natural and right for you.

There is a great deal of exciting work to be done to understand our awesome female body and these intricate interconnections. The need is great, and the list of unanswered questions is long. At *HER Place*, we strive to be among the leaders in these endeavors with an integrated approach to women's health care encompassing Preventive Medicine, Gynecology, Endocrinology, Psychiatry/ Psychology, Nutrition, Complementary Medicine, physical therapies ("body work") and spiritual awareness. Speak out in your community and encourage the development of such integrated services for women. All of us working together can make a difference. It is crucial, in my view, that instead of focusing on fragmented treatment of women's body parts, we must combine our therapeutic approaches in ways to provide effective and safe symptom relief and health *enhancement* (not just treatment) for women of all ages. Our goal is to have healthy, enjoyable, and productive lives for the additional years we now have the opportunity to live.

CHAPTER 4

Hormones of Pregnancy and Stress: Progesterone and Cortisol

We are inundated with health information today—books, news articles, internet sites, tapes, support groups, newsletters, and many others. I enjoy having my patients bring in articles that have stimulated questions and we often discuss these new findings and approaches. One of the topics that comes up daily in my medical practice is "What about wild yam/progesterone creams?" There has been an exponential increase in over-the-counter progesterone creams and multilevel marketing schemes in the marketplace today, with incredible claims touting progesterone as a "wonder hormone" to prevent osteoporosis, lose weight, increase sex drive, and solve all of women's problems.

What's the scientific truth behind those claims? There is a wealth of good solid medical and basic science research going back fifty years to draw on in answering this question, and I think it is important to clarify these issues. There is so much emphasis on using progesterone for treatment of PMS, menopause, and pain problems that I think people who recommend such broad use of one hormone have forgotten that women have a variety of hormones with different functions, and each one has to be taken into account in our evaluation and treatment approaches. In this chapter, I have presented both the historical and the current worldwide research from reputable medical centers, menopause and PMS researchers, and neuroendocrine basic science researchers to describe which functions are known to occur with each of these major hormones. My goal is to give you a reliable "road map" through the maze of conflicting information out there.

Progesterone's Discovery

In 1573, Volcherius Coiter first observed the presence of a yellowish body in the mammalian ovary, later called the *corpus luteum* in 1686 by Malpighi. Then Dr. Born first suggested that perhaps it was an endocrine organ concerned with maintaining pregnancy, and it was his student, Loeb, who showed in 1907 that the corpus luteum specifically prepares the uterus to receive a fertilized egg; that is, it is the cause of the "progestational" changes in the lining of the uterus whether followed by pregnancy or only by menstruation. It was in 1928 that Weichert demonstrated the actual existence of a hormone from this "yellow body" by injecting extracts of corpora lutea into uterine tissue, and this injection produced the changes described by Loeb. Then the pure hormone was isolated by Wintersteiner and Allen and others in 1929 and named "progesterone" for its pregnancy-promoting ("pro-gestational") effects.

Since the quantity of this new hormone present in nature was so remarkably small—perhaps one part in 40,000 in the human corpus luteum or one part in 750,000 in the placenta (Duuyvene, 1939; Pratt, 1936), the greatest practical importance lay in finding a way to make this hormone by synthetic means. It was a significant advance for clinical medicine when Butenandt and Fernholz, in 1934, first prepared the pure corpus luteum hormone from the precursor *stigmasterol* found in soybeans. Allen found that diascorea, a precursor found in the wild Mexican yam could also be synthesized in the laboratory into the molecule of progesterone. Prior to these discoveries, the natural sources were quite limited. Finding "building block" substances in soybeans and yams meant that we now had a renewable natural source from plants that could be cultivated to provide the quantities needed for production of progesterone, and later synthetic progestins and various estrogens, for clinical use.

Natural Body Cycles and Progesterone's Roles

Progesterone is the primary hormone designed to prepare the female body to support a pregnancy. In the first half of the menstrual cycle (follicular phase) there is no significant amount of progesterone produced, and levels in women are about 0.3–0.9 ng/ml. When ovulation occurs, the ovum is released and becomes the corpus luteum ("egg"), which begins to secrete progesterone. Levels of progesterone in this half of the cycle (luteal phase) rise to about 15–30 ng/ml, or up to thirty times the level of the first half of the cycle. Levels in pregnancy are about *fifteen times greater* than luteal phase progesterone levels.

Studies done in the 1970s showed that an oral dose of 300 mg micronized progesterone given daily for one week would produce blood levels of progesterone equivalent to third trimester of pregnancy. Oral doses of 200 mg daily for ten to fourteen days are used in HRT to prevent endometrial hyperplasia. The progesterone secreted by the corpus luteum stimulates the lining of the uterus to thicken and become secretory in preparation to receive a fertilized egg and help it grow. If there is fertilization and pregnancy, the placenta becomes a hormone-producing factory, with increasing progesterone production throughout the months of pregnancy. With so many changes needed in a woman's body for her to sustain a pregnancy, it is not surprising that progesterone has a wide range of metabolic effects on the whole body, not just the reproductive organs. Think about it. For a female to get enough nutrition for the growing fetus, she has to eat more. Progesterone is the hormone that stimulates appetite and drives the individual to eat more (both in a nonpregnant menstrual cycle, as well as throughout pregnancy). It also stimulates the desire for carbohydrates, which are more quickly converted to useable fuel.

In addition, progesterone relaxes the smooth muscles of the intestinal tract, which slows down the movement of food and allows greater absorption of nutrients. For a pregnancy, this is a beneficial effect. If you are not pregnant, you may experience this "slowing down" of the intestinal tract as constipation (especially if you don't get enough fiber). Progesterone has been shown to have marked effects to increase total body fat, and this occurs in many different species studied, not just humans. This fat-storing effect has an obvious evolutionary advantage for survival to ensure that pregnant women have adequate fat stores to provide fuel for mother and baby through nine months of gestation. Another important effect of progesterone is to suppress the mother's immune system so that the mother's body will not "attack and destroy" the foreign protein of the developing fetus that contains the father's genetic makeup and protein coding systems. This is a crucial function of progesterone for a pregnant woman, but not one that we want *all* the time.

The chart that follows shows how the body makes progesterone and other ovary hormones from cholesterol. You have probably seen this chart in other health books, and I wanted to clarify some of the basic biology of how this works. Looking at this sequence, you may be tempted to believe some of the current books and tapes that say progesterone is the "mother" hormone women should be taking because it comes at the beginning of the pathway and all of the other hormones, including testosterone and estradiol, are made from this compound. Think about it. If that logic were really correct, we should be suggesting that *men* take progesterone, too, as they get older and their testosterone declines. But we clearly don't do this for men. Why not? There are several aspects of this whole line of reasoning that are incorrect based on reputable medical science and reproductive hormone endocrinology. First of all, most of the conversion of progesterone down this pathway to the end products of testosterone and estradiol require the presence of *functioning* ovaries. If you have reached menopause, your ovaries are no longer functioning to handle these conversions.

If you had a severe viral illness, a prolonged stress that disrupted menses, a tubal ligation, or one of many other causes of gradual decline in ovarian function, then you may not be able to convert a load of precursor hormones to the end-product hormones. If you have had a hysterectomy with the ovaries removed, well . . . it is obvious you don't have the ovaries to convert progesterone to the end hormones (estradiol, testosterone) that you need for optimal well-being. I think the important point here is that Mother Nature gave us a series of steps for the body to go through to get to the end result . . . we can't assume that we can simply load up on one beginning step in the process and accomplish the same results as the body does when everything is working the way it is supposed to.

Another metaphor for this process comes to mind. Think about the many stages of growth and development that have to occur for a baby to become a child, then an adolescent, then an adult. I think of progesterone as the "baby" in our hormone-development process. It can't carry out all the functions of the "adult" hormones estradiol and testosterone until it has been shaped and altered by the changes of this entire cascade of steps. Progesterone can't be made into testosterone or estradiol directly; it *has* to undergo further changes to become the molecules that are the direct building blocks for testosterone and then estradiol. It's very much like the life process—a baby can't become an adult without going through the stages of childhood, and then adolescence. And without our ovaries to facilitate this "growth" of the "baby" progesterone so it can become the "adult" testosterone and estradiol, we are stuck with a molecule that doesn't have the specific shape of estradiol or testosterone to activate the receptors for normal function. Remember, each of these molecules acts like a different key in various receptor locks throughout the body, so the proper shape to the molecule key is crucial to create the proper results.

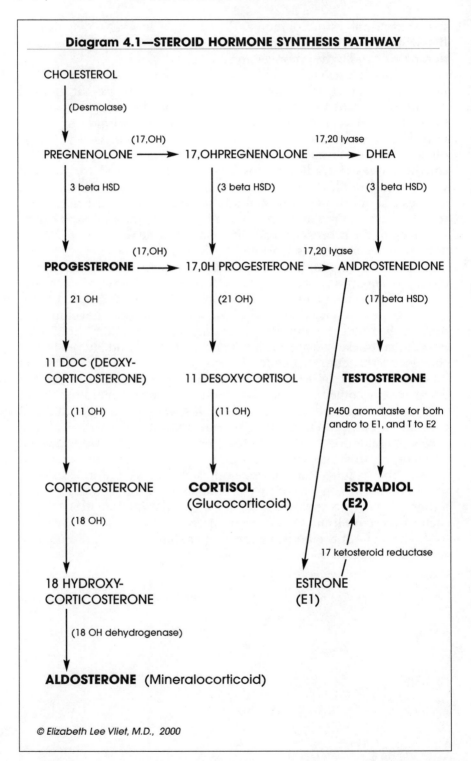

Diagram 4.1—STEROID HORMONE SYNTHESIS PATHWAY

CHOLESTEROL

(Desmolase)

PREGNENOLONE —(17,OH)→ 17,OHPREGNENOLONE —17,20 lyase→ DHEA

3 beta HSD   (3 beta HSD)   (3 beta HSD)

PROGESTERONE —(17,OH)→ 17,0H PROGESTERONE —17,20 lyase→ ANDROSTENEDIONE

21 OH   (21 OH)   (17 beta HSD)

11 DOC (DEOXY-CORTICOSTERONE)   11 DESOXYCORTISOL   TESTOSTERONE

(11 OH)   (11 OH)   P450 aromataste for both andro to E1, and T to E2

CORTICOSTERONE   CORTISOL (Glucocorticoid)   ESTRADIOL (E2)

(18 OH)   17 ketosteroid reductase

18 HYDROXY-CORTICOSTERONE   ESTRONE (E1)

(18 OH dehydrogenase)

ALDOSTERONE (Mineralocorticoid)

© Elizabeth Lee Vliet, M.D., 2000

Progesterone and Progestins: Understanding the Important Differences

Over the many years of research into steroid hormones and their function in the body, it has been known that relatively small changes in the molecule—number of carbons, side chains, number of unsaturated chemical bonds, other atoms added—can make an enormous difference in the way that molecule works in the human body. These small changes in the molecule can affect everything from desired effects to unwanted side effects. For example, once the progesterone molecule is changed in metabolism to a different arrangement of the molecule called pregnandiol, it is now completely inactive. Conversion to pregnandiol is one of the ways that the body clears excess progesterone and makes it possible to be excreted in the urine. Other breakdown products of progesterone (allopregnandiol, epiallopregnanolone) are also inactive and are excreted in the urine.

On the other hand, some metabolic changes in the molecule of progesterone lead to compounds that are even more potent, particularly at brain receptors, than even progesterone itself. This is seen with 3-alpha, 5-alpha THP (allopregnanolone), a highly potent sedative and depressant metabolite of progesterone. We see this issue of different effects happening with small changes in the molecule occur quite strikingly when the molecule of progesterone, as found naturally in the body, is chemically changed to make a synthetic group of compounds called *progestins*. There are several terms that many women find confusing, so I will clarify these to help you understand various options.

Progestogen is the broad term used to describe *any substance* that has chemical effects to sustain a pregnancy, called "progestational" activity.

Progesterone (found in humans and all vertebrate animals) is a biologically natural *progestogen*. *Human* progesterone is produced by the corpus luteum after ovulation, and to a much lesser extent by the adrenal gland (though adrenal production is not sufficient to prepare the body to sustain a pregnancy). *Progesterone USP* is the form of natural progesterone derived from "building block" molecules in soybeans and wild Mexican yams. These "building blocks" (stigmasterol, diascorea, and others) are changed chemically in the laboratory with a series of steps and purified to meet FDA standards for use as a medication. USP progesterone may be dissolved in oil to make an injectable form of medication, which has been available to physicians since the 1940s. USP progesterone is also available as a powder that is made into tablets (Prometrium), or vaginal gel (Crinone), as well as used by pharmacists to compound individual prescriptions of tablets, suppositories, and creams for patients. USP Progesterone is *identical* to the chemical molecule made by the ovary. When used for hormone therapy, it generally has far fewer unpleasant side effects than the progestins (such as Provera and others).

Disogenin (and others) is a plant precursor molecule found in wild yams, soybeans, and a variety of other foods, that has some very mild effects similar to both progesterone and estrogen. This is used in many nonprescription creams. These plant precursors are not the same chemical molecule as either progesterone or estradiol, and do not have the exact same effects in the body—even though the marketing hype will try to make you think otherwise. These *phystosterols* (phytoestrogens, phytoprogestins, etc.) can be made into progesterone or estradiol by chemical changes that are done is a laboratory. Our bodies do not have the enzymes needed to make these changes in the molecule, so our bodies cannot take the wild yam or soybean precursors and make them into the exact same molecules the ovaries make before menopause.

Progestins are man-made chemical molecules that have a different chemical structure from the molecules naturally found in the human body. They have many properties and actions *similar to* progesterone but because their molecules are "rearranged" slightly from progesterone, they have a number of *different* actions as well, and are many times *more potent* than natural progesterone. As a result, progestins can produce very different effects in the body that are at times quite desirable and needed, and other times quite bothersome and undesirable.

Progestins are technically a member of the larger group of *progestogens* because they all have some degree of progestational activity, but they are *not* compounds normally found in the human body. Progestins may be made from progesterone and are then called *progestational* progestins, such as Provera, Cycrin, Amen (generic name: MPA or medroxyprogesterone acetate). MPA was originally approved by the FDA in the 1960s for contraceptive use under the brand name Depo-Provera and has since been used to treat abnormal uterine bleeding and some types of amenorrhea. In more recent years, MPA and other progestins have been used for protection of the uterine lining in menopausal regimens.

Another group of progestins is made from the naturally occurring ovarian molecule of testosterone, and these are called *androgenic* progestins. This group includes medications like Aygestin and Micronor (generic name: norethindrone) as well as products that contain the androgenic progestin *levonorgestrel* (Norplant implant, some combination oral birth control pills). In addition to its progestational activity, this group has effects similar to testosterone and is often used when women are experiencing a loss of libido. The androgenic progestins have generally caused fewer problems with depressed mood and decreased libido than we see with Provera or other progestational progestins. Newer progestins like norgestimate and desogestrel are the *most progestational* and *least androgenic* of the synthetic progestins. This means they are less likely to cause acne, but *more* likely to cause weight gain, loss of libido, or depressed mood.

Synthetic progestins, whether in birth control pills or given in post-menopause, are the most common cause of unpleasant side effects associated with "hormone therapy." Some of these are irritable mood, depressed mood, headaches, decreased energy, weight gain, bloating, and breast tenderness, among others. Two major factors are important in determining the balance of desirable therapeutic effects and undesirable side effects: (1) the relative balance of progestational and androgenic activity, and (2) the balance of progestin relative to estrogen in the preparation. Progestin-only products (that is, contain no estrogen) like Norplant and Depo-Provera, as well as pills such as Micronor, typically have the worst side effect profile of all, because you get all the negative effects of the progestin without any compensating benefits of the estrogen unless estrogen is added as a separate pill or patch.

Progestin-only options are particularly hard to use for women with FMS, vulvodynia, interstitial cystitis, or migraines because they tend to increase pain to a marked degree. This is especially true of the long-acting progestin-only contraceptives like Norplant and Depo-Provera. If I prescribe Micronor, for example, I always balance it with estrogen to avoid making FMS pain worse. My patients tell me that the androgenic progestins cause less bloating and breast tenderness than Provera and other ones in this group. The more androgenic progestins, however, may cause more acne and are not recommended for women with high cholesterol and low HDL, since the androgenic effects can worsen the risk of cardiovascular disease and decrease the benefits of estrogen. Finding the one that works best for your body is both an art and a science!

What about natural progesterone, chemically identical to what the body makes? Why even use the synthetic progestins if they tend to cause so many side effects? There are some situations and some women for whom the synthetic progestins actually work better or have fewer side effects. But there is another practical reason we haven't had widespread use of natural progesterone in this country until more recently. It has to do with technology of delivery of the hormone, as well as expense. Progesterone itself is quickly inactivated by stomach acid and then isn't absorbed into the bloodstream when taken by mouth. So it simply didn't work to give progesterone *orally* until a new process, called micronization (which means making the hormone particles tiny enough to be absorbed before being inactivated), was developed in the 1960s. Only then could we provide more reliable absorption and the desired therapeutic effects of progesterone. The *injectable* form of progesterone is put in oil to promote absorption into the bloodstream and has been available in the United States since the 1940s. It is made by Upjohn, the company that also makes Provera and Depo-Provera, which were originally developed trying to find a tablet form that would be active when taken by mouth. The injectable form of progesterone USP in oil has been widely used by gynecologists for years, but most women understandably did not want to have to get an injection on a regular basis.

By the time micronization processes were developed, doctors were used to using Provera, and it was much cheaper for patients to buy than the newly invented micronized progesterone. From the 1970s through about 1998, micronized natural progesterone was primarily available through specialty compounding pharmacies in various forms (tablets, creams, suppositories). Since these forms were made according to individual prescriptions and not manufactured in huge quantities, they typically were not covered by health insurance plans and were significantly more expensive than the commercially available progestins like Provera. In addition to habit, the higher cost to patients was another reason more doctors continued using the synthetic ones. Then in 1998, the FDA approved Prometrium, a tablet form of micronized progesterone, and Crinone vaginal gel (also micronized progesterone), so more and more physicians are now using natural progesterone for menopause, PMS, and bleeding problems. These new commercial products of natural progesterone are advantageous since they are usually covered by health insurance plans, unlike compounded prescriptions. If Prometrium or Crinone don't quite fit your body's needs in terms of dose and form, then you can still get micronized progesterone tailored to your needs by compounding pharmacists. I have used natural progesterone in a variety of forms since I was a medical student in 1975. I have found that natural progesterone generally works well, when used properly, and has far fewer side effects than do the Provera-type medications.

Progesterone Effects on Sleep

I described in chapter 3 how estradiol produced before menopause is one of the primary hormones regulating the brain's sleep center and facilitating the normal stages of sleep. When estradiol declines, the normal stages of sleep, especially periods of Stage IV deep sleep, are disrupted. So it is crucial for women to have adequate estradiol to regain normal deep sleep and muscle repair. But there are a number of metabolites of progesterone that have potent sedative effects, very similar to barbiturates and benzodiazepines. Remember the compound I mentioned in chapter 3 called 3-alpha-OH-DHP? It is about *eight times more potent* than the sedative methohexital, a potent barbiturate used for anesthesia. The liver provides most of the conversion of progesterone to these sedative compounds, so the sleep-inducing effects of progesterone will be increased if it is taken orally and goes through the liver "first pass" metabolism. So progesterone does have effects on brain receptors that help sleep, by acting like the medications you may already know: Klonopin, Ativan, Valium, and others in this group.

Progesterone's effect on sleep is quite different from estrogen effects, so just taking progesterone doesn't *eliminate* the need for estradiol to restore sleep pathways, as some books claim. Since progesterone can make you sleepy like Klonopin does, there may be times when it can be a useful addition to hormone therapy even if women do not have a uterus. But this has to be balanced against the unwanted, potentially negative metabolic effects of progesterone that I have discussed elsewhere in this chapter and in chapter 3. Some of the metabolites of progesterone have *greater* sedative effects on brain receptors than does Klonopin. If progesterone is used to improve sleep in a woman with FMS, I find that lower doses can be effective *if* estradiol has been restored to optimal levels. If you have a uterus, however, you and your doctor have to be certain that you are taking an appropriate dose of progesterone for the desired protective effects on the endometrial lining.

Progesterone Effects on Pain Regulation

Both estradiol and progesterone have important effects on pain regulation in women. In this chapter I will review aspects of progesterone's effects and talk about estradiol in chapter 5. As I mentioned earlier, several of progesterone's metabolites act as central nervous system *anesthetics*, both by increasing endorphin production (such as late-stage pregnancy) and by enhancing the action of the inhibitory neurotransmitter, GABA. The analgesia of pregnancy has been extensively studied and has been shown to involve central nervous system opioid systems rather than peripheral (body) ones. Since opioid compounds from the body have only limited ability to cross the blood-brain barrier, it has been hypothesized that the estradiol-progesterone-triggered increase in analgesia seen in pregnancy primarily results from a direct effect of activating a brain endorphin system. In addition, the *dynorphin* system has also been shown to be activated in the analgesia of actual pregnancy. Giving estradiol and progesterone peripherally (oral, transdermal, etc.) has been shown to increase several measures of brain opioid activity; increases in opiate receptor density as well as the concentration of beta-endorphin in brain centers have been demonstrated.

In support of this theory of the female sex hormones as activators of pregnancy analgesia systems, it has been shown that the pregnancy concentration of progesterone in cerebral spinal fluid (CSF) increases eight fold, with a rapid decrease in the immediate postpartum period, along with the rapid drop in estradiol levels. In addition, there is more *biologically active* progesterone present in the later stages of pregnancy, since the percentage of unbound or free progesterone *in spinal fluid* was found to be *three times greater than* that in the *blood* in all three types of patients: pregnant, postpartum, and nonpregnant women. The abrupt drop in both progesterone and estradiol with the delivery of the placenta leads to an abrupt drop in the endorphins as well, which is one of the many changes contributing to the irritable, depressed mood, fragmented sleep, and increased pain in the early postpartum weeks. If the estradiol and progesterone levels remain low over a prolonged period of time following delivery, such as with nursing or due to a postpartum thyroiditis or postpartum viral illness, the low levels trigger increased sensitivity to pain. I am convinced that this is a primary factor triggering the postpartum fibromyalgia syndromes, along with the loss of important effects on sleep, muscle repair, and nerve tissue itself from the ovarian hormones. I have treated quite successfully a number of postpartum fibromyalgia patients with just proper hormone balancing, which would fit with the basic science data on these hormones' multiple effects on pain pathways.

Frye and Duncan (1994) showed that, in rats, diminished pain sensitivity correlated well with the relative binding actions of various progesterone metabolites at the GABA receptor complex. They looked at several different compounds, and those that were strongly bound to GABA receptors showed the greatest reduction in pain, while the GABA *antagonist* compounds such as DHEA-S did not improve pain sensitivity. Both the sedative and analgesic effects of progesterone are *gender-independent* effects: They can also be observed when progesterone is given to men. It's just that under normal conditions, the adrenal glands in men normally make only a tiny amount of progesterone, about a third of the lowest concentrations found in women during their bleeding days.

Even in nonpregnant women, progesterone, and estradiol as you saw in chapter 3, play roles in the brain endorphin pathways. When progesterone and estradiol levels both fall in the days just before bleeding starts, the drop in both hormones triggers a fall in brain-body endorphins as well as a lowering of our pain threshold that makes us more sensitive to pain. A cyclic variation in pain threshold in menstruating women has been found in a number of recent studies, which confirms the intuitive wisdom of my patients who have noticed this. Science finally catches up with women's wisdom. This appears to be one of several reasons that women with FMS, vulvodynia, and IC have "flares" with the onset of menstrual bleeding. It is also one of the reasons I try to help my patients keep the estradiol level steady during these days. Progesterone *has* to drop in order to trigger bleeding, but I can help offset the drop in endorphins if I keep estradiol levels steady so that both hormones are not so low. This approach has been one that my patients tell me works really well to help keep the menstrually related pain "flares" in check. So, together the two primary ovarian hormones, estradiol and progesterone, play a significant role in modulating pain in women. It has also been found that for progesterone to exert some of these effects, the receptors need to be "primed" estradiol in the first half of the menstrual cycle. This is another reason to take hormones in a manner that closely mimics the sequence and ratios of a healthy menstrual cycle.

Progesterone Interaction with Other Hormones: Insulin and Cortisol

Numerous studies over the last three decades have shown that progesterone *decreases* growth hormone (GH) and *increases* insulin levels. This metabolic pattern is the same one seen in obese people, in Cushing's disease (excess cortisol), and after starting corticosteroid medication (such as for arthritis or asthma); it clearly isn't a very desirable pattern to maintain. Higher levels of progesterone, such as in pregnancy or when taking large doses for PMS or menopause therapy, are associated with greater amounts of unbound, or free, cortisol in the blood, which further decreases GH and causes higher insulin levels with more insulin resistance. This is another reason that using progesterone regularly, in doses that give blood levels similar to pregnancy, can have negative health effects on a nonpregnant woman. Most of the women I have been treating for hormone imbalances aren't pregnant and don't want to be, so artificially creating high progesterone levels simply doesn't make sense. The brain-body changes triggered by high progesterone levels can wreck havoc with maintaining healthy production of GH, insulin, and cortisol, leading to excessive weight gain and many other problems.

Progesterone Effects on Muscle and Connective Tissue

Muscle protein metabolism is affected by the hormone changes of the menstrual cycle. Studies of exercise effects on protein breakdown in women have been done, with calculations of the amount of breakdown products (urea and others) excreted in the urine based on whether the women were in the mid-follicular (high estradiol) phase or mid-luteal (high progesterone) phase. Such studies showed marked differences in the excretion of muscle breakdown products in the urine by cycle phase, with highest levels of urea in the urine occurring during the mid-luteal phase. Researchers have concluded that the high levels of progesterone in the mid-luteal phase of the menstrual cycle suggest that an elevated progesterone-to-estradiol ratio exerts a catabolic (breakdown) effect on body proteins. If this effect continues to be supported by future studies, it would suggest that women with muscle pain syndrome should be cautious about using progesterone on a regular basis to avoid any excess breakdown of protein and muscle tissue.

Another series of Canadian studies of muscle strength in women showed that in women between twenty and thirty years old, voluntary isometric muscle strength is highest around the time of ovulation, when estradiol levels are at their peak than was muscle strength at other times of the menstrual cycle (lower estrogen phase of bleeding or progesterone dominant luteal phase). At menopause, a significant decline in muscle strength was observed, but this decline was not found in women taking postmenopausal estrogen therapy. Again, these findings suggest that women who are having muscle pain syndromes may want to be careful about using daily progesterone to avoid loss of muscle strength.

Progesterone has interesting effects on connective tissues that make up our body's ligaments and tendons. In pregnancy, as the mother's body prepares for the baby's body to be delivered through the birth canal, high levels of progesterone relax or loosen the supporting ligaments of the back and pelvis. This is an adaptive and desirable effect of progesterone to allow the pelvic bones to separate enough for the baby's head to get through the birth canal. Relaxed ligaments have the unwanted effect of causing backaches in women who are on their feet a lot toward the end of pregnancy. The higher levels of progesterone during the luteal phase of the monthly menstrual cycle has a similar effect on ligaments of the back, hips, and knees, which is one reason we think women athletes have more exercise-related injuries in this phase of the cycle compared to the first half when progesterone is lower.

I recently did a consult for a woman with FMS who had low back pain due to laxity (excess relaxation or looseness) of the ligaments in her sacroiliac joints and pelvis. She had been getting *prolotherapy* to strengthen these ligaments. This is a series of injections using a sclerosing, or scar-forming, solution to make the ligaments form scar tissue to strengthen them. While prolotherapy can be quite painful, it has clearly helped some people by providing stronger ligamentous support and reducing back pain. The irony was that this woman had been using a daily progesterone cream, incorrectly prescribed at ten times the recommended dose. Here she was, getting painful and expensive injections that were being counteracted by the progesterone high-dose cream she was using. Until our consult, no one had talked to her about these effects of progesterone on connective tissues. She was aghast, and understandably, quite upset to find this out. But since her dose of progesterone cream was so high, she still had a month or more to slowly taper off the progesterone to avoid triggering withdrawal symptoms.

Progesterone Effects on Metabolism

The menstrual cycle ebb and flow of hormones, and balance of progesterone relative to estradiol and testosterone, has effects on multiple metabolic pathways: glycogen storage, caffeine metabolism, protein metabolism, food selection, interleukin concentrations, to name a few. Progesterone and estradiol work together to regulate tissue mass and body composition, in part by altering the enzyme lipoprotein lipase (LPL) activity in fat cells (adipocytes). Estradiol acts to *lower* body fat (adiposity) by lowering LPL activity, while progesterone *increases* body fat storage by increasing the activity of the LPL enzyme. Progesterone's effects to enhance fat storage help the expectant mother store enough fuel to nourish her and the developing baby. And you wondered why it is harder for women than men to lose weight, even with a good exercise program!

Estrogen and progesterone also play a role in insulin response to glucose. Multiple studies, in animal models as well as humans, have confirmed that both hormones increase the pancreatic insulin response to glucose, but estrogen and progesterone have very different effects on insulin sensitivity in other tissues. Progesterone has been shown to *decrease* insulin sensitivity and to cause resistance to the glucose-regulating effects of insulin. Progesterone's effect on insulin is quite rapid and can be detected within ten minutes of administering the hormone. It appears to be a direct effect of progesterone on the pancreas itself. This is one of the reasons women often experience increased cravings for sweets in the second half of the menstrual cycle when progesterone rises. Estradiol, on the other hand, has been demonstrated in humans and a variety of animal species to *increase* insulin sensitivity and improve glucose tolerance. The effect of estradiol on improving glucose handling by the body occurs in both menstruating and postmenopausal women (if the latter are on the patch form of estradiol), as well as in diabetic women. The estradiol-induced improvement in insulin sensitivity has been shown to occur at both fat cells (adipocytes) and skeletal muscle and appears to occur by multiple pathways rather than a direct effect on the pancreas. In order to avoid making glucose control worse, women with diabetes need careful attention to optimal estradiol and the least amount of progesterone that will protect the uterine lining from hyperplasia.

In a normal menstrual cycle with optimal hormone ratios, the opposing actions of estradiol and progesterone on insulin tend to offset each other, which suggests that the *E:P ratio* is more influential in determining the net effect metabolically. This has been one of the key factors in determining degree of symptoms in the women whose hormone levels I have evaluated in my practice. When their premenstrual (luteal) phase hormone ratios are shifted toward progesterone dominance, and lower than optimal estradiol, they typically have more intense sweet cravings and more weight gain. Prolonged use of progesterone without adequate balance of estradiol has effects on insulin that result in a problem called *insulin resistance*, which causes weight gain around the middle of the body, increased total cholesterol, lower levels of good cholesterol (HDL), higher levels of bad cholesterol (LDL), and triglycerides (TG). Insulin resistance also causes high blood pressure and significantly increased risk of heart disease from plaque building up in the arteries. The potentially severe complications that occur with insulin resistance make it a crucial factor to consider in determining which hormones are given, and whether they are given orally or should be given in a way that allows them to be absorbed through the skin. I will talk more about insulin resistance in chapter 17, and I will explain how to help reduce this problem with the types of hormone and dietary approaches you select.

Laboratory Tests

Current blood serum tests for progesterone are quite accurate and reliable. The amount of progesterone in the serum reflects the balance, or equilibrium, between the bound and free hormone and gives a total picture of the amount available for the body to use. Since there is a constant dynamic process between the part that is "free" (i.e., biologically active) and the part that is "bound" to carrier proteins, I have found it is important to measure this total amount. A few years ago, I tried using the saliva tests that are now being widely promoted for hormone testing. I initially thought this sounded like a good idea and would be easier for the patients to check at home. For a while, I did both saliva and blood serum tests at the same time in a number of patients to see how well the serum and saliva correlated, and to see if I could just use the saliva tests. I was surprised and quite disappointed to find that these saliva tests turned out to be almost useless. The serum levels were quite consistent and correlated very well with what the women themselves described about body changes that clued them into ovulation and rising progesterone. But the saliva levels were all over the place—from very high to very low and everywhere in between. The saliva results didn't seem to have *any* connection with what symptoms the women were describing. I also have many patients who had already had the saliva tests done before coming to see me. Most of these women had been very good at keeping their own records of menstrual cycles and symptoms and had noticed that the saliva results typically were quite different from the body changes that suggested certain hormone levels.

I tried to get information from the companies that provide this testing to account for these differences, and neither Aeron Labs or Diagnos-Techs biochemists would provide the data I requested correlating serum and saliva hormone levels. As a result, I stopped using the saliva tests several years ago. I have continued to use the serum tests that are much more reliable and clinically useful in helping women design appropriate hormone strategies. My approaches are in keeping with the gold standard of using serum levels that is used in worldwide hormone research.

Current Issues Concerning Progesterone

With all the books and multilevel marketing companies trying to sell you on progesterone, I know it is confusing to you as a layperson to sort it all out and determine who has accurate information. You have to remember that many people selling products may have a financial stake in selling you on the idea of using progesterone. You may have heard or read that progesterone has all these wonderful effects in a woman's body and can be converted into all the other hormones we need. Then I come along and say something different. How are you to know who is right? Let me emphasize, I receive *no* financial gain from sales of *any* hormone product. My only desire is to present the most up-to-date, reputable medical research findings to help you "connect the dots" in your health picture. I have presented both the historical and the current worldwide research from reputable medical centers, menopause and PMS researchers, and neuroendocrine basic science researchers to describe in these chapters which functions are known to occur with each of these major hormones.

What you can do to sort out confusing and contradictory information:

First: *Pay attention* to your own body rhythms, look at a menstrual cycle chart of when each hormone is dominant, and ask yourself "When do I feel the best in my cycle each month?"

That will give you an important clue as to whether you feel best when progesterone is the dominant hormone after ovulation until a few days before menses, or whether you feel best in the first half when progesterone is minimal and estradiol is the highest. Based on when you felt your best in the years of healthy menstrual cycles, you can know generally what balance of hormones gave you those good feelings.

Second: *Check Medline* on the Internet and look up copies of the research I have described and read the conclusions yourself to verify what I have said. Ask other practitioners to give you references and check them out, too.

Third: *Ask* your local public librarian to help you find a basic medical textbook as a reliable reference to check the list of body functions for these key hormones. There are lots of good ones available.

Fourth: *Be skeptical.* As in anything, if someone is trying to sell you a product and tell you something that sounds too good to be true, it probably is! I continue to be dismayed and alarmed about the grossly incorrect physiological effects listed in various consumer-oriented books and tapes. The health consequences for women can be disastrous, as we see daily in our practice.

Fifth: *Don't expect a "magic bullet"* solution to complex health issues. Rubbing on a body cream containing progesterone simply isn't adequate for something as complicated as all the metabolic changes that are going on in the premenopausal and menopausal years. I am certainly not recommending that estradiol is the only approach either. There are many complex issues to address, and you need/deserve a thorough medical evaluation with an integrated treatment approach tailored to your individual needs.

Sixth: *Use common sense.* A recent sales flyer a patient sent me from Florida had this headline: "Estrogen's Lethal Effects." Now really . . . would Mother Nature have given us women a hormone that was "lethal" for our entire reproductive lives? Of course not. As you may have guessed, this newsletter was selling . . . progesterone cream as a hormone cure-all. We women live with estrogen all our lives, and most of the serious health problems that affect our quality of life and our longevity don't start to show up until the primary active estrogen (17-beta-estradiol) is *decreasing*. So if estrogen were truly "lethal," most women would be dead long before menopause, since estrogen levels are their *highest* from puberty until perimenopause. I found the newsletter so ridiculously inaccurate as to be humorous, but the tragedy is that too many women believe it.

Obviously, progesterone is an important hormone that plays a critical role in preparing the uterus each month for a possible fertilized egg to implant and in sustaining pregnancy, but being pregnant is not a woman's *only* function.

There is so much emphasis on using progesterone, I think people who recommend such broad use of one hormone have forgotten that women have a variety of hormones with different functions, and each one has to be taken into account in our evaluation and treatment approaches. I have found through many years of testing hormone blood levels according to menstrual-cycle phase that the majority of women I have seen actually have *low estradiol*/high progesterone causing their symptoms. Obviously, if this ratio is the problem, adding more progesterone won't help and will actually make matters worse. A smaller percentage of the women I have evaluated, perhaps about 5 percent, are found to have the high estradiol/low progesterone levels that were proposed by Dalton and others as the cause of PMS. These are the women I find that do quite well with just supplemental progesterone.

In addition, we have to also keep in mind that many of the same symptoms can be caused or aggravated by loss of thyroid hormone. It certainly doesn't make sense to give progesterone to these women if the problem really lies in low thyroid function. I think there is a place for use of progesterone in some patients, but I think it has to be individualized, based on the type and pattern of the woman's symptoms, and what her actual hormone levels show. As every *woman* knows, what's crucial for our sense of well-being is the *balance* of our primary hormones.

Cortisol and Stress: Interactions with Our Ovary Hormones

> Disease in man or woman is never exactly the same as disease in an experimental animal, for in humans the disease at once affects and is affected by what we call the emotional life.
>
> Sir Francis W. Peabody, M.D.
> Harvard Medical School, Boston, 1927

STRESS. For most of us, it conjures up awful images of body-wrecking effects: cancer, heart attacks, high blood pressure, infertility, allergies . . . the list goes on and on. But all of us live with stress, all of the time, both the stress of constant change going on within the body systems, and the stress of constant interchange with the outside world. Stress is a constant, necessary part of the life process itself. But what accounts for the fact that some people seem to thrive on the very stress levels that others would find overwhelming? What makes some people able to cope with catastrophic stress and others cave in with what appear to be rather trivial events? Physicians and scientists have debated these questions down through the ages. Louis Pasteur developed the germ theory of illness and believed that our exposure to external agents triggers disease. A physician and contemporary of his, Claude Bernaud, believed that the "soil" or environment of the body was the crucial factor. The two often debated who was right, but on his deathbed, Pasteur murmured, "Bernaud was right, it is the soil."

Today, we are even more aware of the role our individual vulnerability brings to the question of who gets ill. Viruses, bacteria, carcinogens alone do not cause illness in every individual exposed to them. We now know that many other factors are involved: our attitudes, our diet, our hormone balance, how tired we are, our feelings of choice and control in our lives, our degree of social support, our faith—to name a few. A few diseases, such as cystic fibrosis, are almost entirely genetic, but most of the diseases we "moderns" develop are predominately affected by the physical and psychological environment of our bodies. Have we made our bodies a compromised host, a fertile "soil" for viral and carcinogenic invaders? Or have we developed lifestyle habits and thought patterns that serve as an inoculation against the development of disease? The balance between the risk factors we have and the "resistance resources" helps determine whether we stay healthy or develop an acute or chronic illness. So, as we shall see in later chapters, there is a lot we can take charge of now that will improve our ability to resist the ravages of stress causing adverse effects on our health. But now, let's explore this idea of stress further, and understand how it plays a role with women's overall hormonal health.

What Exactly Is Stress?

For both men and women, stress of whatever form—external situational and environmental stressors or internal body changes (physiological stressors)—that requires the body to continually adapt, affects the brain and body. Our body is the "final common pathway" through which all of these changes act and operate to produce necessary responses. Our brain constantly perceives and processes information coming to it from the world around us and also from moment-to-moment changes inside the body. Our brain is a *physiological* organ, as well as the *psychological* organ of "mind" expressing our personality and guiding our behavior. Since the brain is affected by outside stimuli (stressors) and by internal stimuli (stressors) or changes in the body, that means thoughts, moods, and behaviors governed by the brain can be caused by both physical and psychological causes.

I find that many times patients have been told that they have a psychological or psychiatric disorder simply because of changes in mood or behavior and such symptoms are *assumed* to have a psychological cause. But these same mood/behavior symptoms may in fact be caused by biochemical changes in our body's physiological balance, and therefore have a physical cause. Likewise, psychological stress causes profound changes in every cell in the body, including our immune cells, pain-regulating neurotransmitters, nerve endings, brain chemistry, and so on. With prolonged stress of any kind—physical, environmental, situational, psychological, spiritual—the body's balance, or homeostasis, is disrupted and we see symptoms that relate to overactivity of the "fight-or-flight" (adrenaline) pathways, such as headaches, acute muscle spasm and pain, high blood pressure, panic attacks, irritable bowel, colitis, angina, eczema, overwhelming fatigue, and many others. Diagram 2.3 in chapter 2 showed these important connections. The interconnections and the ways in which hormonal production may in turn be altered by stress on the body are often overlooked when women seek medical care. The two-way nature of these pathways is crucial to all facets of women's health.

Another aspect of the problem of stress when it affects women is the role of chronic stress in decreasing the normal function and hormone production of the ovaries, as well as the thyroid gland. A variety of studies has shown a correlation between the presence of life stress in women's lives and lower levels of their ovarian estrogen, testosterone, and as well as changes in the cyclic production of progesterone. While one can look at all the data on stress effects and conclude that psychosocial stress and poor coping skills may result in estrogen decline at menopause, it is possible that the opposite hypothesis may also be true about the connection between hormone levels and stress: Declining estrogen levels contribute to alterations in the function of norepinephrine, serotonin, dopamine, and acetylcholine, which regulate pain pathways, sleep, muscle repair, mood, behavior, and cognitive function. I think that the declining estrogen, as well as adverse effects on brain chemical messengers, contributes to the observed difficulty coping with psychosocial stressors by women who have previously been able to cope successfully. Once again, the role of stress is a two-way street: Life stress suppresses the ovaries, which decreases estrogen production, which affects sleep, which increases pain, and then increased pain disrupts sleep, decreases growth hormone production, and leads to further decline in ovary hormones, and so on. Normal declines in estrogen affect brain chemistry, which affects ability to cope with stress. It's another one of those vicious cycles.

Stress also has adverse effects on the brain and body through mechanisms beyond the ovary hormones. Chronic persistent stress causes excessive outpouring of cortisol and other stress hormones from the adrenal glands. High levels of cortisol over time have many adverse effects: (1) suppression of normal immune function, (2) weight gain around the middle of the body ("apple" shape), (3) increased risk of heart disease by promoting plaque build-up, higher cholesterol and triglyceride levels, (4) increased risk of diabetes by stimulating high levels of blood glucose, (5) negative effects on pain pathways, such as increasing brain excitability, via release of excitatory amino acids (EAAs), glutamate, and aspartate. This effect occurs by the action of adrenal stress hormones on sodium, potassium, and calcium ion transport into and out of cells. Cortisol overactivity causes excessive buildup of the EAAs, which then mobilizes calcium in the postsynaptic neuron and leads to overactivation of calcium-dependent enzymes and free-radical-producing cascades. The end result of all this is that neurons begin to die, leading to impaired nerve conduction, abnormal pain regulation, and impaired memory, attention, and concentration. Sound familiar? As stress persists, cortisol effects continue to build up over time, further damaging astrocyte nerve cells in the hippocampus of the brain (memory center). This whole sequence is thought to be one way that memory loss gets worse in chronic pain sufferers, leading to what's euphemistically called "fibro-fog" or "brain fog."

In addition to toxic effects on neurons of the brain, excess cortisol impairs normal metabolism of collagen, which is the basis of healthy connective tissue, or fascia. This adverse effect on connective tissue is part of an overall response of the body to stress that leads to hyperglycemia or elevated blood sugar that over time can increase risk of diabetes. The accumulation of cortisol effects further disrupt the sleep cycle, which in turn means less muscle repair at night, aggravating the damaging effects of declining estradiol. Excess cortisol also interferes with normal thyroid function, leading to *less* of the available T3 that is so important for cellular metabolism in skeletal muscle, the brain, and other organs. High cortisol levels and prolonged stress also increase the body's need for antioxidants, vitamins, and minerals as well as all the macronutrients. But when we are stressed and don't feel well, we pay less attention to getting what we need nutritionally.

It is a complicated picture, and one that has profound implications for all aspects of women's health. The cumulative effects of persistent high cortisol levels and chronic stress adversely affect practically every pathway in the body. I don't have the space in this book to go into more detail on all the potential health consequences of chronically elevated cortisol and ongoing stress, but if you would like more information, I recommend the book *Why Zebras Don't Get Ulcers*, by Robert M. Sapolsky, W. H. Freeman and Company, 1998. It is an excellent, and humorous, review of the damaging effects of excess corticosteroids over time.

Chapter 5

The Big Question:
Has Anybody Seen
My Estrogen?

. . . And Will Someone Help Me Look for It?
What about Blood Tests for Hormones?

Women have been asking me these questions for years. It makes so much sense to measure a baseline level of almost anything before starting a medication designed to *change that particular parameter*. Clearly, one of the important advantages of modern medicine is our ability to measure objective parameters in the laboratory, with X-rays, MRI, bone-density tests, and other techniques. We then combine this information with the clinical description from the patient about what she is experiencing to determine a diagnosis and a meaningful course of action or treatment plan. For example, if you have clinical symptoms that suggest low thyroid function, we measure the level of thyroid hormones in your blood, both those produced by the gland (T3, T4) and the brain (TSH), and possibly thyroid antibodies. If you need thyroid medication, we then prescribe a low dose and gradually increase it. Then we check a follow-up blood level of TSH to see if the dose is right for you and if not, make further adjustments in the amount you take. This process is done routinely with diabetics on insulin by monitoring the blood levels of fasting glucose and postprandial (after meals) glucose. It is also used in patients on heart medicine, such as digitalis, by monitoring blood levels of the medication at a certain number of hours after a dose. By monitoring blood levels of hormones or medications, doctors are able to use the right amount for your body and minimize the possibility of unwanted side effects. Makes sense, right? So why isn't this same standard of medical practice used in helping postmenopausal women find the right dose of estrogen therapy?

Why have we had in the United States this "cookbook" approach, with the same Premarin-Provera "recipe" for all postmenopausal women? We do not use the same dose of blood pressure medication for everyone with high blood pressure or the same dose of insulin for all diabetics. Yet, I estimate that over the last fifteen years of my medical practice, *nine out of every ten* women I've seen who were already taking hormone therapy were on 0.625 mg of Premarin for twenty five days a month, and 5 or 10 mg of Provera for Days 16 to 25 every month. Some women said they felt wonderful; others described having "nothing but problems" since starting on these hormones. I was bothered by the fact that almost every woman I saw was on the same dose and type of hormones, and since not everyone was feeling *well* on them, I began to ask more questions. Why the same dose? *"That's the amount that's needed."* Why always the same type of estrogen? *"That's what we've always used."* Are there any others? *"Don't know of any."* What if women are having side effects? *"She can stop, or just take less."* What about rechecking FSH after a woman is on her therapy and see if she has the right amount? *"That's not needed, the FSH never comes back down to normal after menopause."* How do we know; are there any studies on this? *"No, there aren't any studies, we just* know *that's the way it is."* Can't we check blood levels to see if the amount is right? *"No, blood levels are useless, hormone levels vary."* **That's my point!** They *do* vary, and we need to know *how* they vary in relationship to what a woman is experiencing.

I wanted to scream, it was all such nonsense. How could we *know* if there aren't any studies? Why doesn't FSH come back down when a woman is on the right amount of estrogen? That's how *other* hormone feedback systems in the body work. This "reasoning" (or lack of it) simply did not make either physiological or medical sense to me. With my patients who were taking hormones and yet were still not feeling well, I started letting them know that checking FSH, estradiol, and testosterone blood levels was an option for them. Even though at that time, we did not have a lot of good information about correlation of blood levels and physical symptoms, I thought it was critical to try and sort this out in order to help my patients feel better. Many women elected to have this done—it made intuitive sense to them. Well, amazing results began to unfold. I found that there was a very *good correlation* between desirable blood hormonal levels in women who were doing well on their particular regimen. I usually found suboptimal hormonal blood levels in women who were still having a lot of symptoms and/or side effects.

As I continued to research this issue, I found that Dr. Philip Sarrel at Yale had been finding the same thing, as had some European researchers. Dr. Sarrel studied the women who came to the Yale Menopause Center and tabulated the percentage of women who described problems with sexual function as one of the reasons they were seeking a consultation. The numbers speak for themselves as to the magnitude of the impact on women's lives:

SEXUAL DYSFUNCTION AFTER MENOPAUSE: YALE MID-LIFE STUDY	
Problems Patients Reported:	**Patients Experiencing It**
Decreased sexual desire	77%
Reporting of sexual problems	68%
Bothered by sexual problems	64%
Intercourse (less than/=)1/month	50%

Ref: Sarrel: *Obstet Gynecol* 1990; 75 (suppl. 265–308)

Dr. Sarrel further showed that there seems to be a threshold level of about **50 pg/ml** for estradiol with women having sexual problems at menopause: Women with estradiol levels **greater than** 50 had *minimal* reports of adverse changes in their sexual function. Women whose estradiol levels were **below** 50, however, had a dramatic *increase* in sexual problems of all types, including decreased lubrication, burning and pain with intercourse, difficulty having an orgasm, and diminished quality of orgasm. This was one of the few studies I could find in the literature at that time to clearly demonstrate a relationship between estradiol blood levels and the clinical problems women were describing. Someone else had *listened* to the patients. I felt validated in my own observations and clinical correlations. In 1998, a study by Drs. Vihtamaki and Tuimala was published in *Maturitas,* the journal of the International Menopause Society at that time. They found that as many as 45 percent of patients whose self-assessment had been that symptoms were gone, still actually had serum estradiol levels below the currently accepted thresholds for the various protective effects of estradiol on brain, bone, and other target tissues. The authors concluded, as have I in working with thousands of women over the years, that reliable assessment of serum hormone levels is a crucial method to ensure that adequate levels of estradiol are reached to provide the benefits women (and their physicians) are seeking.

The more I listened to my patients and tried to help them feel better, the more I found that blood-level information helped guide me in my recommendations for each individual woman. It also helped *her* feel that a more rational, logical approach was being used to determine her individual needs. I decided that taking the systematic approach of making treatment decisions based on *both* clinical symptoms and objective laboratory results made good sense and provided better medical care for my women patients. This approach means that the doses are then designed for the individual woman, and we have objective measures of what is the right amount for her. Women quickly discover that many vague symptoms, for which they may have had to see multiple physicians, often went away when the type and amount of estradiol was right for their individual needs.

Estradiol Tests: Target Ranges

If you want to request these blood tests from your physician, what should you be looking for as a desirable target range for estradiol? In my clinical experience, women typically experience their usual energy level, mood, sleep, and memory when serum (blood) levels of estradiol are *above* **90–100 pg/ml**. Levels above this range, up to about 200 or so, are the normal estradiol levels in the first half of the menstrual cycle before women reach menopause. Levels below this are generally too low to maintain a normal feeling of well-being. Recent research has found that estradiol levels below 70–80 pg/ml result in *increased bone loss after menopause*. There now appears to be a minimum threshold level of about 80–90 pg/ml for estradiol to maintain healthy body function. Below this level, women lose more bone, lose the cardiovascular and brain benefits of estrogen, have more problems sleeping, and also have more loss of bladder and sexual function. I describe what to look for with testosterone levels in chapter 6.

I have been criticized by other physicians for recommending that women have both FSH and estradiol levels checked. They have often said to me that it is "too expensive," "unreliable," or "doesn't tell us anything." **I disagree.** This information has made an enormous difference to the women who had been told their symptoms were "all in their head" and who now have a hormone regimen tailored just for them. Many of my patients have also been able to stop the expensive medications for lowering blood pressure and cholesterol, as well as eliminate psychotropic medications when their estradiol levels were again in the optimal ranges. Furthermore, it is difficult to put a price tag on improving someone's quality of life. I think in the long run it is less expensive and more cost effective to check hormone blood levels than to do all the myriad tests and evaluations that end up being done when hormone problems are *not* recognized, or for women to undergo a long series of psychotherapy sessions, thinking that the mood changes are just stress or an empty nest or a bad relationship. In my opinion, these blood tests are efficient, informative, and psychologically helpful in identifying a physical cause of disturbing symptoms women frequently experience at midlife and around menopause. I feel strongly that such tests of hormone levels should be available to all women, especially those who have had their ovaries removed.

I am in the process of collecting outcome data on larger numbers of patients to be able to demonstrate to insurance companies that such tests are in fact useful and cost-effective. This research, underway at both 𝓗𝓔𝓡 𝓟𝓵𝓪𝓬𝓮 centers, will help clarify these important issues and, I hope, change the way health services are offered to midlife women. Instead of operating on **unproved assumptions** and old myths, we really need to look at the whole woman and evaluate her endocrine system carefully to rule out hormonal factors contributing to her symptoms as well. **If your doctor isn't listening to your requests, find one who will.**

The Three Types of Estrogen for Human Females

There is so much confusion about *estrogens,* I would like to describe some of the differences between various types. Bear with me for the chemistry lesson. There are *three* estrogens found in human females, and the relative amounts of each one present is determined by several factors: genetic makeup, age, amount of body fat, pregnancy, diet, and the presence of any medical condition or lifestyle habits that alter ovarian function. Many women at my seminars think "estrogen" equals "Premarin." This is not the case. Premarin is only *one* brand of estrogen among many brands available. I will describe the estrogens commercially available in the U.S. First, some definitions:

Human Estrogens

17-BETA ESTRADIOL (E2)

This is the predominant natural human estrogen produced by the ovary *prior to menopause*; it is the primary *biologically active* estrogen at cell surface receptor sites and also inside the cell at the nucleus receptor sites as I described in chapter 3. It is the major *functioning* estrogen for our bodies from puberty until menopause, and it is the one responsible for over four hundred functions in the female body. After menopause, we lose the ovary source of **17-beta estradiol**, and other body tissues can't make up for this loss of the most active form of the hormone. We are left with only the estrone made in fat tissue as a poor substitute! Losing the 17-beta estradiol results in the postmenopausal changes in skin, bone, hair, heart/ blood vessels, brain, and other organs. Ideally, if you decide to take estrogen therapy after menopause, you would choose a form of 17-beta estradiol to provide exactly the same chemical molecule your ovary had previously made.

There are several brands of 17-beta estradiol commercially available in this country, and all of these brands use a form of estradiol that is derived from soybean or wild yam precursor molecules. These are as follows: **Estrace** tablets and vaginal cream (FDA approved in 1976), **Gynodiol** tablets and **Alora, Climara, Vivelle, Estraderm** transdermal patches (all FDA approved between 1985–1997). Even though some of these have been around a long time, many women and still some physicians seem to have heard about only Premarin. That's more a testament to effective marketing and prescribing habit than to Premarin being a better estrogen source. There is some 17-beta estradiol in Premarin, but a small amount in comparison to the other ingredients in each tablet. The comparative studies that have been done, although not many, do show that the bioidentical human form of 17-beta estradiol is much better tolerated, with fewer side effects and better improvement in outcome measures (lipids, bone markers, and others).

ESTRONE (E1)

This is the predominant estrogen found in *postmenopausal* women. Before menopause, estrone is made by body fat, the adrenal glands, the liver, *and* in the ovary. Estrone is also produced from conversion of estradiol, and vice versa. It serves primarily as a reservoir for the body to make the biologically active 17-beta estradiol, but most of this conversion takes place in *functioning* ovaries. Estrone (E1) is the form of estrogen that many researchers think may be related to the higher risk of endometrial and breast cancer in older women who are obese. Estrone continues to be produced in the liver and body fat (adipose tissue), and to a smaller extent the adrenal glands, after menopause. The more body fat a woman has (before or after menopause) the more estrone is present. One synthetic brand of estrone is commercially available in the United States for postmenopausal therapy: **Ogen** (piperazine estrone sulfate). It is not the same chemical structure as estrone made in the human body because it has the *piperazine* ring structure attached to it. This makes Ogen *chemically **similar** to, but **not exactly** the same as,* human estrone. If you are taking a form of estrone for a postmenopausal estrogen, you may still have some residual symptoms due to the lower amount of estradiol present, and the different chemical ring from the *piperazine* part of the molecule. I don't recommend Ogen for women with any kind of muscle or bladder pain syndromes because I have found clinically that this difference in its chemical structure makes it more likely to aggravate the pain prob-

lems. The estrogen products that give high levels of estrone and relatively little of the 17-beta estradiol are **Premarin, Prem Pro, Prem
Phase, Estratab, Estratest, Cenestin, Menest, and Ogen.**

ESTRIOL (E3)

This is the weakest of the human estrogens, and is produced by
the placenta during pregnancy. Estriol is **not** normally present in
measurable amounts in **non**pregnant women. Estriol is biologically
the weakest estrogen and has been studied extensively. It really isn't
the "forgotten estrogen" as marketing hype would have you believe;
it has been extensively studied in Europe over the last fifty years.
Estriol just isn't used much for menopause therapy because it hasn't
been found to provide the degree of protective effects on bone,
heart, brain, and nerves as does our premenopausal 17-beta estradiol. In addition, there are no reputable medical studies showing any
protective effect of E3 on breast cancer development, *other than* the
known effect of full-term pregnancy prior to age thirty in reducing
breast-cancer risk. Whatever role estriol plays in reducing breast
cancer risk is not an independent effect of estriol but rather is
thought to occur *along with other factors from a full-term pregnancy before age thirty.*

For some women, estriol relieves milder *symptoms* (e.g., vaginal
dryness, mild hot flashes), and I describe its use for vaginal symptoms in chapter 12. Estriol has clearly been shown in many studies
to have very little benefit on sleep, quite a contrast to what has been
shown with 17-beta estradiol. Estriol also does not have the significant beneficial effects found with 17-beta estradiol for improving
pain, memory, mood, and the "brain fog" symptoms that are so
common in mid-life. I have treated a lot of women who had been
put on estriol and suffered from "brain crash" when it didn't work
as well as estradiol on these crucial brain pathways. If you are told
that your estriol level is low, that's a normal finding if you are not
pregnant. Another concern that is emerging with more "natural hormone" practitioners recommending estriol is that studies by
Whitehead and a number of others over the past twenty years have
found that higher doses of estriol (needed to give much symptom
relief) will *also stimulate the endometrium of the uterus to prolifer-
ate* just as other estrogens do. Thus, if you take enough estriol to
really help your symptoms, you have to still watch for endometrial
hyperplasia just as you would if you took any of the estradiol
products. Adding estriol to menopause therapy really isn't "natural"
hormone therapy as many compounding pharmacists and alternative practitioners are now promoting; it is simply their desire to sell
a product.

Animal Estrogens

EQUINE ESTROGENS

Extracted from the urine of pregnant mares to produce a mixture known as *conjugated equine estrogens*. The most commonly used brand is **Premarin** (*pregnant mare's urine*). It is interesting to notice that the company making Premarin stopped using the word equine several years ago after PETA (People for the Ethical Treatment of Animals) began their campaign to make consumers aware of the inhumane way pregnant mares are confined during the long periods of urine collection and their foals sold for slaughter. But dropping the equine from the PR materials didn't change the composition of the product or the way it is collected, so it still contains many estrogens not natural to a woman's body. I think we should be at least as concerned about what effects occur in human females from these "unnatural" estrogens in our bodies as people are worried about the treatment of the mares.

Actually, the equine estrogens are *not* just one estrogen as many women think; "conjugated equine estrogen" refers to the entire group of about ten or more different chemical molecules that have different "attachment strengths" for the estradiol receptor sites. Many doctors consider that Premarin is the gold standard for estrogen therapy because it has been on the market longer, and most of the research studies have used only this one type of estrogen to determine estrogen benefits, side effects, and risks. But many people don't realize that the manufacturer of Premarin is the company that funded much of the research, which is one reason we don't have more comparative studies using other estrogens. Since the equine estrogens have several components that attach more strongly to the estradiol receptor than does human estradiol, and some of the equine estrogens stay in the body far longer than does estradiol (up to 2–3 months after the last dose), it only makes sense to me that we should study the potential for different effects of horse-derived estrogens on human females. There are many reasons I don't recommend Premarin, and I will elaborate on these later in this chapter.

"Synthetic" Estrogens

All of these estrogens have slightly different chemical structures from the three human forms (estradiol, estrone, estriol), and are therefore more potent, as well as having somewhat different effects and side effects on the body.

ETHINYL ESTRADIOL

The most common form of estrogen found in the birth control pill. Although the ethinyl estradiol in birth control pills is widely used in perimenopausal women who may need better control of irregular cycles and erratic bleeding, it is not widely used in the United States for postmenopausal ERT because it has far greater potency and hepatic effects than does 17-beta estradiol and provides more estrogen effect than is generally needed after a woman reaches menopause. Ethinyl estradiol is also available alone as the brand **Estinyl.** It is not a birth control pill since it contains only the estrogen and no progestin.

ESTRADIOL VALERATE

About **one hundred times more potent** than 17-beta estradiol, it is rarely used in the United States, but it is common in Europe for post-menopausal ERT. Estradiol valerate is available for oral or intramuscular delivery. Estradiol valerate was the type of estradiol used in the 1979 Swedish study initially reporting a higher risk of breast cancer in estrogen users. Subsequent analysis and update of the data in 1992 from this group in Sweden did not support the earlier conclusion of higher risk. I elaborate on the flaws in that study in chapter 14.

You need to keep in mind that the *estradiol* referred to in European research can be *either* the native human form (17-beta estradiol) *or* the synthetic and more potent estradiol valerate. It is important not to confuse 17-beta estradiol with estradiol valerate, given their marked differences in potency and estrogenic effects.

Plant Estrogens

PHYTOESTROGENS

These are estrogenic compounds found in several hundred different plants, including soybeans, red clover, grains, and many others. Phytoestrogens are biologically weaker than the native human estrogens and have quite a range of activity at the human estrogen receptors, varying from pure *agonist* to mixed agonist-antagonist, to full antagonist effects. Some of these different actions are dose and concentration related, and others are related to small chemical changes in the molecular configuration of the molecules. These potency differences may help explain the apparent discrepancy in reports that in China and Japan, where diets are high in phyto-estrogens and herbal sources of estrogen are widely used, women do not typically describe hot flashes but *do continue to have bone loss* after menopause. Japanese menopause researchers have shown clearly that there is an epidemic of osteoporosis in their country; their research indicates that phytoestrogens alone do not provide enough estrogen effect to protect against osteoporosis and decline in cognitive function, even though the plant sources may be helpful for mild symptoms. I describe more aspects of current research on phytoestrogens in chapter 16. Ginseng is often recommended by herbalists as a "natural" source of estrogen. Ginseng, however, can cause high blood pressure, insomnia, anxiety, or agitation if taken in large amounts and, according to current controlled studies, gives little measurable estrogenic effect.

Several recent double-blind, placebo-controlled, prospective studies from the international menopause literature have found that phytoestrogen products were no more effective than placebo even for controlling hot flashes. Although the phytoestrogens are less potent than 17-beta estradiol, it is quite easy with the use of many supplements currently available to produce much higher serum concentrations of the phytoestrogens that competitively inhibit the action of 17-beta estradiol at cellular receptor sites.

Phytoestrogens from soy and wild yam are used in the pharmaceutical industry as the precursor molecules for producing 17-beta estradiol to use in tablets, patches, and creams and also to make the conjugated plant estrogens, **Estratab** and **Cenestin**. All of the phytoestrogen precursors require chemical conversion in the laboratory to make the bioidentical human form of 17-beta estradiol, since the human body does not have the enzymes needed for these changes. So just taking phytoestrogen supplement is not going to provide you with the critically necessary 17-beta estradiol.

Xenoestrogens

A group of synthetic organo-solvent, pesticide, and other compounds that mimic some of the actions of estrogen in humans but are not native to the human body and also produce toxic effects. These chemicals, such as DDT, PCB, and a variety of others not normally found in nature, are as a group responsible for a great deal of environmental damage to animals, plants, and water sources. Their potent effect on living organisms is one of the factors responsible for reproductive abnormalities in wildlife and is also postulated as a cause of lower average sperm counts found in human males in recent years. I talk more about these compounds in chapter 14 and what we know about their potential carcinogenic effects. The important thing to keep in mind is that although these chemicals may have some *estrogenic* effects, their effects are generally negative, and they are *not* the same estrogen produced by our bodies.

What Do We Mean By Natural or Synthetic?

I hear a lot of women talking about wanting to only take *natural* hormones, and this is the reason often given for wanting to use the wild yam skin cream advertised as a source of progesterone, or dong quai (an herb with estrogenic compounds), or estriol (weakest of the three primary human estrogens) instead of "drugs," which are "synthetic." Use of the words natural and synthetic can be very confusing, to patients and doctors alike.

Actually, something *synthetic* can also be *natural*, while something *natural* may be *foreign (not native to)* the human body. One example is Premarin. It is a "natural" mixture of estrogens because it is made by a biological organism, in this case the horse. But as I said earlier, it contains types of estrogen that are *not* found in the human body, so it is an "**un**-natural" estrogen for women. Another example is the "natural" estrogen-type compounds (genistein and others) found in soy and red clover, among others. These are "natural" substances since they come from a biological source, the soy plant. These compounds are "un-natural" for our bodies, however, since we don't make these same compounds and don't have the enzymes to change the genistein into 17-beta estradiol.

Making "natural" hormones like what the human body has is a process called "systhesizing," which must be done in the laboratory. The term *synthesis* comes from the Greek meaning "a putting together, composition." In other words, it means "to make something." *Synthetic* simply means "produced by synthesis." In common usage today, *synthetic* has *come to mean "artificial,"* but that is not always correct. Synthroid and Estrace are "synthetic" in that they have been made in the laboratory rather than within a biological organism, but they are "natural" in being the exact molecules made by the thyroid and ovary, respectively. Other examples of **exact** copies of our bodies' hormones synthesized in the laboratory are Humulin (insulin) and cortisone (cortisol).

The sources for most of these "natural" human hormones are actually plants such as soybeans and yams, with the purified, concentrated extract producing chemical molecules *identical to those made in the human body.* This resulting 17-beta estradiol, progesterone, or testosterone is then compounded into standardized tablets to regulate the amount of hormone given. Standardization of the dose in each tablet also allows for tailoring the amount given more closely to each individual woman's needs. I feel this approach is better than trying to get enough active hormone from plant/herbal sources alone, since you really are not able to *determine how much you are taking and whether the amount is right for you.* There is also the question of whether you are getting additional chemicals *native to plants* that your *human* body may not need.

So, when you read ads, newsletters, and books, be an educated consumer, and keep in mind: The important point is not whether a compound is "natural" to plants or horses or whatever, but whether the molecule shape, makeup, and structure is exactly **identical to what is made in the human body** so that it will fit properly as a "key" in the body's receptor sites. A compound that meets these requirements is called "bioidentical," and it becomes like a duplicate key to your car that you have a locksmith make in case you lose the original key. If the locksmith did the job correctly, the duplicate key works exactly the same way as the original. In the case of your hormones, the manufacturer (the ovary) stops making your own hormone at menopause, so a "locksmith" (the laboratory) makes an exact duplicate hormone molecule for you to have to use if you choose to.

I hope this helps clear up some of the confusion. Don't be misled by clever wording in advertising. Everyone is doing it these days—some pharmaceutical companies are calling their products "natural" because they come from soy plants, since they now know that women want "natural" hormones. Alternative medicine practitioners and compounding pharmacists are calling many things "natural" hormones, including soy compounds that your body has never, ever made. Again, they all are engaging in clever marketing to sell you a particular product. I made up a chart, based on information from various manufacturers, about what is in the various products and what the sources are. If you aren't sure about what you are taking, or considering taking, check the chart on page 120 to guide you.

Sources and Components of Various Estrogen Products

We previously used insulins derived from cows (bovine) and pigs (porcine, or pork insulin) to treat diabetics who needed insulin, because we did not have a way to obtain human insulin. These animal insulins were "natural" in that they came from biological sources, but they were not native molecules for the human body, and many times, human diabetics developed allergic reactions or a resistance to the animal insulins. In recent years, scientists have determined the makeup of the human insulin molecule and have been able to synthesize the exact same molecule of human insulin in the laboratory, so that we can now give human diabetics the *native* human insulin (one brand is Humulin). So, here is one example of a synthetic medication being used because it is the natural one for humans and, therefore, is better tolerated, more effective, and has fewer side effects.

The same is true with estrogen. In the past, we did not have a way to give estrogen orally, because it would be broken down and lost in the digestive process before getting into the bloodstream. About fifty years ago, scientists developed a way to extract estrogens from the urine of pregnant mares, purify the extract containing "conjugated equine estrogens" (CEE), and then coat the estrogens in a matrix of binders (called enteric coating) that allowed the tablet to survive digestion in the stomach, reach the small intestine, be absorbed into the bloodstream, and then produce an estrogenic effect on the body organs. This product, Premarin, has been the primary type of estrogen used in the United States since that time, accounting for about 85 to 90 percent of the prescriptions written for estrogen in the United States. An oral dose of Premarin produces blood levels of the two primary estrogens also found in humans, estradiol and estrone, but it also produces *high blood levels of equine estrogens native to horses, also called equilin estrogens*. A typical oral dose of 0.625 mg Premarin produces about two thirds of the total circulating estrogens as equilin compounds; only about one third of the total estrogen present is the estrone and estradiol found in humans. I have shown some comparisons on blood levels in the graphs below.

In 1976, the FDA approved a new product (brand name: Estrace) that had been developed as a form of native human estrogen, 17-beta estradiol (derived from soybeans), in a *micronized* form, which survives digestion and is well absorbed into the bloodstream. Micronization means making the molecule particles small enough that they can be rapidly absorbed into the bloodstream before being broken down by digestive acids and the liver. Many recent studies have shown that the smaller the particle size, the better the absorption and the more reliable the blood levels obtained. Micronization is used to make many therapeutic medications and has been particularly helpful in developing native human forms of estradiol (estrogen), progesterone, and testosterone because these hormones typically were inactivated or destroyed by digestion when taken orally.

The various brands of transdermal estrogen patches listed earlier above are recent innovations to deliver the human 17-beta estradiol in a way that is the most "natural" of all. The patch system allows the estradiol to be absorbed through the skin, directly into the bloodstream, bypassing the "first pass" metabolism in the liver (which breaks down some of the hormone and changes it into other metabolites, making it unavailable for its normal functions). Using the patch means the hor-

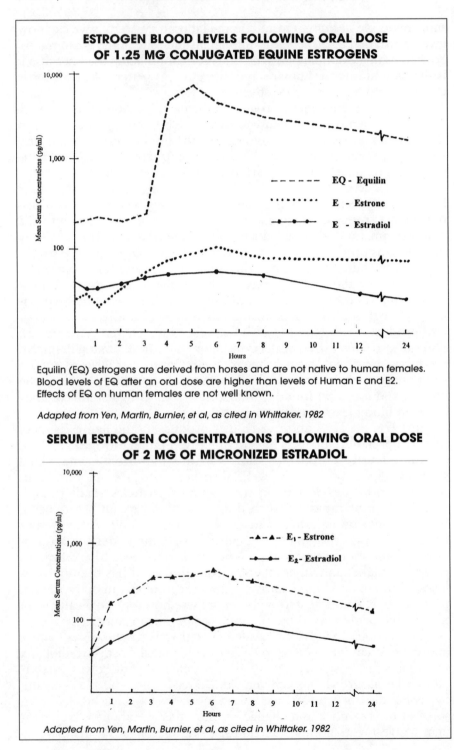

ESTROGEN BLOOD LEVELS FOLLOWING ORAL DOSE OF 1.25 MG CONJUGATED EQUINE ESTROGENS

Equilin (EQ) estrogens are derived from horses and are not native to human females. Blood levels of EQ after an oral dose are higher than levels of Human E and E2. Effects of EQ on human females are not well known.

Adapted from Yen, Martin, Burnier, et al, as cited in Whittaker. 1982

SERUM ESTROGEN CONCENTRATIONS FOLLOWING ORAL DOSE OF 2 MG OF MICRONIZED ESTRADIOL

Adapted from Yen, Martin, Burnier, et al, as cited in Whittaker. 1982

mones are delivered to the bloodstream as the ovary did it before menopause, not going through the stomach and liver first. The estradiol patches look like clear circular, oval, or rectangular Band-Aids that stick to the skin and are left in place for several days for the hormones to be slowly absorbed. Then as the hormone delivery is falling, a new patch is put on. Each brand of patch lasts for a slightly different period of time, and women metabolize the hormones at different rates, so it may take a little experimenting to find the change schedule that is right for you.

The patches have several advantages that I will elaborate on in chapter 15, but generally they keep blood levels of estradiol fairly steady, similar to the hormone production by the ovary. Patches are a very good option for estrogen therapy, with only two primary drawbacks to this form of estradiol: (1) the skin irritation from the adhesive may bother some women, and (2) if you have a very low level of HDL, you may want the extra "plus" of having the oral estrogen stimulate the liver to make more HDL. The patches used in the United States (skin gels and patches in Europe) still give you the beneficial *physiological* effect of estrogen to maintain the normal level of HDL cholesterol, they just don't give you the *pharmacologic* effect of extra liver stimulation to make more HDL that we see with the oral estrogens. The patch may be all that is needed for women who have a normal cholesterol profile. For women who have *high* total cholesterol and *low* HDL, however, an *oral* form of estradiol provides more *decrease* in total cholesterol and a more significant *increase* in HDL for cardiovascular protective effects.

COMPONENTS OF ORAL MIXED ESTROGEN PRODUCTS

COMPONENT	PREMARIN[a]	ESTRATAB[b]	CENESTIN[c]
estrone	49.9%	88.8%	58%
equilin	22.8%	5.9%	28%
17-alpha dihydroequilin	13.5%	2.6%	15%
delta 8, 9 dehydroestrone	3.7%	——	x
17-alpha estradiol	3.6%	1.2	x
equilenin	2.8%	1.1	x
17-beta dihydroequilinin	1.4%	——	x
17-alpha dihydroequilinin	1.4%	——	x
17-beta estradiol	**0.5%**	x	

a - conjugated equine estrogens
b - esterified estrogens
c - conjugated estrogens from soy

© Elizabeth Lee Vliet, M.D., 2000

Estrace (17-beta estradiol) gives only estrone (made in the liver) and 17-beta estradiol; it does not contain any of the other compounds shown above, thereby reducing the overall estrogen amount delivered per dose when compared to the above types.

SOURCES OF ESTROGENS

Pregnant mares urine	Premarin
Soy	Climara, CES (Canada)
Yam	Vivelle, Alora, Estraderm, Estring,
Yam and soy	Estrace and Gynodiol (17-beta estradiol), Cenestin (estrone, equilin)
Plants (incl. soy)	Estratab (estrone, equilin)
Plant + Synthetic	Ogen, generic conjugated estrogens
Synthetic	Estinyl, Estrovis, Tace, Dienestrol ethinyl estradiol (in birth control pills)

© Elizabeth Lee Vliet, M.D., 2000

New Research on Estrogen and a Woman's Body

I have talked about the concept of the body's chemical messengers (hormones, neurotransmitters, etc.) acting like "keys" in special receptor-site "locks" on the cell membrane. The molecules made by the human body are the specific keys that fit our cell receptor sites. Similar chemical molecules, either from other animals or made in the laboratory, may also work the locks, at least partially the same as the human molecules do. But some of these other chemical molecules may get stuck in the lock and actually block the action of our own human molecular keys. That's why it is important to understand the different types of hormone preparations and know that the different forms available may have very different effects in your body.

For the steroid hormones, there is an additional receptor site located in the cell nucleus. These receptor sites have been identified for all three primary ovarian hormones. In particular, estrogen receptor sites are found throughout the brain and all organs of the body—skin, blood vessels, bone, heart, intestinal tract, urinary bladder—not just the organs of reproduction. The blood levels of human estrogens include predominately estradiol and, in lower amounts, estrone. Most of an oral dose of estrogen is converted in the blood to estrone or estrone sulfate. But there are important differences between the estrogen circulating in the blood and the estrogen that acts at the cell receptor site. 17-beta estradiol is needed at the receptor site to actually work properly. *Estradiol* is the estrogen in humans that declines so rapidly after menopause, causing the *symptoms* of declining estrogen. Estrone is still present in postmenopausal women since it is made in the adrenal glands and in the fat tissue. If estrone were the primary hormone activating the receptor site, then we would NOT expect to see postmenopausal women having the symptoms of estrogen decline. Make sense?

So far, researchers have identified three types of estradiol receptors (ER) in the body: two (ER-alpha and ER-beta) inside the *nucleus* of cells, and another on the *membrane* surface of cells. The body's estrogen receptors need the proper keys of 17-beta estradiol molecules to fit in the locks but the nucleus and membrane receptors each act by a different mechanism to influence the biochemical processes of cells. ER-alpha and ER-beta receptors are found in different types of organs and target tissues throughout the body. They interact in very complicated ways we are just beginning to unravel.

The estradiol receptors in the nucleus works in a more complex manner than the membrane receptors. The estradiol molecule fits into the nuclear receptor and then binds with the cell's DNA to regulate gene expression. These genes are involved in the synthesis of particular proteins that make up neuropeptides, crucial enzymes, and other chemical messengers. This process is called the *genomic* hormonal action. An example important in memory regulation is the action of estradiol to trigger the formation of *choline acetyltransferase*, the enzyme that makes the memory-enhancing chemical messenger, *acetylcholine*. This effect cannot be investigated in living humans with our current techniques, but it has been shown in studies of rat brains. Estradiol also acts at the nucleus receptor to stimulate messenger RNA inside cells so that neurons in the brain can make *proenkephalin*, an opiate "messenger" peptide important in pain-reducing pathways. These are just two of many examples of estrogen action at the *genomic receptor*. Many of the sites of estradiol's action in the brain, as well as other body organs, work by this process.

Another mechanism of action for estradiol and other hormones is called the nongenomic process. Here, the estradiol binds with a specific "lock" or receptor site on the cell membrane rather than inside the cell. We have not yet discovered the many ways in which these membrane receptors work, but we do know that this mechanism produces much more rapid effects than does the process of gene regulation directed by the nucleus estradiol receptors. Examples in this category seem to be the estradiol stimulation of various neurotransmitters, such as serotonin, dopamine, and GABA. Recent studies in mice indicate that pain pathways in males and females are functionally distinct, and that estradiol is an important regulator of these pathways. Such a significant finding means that we now need to take into account the sex differences in nerve mechanisms regulating pain when we are treating women patients, as well as when doing basic scientific research on pain mechanisms.

SUMMARY: Estradiol Receptors in the Nervous System

- CNS: Concentrated in limbic system
- PNS: Found in spinal cord, peripheral nerves
- Specific for 17-beta estradiol (E2)
- Nerve function is affected by *changing E2 levels*
- 17-beta estradiol is the *active* form at E2 receptor
- equilin estrogens: higher affinity at receptors *than human E2*
- equilin estrogens *may displace* 17-beta estradiol at receptors

© Elizabeth Lee Vliet, M.D., 1995

Different Estrogens, Different Effects

Although many physicians think all the estrogens for ERT are essentially the same, and the manufacturers of the leading products would like you to *think* they are all the same, **they are not.** Over two decades ago, two leading menopause researchers in England, Dr. Malcolm Whitehead and Dr. Campbell, did studies of the potencies of the different types of estrogens and the effects of the various estrogens on different target organs in the body. What they found was quite disturbing and has profound implications for women taking various products. They raised some critically important questions back then (1978–1982), but practically speaking, *none of their questions and concerns* have been addressed with further studies in this country. In fact, as I travel and speak to physician groups, very few of them even know these studies were done and what the outcomes were. Dr. Campbell and Dr. Whitehead's work has languished in the literature, and their questions are left unanswered.

How does this issue relate to women at risk for heart disease? The work done by Campbell and Whitehead shows that the conjugated equine estrogens are about *three times more potent* in stimulating the liver production of *renin substrate*, which is used to make angiotensin in the body, a factor that causes *increased blood pressure.* Increases in the circulating levels of renin substrate have been proposed as the possible mechanism by which conjugated equine estrogens may elevate blood pressure in some women. Two other estrogens used in this study, micronized estradiol (brand name:

Estrace) and piperazine estrone sulfate (Ogen), did **not** show this elevation of renin substrate. This finding also fits with work published by Geola in 1980, who observed that 1.25 mg of conjugated equine estrogens (brand name: Premarin) daily, caused *supraphysiologic* (greater than normal) effects on the liver synthesis of renin substrate, physiological (normal) actions on the vagina lining tissue (epithelium), and *subphysiological* (less than normal) effects on the brain hormones FSH and LH. This correlates with what I have been seeing clinically: The dose of equine estrogens that is adequate for vaginal lubrication may produce a rise in blood pressure, and inadequate effect on brain phenomena like memory. It has to do with *different target organs* (in this case, liver, vagina, and brain) having very *different sensitivities* to the various molecular types of estrogens. The findings from studies such as those by Campbell and Whitehead are an additional argument for *individualizing* the estrogen options for women, rather than using one kind of estrogen and one dose *for every woman.*

Based on work such as that done by Campbell and Whitehead, it appears that women with existing hypertension would be better served to use one of the native human forms of estrogen, rather than the equine estrogens, in order to avoid the potentially harmful production of high levels of renin substrate. I recently presented this information at a Grand Rounds program for Internal Medicine and Family Medicine physicians at a major medical center. The physician who was head of the hypertension clinic was shocked to hear about these differences in various estrogen potencies on angiotensin. He had not heard about the studies from England and now wants to design a research project in his clinic that will compare blood pressure effects of several types of estrogens. This is the important kind of cross-fertilization of ideas and questions that helps us find better approaches for women.

I have seen many women for evaluation who clearly have had allergic-type reactions to the horse-derived CEE. I also have a significant number of patients who had had problems with vague joint pain syndromes that resolved when I took them off the CEE and prescribed a native human form of 17-beta estradiol. These women had already been evaluated by rheumatologists for possible rheumatoid arthritis, osteoarthritis, lupus, and other diseases that cause joint pain, and had been told "there was nothing wrong." To me, that statement means simply that there were *no laboratory abnormalities* that provided a diagnostic label for the joint pain. The joint pain was definitely real for these patients, and it improved with the change in type of estrogen. Whether the pain was due to an adverse allergenic or autoimmune reaction to the horse-derived estrogens, or whether it represented the kind of joint pain that is seen with estrogen deficiency, I cannot say at this point in time. I am suspicious that the joint pain syndrome I have seen so commonly in women on CEE is related to an immunologic reaction to the equilin estrogens, similar in theory to the immunologic reactions seen in diabetics on the animal-derived insulins. Until more physicians and basic science researchers take seriously the descriptions women give about their body experiences on different estrogens, we will not be able to answer these questions.

The data from Campbell and Whitehead, as well as other researchers, has indicated that the equilin (horse) components of conjugated estrogens (equilin and 17-alpha-dihydroequilin) in themselves possess estrogenic activity in the human female, but this has not been studied further to determine whether this activity is beneficial or adverse. I find it incomprehensible that the Campbell–Whitehead research has not prompted more investigation in this country on the potential adverse effects of the equilin estrogens. Even the recently published PEPI studies (Postmenopausal Estrogen and Progestin Intervention trial) *used only Premarin as the estrogen,* even though this important study compared *natural micronized progesterone* with a *synthetic progestin* (Provera) for the first time in the United States. *Why aren't such studies also including a native human form of 17-beta estradiol?*

More Food for Thought: Horse Estrogens and Your Body

A few years ago, media attention focused on reports of an increased risk of breast cancer in women in the Nurses Health Study who had been on estrogen longer than five years. Another study published in January 2000 showed an increased risk of breast cancer in women taking combination estrogen-progestin therapy compared to estrogen alone. What was never addressed by any of the physicians or health writers commenting on this disturbing information is that the overwhelming majority of women in both of these large-scale studies were using Premarin, alone or with a synthetic progestin (Provera), not 17-beta estradiol. With what we know about (1) how long the equine estrogens stay in the human body (anywhere from eight to fourteen weeks after the last dose), and (2) the stronger "attachment strength" (affinity) of the equine estrogens for the body estradiol receptors (especially the breasts, where estrogens may concentrate in the fat tissue), and (3) the much higher total blood level of equilin estrogens following an oral dose of Premarin, it seems incredible to me that *no one is talking about* a possible link between accumulations of equine estrogens in breast tissue and the observed higher risk of breast cancer with long-term use. I think this is such an important question that it deserves careful attention and research, but prescribing habits and research protocols are so dominated by the use of one type of estrogen that no one seems to even consider that there may be crucial differences that women need to know.

Then there is just the dimension of women *feeling better* when they use something more like what their bodies make. Listen to what this young woman had to say after I changed her from PremPhase to natural forms of 17-beta estradiol and progesterone:

> *Being off the PremPhase has really helped. I feel lots better—have more energy, my sex drive is back, I am not as moody as I was, my memory is definitely better, and I am doing better in school.*

She was now taking Estrace 0.5 mg twice a day, and then cycling with natural progesterone orally 200 mg a day for twelve days a month. The additional interesting aspect about her situation is that she was only thirty-four years old, and had been diagnosed with premature menopause by her gynecologist and begun on the PremPhase about two years earlier. No one had done any hormone levels or a check of her bone density, urine bone markers, or lipids to see whether the hormone therapy was doing what it was supposed to do in providing the benefits of estrogen. When I checked all of these measures at her consult, she was shocked to find that on PremPhase (1) her estradiol was far too low at 38 pg/ml (certainly a reason she didn't feel very good and was having trouble with memory, sleep, and concentration affecting her school performance), (2) her urine bone marker (NTx, 65) was *double* what it should have been to preserve bone (this should come down to less than 35 if the estrogen therapy is doing its job), and (3) her 8 A.M. cortisol was too high at 17.9, and her fasting lipid profile showed elevated triglycerides. These were ominous findings, especially since she was so young. I wasn't surprised by this, however, since I commonly find that the progestin in PremPhase and PremPro causes problems with increased triglycerides and higher cortisol. Her low estradiol level helps to explain the "brain fog" and her continuing bone breakdown.

Six months after the change to Estrace and natural progesterone, her 8 A.M. cortisol was completely normal at 9.5, her serum estradiol was 115 pg/ml (drawn at our standard ten to twelve hours following a dose, which is the level we look for), her NTx had come down to 28, and as you saw from her comments, she just *felt* better!

This is why our work with fine-tuning women's hormone balance is so rewarding. I can see the "objective" measures change in positive ways, and I enjoy hearing that they feel better and are finding their vitality, energy, and enthusiasm coming back.

Effective Evaluation of Hormone Levels to Assess Therapy

Current international menopause research has verified in a variety of settings that it is more important to assess serum estradiol levels than we had previously been taught. Recent studies have shown that as many as 45 percent of patients whose self-assessment had been that symptoms were alleviated, actually still had serum estradiol levels below the currently accepted thresholds for the various protective effects of estradiol on brain, bone, and other target tissues. Reliable assessment of serum hormone levels is one method to ensure that adequate levels of estradiol are reached. Problems as I described with the young woman above could be reduced if we verify adequacy of the hormone replacement our patients are taking and do so with reliable, systematic approaches. Monitoring therapy at appropriate intervals with serum estradiol levels is cost-effective in that it helps to reduce the likelihood of additional medications, or more involved and costly treatments, and helps reduce unpleasant side effects.

Beyond Bones: Estrogen Effects on Skin, Hair, Eyes, and Other Fun Facts

Women often comment that they hit their forties and suddenly their contact lenses don't seem to be tolerable any more, or their hair is falling out, or their skin is so much drier, or they now get "zits" like a teenager. "I'm getting pimples and wrinkles, what's going on?" said one forty-two-year-old mother. "What's happening?" Remember, estrogen is Mother Nature's moisturizer for our body. That means everything from skin to scalp to eyes to mouth to nose to intestinal tract, bladder, and vagina are all affected by increasing dryness as estradiol declines and we are left with more estrone and androgens. How does this show up for you? Dry eyes are the result of loss of estradiol effects on the moisture of the tissue that covers the eyeball, along with other changes as we get older. To fit properly, contact lenses "float" over the eye on a thin film of water. If the surface of the eye isn't as moist, contact lenses don't have their usual "floating pad" to ride on, and they burn or feel scratchy. If your eyes are dry, your wearing time decreases. Doctors suggest such dramatic steps as surgically blocking tear ducts without ever thinking about a woman's hormone balance and its effect on the eye. And it is not just the dryness of your eyes that we need to watch. Current studies have also shown that declines in estradiol are associated with increases in age- related macular degeneration (ARMD), and with the development of glaucoma and cataracts. Research from medical centers in many different countries has shown that estrogen replacement therapy helps to reverse all of these adverse changes on the eyes.

Dry skin is obvious. But less obvious is the loss of collagen as estradiol declines. Collagen gives your skin its elasticity and firmness. When you combine the dryness with loss of collagen, you get the dry, wrinkled, sagging appearance that is associated with aging. It turns out that these changes are not just due to getting older. They are accelerated by loss of the active form of estrogen, estradiol. Since no ones dies of old age of the skin, estrogen effects on skin aging have not been subjected to as many clinical studies as we have seen in more crucial areas, such as estrogen effects on heart, bone, and brain. A carefully designed study from Spain, published in *Maturitas* in 1992, evaluated the effects of time after menopause on skin collagen content, and the effects of three different estrogen regimens on skin collagen. The researchers showed that skin collagen decreased markedly beyond the forties and after menopause, no matter what age menopause (surgical or natural) occurred, and even if menopause occurred in women younger than forty. This decrease in skin collagen was preventable by the use of all of the estrogen approaches studied, but the transdermal estradiol therapies showed a greater degree of preservation of skin collagen compared to that seen with the conjugated oral estrogens. If you have noticed marked changes in your hair and skin quality as you experience other hormone-related changes, maybe it is time to have your hormone levels and bone density checked. The outer changes you can see may well be a clue to unwanted *inner* body changes as well.

Thinning, brittle, dry hair is not life threatening, but it certainly is a source of major distress to many women. In fact, losing hair is one of the more common problems women report, right up there with insomnia, fatigue, mood swings, and loss of sex drive. I don't have space to go into all the causes of *alopecia,* or hair loss, but some of the common overlooked *hormonal* causes for women are loss of estradiol, excess testosterone *as well as* low testosterone, excess DHEA, hypo- *and* hyperthyroidism. Again, it is surprising to me that dermatologists diagnose "menopausal alopecia" and will prescribe Rogaine for women without even suggesting that hormone levels be checked, or supplemented. Before you go off on tangents of expensive hair loss evaluations, supplements, and medications, at least get a careful and reliable measure of your ovarian and thyroid hormone levels, including thyroid antibodies. In order to be certain of the complete picture with regard to your hormones and hair loss issue, you cannot depend on saliva hormone levels. They simply do not correlate very well with actual hormone delivery to the hair follicle. We have had too many patients whose saliva tests have said they were high in estrogen and low in progesterone, but when I checked the more reliable clinical findings and serum levels, I found the reverse: low estradiol and continuing normal levels of progesterone. The serum hormone tests are what I want to trust in making recommendations for treatment options.

What about those "sinus problems" you have suddenly started having as midlife hit? Remember, the nose and sinus cavities of the face and forehead are lined with a mucous membrane. Similar to the way the loss of estradiol causes dryness of the lining of the vagina, we also see a loss of moisture and healthy mucous lining of the nose and sinuses when estradiol declines. The production of mucous by this lining helps to clear out allergens, bacteria, and viruses from the air you breathe. When estradiol declines, the mucous membrane becomes drier and then doesn't function as well to clear out all these invaders. Blood flow is decreased as well, due to the constriction of small arteries when estradiol levels fall. If blood flow is diminished, the immune cells and proteins carried by the blood aren't as available to the tissues to ward off or destroy the invader particles. Taking antihistamines and decongestants every day just makes all this worse, since together they dry the membranes even more and cause more constriction of the blood vessels. A better option is to use natural saline nose sprays to provide needed moisture, and several times a week, do a steam bath (easy—just hold your head, covered with a towel, over a sinkful of hot water and let the steam clear your sinuses and moisturize your face at the same time). Then, get your hormone levels checked and look into whether hormone therapy is more appropriate for you than taking lots of decongestants and antihistamines every day.

I will talk more about estrogen effects on sleep in chapter 11. For now, let me just say that you are not imagining changes in your sleep quality as hormone change hits. Sleep becomes more elusive, it gets more fragmented once you do fall asleep, there are multiple awakenings that you didn't use to have, you may notice less dreaming and more "restless legs" or muscle twitches, and you wake up feeling exhausted. Sound familiar? Menopausal women commonly develop abnormal breathing during sleep and suddenly start developing *sleep apnea syndrome* (SAS), a potentially serious sleep disorder, at rates about equal to those seen in men. Prior to menopause, sleep apnea in women is much less common than it is in men.

Chronic sleep disruption and loss of sleep leads to daytime fatigue, memory and concentration difficulties, mood problems, muscle pain syndromes and other health problems. If the sleep disturbance is severe, prolonged, and includes significant apneic (stop breathing) spells that cause oxygen loss, the consequences can be even more severe. Sleep apnea is already known to be a significant contributing risk factor for high blood pressure, cardiovascular disease, early morning fatal heart attacks, onset of major depression, and erectile problems in men. The reason such serious consequences of sleep apnea occur are the dangerous drops in oxygen (O_2 saturation) of the blood when sleep apnea causes you to stop breathing. This drop in oxygen saturation to dangerously low levels happens in both men and women. Menopausal women, however, have an even greater vulnerability than men to sudden death or heart attack during sleep because the estradiol drop in women causes combined effects that make the situation worse. There is the oxygen drop when you stop breathing, added to the effect of nighttime hot flashes causing a rise in catecholamines and instability in heart rate and blood pressure that also affect blood delivery to the heart.

Since our current therapeutic options for sleep apnea are limited to weight loss, surgery, and/or continuous positive airway pressure (CPAP), it would be helpful to know whether hormone changes at menopause, and the use of hormone therapy, play a role in women's risk of this serious sleep disorder. Drs. Keefe, Watson, and Naftolin conducted a pilot prospective crossover study of the effects of hormone replacement therapy on sleep apnea that was published in 1999 in the *Journal of the North American Menopause Society*. They performed detailed sleep studies and serum hormone levels both at baseline before hormone therapy and three to four weeks after the women had been on either 17-beta estradiol (E2) 2mg daily alone or together with ten to twelve days of medroxyprogesterone acetate (E2 + P). They did not include a progestin-only group because earlier studies had found no effect on sleep apnea from giving progestin without estrogen. Both E2 alone and with E2 with P regimens were found to decrease sleep apnea to a statistically significant degree in all subjects tested. The investigators concluded that hormone therapy for menopause has a potential role in reducing SAS and its many associated health risks. They also reported another interesting finding: 40 percent of the waking episodes these women had were *not* associated with vasomotor flushing ("hot flashes"), which suggested that vasomotor flushing and waking episodes are separate and *independent* manifestations of estrogen decline. It was previously thought that fragmented sleep around menopause was due only to hot flashes at night.

The study confirmed what many other sleep studies have suggested: Ovarian sex steroids, particularly estradiol, have a variety of effects on normal sleep regulation, including direct effects on sleep apnea. It is also significant that patients with SAS, the most severe form of sleep disorder, were used for this study and had the degree of benefit shown. These findings are all the more promising from women with milder forms of sleep disruption, and fit with basic science studies showing that there are many mechanisms by which estradiol with progesterone/progestins interact with neurotransmitters and regulate brain centers involved in sleep pathways. Formal studies like this give further support to "anecdotal" reports from women themselves that their sleep is better when they start a hormone therapy that includes estradiol. With new evidence that hormone therapy containing estrogen can reduce sleep apnea, I think it is even more important for physicians not to dismiss sleep problems in women as "just stress," and prescribe sleeping pills, such as Ambien, Klonopin, Dalmane, and others. If women actually have sleep apnea, sleeping pills can make the situation even more dangerous by further suppressing breathing during sleep. If your bed partner tells you that you have started snoring at night, or maybe that you seem to stop breathing at times and then "jerk" back in to a loud breathing, I urge you to talk with a physician about having sleep studies to check for sleep apnea, and again, have your estrogen level checked.

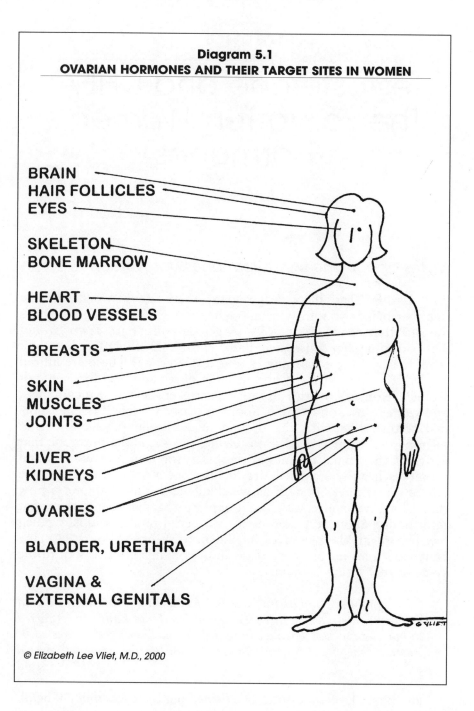

Diagram 5.1
OVARIAN HORMONES AND THEIR TARGET SITES IN WOMEN

BRAIN
HAIR FOLLICLES
EYES

SKELETON
BONE MARROW

HEART
BLOOD VESSELS

BREASTS

SKIN
MUSCLES
JOINTS

LIVER
KIDNEYS

OVARIES

BLADDER, URETHRA

VAGINA &
EXTERNAL GENITALS

© Elizabeth Lee Vliet, M.D., 2000

Testosterone and DHEA: The Forgotten *Women's* Hormones

Myths about "The Male Hormones" for Women

Testosterone? That's the *male* hormone isn't it? *Testosterone?* That's the one that makes you grow a mustache, isn't it? *Testosterone?* That's the one that causes your voice to get deep, isn't it? *Testosterone?* That's the one that causes liver damage, isn't it? How often have you read or heard these warnings about testosterone? These are all old myths, based on synthetic hormones in doses designed for men, not women. Women's **ovaries** also make testosterone before menopause, and women lose, on average, about at least 50 percent of their normal testosterone with the decline in hormone production after menopause. Women need testosterone, too—it is the hormone that activates the sexual circuits in the brain for men **and** women and promotes healthy sexual desire. It also has a lot of other positive effects on women's bodies, as we shall see in this chapter. So now that I have your attention, we'll explore together some important information about testosterone for women. I find that most women have heard all the negatives but know very little about the many beneficial roles testosterone plays in a woman's body. Listen to the voice of this young woman:

> I just don't have any desire for sex. I feel terrible about this. I would like to be interested in it, I love my husband and I am very attracted to him. I enjoy sex when we have it, but I just don't feel interested. It frustrates me and it frustrates my husband. It's like somebody turned off a switch.   —MG, 33 years old

Her blood level of testosterone turned out to be *less than* 10 ng/dl. Her low blood level corresponds with the way she described feeling. For women to have an optimal sex drive and interest in sex, testosterone blood levels need to be about 40 to 60 ng/dl, although the range of what is "normal" for a given woman can vary quite a bit within, or even below, this range. For comparison, men's testosterone levels normally run about 500–1200 ng/dl. Most men don't experience a loss of libido until testosterone drops down to around 500 or less, although this may vary slightly depending on what is "normal" for a given man. Because women's optimal ranges for testosterone are so much lower and narrower, women are more sensitive to a smaller degree of change: A slight drop of only 10–15 ng/dl can make an enormous difference in whether a woman will feel her usual sexual spark. A comment about the numbers I have given above: You may find different books quoting ranges for testosterone that will seem quite different from those I have given here. The differences occur because laboratories may use different units of measure. Throughout this book, I use *nanograms* per deciliter in the testosterone ranges I give; ranges that are reported in units per milliliter will appear to be different, when in fact, they simply need to be converted to the same scale.

When the young woman above talked with her primary physician about her loss of libido, she said he told her: "Well, I guess you'll need some marital therapy. It must be a problem in your relationship." When she asked about having her hormones tested, she was told "there's no way to do that, and it doesn't mean anything anyway." When she had her consultation with me, an integral part of my evaluation was to measure her blood levels of testosterone. I check serum levels of *both* total testosterone and *free* testosterone together. I'll explain more about what this means later in the chapter. Not only is the actual blood level very helpful in determining *whether* a testosterone supplement may be indicated, it also helps guide me in planning the appropriate amount for each patient. This all made a great deal of sense to MG and helped her see that there is a systematic way to evaluate her needs. She was quite willing to consider the necessity of marital therapy, but not until the *hormonal* aspects of her problem were at least checked. In her body wisdom, it appeared more likely to her that the problem was a physical change, since she honestly felt her relationship was a good one, there weren't any marital problems that had occurred, and her previous enjoyment of sex had been high.

Women's Sexuality: An Overlooked Concern in Health Care

A patient recently wrote me that she asked her doctor about checking her testosterone level. He told her that it "couldn't be done," and anyway, it "didn't matter," since her level would be normal for a fifty-five-year-old. Her letter to me commented, "I said to him,

'What if I want a level of a 25 year old woman?' He then said to me 'That's ridiculous!' At that point, I realized this discussion wasn't going anywhere at all and I gave up." It may appear from experiences like this that the men who have dominated the hormone decisions, medical research, and the rest of women's health have been a little *afraid* for us women to have access to testosterone and a vital, normal, healthy, active sex drive as we grow older. After all, *their* testosterone, and erectile function, is often declining as they grow older, and they are quite often ashamed to discuss this problem with *their* doctors. And, for generations, the standard medical teaching was that it was *abnormal* for women to have a sex drive. Women ("good girls" and "ladies") were supposed to be passive recipients of the sex act and were considered "loose" if they appeared to actually desire sex.

Myths and Stereotypes Still Affect Your Health Care

Many of these myths and age-old stereotypes lie just beneath the surface in women's encounters with health professionals today. I know that seems like a strange idea, given the relatively open sexuality of our culture today. But these hidden messages about women's sexuality and how women are "supposed" to act are deeply embedded in our culture and especially in the traditional medical teachings. If you doubt me on this, just notice the mixed messages about women's sexuality in many ads—women are portrayed as "innocent" and sexy at the same time. Take a look at these examples, some from a long time ago and some more recent.

Dr. W. W. Bliss (1870), in keeping with the thinking of the times, made a rigid distinction between a woman's *reproductive* ability and a woman's *sexuality*. Female sexuality was seen as unwomanly and detrimental to the supreme role and function of reproduction. Dr. Bliss in his writings warned against "any spasmodic convulsion" (i.e., orgasm) by a woman during sexual intercourse to avoid interfering with conception.

Dr. Mary Wood-Allen, a woman physician of the same era, wrote that women should embrace their husbands "without a particle of desire." Doctors were taught that women were not meant to enjoy the sex act, and a "ladylike" woman should certainly never *initiate* the sexual act. Even though the physicians of the time denied that there were female sexual feelings and desires, there still appeared to be an undercurrent of male fear of women's potentially *insatiable lust*, which, if ever aroused, might then become uncontrollable.

Things haven't gotten much better in more recent medical textbooks. Consider this quote from a textbook of gynecology used when I was in medical school in 1977 (and think about all the physicians practicing medicine today who were trained when such textbooks were in use):

> *There seems to be little doubt that libido, which is well-developed among normal males, appears to be less highly developed among females. Certainly the majority of cases of dyspareunia [painful intercourse] or frigidity, or both, undoubtedly fall into the psychogenic category. The treatment for frigidity must usually stress the educational and psychotherapeutic aspects rather than the patient's pelvic or endocrine [hormonal] status. The female should be advised to allow her male partner's sex drive to set their pace and she should attempt to gear hers satisfactorily to his. . . . The importance of the [sex] act to her husband in both physical and emotional aspects should be stressed [i.e., by the physician].*

The emphasis on the man's sexual needs being met, and a woman's sexual problems as primarily psychogenic, viewed from our perspective today seems quite strikingly unbalanced. As a third-year medical student, I was, like the rest of my classmates, appropriately deferential to the teachings of the "authorities," the "experts in the field," even though these teachings did not fit with my own experience or what I was hearing from my patients. Yet, these attitudes persist when women seek help for sexual problems from many gynecologists (male and female) in practice today. Daily, even in the year 2000, I hear such stories from women seeking hormone evaluations in our offices. Last week, a woman told me that after getting the results of the lab tests I had ordered, she asked about improving her testosterone level to a more range to improve her libido. Her male gynecologist said "Why do you want to have a high level like that? You are fifty-four, not thirty!" Needless to say, she was furious at this attitude.

Listen to the voice of this *recently married sixty-seven*-year-old woman who had a consultation about her problems with vaginal dryness and decreased sexual desire:

> *My gynecologist just seemed to dismiss my concerns. He just told me that's what happens when you get older. I don't want to lose the sexual part of my life. I have a new husband, I love him, and we want to enjoy our sex. I just don't seem to have the interest I used to, and it hurts because I'm so dry.*

She reported that she had been offered a vaginal estrogen cream and marital counseling had also been recommended. When she asked about having her hormones checked, her physician's reply was, "That's not necessary. It won't tell us anything." When I evaluated her, her estradiol level was *less than 30* pg/ml (a desirable level would be at least 80–90 pg/ml), and her testosterone level was reported as "nondetectable," which means below the sensitivity of the test at about 10 ng/dl. You may recall that I said testosterone is optimal for women from about 40–60 ng/dl). It helped this woman and her husband to find out that her hormone levels were so low, because it confirmed that the sexual difficulties were not due to a relationship problem or her dissatisfaction with her new husband. You can imagine how much relief they both felt with this news.

Now, I ask you, is it reasonable to ignore these concerns and to dismiss a patient's request for a perfectly appropriate blood test? Particularly when, in this case, the patient has concerns that may be so easily alleviated with readily available natural forms of hormones to restore her premenopausal balance. Before sending her to a therapist, this woman should have at least been given the information that (1) we do have reliable and useful tests to measure hormone levels, and (2) we have a variety of bioidentical hormone options to enhance her sex life for this new phase of her life. After being started on a low dose of supplemental testosterone and estradiol, she came in a month later and described, *"I feel like a new woman. I have my old spark back, and now I want—and enjoy—sex again."* She also told me that her quality of orgasms had improved, it was easier to have an orgasm, and she now had no difficulty with arousal and lubrication. Her estradiol level at the three-month follow-up visit was 98 pg/ml, and her testosterone level was now 25 ng/dl, which were good levels for her, based on her self-reports of restored libido and healthy sexual responses.

Women's Bodies Do Make Testosterone

Testosterone is one of a group of hormones called *androgens*, from the Greek "andros" meaning malelike. The word androgen refers to any steroid molecule with nineteen carbon atoms that is able to bind to the androgen hormone receptor sites in the brain and body. All of the androgens are made from cholesterol by the female ovary, the male testes, and, to a lesser extent, by the adrenal glands in both men and women. Androgens are also made from chemical "building blocks," or precursor molecules, in body-fat tissue, muscle, the liver, skin, and the brain. But these precursor molecules are produced in the ovaries and adrenal glands, so it really ends up that the ovaries and adrenal glands together are responsible for either directly or indirectly making all of a woman's testosterone. In a Gallup poll of American women, conducted for the North American Menopause

Society in 1993, only 5 percent of the women polled knew that their bodies make androgens and that the amount made declines after menopause. Doctors used to think that testosterone isn't very important for women, so the whole issue of testosterone therapy for women is relatively new. The amount of circulating active androgens in women is obviously much lower than in men, but these compounds are important for quite an array of vital functions in women's bodies. Many studies over the last thirty years or so have shown what powerful effects testosterone has on a woman's sexuality, mood, zest, and vitality, and on maintaining healthy muscle and bone, to name a few of its functions. Fortunately today, more women are aware of the importance of androgens like testosterone and DHEA and are asking physicians for more information about how to measure them and what options there are for adding back what the body formerly made.

TYPES OF ANDROGENS

- *dihydrotestosterone* (DHT)
- *testosterone*
- *dehydroepiandrosterone* (DHEA)—ovary
- *dehydroepiandrosterone-sulfate* (DHEA-S)—adrenal
- *androstenedione*

© Elizabeth Lee Vliet, M.D., 1955

Over the course of a woman's life, the ovary makes on average about one-third of a woman's total circulating androgens, in addition to producing the female hormones estrogen and progesterone. But beginning several years before a woman's ovary becomes menopausal, the adrenal glands have already decreased androgen production by about 50 percent, and the ovary levels of testosterone have already started to decrease. That means your sexual desire and ability to become sexually aroused can be significantly diminished several years before you actually stop menstruating at menopause. If you have a hysterectomy *with* removal of the ovaries before you are actually at menopausal hormone levels, the change is even more drastic. Concentrations of testosterone in the bloodstream fall markedly *within twenty-four to forty-eight hours* after surgery. Since you no longer have the ovaries to make more testosterone, or to efficiently convert adrenal DHEA to testosterone, there is an abrupt loss of this important hormone. That's a big shock to the body, and there are potentially major unpleasant effects from the loss of testosterone: loss of sex drive, fatigue, decrease in muscle mass, decreased bone density, depressed mood, achy joints, and changes in feelings of well-being to name a few. Even if one or both ovaries are left in place, newer studies have shown that the hormone production reaches menopausal levels within three to four years in as many as 60–70 percent of women, even if they are only in their thirties when the uterus is removed. This more rapid decline in hormones after the uterus is removed is thought to be due to decreased blood flow to the ovaries as a result of having to cut and tie off the uterine artery during surgery.

In addition, if you are then started on just estrogen therapy, the amount of free, biologically active testosterone falls even further, since estrogen increases SHBG, sex-hormone-binding globulin, that "binds up" more of the testosterone molecules. This is one reason that many women lose sex interest, sex drive, and energy after hysterectomy and then think these losses are due to the surgery. It isn't usually the surgery *per se* that caused the problems. It is generally that you need more optimal hormone replacement to restore the desirable levels of what you had before surgery. And often, women who have had their ovaries removed will need testosterone added to the estradiol prescription. But if your doctor doesn't check the hormone levels, mistakenly assumes you are "just depressed," and prescribes a medication like Zoloft, Paxil, Celexa, or Prozac, the results on your sex life can be disastrous. All of these serotonin-augmenting medications drastically reduce sex drive and orgasm ability in women who have *normal* levels of testosterone, much less women who have lost their testosterone. How do doctors really know what a woman needs after surgery if no one ever checks hormone levels or considers that the loss of crucial hormones may cause these changes I have described?

Women who become naturally menopausal and have decreased ovary production of all the hormones lose about 50 percent of their androgen source, especially the testosterone. I wonder how many men would like to go around for the last thirty or forty years of life with only *half* their normal testosterone! One reason there is *less* of the active form of testosterone after menopause is that an important precursor molecule, *androstenedione*, decreases more than 50 percent when the ovary ceases its hormone production. Many doctors do not realize that when women have a decline in *estrogen* production, it also results in a decrease in *testosterone* production, due to the loss of precursors usually made by the ovary. If you don't have functioning ovaries due to either natural menopause or a condition that causes premature ovarian decline (viral syndromes, tubal ligation, cigarette smoking, excessive exercise, to name a few), or if your ovaries have been removed in surgery, remember that you can't produce optimal levels of testosterone or estrogen by taking DHEA supplements alone, since it is in the ovary that most of the enzymes and pathways exist for us to be able to convert DHEA to testosterone or, to a lesser extent, estradiol.

There are noticeable effects of the changing hormone balance during the climacteric or midlife years: Lower estrogen *relative* to the amount of testosterone present allows for the testosterone effects to be "unmasked," producing changes in facial hair, voice, sex drive, energy level, and distribution of body fat. With loss of estrogen, the androgens that are left will be shifted more into the "free" portion in the bloodstream, and will therefore be more biologically active. So even if you have less testosterone and DHEA present than you did before menopause, you now have more in the active state and will therefore see more of the androgen influences on your body. This means women having more facial hair, losing scalp hair, and experiencing a shift in body fat from the "pear" or gynecoid (female) pattern to the "apple" or male pattern of body fat around the waist and trunk (see chapter 2 for a diagram of these body-shape changes). It may not be just that you "don't have the willpower to lose weight"; it may be that your hormone ratios are now working against you. This is especially true if you are taking over-the-counter DHEA supplements that usually come in doses too high for women to use on a daily basis.

Contrary to the popular myths and incorrect information about hormones perpetuated in a number of books and articles, it *isn't* the *estrogen* that is typically the culprit in weight gain at midlife. There are several bigger culprits in weight gain for women: (a) the changing *ratios* of the ovarian estrogen and testosterone, (b) taking excess progesterone relative to estrogen, (c) the effects of excess adrenal androgens and cortisol relative to estradiol, (d) increased insulin levels as we age and lose the beneficial regulating effects of estradiol, and (e) the gradual decline in thyroid function as we age. All of these hormone changes combine to give us a slower metabolism. A lower metabolic rate combined with less physical activity and usually more food intake than is needed as we age, all add up to excess pounds. In addition, once you start gaining weight, there tends to be more insulin production, which in turn promotes more fat storage around the middle of the body. The characteristic *premenopausal* balance of estradiol, testosterone, progesterone, thyroid hormones, cortisol, and insulin are important in order to reduce these undesirable body changes in later years.

Without the proper balance of estrogen, androgens from the adrenal gland and fat tissue begin to produce even more unwanted body changes for women: *increasing* blood pressure, *increasing* total cholesterol, and *decreasing* HDL ("good") cholesterol, along with *increasing* LDL ("bad") cholesterol. All of these changes contribute to the increasing risks of heart disease, hypertension, and diabetes in women in over age thirty-five. You will read more about this in chapter 13. At first, we thought that testosterone itself was responsible for these negative effects on the cholesterol ratios. Newer studies have shown, however, that when given with the right balance of estradiol, testosterone actually helps maintain the normal mechanisms involved in vasodilatation that serves to help lower blood pressure. Testosterone, and other androgens such as DHEA, if given alone appear to *promote* buildup of artery-clogging plaque (atherosclerosis). If the androgens are given *with* estrogen, however, they have the *opposite* effect on the arterial wall and actually help prevent buildup of plaque in the arteries.

Throughout a woman's life, testosterone has important functions in maintaining muscle tissue—that wonderful "fat burning," machinery—in women. Lower testosterone levels mean less muscle building, even if we are exercising several times a week. Testosterone also plays a key role to help *build bone* and prevent osteoporosis, an even more crucial function as women lose the effects of estrogen in maintaining bone density. Furthermore, testosterone plays a key role in keeping a woman's energy level optimal. Decline or loss of this critical hormone is one of the frequently unrecognized factors in the midlife problem of "chronic fatigue." Many women have multiple medical evaluations and spend hundreds or thousands of dollars on tests and therapies to diagnose and treat "chronic fatigue" (CFS, CFIDS) and *never have a blood-level test for testosterone.*

Mrs. C. Keeps Skiing

Mrs. C., a delightful woman in her early sixties who loved to ski every winter, had noticed a significant decrease in her stamina and energy on the slopes over the past two or three seasons. During her consultation to discuss her questions about hormone therapy, she mentioned that she had experienced a noticeable decline in her strength and endurance for skiing. She had never had anyone check her hormone levels, although she had asked about having this done. Along with an estradiol that was too low in spite of her being on Premarin 0.625 mg, she also had a testosterone level of less than 10 ng/dl. I suggested she add testosterone to her therapy, and I also changed her to a bioidentical form of 17-beta estradiol, using a skin patch delivery. She began using 2.5 mg of natural micronized testosterone oral sustained release capsules, along with the Climara transdermal estradiol patch, 0.1 mg every five days, and has now been on this combination for the past several years. From a medical standpoint (and her preference), she did not need to take progesterone since she had a hysterectomy many years ago. Within the first six months, she described a marked increase in her energy level, and what she described as "my old spark coming back." The next year at her follow-up visit, she gleefully told me that when she returned to the ski slopes the season after starting testosterone, her ski instructor commented on the noticeable improvements in her strength and stamina. He asked her what her new training regimen had been over the summer. She smiled and said *"I never told him what really made the difference, but I know it was the testosterone. I could feel my muscles getting stronger with the exercise, and this was different from the way my muscle strength developed when I was just on the Premarin!"* She didn't have any adverse side effects on this dose of testosterone, and her cholesterol profile has continued to be in a healthy range. She also commented *"I just feel better. It's hard to describe, but I just have such a good change in my overall feeling of well-being and energy again. I didn't realize I had lost some of that until I got it back! I really feel like my usual self."*

Our psychological sense of well-being is also enhanced by testosterone. In some women, what appeared to be a depression turned out to be a deficiency of testosterone. Yes, this hormone does lift moods when the amounts are present at normal levels for women. As testosterone levels rise higher than needed for optimal balance (whether from overproduction in the body or from supplemental hormones), women report increased facial hair usually above the lip, increased dreaming and/or nightmares, difficulty falling asleep, and perhaps more sex drive than usual. At high levels, and in doses used in steroid abuse for muscle building, *both* men and women develop toxic behavioral effects such as extreme irritability, volatile/explosive moods, aggressiveness or assaultiveness. Again, *balance* is key.

Synthetic versus Natural Micronized Testosterone

Remember from my discussion in chapter 5, *synthetic* simply means "produced by putting together," not necessarily "artificial," as it has come to be used. Remember the example of human insulin from the previous chapter? Another illustration is human growth hormone, which scientists have been able to synthesize in the laboratory, so that we can now give the human form to children deficient in this hormone. These are examples of *synthetic* (i.e., made in the laboratory) medications being used because they are the *bioidentical* to the ones found in human bodies. Molecules that are the same as those made by the body, even if synthesized in a laboratory, are better tolerated, more effective, and have fewer side effects. Then there are synthetic hormone medications that are truly artificial in the sense that they are chemically different from the molecules the body makes.

Methyl testosterone is an example of a form of testosterone created in the laboratory and not found in the human body. This compound was developed by scientists trying to find a way to make testosterone able to be used in an oral tablet. In the past, we did not have a way to give natural testosterone orally because it would be broken down and lost in the digestive process before getting into the bloodstream. It is the addition of the methyl group to testosterone that makes it possible to be absorbed orally without being completely lost in the digestive tract first, and then produce its androgenic (testosterone-like) effects at the receptors throughout the brain and body. But, it is also this methyl group that increases the potential for liver toxicity. Methyl testosterone has worked well for the majority of *male* patients needing testosterone but not as well for women, because the commercial doses available were designed for men and are simply too high for most women to use on a daily basis.

In recent years pharmacists began making a form of natural testosterone in a micronized form that produces particles small enough to survive digestion and be absorbed into the bloodstream. Micronization is also used to make native human preparations of progesterone and estradiol as I talked about in earlier chapters, since all of these hormones are inactivated or destroyed by digestion when taken orally. The source for all of these natural, bioidentical forms of human hormones is actually from plants: soybeans and yams. The chemical precursors are extracted, purified, synthesized into molecules *identical to those made in the human body,* and then compounded into standardized tablets so that you know the amount of hormone you are getting. This approach, I feel, allows better fine-tuning of hormone therapy than trying to get enough active hormone from plant/herbal sources, since you really are not able to determine how much you are taking, and whether the amount is right for you.

Testosterone can also be made by pharmacists in a wide variety of other forms: skin cream, skin gel, sublingual tablets (to dissolve under the tongue), and vaginal suppositories. The way that testosterone is given will determine (a) the amount absorbed, (b) the metabolism to different forms, (c) the development of desirable effects, as well as (d) the presence of adverse side effects. I generally don't recommend the rapidly absorbed forms of testosterone, such as gels and sublingual tablets or troches, since these are more likely to make you feel like you have been hit by a Mack truck when the blood levels rise so fast. A rapid rise in testosterone to high levels typically causes marked irritability, edginess, muscle tension, and aggressive, angry feelings. I have found that these unwanted testosterone effects are decreased by using either oral testosterone in a sustained-release capsule or tablet, or a low-dose cream form that is more slowly absorbed. I have listed in Appendix II several experienced, reputable pharmacists who will work with you and your physician to determine the proper amount of natural testosterone for you as well as provide educational resources and telephone question/answer services to assist patients and physicians in determining the most appropriate options.

My Response to the Myths about "Male Hormones" for Women

Most of the women I see have already heard comments like those I made at the beginning of this chapter: Testosterone causes a mustache, a beard, a deep voice, liver damage, and "oversexed women." A key factor most women don't know is that all of these problems are related to the *dose* and *type* of testosterone used, not just testosterone itself. In the United States, until very recently, we have had only synthetic *methyl* testosterone or other androgen compounds that are not made in the human body. These synthetic androgens are chemically different molecules and are far more potent than the natural hormones made by the ovary and adrenal gland.

Until more recently, doctors did not realize that women needed *much* lower doses of testosterone than had been thought, based on doses used for men. In the United States, we have not even had commercial tablets available in doses *low* enough for women. As an example, in the past, 10–15 mg has been a typical dose of methyl testosterone prescribed for women. On average, I am using doses of 1.25 mg to about 3 mg a day of the natural micronized testosterone. Obviously, this is quite a difference. These lower doses are based on the physiologically natural range of testosterone production in women. When using a more appropriate *woman's* dose, my patients tell me they feel more energy, have a return of their normal sex drive, and do not have the unwanted side effects described above. In addition, I monitor cholesterol blood levels and have not had any patients who have had a negative effect on their cholesterol levels if we keep the dose in the usual range for women, and check to see that blood levels are not getting too high.

Currently, there is a natural testosterone patch in a dose designed for women being developed with the same technology that has made estrogen and progestin patches available. It is not yet on the market, and the testosterone patches for men are far too high a dose for women to use. Future directions for androgen research in the United States are focusing on the role of testosterone in

Alzheimer's disease, in improving cognitive function in older people without dementia, in treating bone loss for men and women, in lipid disorders and breast cancer. With greater recognition of the important role testosterone plays in our health as both men and women get older, and the benefits documented with the transdermal testosterone patch for men, it would be quite helpful if we had a patch form of testosterone suitable for women to use.

DHEA: Promises and Pitfalls

DHEA has had a great deal of publicity in recent years, and is available in the United States in a wide variety of over-the-counter products of varying quality and potency. Since the over-the-counter DHEA is not regulated by the FDA, it is difficult for you to know exactly what you are getting when you buy it, and most of the doses are much more than women need for daily use. DHEA is also recommended by many alternative and "natural hormone" practitioners as the "Mother Hormone" precursor for the body to make estradiol and testosterone, and is suggested by some fibromyalgia specialists as a way to treat FMS or chronic fatigue. But remember what I said earlier: You have to have *functioning* ovaries for the "Mother Hormone" to be made into estrogen and testosterone. Behind the headlines touting the benefits of DHEA on everything from brainpower to sex, there is very little good science to back up the claims. This situation is very different from the extensive body of science showing the many beneficial effects of estrogen for women, and good data on the risks that may occur with long-term use of various estrogens. What dose of DHEA is safe is also a critical unanswered question. This is far different from having such good information available about doses and routes for estrogen. So, before you jump on the bandwagon and buy your "superhormone" at the grocery store, remember this is a potent steroid with profound effects throughout the brain and body. Make sure you have done your homework before you swallow all the claims . . . or the pill!

DHEA use has some special concerns and cautions for women that I want to briefly address here. I don't have space to go into all the pros and cons, or to describe in detail the research findings. I will cover the highlights, and if you would like to read more about DHEA from a well-respected DHEA researcher, I recommend the review article *"Dehydroepiandrosterone Replacement in Postmenopausal Women: Present Status and Future Promise,"* by Peter R. Casson, M.D. and colleagues. This excellent article was published in *Menopause: The Journal of the North American Menopause Society, vol. 4, 1997, pp. 225-231.* While this is a medical article for a medical audience, it will give you a balanced and reliable view of what we know and what we don't yet know about the safety and effectiveness of DHEA for women. Dr. Casson has been systematically researching DHEA for many years and has published a wide variety of well-balanced and carefully done studies, so his articles are a reliable resource for you to read if you want more in-depth information than I have provided here.

DHEA, like other precursor hormones, requires enzymes found in healthy ovaries for the DHEA to be changed into testosterone or estradiol by the body. If for whatever reason, your ovaries are not functioning optimally, you won't be able to adequately convert DHEA to the other hormones further down the pathway. When that happens, women tend to have the "excess androgen" side effects I showed in the summary chart for testosterone effects later in this chapter. Too much DHEA can cause exactly the same side effects as too much testosterone. In addition, neuroendocrine research has found that women's testosterone receptors need to be "primed" with estradiol in order for the androgens to have optimal effects. So if you are given DHEA, but your estradiol levels are too low, you again have the risk of adverse side effects as well as increased irritability and restless sleep seen with excess testosterone. In FMS and CFS the issue is even more problematic: Women tend to experience *worsening* muscle pain and spasm if the androgens (either DHEA or testosterone) are replaced *prior to* having optimal estradiol. Remember your basic body chemistry and the differences between men and women . . . you need a *woman's* balance restored.

Both men and women lose DHEA with age, and by the time we reach about age seventy, DHEA levels are only about 10 percent of what they were in our peak reproductive years. We don't yet know for certain whether this decline in adrenal androgens, called *adrenopause*, represents just an effect of getting older, or whether the *decline itself* causes the problems we thought were due to aging, such as loss of muscle strength, loss of optimal immune function, loss of cognitive "sharpness," loss of bone, and many other effects. Most of the current studies available showing benefits of DHEA have been conducted on animals, and there are problems with using animal models: doses used are often much greater than what would be appropriate "replacement" for humans, and the animal model itself is flawed, since animals don't go through the same adrenopause as humans do. But, in spite of these difficulties, a lot of what you read about DHEA's benefits has been the result of studies done on animals.

In human studies, important differences for men and women are emerging. A 1988 study on five young men by Nestler and colleagues showed that these young men given high-dose oral DHEA over a month had a decrease in body fat and a decrease in "bad"

(LDL) cholesterol. The same study was then conducted in women by Mortola and colleagues: *No benefits* were seen for the women. In fact, the women became "androgenized" with increased facial and body hair, acne, decline in good (HDL) cholesterol and increase in bad (LDL) cholesterol, decreased sex-hormone-binding globulin, and increased insulin resistance. Remember, insulin resistance helps make you fatter around the middle of your body—not a good thing cosmetically or from a health standpoint. Dr. Casson did a subsequent study using a much lower dose of DHEA (50 mg) for women and found that even this dose (commonly seen in over-the-counter products) caused excessively high testosterone serum levels in women. He reported that this finding indicated the need for further dose reduction if DHEA was being given to women. Earlier studies have suggested a cardio-protective effect of DHEA, again, this was in men and the positive effects were not seen in women. The data on this point continue to be conflicting. In addition to the possibility of weight gain with excess DHEA, there is a concern emerging from animal studies about possible adverse liver effects of long-term oral DHEA use, particularly at the high doses being promoted for women in the over-the-counter products.

Now that I have pointed out some pitfalls to watch for, what about promises for DHEA? DHEA has been promoted as the "feel-good" hormone, improving one's sense of well-being, energy, memory, and mental sharpness. Unfortunately, the few carefully done, placebo-controlled studies of possible cognitive benefits with DHEA have also been disappointing, with no clear evidence of improved mental function, sense of well-being, or memory increase. Some clinicians have proposed that DHEA may help prevent osteoporosis, but again, we don't yet have good data on a bone-sparing effect from using DHEA. Dr. Casson's group studied DHEA replacement effects on various markers of bone, and found no change in urinary hydroxyproline, hydroxylysine, or collagen crosslink excretion, and no improvement in bone mineral density on DEXA testing at the six-month point.

Evidence to date does not support DHEA being given *routinely* to healthy postmenopausal women for hormone replacement, but there are some situations in which DHEA does appear to have an important role. One of those is systemic lupus erythematosis. Studies at UCLA using DHEA replacement for lupus have been promising in reducing pain and other manifestations of the disease, but at the high doses used, many of the women in the studies developed unwanted side effects (facial hair, acne, irritability, for example). It may be that future studies will show that lower doses maintain the benefits without causing so many side effects. In a 1999 study published in the *New England Journal of Medicine*, Arit and colleagues in Germany studied the effects of DHEA supplementation in twenty-four women with adrenal insufficiency (AI) to determine effects on sexuality and well-being. Fourteen of the women had primary adrenal insufficiency, and all were taking corticosteroid replacement. Of the group, there were seventeen women who were either hypogonadal (estrogen-deficiency) or postmenopausal, and thirteen of these women were also taking estrogen-progestin replacement therapy. The women were given either 50 mg DHEA or a placebo for four weeks and then crossed over to the opposite treatment to compare responses. The women were not told which treatment they were receiving.

These investigators from Germany found that supplemental DHEA produced increases in serum DHEA, DHEA-sulfate, and testosterone, but no increase in estrogen levels. Sex-hormone-binding globulin was *decreased* (which meant more of the sex hormones were pushed into the free fraction in the serum). Total cholesterol decreased, but an *unwanted* finding was that HDL cholesterol also decreased on DHEA therapy. Objective measures, as well as the women's self-reports, showed improvement in overall well-being, depression, anxiety, and sexual thoughts, sexual interest, and sexual satisfaction. Side effects that occurred were the well-known ones of excess androgens: acne, oily skin, increased body/facial hair, and loss of scalp hair (alopecia) during the time of active hormone treatment. Decreasing the dose of DHEA helped to minimize or eliminate these unwanted side effects. The researchers concluded that DHEA replacement was an appropriate therapeutic option for women with well-documented adrenal insufficiency, even though this is an uncommon condition. Regular daily use of corticosteroids is much more common than is adrenal insufficiency, since these medications are given to people who suffer from osteoarthritis, rheumatoid arthritis, lupus, asthma, and other medical conditions. Taking corticosteroids daily will suppress the adrenal (and ovary) production of DHEA, so women who are taking corticosteroids over a long period of time may also benefit from DHEA supplementation.

I recommend that if you want to take DHEA, you should have a thorough evaluation by your physician, and have the appropriate blood tests done for hormone levels, lipids, and liver function. Then, work with your physician to determine an appropriate dose formulated to your needs by your physician and a compounding pharmacist, and be sure you use *prescription-grade* DHEA. You should keep in mind that over-the-counter DHEA is *food*-grade, not the *pharmaceutical grade* quality that is used in research studies. Not all over-the-counter brands deliver the amount they state on the label, and many products contain excessive doses for women. Since there is the potential for significant adverse side effects and long-term risks of DHEA use, it should be monitored by a physician who checks your serum levels of hormones, fasting lipids, and liver function at appropriate intervals. You need to pay attention also to what is happening to your quality of sleep and scalp hair—both of which can be disrupted and lost by too much DHEA. And if you start taking DHEA and are gaining weight around the middle of your body or craving sweets, you need to talk with your physician and cut back on the dose. A key point with DHEA is to *start low and go slow* with the amount you are using.

Finding What's Right for You: Options Available

To help you make the important decisions about what is best for you and your health needs, I have summarized in the following table benefits of adding testosterone to a hormone therapy regimen. I have also given you some pointers on what to look for as effects of too little and too much testosterone, or DHEA. Most women need only very small amounts of testosterone to achieve these benefits. I generally start my patients on 1.00–1.25 mg of oral sustained-release micronized testosterone, and then gradually increase the dose based on the woman's description of how she is feeling and what we are achieving in her serum levels. I find that most women I see will achieve the desirable response at a dose somewhere between 2–4 mg a day. I recommend rechecking the testosterone blood level before going higher on the dosage. Sometimes oral doses may still not be absorbed well enough to give desirable blood levels or will cause adverse changes in cholesterol, and I will suggest changing to a transdermal, gradually absorbed cream to improve the overall response. The transdermal cream form of testosterone (and DHEA, when appropriate) is less likely to cause the negative changes in HDL cholesterol, since absorption into the bloodstream through the skin bypasses the liver "first-pass" metabolism. Cream forms are an option for testosterone therapy that I find useful for women with high cholesterol or low HDL who still need to have the other benefits of testosterone. Cream forms require much lower doses than the oral route, since more is absorbed and less is lost by liver conversion to other compounds. A safe rule of thumb for a starting point is that a dose of the cream form of the hormone should be about 10 percent of an oral dose. The amount should then be adjusted based on your response and your serum hormone levels.

Options for Testosterone Supplementation

In addition to the natural micronized testosterone that can be compounded for you by pharmacists who provide this individualized service, there are a number of commercial methyl testosterone products available in the United States. These are summarized in the table below. A word of **caution** about the **injectable** testosterone preparations: It is more difficult to achieve the right dose for women with these, and as a result, they are more frequently associated with the unwanted side effects I have described. Injectable forms also give high levels at the beginning and wear off rather unpredictably, making it difficult to feel like you are on an even keel when you are using these forms. Testosterone pellets can be prepared to give a lower dose and more gradual absorption than the injectable forms, but the pellets also wear off unpredictably and make it harder to keep you feeling "even" without getting too much testosterone at the beginning and too little at the end. An even more important reason I don't use these preparations for women is that I *like to use methods that the woman herself can easily control*, based on how she is feeling. With pills or creams (or patches when available), each woman decides whether to use it that day; with the pellets and injections, you are stuck with them until either you go back to the doctor and have the pellet taken out or the injection wears off. In my opinion, *you* need to be the one with more flexibility and control over your hormone management!

SUMMARY OF TESTOSTERONE AND DHEA EFFECTS

Too Little	Just Right	Too Much
• low energy	• normal energy	• hyper feelings
• loss of sex drive	• normal libido	• increased libido
• slowed down	• alert, interested	• "scattered" thoughts similar to A.D.D.
• mildly depressed mood	• positive mood	• irritable, anxious, edgy, tense, agressive
• fewer dreams	• normal dreams	• intense dreaming
		• aggressive dreams
		• violent dreams
		• disrupted sleep
• thin, fine hair	• hair thicker	• facial hair
• hair loss (alopecia)	• normal hair growth	• hair loss (alopecia)
• dry, thin skin	• normal skin	• acne, oily skin

© Elizabeth Lee Vliet, M.D., 1995, revised 2000

COMMERCIAL TESTOSTERONE PREPARATIONS

TESTOSTERONE ALONE:	Doses Available
Oreton, Metandren, Test-Red (methyltestosterone)	5mg, 10mg, 25 mg (oral tablets)
Halotestin, Ora-Testryl (fluoxymesterone)	5 mg, 10 mg (oral tablets)
Testopel (Testosterone pellets)	75 mg (inserted under skin)
Delatest, Testone LA, Depo-Testadiol (testosterone enanthate)	100 mg/ml (injectable)
Depo-Test (testosterone cypionate)	50 mg/ml (injectable)

NOTE: Injectable steroid hormones are now more difficult to obtain since Steris Pharmaceuticals closed approximately 1998; generally are now made by appropriately equipped compounding pharmacies.

TESTOSTERONE-ESTROGEN COMBINATIONS:

Estratest: esterified estrogens . . . . 1.25 mg (oral tablets)
     and methyltestosterone . . . . 2.5 mg

Estratest HS: esterified estrogens   . . . . . . 0.625 mg (oral tablets)
     and methyltestosterone 1.25mg

Depo-Testadiol: estradiol cypionate . . . . 2 mg (injectable)
     with testosterone cypionate . . 50 mg

Discontinued by the manufacturer, approximately 1997:

Premarin with methyltestosterone (MT) . . 0.625mg E, 5 mg MT and
     . . . . 1.25 mg E, 10 mg MT

© Elizabeth Lee Vliet, M.D., 1995, revised 2000

In my opinion, Premarin with methyl testosterone had **far too much testosterone** for most women, particularly when you consider the much lower dose of estrogen included in the tablet, and the fact that Premarin delivers such a small amount of the most active form of estrogen, 17-beta estradiol. Since these high doses of testosterone were commonly used in the past by the dominant estrogen manufacturer, I think this is one of the primary reasons that oral testosterone therapy got such a bad name and was associated with so many unwanted and potentially serious side effects. As you see from the table, one tablet strength had 5 mg methyl testosterone, and the other had 10 mg methyl testosterone. I have *never* used even 5 mg of methyl testosterone, much less 10 mg of this more potent form of testosterone, in prescribing androgen therapy for women. Doses this high of oral methyl testosterone for women may commonly cause development of facial hair, acne, voice changes, loss of scalp hair (male pattern baldness), elevated total and LDL cholesterol, decreased HDL cholesterol, elevated triglycerides and insulin, as well as more body fat deposited around the waist. If your doctors are concerned about such side effects when you ask about testosterone therapy now, it is likely that they are remembering what happened with the older forms and higher doses of testosterone therapy. They may not realize that micronized testosterone, in the bioidentical ("natural") form the ovary made, is only about one third to one quarter the potency of methyl testosterone, and we are using even lower doses today as well.

Although the brand Estratest has become much more popular and widely used in recent years, thanks to increased awareness by physicians and consumers of the importance of testosterone for women, I think there are problems with this product you need to keep in mind. Estratest contains esterified estrogens that are converted primarily to estrone and very little of the 17-beta estradiol, which means less than optimal estrogen effect, and it contains the more potent methyl testosterone. Acne or oily skin, flare-ups of fibromyalgia pain, irritability, insomnia and feeling anxious or tense, not sleeping well, and hair loss are common side effects women tell me about their experiences with Estratest. Since it doesn't have an adequate amount of 17-beta estradiol to properly balance the amount of testosterone it contains, in my experience, I am not surprised to hear these negative comments from women who try it and decide not to continue.

Estratest illustrates a common problem with any medication that comes in a fixed-dose combination of different hormones or medications. There may not be enough of one thing and too much of the other for everyone to have the right blend. As a result of these problems, I rarely use the *fixed-dose* combination estrogen-testosterone such as Estratest. In my opinion, these fixed-dose products do not allow for individualized adjustments of hormone therapies tailored to each woman. I find it works much better to adjust each hormone separately so that you get exactly the right amount of each hormone for your body needs. Taking each one separately also allows you to make changes in only one at a time, based on what you are experiencing with desirable or undesirable effects, or interactions with other medications (such as antibiotics, asthma meds, etc.), or effects of situational stresses on your hormone metabolism.

If, however, you want to have the convenience of a combination estrogen-testosterone tablet available at your local drugstore or you want a prescription that is more likely to be covered by your health insurance, I have found that it can work fairly well to start first a 17-beta estradiol prescription (patch or tablet) and then use the combination estrogen-testosterone tablet (i.e., Estratest HS) just two to three times a week rather than every day. This approach minimizes the adverse side effects of the higher dose, more potent methyl testosterone and yet provides a more consistent level of 17-beta estradiol than is provided by Estratest. This option seems to work well for some women. Other women can use these combination products daily and find that they provide the desired benefits without unwanted side effects. The key is finding what is best for you. I would expect your "recipe" would likely be slightly different from what works for your friends.

If you decide to take testosterone, remember that each woman's body is different. Trust *your* body wisdom, and what *you know* about how you feel. You may also check the summary chart on indications of too much versus too little testosterone, ask your doctor to check a blood level and to work with you to adjust your dose to one that feels good for you. You and your physician need to be effective partners in the process of *maximizing* your benefits from hormone therapy and minimizing any undesirable side effects. There are good options available now to help you achieve your goals for enhanced well being and improve your sexual zest, too!

The Role of Hormone Testing: Blood versus Saliva

Objective laboratory testing allows hormone doses to be specifically tailored to meet your needs as an individual. What should you be looking for as a desirable target range for testosterone? In my clinical experience, women typically experience their optimal normal energy level and libido when serum levels of *total* testosterone are between 40–60 ng/dl, with a free testosterone serum about 1 to 2 percent of the total testosterone. I now regularly check the blood level of *free* testosterone as well as the *total*. Free testosterone is the biologically active, unbound portion circulating in the blood, and the ratio of total to free is important in helping to determine the amount needed and the effects of other hormones on the testosterone balance. Imbalances between total and free testosterone give clues as to the direction to take in making dose adjustments to improve response or reduce side effects. Levels below about 20 ng/dl are generally too low to maintain your usual libido and energy. The majority of menopausal women I have evaluated, particularly those who have had surgical removal of the ovaries in their thirties and forties, have had testosterone levels of less than 10–15 ng/dl. This is certainly an understandable factor in fatigue or low energy, loss of muscle strength, and marked decrease in sexual desire.

As I said earlier, I haven't found the saliva tests to be very reliable or useful, particularly for testosterone. The most current research has shown that it is *not only* the *free* testosterone that is biologically active at the receptor sites. The portion that is *weakly bound* to serum albumin is also now known to be active at certain of the testosterone receptors. So, if you just measure the free portion in the *saliva* (which is all this test can measure), you miss having the important added information provided by the *serum* test: *total* amount available for immediate release to the receptors as needed, *weakly bound* portion available for activating certain receptors, and the *free* portion that is most biologically active. If you don't know all of these dimensions of your "testosterone account," it is difficult to determine the correct dose and avoid side effects. In the patients I have tested saliva and serum at the same time, the results are so far apart that it is a major concern to me that women are making important hormone decisions based on only the saliva test of free hormone.

If you are going to the expense and effort of having your hormone levels checked, I encourage you to work with your physician to have the gold standard serum tests. This approach will give you the best picture possible of your hormonal balance. In my opinion, serum hormone tests are helpful, efficient, cost-effective, and provide psychological benefit by identifying a physical cause of the disturbing symptoms women may experience at midlife and around menopause. I feel strongly that such tests should be available to women, especially those who have had their ovaries removed. There are too many "hidden" medical, psychological, and relationship costs if you don't know your physiological measures. You may find that it is too expensive **not** to have this information as you plan how to best achieve your health goals.

Keeping Your Sexual Vitality As You Age

A healthy, vital, invigorating sexual responsiveness is an important dimension of your optimal well being throughout your adult years, whether it results from having a partner or self-pleasuring if you are alone. There are many books totally devoted to this subject, so I will hit only the highlights in my discussion of sexual vitality here.

Lifestyle habits are really important to review. Thieves of sexual vitality abound in our modern lifestyle. **Cigarette smoking** (and use of chewing tobacco) is a big culprit robbing you of sexual vitality. **Nicotine** in all forms of tobacco products constricts blood vessels and decreases blood flow to the pelvic organs in men and women, which causes impaired sexual arousal and performance. Vasoconstriction from nicotine affects men by decreasing blood flow to the penis, which markedly diminishes fullness and firmness of erections, especially as men get older and vascular damage from use of nicotine increases. Talking with men about this effect of tobacco has been one of my effective motivators to get men to stop smoking. Most of my male patients had never had a physician tell them that cigarette smoking adversely affects quality of erections as men grow older.

Alcohol is another thief of sexual vigor. Too much alcohol robs you of your sexual desire and your ability to respond normally. Alcohol is a *depressant drug* that dampens down the brain centers for arousal and orgasm. A small amount of alcohol may initially release your inhibitions and make you feel relaxed and "in the mood for sex." After that, alcohol begins to make it harder to reach full arousal and orgasm. Men who have had too much alcohol often have difficulty achieving an erection that is full and rigid enough to allow satisfying intercourse.

Stress is another frequently overlooked thief of sexual interest and responsiveness when you have a hectic lifestyle. You may be simply too exhausted to relax and become aroused. Remember, the "flight or fight" adrenaline response evolved to help us *escape danger,* not to relax and become aroused for sex. If your adrenaline system is working overtime to keep up with the demands in your life, your sexual drive will be nil. Take time out to "get away," slow down, relax, and enjoy the physical pleasures of relaxed foreplay and sexual exploration. Notice I said **take** time, not **find** time. You have to establish your priorities and *take* the time for what is important to you—it doesn't just happen, given the busy lives we all lead today. And another thing: *Get up and move your body*. Exercise has a lot of well-publicized health benefits, including revving up your sexual energy and clearing away the sluggish feeling from stress overload. Besides, a fit body just feels sexier, to you and to your partner.

Medication side effects and **medical disorders** are other thieves of sexual vitality, sexual desire, and ability to have orgasm. Medicines such as serotonin-boosting antidepressants, mood stabilizers, beta blockers, blood pressure medication, diuretics, high progestin birth control pills, high dose progesterone creams, antianxiety and sleeping medications may all cause reduced sexual desire and difficulty having an orgasm. Unrecognized medical disorders such as diabetes are other causes of loss of sexual desire and problems with orgasm. It really is important to have a thorough medical checkup and appropriate laboratory tests if you have noticed a significant change in your sexual desire; painful intercourse; vaginal dryness, burning, or itching; or diminished ability to have an orgasm (or for men, diminished ability to achieve an erection). This checkup should include a physical examination by your primary care physician or specialist, laboratory tests of general blood chemistries, blood glucose, liver function tests, tests for sexually transmitted diseases, and hormone blood tests (especially thyroid, estradiol, and testosterone). If your hormone levels are too low, talk with your physician about an appropriate hormone regimen to help you regain your sexual vitality. More information on hormone therapy regimens is found in chapters 5 and 15. Healthy lifestyle changes I described above are your primary foundation, so be sure to address these. Hormones do help many women immensely, as my patients tell me after they experience the balance right for them: "It's like someone turned the light switch back on! I just feel better."

Beware of Sexually Transmitted Diseases (STDs)

Relationships often change at midlife, and many women find themselves back in the dating arena after many years in a stable relationship. I feel it is important to address the issue of sexually transmitted diseases (STDs), all of which are far more common today than when many of us baby-boomers were becoming sexually active. Bacterial vaginitis, trichomonas, chlamydia, herpes, human papilloma virus ("venereal warts"), gonorrhea, syphilis, and now AIDS. The list is daunting. While AIDS is the most feared STD, the others are many times more common and may result in a variety of symptoms that rob you of sexual pleasure and vitality. And yet, women are still frequently too shy about asking male sexual partners to wear a condom for fear of hurting their feelings. Women wake up! You are the only one who can take steps to protect yourself. I will tell you bluntly that if a man is worth sharing your body with, he should be concerned enough about *your* health to wear a condom. This is particularly true in new relationships, or even in long-standing relationships if there is any indication that your partner has had sexual encounters outside of your relationship. With *proper* use of a latex condom, you markedly decrease your risk of getting STDs, unless you have unprotected oral sex with a partner who has an active infection. For best protection against STDs, use of a high-quality *latex* condom should be combined with use of a spermicidal foam or jelly. In recent studies, the most widely used spermicide, *nonoxynol-9,* has been shown to kill all of the bacteria and viruses listed above. If you are concerned about whether your partner will have a condom available, you can always carry your own supply and be in control of having one when you need it.

The incidence of AIDS *in women* in this country has been largely underestimated until recently due to the fact that women in the early stages of the disease suffer different manifestations such as chronic vaginal infections. This wasn't even initially included as one of the criteria symptoms of AIDS. Another factor is that virtually all the research on AIDS has been done on homosexual *men,* the population in which it first developed. Women with AIDS also frequently die of different causes and infectious illnesses than do men. Men with AIDS have been twice as likely to get AZT as women, a drug that clearly prolongs survival. Not surprisingly, the survival rate of women with AIDS is significantly lower than that of men, according to a study conducted by the Maryland Department of Health in Baltimore. If the current trends continue, AIDS will be the fifth leading cause of death next year for women between the ages of fifteen and forty-four. Not using a condom may be potentially life threatening. Be aware, and be prepared.

Resources to Help You Rekindle the Sexual Fires

Often, patients tell me that their doctors have never asked about their sexual activity or changes in sexual function. Many physicians are still embarrassed to initiate this discussion with patients, particularly women in midlife and beyond. Then I hear physicians say that they assume their patients will tell them if they are having sexual problems, but most women tell me *they* are too embarrassed to bring this issue up when they see their doctor. So it ends up being a stand off, and the discussion doesn't happen. I urge you to be proactive and bring up your sexual questions and concerns when you see your physician. Take responsibility for your health and ask. If sex has become painful, you may want to consider using one of the nonhormonal lubricants such as Astroglide or Replens. If these don't do the trick and sex is still painful, it would help to read chapter 12 about the effects on the vagina and bladder as we lose estradiol and testosterone. I have outlined a number of ways to use topical hormone preparations to improve the health of the vagina, reduce vaginal and bladder infections that make sex painful, and also help alleviate the pain of vulvodynia and vestibulitis.

One of the most common problems I encounter in my medical practice is primarily a lack of knowledge about the human sexual response in men and women; concerns over what is "normal" and culturally derived unrealistic performance expectations. Consequently, I have included a list of resources in appendix II that will give you additional ideas for enhanced sexual vitality and rekindling the sexual fires. My patients, men and women of all ages, tell me that the ones listed have been helpful, well written, and beautifully descriptive of the wide variety of sensual pleasures. Dr. Miriam Stoppard's book, *The Magic of Sex,* is the best I have seen as a comprehensive, beautifully illustrated, and sensitively written guide for sexual enjoyment for men and women.

Another resource you may find helpful is the *Sensate Focus Experience*. This series of sexual pleasuring exercises is designed to help you and your partner explore each other's bodies and communicate your feelings to each other so as to help each of you learn what is most pleasing, arousing, and desirable for the other. You may also do this alone if you do not have or want a partner. This series of exercises is described in more detail in many of the books I have included on the resource list. Briefly, the Sensate Focus Experience establishes a structure to help both of you relax and not feel pressured to perform sexually. You and your partner commit to a specified amount of time, for example thirty minutes or an hour. Select a time and place when you won't be interrupted and are able to "tune out" stressful stimuli. You may want to help create the desired mood with music, candles, pleasant fragrances, and sensuous fabrics. One person begins as the *receiver* of the sensate pleasuring, and the other person is the *giver*. In the next time together, you alternate roles. During the entire time of the session, the giver caresses, touches, and explores the receiver's body. The receiver gives positive feedback about what feels pleasurable, what is less desirable, and what is uncomfortable. What does one do during these pleasuring times? Be creative! You may also have to redo the "mental tapes" from childhood prohibiting touching various body areas. Nothing is off limits for you as an adult unless it causes discomfort or pain for the partner. You may find ideas in some of the resource books in appendix II.

I encourage couples to proceed, *at your own pace*, through the following levels of Sensate Focus Experience:

Level I: nonerotic, nongenital pleasuring
Level II: erotic, nongenital pleasuring
Level III: erotic and genital pleasuring
Level IV: pleasuring that proceeds to intercourse

Prior to reaching Level IV, couples agree to abide by the guidelines of no intercourse, no matter how sexually aroused you become. Keeping this agreement helps build trust and reduce performance anxiety. If you commit to this process, and communicate with each other positively and sensitively, you will likely find the "fires" rekindled in your sexual encounters.

Sexuality does not have to decline as we age. There are many avenues for keeping your sexual interest and vitality alive and well. Some of these approaches you control, and some of these options are ones you will need to explore with your physician. Before you visit your doctor, you may find it helpful to explore your feelings about your sexuality in the self-check questionnaire in appendix III:

"How's My Sexuality?" Jot down whatever comes to mind about each of these questions. This will give you a list of topics when you go in for your medical visit and may help you focus your questions in the time you have with your doctor. If your physician doesn't seem interested or knowledgeable in these areas, then seek other resources for help. Don't just suffer silently. Know that help is available and that you deserve to enjoy your sexuality, whatever your age!

Chapter 7

The Persnickety P's:

PMS, PCOS, Premature Menopause, Perimenopause, and Postpartum Depression

Listen to the voices of these women who have called our center for a medical consultation. Each of these women had seen other physicians (both male and female physicians, I might add). Each woman described on our initial health form that she had felt dismissed, like her problems were trivial, and had felt that the physicians "just weren't listening to me, he/she just seemed to want to get me out the door, I felt like I was on an assembly line, I felt like I was just being patted on the head like a little girl and my problems weren't important." I know there are good, competent, caring physicians out there—both men and women—but I am greatly concerned with the overwhelming frequency with which I hear comments like those above. The trend seems to be getting worse, not better, as more and more patients are thrust into HMO settings where many physicians are on quotas as to how many patients they have to see in an hour. Do any of these descriptions sound familiar?

> "I hit thirty-nine and all of a sudden I'm a witch before my period. I never used to have PMS, and this is terrible. My mood! What's happening to me?"

> "I used to sleep so soundly a train coming through the bedroom wouldn't wake me up. Now, I wake up five or six times a night, wide awake, my heart racing, and I get up in the morning feeling like I never went to bed. I'm just forty-two, and I asked my doctor if I was starting into menopause, but she said I'm too young."

"Could I have PMS? I go through these awful moods—bitchy, cranky, irritable, yelling at my kids—the week before my periods, and then it seems to go as quickly as it came on after my period starts. And my hip joints, knees and shoulders seem stiff and achy so much. Am I beginning to get arthritis?"

—FORTY-ONE-YEAR-OLD MOTHER OF TWO

"I never had headaches, and last year I started getting fierce, stabbing, pounding headaches the day before my period. I feel like my head is coming apart, and I've missed work more, I just can't function when a headache hits. I've seen three doctors. They tell me there's nothing wrong to worry about, but nothing has helped stop these headaches. What can I do to get some relief?"

—FORTY-SEVEN-YEAR-OLD WOMAN

"My bladder is acting up, I have more problems with infections, and I want to see if you have any ideas to help me. I've been having these strange times each month before my period when I feel like somebody pulled a curtain over my brain. I feel foggy, my memory is shot, I can't sleep and wake up a dozen times a night soaking wet, I don't have any energy and I feel really blue and bad about myself. Is this stress or am I getting depressed? My doctor told me it's just PMS and not to worry about it, but I never had this before. Is there anything that will help?"

—THIRTY-EIGHT-YEAR-OLD WOMAN

"My sex drive is gone. Zip. Zero. Just nothing there. I love my husband, we have a great relationship, I enjoyed our sex life. I have less stress in my life than I have had for years. Things should be good. I don't understand it. My periods are getting lighter. Some months I don't have one. My hair is falling out in clumps and I always had such great hair. I'm not sleeping very well, my energy seems shot. I feel like I've been run over by a truck. I try to keep going, but inside I'm worried about what is going on. My doctor said I couldn't be starting menopause because I am too young, and she said my thyroid was normal."

—THIRTY-SEVEN-YEAR-OLD WOMAN

PMS. PCOS. Perimenopause. Panic. Premenopause. Stress. Uncertainty. What does all this mean? One thing is clear. There are a lot of unanswered questions out there. There are a *lot* of women who are confused by the terms, unsure of when to be aware of changes that might mean menopause is beginning. There are also a lot of women who are experiencing premenstrual problems, who are seeking help and having difficulty finding it. I hope you will find the beginning of some answers as you read this chapter, and I also hope that if you are having problems like this, you will learn some options for feeling better.

Is It PMS, PCOS, or Perimenopause?

Premenstrual syndrome (PMS) was first described in *modern* medical writings in 1931 by Dr. Robert T. Frank, an American gynecologist. (Unfortunately, his work appeared in the *Archives of Neurology and Psychiatry*, a journal not widely read by the rest of the medical profession.) Incredibly, these kinds of problems were also described in the writings of Hippocrates in ancient Greece. In the new millennium, medical science *still* says we aren't sure what the causes are, or what helps, or even *if* the mood and physical changes are caused (or contributed to) by hormonal changes. Of course, most women who suffer with these problems are pretty certain there is a hormonal connection, and I would definitely agree.

An overlooked serious metabolic endocrine condition affecting about 6 percent of premenopausal women, *including teenagers,* called polycystic ovary syndrome (PCOS), often causes premenstrual mood and physical symptoms similar to PMS, but there are other changes with PCOS as well. These are described in more detail in chapter 13, but briefly, PCOS causes excess hair growth, irregular menses, waistline weight gain, high blood pressure, high androgen levels, insulin resistance with glucose intolerance, and marked increase in risk of diabetes mellitus later in life. A sixteen-year-old young woman I saw recently had severe hormonal imbalance typical of PCOS, with a very high level of free testosterone, low estradiol, and had gained fifty pounds over six months in spite of a very healthy diet and extensive exercise regimen. She had PCOS, but her gynecologist had not recognized it, because he saw her as simply a teenager obsessed with weight gain and complaining of PMS. Many physicians don't realize that PCOS has potentially devastating consequences for the rest of a woman's life, and could lead to early death from heart attacks or diabetes complications long before menopause. So it isn't just a cosmetic issue—your life may be at stake. That's why I am addressing these issues together in this chapter. For more information on the specific ways PCOS increases risk of heart disease, see chapter 13.

As I have listened to women's descriptions over the years, I have to say it seems pretty obvious that there *has* to be *some kind* of hormonal connection in something that happens cyclically before menses on a consistent basis and resolves after the period is over. Just because we physicians and scientists may not have *found* the connection doesn't mean it isn't there. I do find it curious, however, that medical science has considered the hormonal-mood connection "controversial." Most studies I have reviewed do not even measure hormone levels—the reason given is usually something inane like hormone levels aren't reliable (they *can't* be if you don't check them), or hormone levels vary. Of course. That's the point. They *do* vary, throughout the menstrual cycle! I think the question is: HOW do they vary, and in what relationship to the pattern of mood changes and physical symptoms?

"All these women can't be wrong!" I said to myself. I knew that what I was seeing, and hearing my patients describe, was clearly different from the biological disorder of major depression. So I began to try and figure it out based on what I was hearing, and what I knew *could* be measured. I systematically checked hormone levels at specific times in the menstrual cycle, and used daily mood rating scales, depression inventories, and other measures. The patterns of hormonal change I have identified as being connected to the premenstrual mood and physical changes are:

1. Declining estradiol levels in the luteal phase (relative to levels seen in women without PMS), yet normal ovulatory levels of luteal phase progesterone being maintained, even when estradiol is significantly below optimal ranges
2. Changing ratios of estradiol and progesterone in the luteal phase
3. Lower-than-expected levels of testosterone, or in the case of PCOS, higher-than-expected levels of androgens (testosterone and DHEA), particularly the free, biologically active fraction
4. In women in their mid-thirties to mid-forties, lower-than-expected estradiol levels in the first one to three days of menses, but with FSH levels still in the premenopausal ranges

Women in this last category are still menstruating (unless they have had a hysterectomy) and most are still ovulating, but their estrogen is declining and appears to have a marked and consistent connection with the symptom clusters such as those described at the beginning of this chapter.

Now, do we call it PMS, PCOS, premenopause, or perimenopause? One of the reasons this becomes confusing is that these terms are used in many different ways in the media and in scientific articles. Generally, but not always, **premenopause** refers to a woman *still menstruating* regularly; **perimenopause** refers to a woman who has begun to have *erratic, inconsistent periods* with changing flow-patterns (may be heavy one month, lighter and shorter the next), and she is also beginning to skip periods; **PMS** refers to the *symptom cluster* of physical and emotional changes occurring *between ovulation and menses*, which then clears for a symptom-free interval each month. PMS may occur in both pre- and peri-menopause, since women are still having their ovary cycles. *Menopause* technically means "cessation of menses" and loss of the ovary cycles. I pointed out earlier, however, it is difficult to know when the last period is until a woman has gone an extended time without any menstrual periods, usually at least a year. If we use the commonly accepted definition of PMS, it doesn't occur after menopause because there are not any more ovary cycles. In menopausal women taking cyclic progesterone or progestin hormone therapy, however, there may be PMS-like symptoms that still occur. **Postmenopause** refers to the years after the complete cessation of menses. Now that I have defined the terms, they may not really tell you all that much, because they aren't always used the same way in all settings. The other problem is that rarely is there a discussion of age ranges, or the fact that *chronological* age doesn't necessarily correlate well with the *endocrinological* age. You will typically see health books and articles write as if the chronological age were the *primary* indicator of what to expect with menopause changes. What we really must assess is the *endocrinological* age to determine whether you are menopausal or not.

The climacteric, pre-, or perimenopausal years are a normal phase of a woman's reproductive life cycle. Many women make this transition to menopause without difficulty; however, approximately 60 to 80 percent of women DO experience mild to moderate symptoms such as PMS, insomnia, worsening premenstrual tension, irritability, mood swings (lability), and tearfulness during their thirties and forties. How serious are such symptoms? They are usually not serious enough to cause significant disruption in home, work, and social relationships and activities. Another 15 to 20 percent of women, however, experience *marked* luteal phase (PMS) symptoms, which are severe enough to disrupt optimal function at home and work, and are a significant source of distress for the individual woman. Several recent studies have shown that these brain-mediated symptoms are actually more numerous during the premenopause (typically, ages thirty-nine to forty-nine years) than after menopause. When articles say "there's no evidence that women become more depressed at menopause," they are missing the important *time frame* in which to look for these mood changes, as well as to look for major depression. Based on the *existing* studies that have asked this question, and included women in their late thirties and early forties, such distressing symptoms are extremely common and do appear to correlate both with *declining* hormone levels and with *widely fluctuating* hormone levels. Many women know or suspect this connection, but have had their observations devalued and discounted.

Early effects of estradiol decline usually manifest as restless sleep, premenstrual migraines, chronic fatigue, declining libido, the premenstrual mood changes I listed above, and irregular menstrual cycles with changing flow (lighter *or* heavier). While women in midlife may also be experiencing many *life* changes—balancing home, career, children, aging parents, community roles—I find that their changing *physiological hormone balance* often increases their susceptibility to situational stressors and contributes to an increasing degree of bothersome symptoms, as well as to increasing health risks for future problems like bone loss. This can become a vicious cycle in that physiological and psychological stressors further suppress ovarian function, which then exacerbates bone loss, particularly if the woman is a smoker or lacks adequate dietary calcium and weight-bearing exercise.

These are not just the "worried well" women, as they have been labeled in some settings when health professionals (and sometimes other women) perceived these kinds of symptoms as minor. I have not encountered many women who want to take time off from work or away from their families and busy lives to come for a medical appointment just because they are "worried but well." I think this is another paternalistic attitude about women, whether it's a male or a female physician who voices such a view. In my experience, the women who come in are having health changes that are a significant source of distress, or they wouldn't be making the effort and spending the money (and time, which may be even more valuable to many women these days) to come and see a physician. I think we in medicine sometimes forget that point and think women have nothing better to do than come see the doctor. I do think there is something important going on; I just don't think our present healthcare settings have *really listened* to what our midlife women have been trying to tell us. This next woman's story will give you some insights as to why I think these issues should be taken seriously.

Sue was a thirty-six-year-old married woman, with no prior history of depression, who came in for an evaluation of "worsening PMS" over the past several years. She was very concerned that her mood changes and angry outbursts were getting out of hand, both at home and at work. She was worried that because she had gotten angry at her boss several times, and had "popped off" at a coworker, she might be in danger of losing her job. She was also beginning to realize that during her PMS time, she was craving alcohol in a way that she had never experienced before, and was consuming more alcohol during that week than she felt was healthy. She had not had any pattern of daily alcohol abuse and had not experienced any alcohol withdrawal episodes, but she was worried about her increasing tendency to drink too much in the week before her period. She also described herself as "a raving maniac for chocolate" during the premenstrual week, and had even gone to the store at 2:00 A.M. to buy chocolate candy. She knew that wasn't particularly safe, given where she lived, but she said "it was such an overwhelming urge, I thought I would fly out of my skin if I couldn't get some chocolate right then!"

In getting a complete and more detailed picture of her symptoms, both at the initial visit and then with the daily symptom logs she kept for the next two cycles, it was clear that she had a well-documented, progressively intensifying pattern of premenstrual (luteal phase) mood changes (lability), tearfulness, anxiety, irritability, anger outbursts, depressed mood, decreased energy, restless sleep, nightmares, cravings for sweets and alcohol, breast tenderness, bloating (with a three- to five-pound weight gain), and constipation. She described feeling "almost suicidally depressed" just prior to her menses, although she had never made any suicide attempt and had not been treated for a primary depressive disorder. She said "the weird thing is, once my period starts, the feeling of wanting to die seems to vanish almost as fast as it came on, and it's gone completely until next time before my period, and then it all starts again." She also described difficulty functioning at work the week before menses, due to her mood changes, diminished energy, and a decreased ability to concentrate, along with changes in her short-term memory and word recall.

She did not have a sustained pattern of depressive symptoms present throughout her menstrual cycle, and described feeling "my mood lifting, and I felt normal again" soon after menses began. In her words, "I hate this merry-go-round of being this way . . . two weeks of the month I'm fine, and ten days of the month I'm a lunatic. Isn't there anything I can do to get this under control and feel better?"

Her past medical history was unremarkable for major medical illnesses. She had a pregnancy at age fifteen, but later was unable to conceive. She was found to have marked endometriosis and underwent laser surgery treatment at age twenty-eight, which appeared to solve the menstrual pain and cramps she had previously experienced. Menses continued to be regular. She took no medications except Tylenol occasionally for premenstrual headache or back pain. She started to smoke cigarettes at about age eighteen and was soon smoking two packs of cigarettes a day. She did not have a history of illegal drug use.

Both parents were alcoholic, and her three sisters had all suffered from PMS. Two sisters had undergone hysterectomies, and it was no longer clear whether they had a cyclic pattern to their symptoms. Neither her sisters nor her brother had ever required treatment for major depressive disorder. Her biological father's medical history was not known, other than that he had been an alcoholic. Her mother was diabetic, not yet on insulin, and had been alcoholic but off alcohol for two years. Her mother had no history of depression. There was a strong history of diabetes in both parents' families.

Her physical examination was normal, including pelvic and pap. She was slender and had a normal blood pressure. Her blood studies showed a normal chemistry profile, normal blood cell count, and normal urinalysis. Her thyroid profile, including TSH, was also normal. Day 1 estradiol was low at 20 pg/ml; her Day 20 estradiol was also quite low at 57 pg/ml (it should have been in the range of 150–250 pg/ml), but FSH and LH were still at premenopausal levels. Progesterone on Day 20 was 10 ng/ml, which indicated an ovulatory level of progesterone even though her estradiol was so low. Testosterone was less than 20 ng/dl, also too low.

Since she had such pronounced sweet cravings premenstrually and a strong family history of diabetes, I thought she may be having progesterone-induced changes in blood glucose regulation in the second half of her menstrual cycle. I suggested a luteal phase five-hour Glucose Tolerance Test, which was done in my office where I could observe any major symptoms and where my staff could help track symptoms in between blood drawings. She developed drowsiness, palpitations, and fell asleep in the first hour and a half of the test; between the third and fourth hours, she became cool, clammy, sweaty, nauseous, had trouble reading, burst out crying, described feeling anxious, and experienced the intense urge for alcohol "to calm me down." About twenty minutes later, these symptoms had passed, and she described feeling extremely tired, "wrung out," and had difficulty concentrating on her magazine. When we reviewed the test results two weeks later, she showed a rapid rise in her blood glucose to 180 mg/dL at the first hour (which had contributed to her drowsiness) and at hour four her blood glucose had dropped sharply to 45 mg/dL (normal is greater than 65 mg/dL). With the adrenaline surge triggered by the dropping glucose (which had caused the symptoms she experienced between hours three and four), her blood sugar had risen to 60 mg/dL by hour five. This was still lower than her initial fasting glucose, which had been normal at 84 mg/dL. I explained that she had a reactive hypoglycemia pattern, which is common in women who have diabetes in their families and is aggravated by the effects of progesterone on insulin secretion in the second half of the menstrual cycle. I thought this was a major factor in her premenstrual craving for alcohol and sweets.

With her long history of smoking and her current low estrogen levels, I recommended she have a bone density test done even though she was still menstruating and was only thirty-six. My goal in recommending the test was to have a baseline evaluation, but it turned out that she was *already quite low for her age* on bone density at the hip. This meant she was at a much higher risk for early osteoporosis.

With all this information, what recommendations did I make for this woman? First, **dietary and lifestyle habit changes were crucial.** She needed to decrease caffeine to help keep her from losing more calcium and making her bone loss worse. I also urged her to stop smoking because of tobacco's many adverse health effects; but the most crucial reason for stopping smoking was the further suppression of her ovaries by smoking, which in turn caused more loss of estrogen and more bone loss. She was clearly much too young to have this much bone loss. She needed to completely eliminate alcohol during her premenstrual week, because this made her blood glucose changes even worse and contributed more to the depressed mood and angry outbursts, as well as additional loss of calcium needed for her bone health. She had not realized how damaging the alcohol was and had thought it helped keep her from having the mood changes and anxiety symptoms. She was willing to eliminate it once she had experienced the effects of the blood glucose changes so dramatically. The nutritionist in my office went over a meal plan to control the reactive hypoglycemia, which consisted of approximately 40 percent complex carbohydrates, 30 percent fat, and 30 percent protein with three smaller meals and three healthy snacks daily during the premenstrual week in particular. She was advised to avoid salty foods that aggravated her fluid retention.

Second, I thought that **hormonal approaches** were important. This is an example of a situation where having information about the hormone levels made a difference in the treatment recommendations. Without such *definite* evidence of low estrogen, I would not have been as likely to suggest she consider adding hormones. If medication had been needed, I would probably have used one of the serotonin-augmenting medications for the second half of her menstrual cycle and encouraged her to make the dietary and lifestyle changes I had described. But given the significant *objective* evidence of early ovarian decline (bone loss, low estradiol), and the severity of the premenstrual hormonal effects on mood and sleep, we discussed the pros and cons of adding estradiol during the premenstrual and menstrual week to boost estradiol levels to more normal ranges.

I gave her several articles to read about these options and encouraged her to think about what she wanted to try. She was aware that, due to her continued cigarette smoking, she was not a candidate for a trial of oral contraceptives. When she came back for her follow-up visit to discuss her choices, she said "my quality of life for the next ten to fifteen years is more important than the remote chance of some dread disease." We also discussed the possibility that adding estradiol might have a slight possibility of triggering her previous endometriosis. She decided she wanted to try Vivelle anyway, since she had no problems with endometriosis since the laser surgery and her PMS was so disruptive for her. Four weeks after beginning the estradiol patch she stated she was feeling better overall, and both subjective and objective ratings of PMS symptoms had improved significantly. She continued to use the estradiol patch premenstrually for another two years, at which time she had successfully stopped smoking and wanted to change over to the low-dose birth control pills. She has continued to do well on her overall program and has maintained a healthier lifestyle in addition to the hormone regimen. She feels that hormonal stability has helped immensely to eliminate the disruptive mood and physical symptoms. I think the dietary changes were also a significant factor in helping her feel better, but I agree that restoring her estrogen level to a more normal range was a crucial dimension of her improvement. I believe this is a good example of the way in which our approaches need to be *individualized*, utilizing objective information combined with the patient's descriptions, to determine how best to create a woman's personalized health plan.

At this point, you may be asking yourself, "Well, did she have PMS or was she perimenopausal?" Technically, by our currently accepted definitions, Sue had PMS and was not yet perimenopausal, because her FSH and LH were still low (premenopausal levels), and she was still menstruating regularly. The window of time chronologically listed as perimenopausal is usually given as four years before menopause and four years after menopause, taken as an average age of fifty-one. Because women are all so different, I really find these arbitrary age ranges rather useless. I also think that what we will come to understand in the future is that the observed pattern of "worsening PMS" in the mid- to late thirties and forties is in all probability the *beginning of ovarian decline* leading to perimenopause, and that the worsening symptoms of PMS are all part of the *continuum* of women's midlife changes rather than *discrete* points in time.

Just What Is PMS?

Some of you may have experienced PMS, or family members with PMS, and it may have looked a little like this:

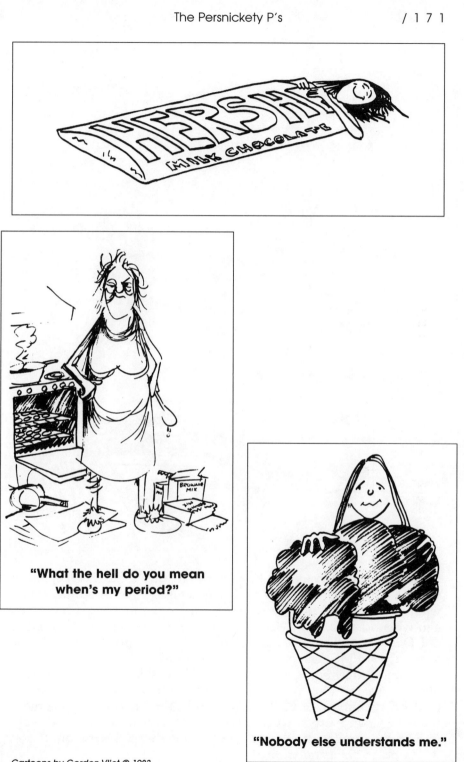

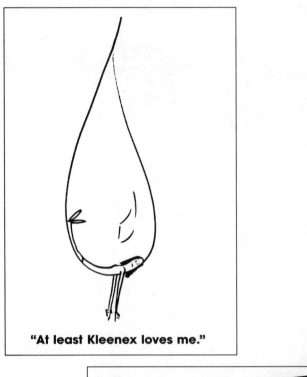

"At least Kleenex loves me."

Cartoons by Gordon Vliet © 1983

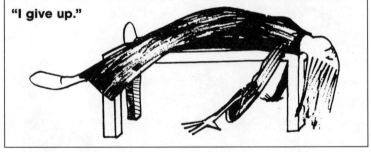

"I give up."

Women at my seminars howl with laughter and self-recognition when I put up the slides of these cartoons. I have to admit, somewhat sheepishly, that these were drawn by my husband a few years ago when I asked him to draw something funny for my talks. Little did I know that he was such a keen observer! So now you know some of my PMS secrets.

I enjoy the humor, but there is a downside to it: If by joking about it, we trivialize the experiences of women who are truly bothered by symptoms of PMS each month, then it doesn't become a focus of medical study to determine the causes of and to find ways to help the significant percentage of women who suffer from PMS.

Look at these statistics:

- 40 percent of all menstruating American women have regular premenstrual symptoms. This figure translates into **27 million women!** The majority of these have a milder form of the disorder, with bloating, headache, irritability, and the "blues."
- 5 to 10 percent of these, or **3 to 7 million women,** have symptoms severe enough to disrupt their personal and professional lives.

Even today, we don't have many answers to the questions I have raised above. The science of the menstrual cycle still is not adequately understood and lags behind our knowledge of body functions common to males and females. Some of the major difficulties in conducting research into PMS are the heterogeneous and amorphous descriptions of menstrually related syndromes, the multiplicity of populations evaluated, and the paucity of adequate rating instruments—among others. Studies that purport to address the question of menstrually related mood disorders have included subjects from PMS clinics; infertility clinics; women who have had gynecological surgery; patients from primary care settings, with and without complaints of PMS symptoms; college populations; "normal" women *without* symptoms; and "normal" women *with* symptoms but not seeking treatment. Some authors have excluded women with irregular menstrual cycles, even though this group is reported to have a greater incidence of symptoms. Such a mixed bag of study populations obviously makes it difficult to come up with meaningful and reliable data!

PMS *primarily* affects women between the ages of twenty-five to forty-eight, but it can affect adolescents as well: My youngest patient with clearly documented PMS was fourteen. I have been asked by pediatricians to consult on a number of cases of girls with PMS, and I think they may well have some parallels with the erratic hormonal balance and fluctuations seen in the perimenopause. PMS does, however, seem to be more common in older women and to worsen with age, generally becoming most marked for women in their late thirties to mid- or later forties.

The symptoms of PMS typically begin in conjunction with a hormonal change such as puberty, pregnancy, starting or stopping oral contraceptive pills, or following surgery that affects the blood supply to the ovaries, such as tubal ligation or hysterectomy without removal of the ovaries. In fact, a common pattern is for a woman to have the onset of her PMS about three or four years after a tubal ligation. This is now recognized to be related to the alterations in blood flow to the ovary resulting from having the tubes tied. Although when they ask about these connections, many women are still told that "this couldn't possibly be happening." This connection between PMS and surgical procedures has been increasingly discussed in gynecology journals. Thus, new techniques for tubal ligations have been developed to minimize any negative effects on ovarian blood flow. Use of oral contraceptives with a *multiphasic* (many are *triphasic*) hormone content has also been found to produce a PMS-like syndrome in a significant percentage of women. A *multiphasic* pill has two or three *different* hormone doses, designed to theoretically mimic the normal cycle using synthetic hormones (some brand names are Triphasil, Tri-Levlen, Tri-Norinyl, Ortho Tri-Cyclen, Ortho-Novum 7/7/7, Ortho-Novum 10/11, Jenest). Aggravation of PMS, as well as migraine headaches, are reasons I *don't* recommend this type of birth control pill, *especially for perimenopausal women* who tend to be more negatively affected by the hormonal fluctuations produced by the multiphasic pill.

I find it fascinating to look back in the older medical literature, when the observations of patients formed the basis of clinical writings and practice. Such observations are now called "anecdotal" information and devalued in importance. I have included Dr. Frank's original description of the PMS syndrome he recognized from *observing and listening to his patients.* I think it is important for several reasons. First, dietary habits in the United States in 1931 included far more fresh fruits and vegetables, and less refined sugar, alcohol, and caffeine than is typical today; yet women are describing the same experiences then and now. So, while dietary factors play a role in *aggravating* PMS symptoms, I do not think they are the primary *cause* of PMS. The language Dr. Frank used in 1931 is somewhat different from words I would use today, but notice how similar his description is to what women continue to describe in 2000. Over the last seventy years since Dr. Frank's article, nothing much has changed in *women's described experiences,* so why would we even question whether PMS is real or not? Yet, you will still hear people arguing over this issue and saying PMS is a psychological problem without evidence of a hormonal cause.

DESCRIPTION OF PMS: 1931

The group of women to whom I refer especially complain of a feeling of indescribable tension, from ten to seven days preceding menstruation, which in most instances continues until a time that the menstrual flow occurs. The patients complain of unrest, irritability, feeling like jumping out of their skin, and a desire to find relief by foolish and ill-considered actions. Their personal suffering is intense and it manifests itself in many reckless, and sometimes, reprehensible actions. Not only do they realize their own suffering, but they feel conscience-stricken toward their husbands and families, knowing well that they are unbearable in their attitudes and their reactions. Within an hour or two after the onset of the menstrual flow complete relief from both physical and mental tension occurs. —ROBERT T. FRANK, M.D.

It is important to note that the key defining characteristic of PMS is the *cyclicity* of symptoms, which then resolve around the onset of menses. PMS alone occurs prior to menstruation, and the bleeding phase itself is usually painless. PMS is **not** menstrual pain and cramps. The medical term for menstrual pain is *dysmenorrhea*, and it is another disorder altogether, although it may coexist with PMS in a small percentage of women. This is the widely used operational definition of PMS now:

CURRENT MEDICAL DEFINITION OF PMS

A pattern of recurring mood, behavioral, and physical symptoms which regularly occurs between ovulation and menstruation (in the luteal phase) and abates by the end of menstruation to then be followed by a symptom-free interval each month. Symptoms are present for at least six months, cause moderate to severe disruption in normal functioning, and are not due to another disorder.

PMS, which is *cyclic,* is also different from major depressive disorder, which is a *sustained* pattern of depressed, dysphoric mood and physical symptoms. I will discuss major depression in the next section. PMS as a recurring pattern of symptoms that may *include anxiety attacks*, is also different from panic disorder or dysthymic disorder, which are ongoing disorders without a clear pattern of relationship to the premenstrual phase of the cycle. Before concluding that a woman has PMS, the physician needs to rule out other medical disorders that may mimic the symptoms of PMS, such as thyroid problems, diabetes, and others.

Common Symptom Clusters in PMS

There have been over 150 symptoms described as part of PMS, but these can be grouped into a few common *patterns* of symptoms. I have designated several major categories: *affective (mood), behavioral, autonomic, fluid/electrolyte, dermatological, cognitive (brain), pain, and an "other" group*. The list below features some of the frequently reported symptoms in each category. Not every woman will have all of these symptoms, but for each woman there is usually a typical pattern, and the same symptoms tend to recur with each cycle. Sometimes the symptoms for one person may begin soon after ovulation and continue until menses; in other women the symptoms begin about the peak of luteal phase rise in estrogen and progesterone (about Day 21 or 22), a week before the period. Pattern of onset may vary from woman to woman but tends to stay about the same in a given person from one cycle to another, which is why symptom logs kept daily for several cycles are so helpful in making a correct diagnosis of PMS.

PMS SYMPTOM CLUSTERS

AFFECTIVE: depression, irritability, anxiety, angry outbursts, tearfulness, panicky feelings

BEHAVIORAL: impulsive actions, compulsions, agitation, lethargy, decreased motivation

AUTONOMIC: palpitations, nausea, constipation, dizziness, sweating, tremors, blurred vision, hot flashes

FLUID/ELECTROLYTE: bloating, water weight gain, breast fullness, hands and feet swelling

DERMATOLOGICAL: acne, oily hair, hives and rashes, herpes outbreaks, allergy outbreaks

COGNITIVE (BRAIN): decreased concentration, memory changes, word-retrieval problems, fuzzy thinking, foggy brain feelings

PAIN: migraines, tension headaches, back pain, muscle and joint aches, breast pain, neck stiffness, and pain

OTHER: drug/alcohol abuse, food binges, hypersomnia, or insomnia

© Elizabeth Lee Vliet, M.D., 1955

What Are Some of the Causes of PMS?

In spite of clinical evidence of *physiological* changes as the underlying disturbance, most medical textbooks, researchers, and physicians have attributed PMS symptoms to *psychological or sociological causes*—such as women's failure to accept the female role. Though psychological factors may *intensify* the patient's suffering, they do not *cause* the syndrome. Dr. Samuel Yen and other current researchers who have systematically studied PMS think that it is a *neuroendocrine imbalance*. The underlying mechanism involves neuroendocrine triggers within the hypothalamus and pituitary that then affect the function of such neurotransmitters as *serotonin (ST), norepinephrine (NE), dopamine (DA),* and *acetylcholine (ACh)* (see chapters 3 and 4).

The diversity of symptoms in PMS is caused by the many different brain centers and the whole series of pituitary and hypothalamic neuropeptide hormones governed by these neurotransmitters (TSH, FSH, ACTH, beta-endorphin, and alpha melanocyte stimulating [MSH] hormone and others). The neuropeptides beta-endorphin and MSH not only regulate the neurotransmitters involved in mood and behavior, but they also modulate pituitary release of other hormones such as prolactin and vasopressin, which produce a number of physical and mood effects on the brain and body. The brain-body regulation of progesterone and estrogen in response to these changes in neuropeptides differs from woman to woman and I think accounts for the various clinical forms of PMS. As better-designed studies are done, I think we will find that **hormone ratios** and **rate of change** are key factors triggering the diverse brain-mediated symptoms of PMS.

Dr. Katharina Dalton, the British pioneer who has studied PMS patients for more than thirty years, *hypothesized* that a deficiency of progesterone relative to the amount of estrogen present before menstruation triggers the syndrome. Dr. Dalton found that some women with PMS respond well to large doses of natural progesterone, but PMS researchers and clinicians have not found this to be consistently true. Dr. Dalton's theory, however, was not based on actual measurements of hormone levels in the manner I have described in my book. In my clinical experience of actually measuring the luteal phase hormone levels in several thousand PMS patients, I have found that the most common pattern is *low* estradiol and normal progesterone levels. Thus, I have found that Dr. Dalton's theory did not hold up under closer scrutiny and use of objective laboratory measures. I think this is one reason researchers and physicians report such mixed results about the use of progesterone to treat PMS: The treatment is applied across the board to all the PMS patients in the study, regardless of whether they actually had low-luteal phase progesterone levels or not.

In the patients of our practice, I have not found progesterone alone to be very helpful, but this is what you would expect if the progesterone levels are normal and it is the estradiol that has declined. If I do find a patient who has low progesterone levels in the luteal phase and has normal estradiol levels, then I would use progesterone, and I would expect it to alleviate the symptoms. But in many women, the declining estradiol is a more crucial factor. The clear pattern of hormone profiles in the majority of my patients is one of *low* estradiol (E2) and relatively normal levels of progesterone (P), so that there is a reduced ratio of E2 to P. If this is the pattern on the laboratory studies, then it only makes sense to boost estradiol back to optimal ranges rather than adding progesterone as a first step. In these women, adding progesterone actually makes them worse. Several recent double-blind, placebo-controlled studies have shown that natural progesterone is not any better than placebo in reducing PMS symptoms, and this has been my clinical experience as well. Consequently, I think there is much more to PMS, than just progesterone deficiency. In addition, the many different responses of women to a variety of hormonal approaches suggest we need a more encompassing theory of cause. I view PMS as a neuroendocrine disorder that begins with physiological hormonal shifts affecting multiple brain centers. The brain events then trigger a variety of physical changes in multiple systems in the body and can be aggravated by diet, substance use, and life stress.

Many women describe their worst days in the cycle as being the day prior to bleeding and the first day bleeding begins. Tearfulness, crying spells, fragmented sleep, anxiety attacks, palpitations, and irritability typically are intensified for these two or three days. What causes the elevated frequency of symptoms on these two specified perimenstrual days is not known with certainty. Based on my knowledge of brain chemistry, it seems most likely that these are triggered by the *falling and low estrogen*. It is interesting that the estrogen levels reach their bottom point of the cycle close to the day before the onset of menses and are still low on Day 1 of bleeding. Low levels of estrogen are known to coincide with both *low endorphin levels* and *high* levels of monoamine oxidase enzymes (MAO), which break down catecholamines, resulting in catecholamine depletion in the brain. Loss of catecholamines is a significant factor in precipitating depressive mood changes. The decrease in endorphins contributes to the irritability, tearfulness, and restless sleep.

Dr. E. L. Klaiber and colleagues found that a series of premenopausal women with regular menstrual cycles who suffered from a major depressive illness had higher levels of plasma MAO activity (which breaks down and inactivates catecholamines and serotonin) than did *nondepressed* women. Dr. Klaiber interpreted these abnormalities as further evidence of norepinephrine/serotonin insufficiency consistent with current biological theories of depression. His study did not attempt to evaluate the therapeutic effectiveness of the estrogen therapy, but all of the patients who received estrogen therapy reported "moderate to marked" improvement in their moods. In another study of women with treatment refractory depression, Dr. Klaiber's group found that oral estrogen therapy was significantly effective in improving mood in women who had not responded to more traditional antidepressant medications. Taken together with the other evidence I have described in chapters 3 and 4, Dr. Klaiber's research lends additional support to the role of premenopausal decline in estrogen as a contributing factor in the PMS-perimenopause continuum of mood and physical symptoms.

There is an additional mechanism by which perimenopausal women may experience anxiety attacks and depressive mood changes: This is related to the drop in estrogen levels, which triggers hot flashes that cause multiple awakenings at night. Nocturnal hot flashes causing waking episodes can be objectively measured in sleep laboratories; these waking episodes caused by surges of adrenaline trigger hot flashes that have been confirmed on EEG brain-wave recordings during sleep. Such waking episodes result in sleep deprivation, a factor associated with irritable, depressive mood changes. Eighty to 85 percent of women experience hot flashes that typically occur at night for several years prior to the beginning of skipped periods in perimenopause. The resulting sleep disturbances, coupled with unhealthy lifestyle habits, could contribute significantly to disturbances in mood (irritability and depression), loss of energy, reduced concentration and memory, fatigue, and diminished sense of well-being. I have listed the four *key* antidepressant actions of estradiol again in the chart below. Unpleasant changes like ones I just described respond best to a *boost in estradiol*, rather than antidepressants, antianxiety medications, or sleeping pills.

ESTRADIOL: ANTIDEPRESSANT EFFECTS

- Increases serotonin levels and receptors
- Increases endorphin activity
- Inhibits MAO enzyme activity, which prolongs activity of ST, DA, NE
- Enhances binding of tricyclic antidepressants at brain receptors

---

PMS, ESTRADIOL, AND SEROTONIN (ST)

- Rate of rise and fall in E2: *crucial* variable in effects on serotonin
- A more rapid rise or fall in E2 causes greater change in ST
- E2 effect on serotonin is a probable trigger for premenstrual migraine and mood changes

(see chapter 10)

© Elizabeth Lee Vliet, M.D., 1955

There are other postulated causes of PMS, but these may also be *results* of the neuroendocrine changes I have already described, so it is unclear whether some of these disturbances are causes of the syndrome or are results of alterations in the reproductive hormone levels:

- altered glucose metabolism perhaps due to alterations in glucocorticoids and/or insulin activity, or the effect of excess progeserone relative to estradiol;
- abnormal fatty acid metabolism resulting in altered tissue sensitivity to reproductive hormones;
- abnormalities in the prolactin, aldosterone, renin, angiotensin, and vasopressin that govern normal fluid and electrolyte balance in the body.

Other factors that may be involved in the rising incidence of PMS in recent years, and *adversely amplify* menstrual cycle hormonal changes, are as follows:

1. The fact that many women are postponing pregnancy and having fewer pregnancies than women did years ago, resulting in more

years of ovulatory cycles, which are clearly associated with a higher incidence of PMS;

2. The significant increase in obesity in our society, which results in increased conversion of androgens in body fat to the estrone type of estrogen in women. This alters the total estrogen-to-progesterone ratio but does not provide the higher level of 17-beta estradiol produced in the ovary, which now appears to be the primary active estrogen at brain receptors. The majority of women suffering from PMS are obese, defined as more than 20 percent over ideal body weight;

3. In addition to the problem with obesity, our cultural emphasis on extreme thinness has resulted in younger, thin women having premature decline in ovarian hormones due to *loss* of the minimum amount of body fat to maintain normal, ovulatory function of the ovaries. Women who are overly thin, *and* eat an extremely low fat diet, furthermore do not have the necessary building blocks of cholesterol needed for the ovary to make its hormones. In these women, we often see a low luteal phase estradiol, even if progesterone levels are still in the normal ranges.

4. For the majority of women today, the typical American diet is high in saturated fat, salt, refined sugars, alcohol, and caffeinated beverages, all of which have been shown to significantly aggravate the symptoms of PMS;

5. Most American women today have a deficit of magnesium in their diets, which also contributes to PMS symptoms, due to magnesium's role as an important cofactor in the synthesis of mood-elevating neurotransmitters and mood stabilization;

6. Inadequate intake of vitamin B6 (pyridoxine), which is also a cofactor in the synthesis of mood-elevating neurotransmitters and is involved in the liver metabolism of estrogen and progesterone.

In summary, I think our current research findings lend more support to the integrated theory of PMS being triggered by the brain effects of ovarian hormones, with multiple brain-body systems then being affected and leading to the wide variety of symptoms. This integrated model makes sense to me physiologically, and approaching it from an integrated point of view helps me to develop a more systematic, and physiological, approach to helping women feel better and deal constructively with the menstrual cycle hormonal shifts.

Is It the Blues, the Blahs, or Major Depression?

Nearly everyone has occasional down, moody times, or bouts of sadness and discouragement that may last for a while. When do the "blues and blahs" become major depressive disorder, a clinical depressive illness requiring professional intervention and possibly medication? When a black mood settles in and remains for several weeks, sapping your energy, appetite, your interest in life and activities you usually enjoy, and altering your sleep, you may be clinically depressed.

Clinical depression is a medical illness that is thought to have a primarily physical cause, that of a chemical imbalance in the neurotransmitter or "messenger" molecules in the brain. The illness of depression is two to three times more common in women, with the gender differences beginning in puberty and ending after menopause, when rates of depression become higher in males. This gender difference implicates a hormonal factor, which has not been addressed as an important connection in women's depression.

In spite of major advances in our understandings of the neurobiology of depression, and the development of new and safer antidepressant medications, physicians and the lay public still labor under the misconception that the "chin up and get through it" approach is all that is needed. In fact, according to a recent poll by the National Alliance for the Mentally Ill, the American public still has many mistaken beliefs about mental illness in general:

- 71 percent believe it is due to emotional weakness
- 65 percent believe it is caused by bad parenting
- 45 percent believe it's the victim's fault, can be willed away
- 43 percent believe it is incurable
- 35 percent believe it is the consequence of sinful behavior
- only 10 percent BELIEVE IT HAS A BIOLOGICAL BASIS and involves brain chemistry (in spite of much publicity on this over the past thirty years!)

Clinical depression is a very common disorder, affecting 20–30 percent of adults sometime during their lifetime. Experts estimate that at any given time, some 10 million Americans are in its throes. Unfortunately, even today with so much good information available, depression is still all too frequently misunderstood by the general public and physicians alike. Many people who suffer from depression are too embarrassed to seek help. A common expression I hear in my medical practice is "I feel like I'm weak. I should be able to handle this by myself." Such self-blaming, negative thought patterns are *often a symptom of depression* but the person doesn't recognize these thought patterns as due to the illness, and so has difficulty asking for help.

Lack of proper treatment causes not only untold suffering, lost productivity, and diminished quality of life, but is also a major risk factor in suicide. Fifteen percent of people with clinical depression commit suicide. This is a tragic loss when we consider that treatment of depression is successful for 80 to 90 percent of sufferers, with *proper diagnosis* and careful use of medication. **The lifetime risk of death from major depressive illness due to suicide is greater than the lifetime risk of death from breast cancer.**

This physical, or biological, form of depression is not likely to be cured by "talk" therapies alone. Antidepressant medication to reestablish the normal chemical balance in the brain is now considered to be the most effective treatment. Proper medical diagnosis is needed to identify this form of depression and rule out other medical causes for the symptoms, such as hypothyroidism, diabetes, lupus, and perhaps a hundred or more medical problems and medications that have been found to cause a syndrome indistinguishable from primary major depressive disorders. Overuse of alcohol, caffeine, nicotine, decongestants, phenylpropanolamine diet pills, herbal products containing *ephedra,* and illicit drugs (cocaine, stimulants, hallucinogens, and others) may also cause biological depressions. Severe and *prolonged life stress,* even though "understandable," may cause enough biochemical changes in the brain and body to result in depressive illness needing medication and psychotherapy. After a careful medical history, physical examination, and appropriate blood tests rule out these other causes, your physician may recommend antidepressant medication, which can alleviate sustained and severe depressions even though they may be clearly related to life stress.

How do you tell if what you are experiencing is just the normal "blues" or a clinical depression? DURATION of symptoms is one important key. If your mood remains down, blue, sad, discouraged, or hopeless for *more than two weeks,* in spite of pleasant events in your life, clinical depression is likely. People with clinical depression may also describe feeling "numb," "leaden," or like "I'm just going through the motions" of life. Women have said to me " I feel like I'm trying to move my body through quicksand." Another woman said she felt like her body "weighed a thousand pounds, it was just hard to even start moving."

Presence of SOMATIC (physical) or VEGETATIVE changes occur, such as significant loss or gain of weight for no apparent reason or changes in your sleep pattern (trouble falling asleep; problems with multiple awakenings at night; or waking up very early, unable to go back to sleep). Loss of energy, feeling "keyed up" and "hyper," or feeling very "slowed down" and "sluggish" are other signs, along with changes in your ability to concentrate on tasks, loss of sex drive, fatigue, menstrual irregularities, marked decrease or increase in appetite with compulsive overeating, GI upset, constipation or diarrhea, and loss of interest or pleasure in your usual activities.

THOUGHTS OF DEATH OR SUICIDE are very serious symptoms and should never be ignored, particularly if you begin to feel that you no longer care about living and think about ways of taking your life.

You *must* seek a qualified professional to help you if thoughts of suicide are present for any length of time. If a friend or family member tells you about such thoughts, even if they try to pass it off as a joke, you should take it seriously and bring it to the attention of someone who can get them to see a qualified mental health professional or physician for an evaluation. Studies are clear in showing that better than 90 percent of people who commit suicide *have told someone ahead of time that they had these thoughts,* but many were just not taken seriously and guided to professional help.

If you find that you have *five of the above symptoms persisting more than two weeks,* it is important that you see your physician for help. Many people come into a physician's office with vague physical complaints and sidestep the real reason they are seeking help. This only leads to misdiagnosis and delay of proper treatment. Be direct. Tell your doctor that you feel depressed. Depression is just as much of an illness as diabetes, high blood pressure, and heart disease are. Depression can have physical, chemical, genetic, hormonal, medication, emotional, and situational causes. Help is available, and the newer antidepressants have typically very few side effects. Depression is NOT "weak character." You should not feel ashamed about having the illness of depression.

If your physician recommends an antidepressant, the serotonin-augmenting ones have few side effects and are quite effective. The serotonin-boosters are especially helpful for women in whom depression may be caused or aggravated by estrogen changes that appear to specifically decrease serotonin. Your doctor may also recommend counseling or psychotherapy to help you deal more effectively with the stresses in your life. I think other effective, helpful approaches are professionally led support groups, healthy eating, regular exercise, relaxation training, and/or meditation.

Since the large majority of patients with depression are seen by primary care physicians (often for vague somatic complaints) *rather than by psychiatrists,* I think it is crucial that YOU know how to recognize symptoms that could indicate the presence of a biological major depression, so you can tell your doctor. I also think it is imperative that we intensify efforts to help primary care physicians recognize milder forms of depression and begin to treat these syndromes appropriately, using antidepressant medications when indicated. Patient education brochures on depression are published by the National Institute of Mental Health and are available free. Simple screening questionnaires, such as the Zung Depression Inventory, are also available free from various sources and are valuable aids to you and your physicians to identify "masked" depression. I have included one of these self-tests for depression in appendix III.

I think it is crucial that we teach women that depression is a highly treatable biologically based disorder, and getting help early greatly reduces suffering and debilitation, as well as helps to reduce the economic burdens of excessive medical utilization and lost productivity in the workplace or at home. Yet, I do think ovarian, thyroid, and adrenal hormone levels should be carefully and completely checked before the diagnosis of major depression is made. If you find yourself feeling overwhelmed by life and slipping into a major depression, don't feel ashamed and withdraw or hesitate to ask for help. Clinical depression is a highly treatable medical condition—one that you should NOT have to suffer through alone.

Stress: Vicious Cycle Effects on Hormones, Anxiety, and Depression

In spite of the fact that we live in a culture that often times acts as if women don't have a brain, WE DO, and the brain is a *physiological* organ, as well as the *psychological* organ of "mind" expressing our personality, psyche, and behavior. It is affected by outside stressors (stimuli) and by internal stimuli or changes in the body, so that many times what are labeled psychological symptoms and *assumed to have a psychological cause* may in fact be *caused by biochemical* changes in our body's *physiological balance*. Likewise, psychological stress causes profound changes in every cell in the body, including brain chemistry.

For both men and women, stress of whatever form, whether it's external stressors or whether it's the internal stressors of physiological changes that require the body to change and adapt, all of us have the body as our "final common pathway" through which these changes act and operate. With prolonged stress the body's balance, or homeostasis, is disrupted, and we see symptoms that relate to adrenaline overactivity, such as headaches, high blood pressure, panic attacks, colitis, arteriosclerosis, eczema, overwhelming fatigue, and many others. We also see illnesses that are the result of long-term chronic stress having an adverse effect on the immune system, producing problems related to *hyperactivity* of the immune system such as asthma and allergies; problems related to a *hypoactive* immune system, such as cancers; and problems that arise when the immune system runs amuck and attacks your own body, such as the autoimmune disorders. All of these are manifestations of the combined effects of stress-induced biochemical changes on the body pathways, occurring over time.

Another aspect of the problem of stress when it affects women is the role of chronic stress in decreasing the normal function and hormone production of the ovaries, as well as the thyroid gland. At a meeting of the North American Menopause Society, Susan Ballinger, Ph.D., of Sydney, Australia, reported on her study addressing connections between women's perception of the presence of life stress and levels of their ovarian estrogens. Ballinger's study assessed life events, clinical depression, and anxiety, together with measurements of urinary and plasma estrogens. This study demonstrated that a high level of urinary estrogens correlated with higher psychosocial stress scores. Her conclusion was that "psychosocial stress, emotional vulnerability, and coping skills may all contribute to estrogen deficiency in post menopause."

From my clinical observations and correlation of the estrogen levels in perimenopausal women, the opposite hypothesis may also be true about the connection between hormone levels and stress, but we don't yet have much information on this half of the equation: Declining estrogen levels contribute to alterations in the function of norepinephrine, serotonin, dopamine, and acetylcholine that regulate mood, behavior, and cognitive function. Declining estrogen, and the subsequent effect on brain chemical messengers, appears to then contribute to the observed difficulty coping with psychosocial stressors by women who have previously been able to cope successfully. Once again, the role of stress is a two-way street: Life stress suppresses the ovaries, which decrease estrogen production, which affects sleep, and so on. Normal declines in estrogen affect brain chemistry, which affects ability to cope with stress. It's another one of those vicious cycles, as I have diagrammed in the next section.

How Are All of These Phenomena Related?

Since I am such a "visual" learner, I decided to give you a diagram (*see following page*) that represents how I see these various stress and hormone factors coming together to cause some of the phenomena, or symptoms, we experience. I see it as a vicious cycle, with one event affecting another until it all snowballs on us. Think about these various pieces of the puzzle as they relate to your life, and your lifestyle habits, and see if it helps you identify some healthy ways to break the cycle.

How Can I Tell What My Problem Is?
Getting Checked Out

PMS is commonly not recognized or is misdiagnosed, so it is important for you to seek a thorough evaluation. There are many diagnoses given to women who, in fact, have PMS: Some of these are dysthymic disorder, manic-depressive illness, major depressive disorder, atypical depression, chronic fatigue, chronic candidiasis, panic

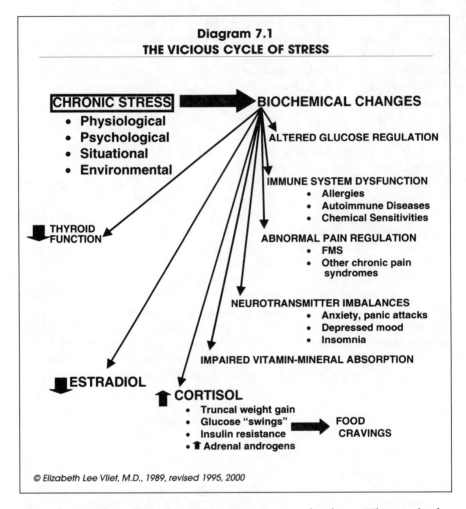

Diagram 7.1
THE VICIOUS CYCLE OF STRESS

CHRONIC STRESS ➡ BIOCHEMICAL CHANGES
- Physiological
- Psychological   ALTERED GLUCOSE REGULATION
- Situational
- Environmental

IMMUNE SYSTEM DYSFUNCTION
- Allergies
- Autoimmune Diseases
- Chemical Sensitivities

THYROID
FUNCTION

ABNORMAL PAIN REGULATION
- FMS
- Other chronic pain
  syndromes

NEUROTRANSMITTER IMBALANCES
- Anxiety, panic attacks
- Depressed mood
- Insomnia

IMPAIRED VITAMIN-MINERAL ABSORPTION

ESTRADIOL

CORTISOL
- Truncal weight gain
- Glucose "swings" ➡ FOOD
- Insulin resistance   CRAVINGS
- ⬆ Adrenal androgens

© Elizabeth Lee Vliet, M.D., 1989, revised 1995, 2000

disorder, anxiety disorder, stress reaction, and others. The goal of a comprehensive evaluation is also to make certain that you do not have another medical problem causing similar symptoms, and to ensure that any previously unrecognized secondary disorders, which may be contributing to your symptoms, are diagnosed and properly treated.

If you are having difficulty feeling that your PMS concerns are taken seriously, you may find a specialty clinic for PMS would provide more helpful resources and suggestions. I have designed the ℋℰℛ Place programs in Tucson, Arizona, and Dallas–Ft.Worth, Texas, to help women get hormone levels properly tested and to identify dietary, lifestyle, hormone, and alternative therapies to alleviate troublesome symptoms. The chart below lists aspects of a complete evaluation, and points to discuss with your physician.

COMPONENTS OF A COMPREHENSIVE PMS EVALUATION

I. MEDICAL HISTORY. Key aspects include:

1. Timing of symptoms (onset, duration, when end)
2. Symptom cluster (types of problems you encounter with your cycle)
3. Onset in relation to some hormonal change (puberty, pregnancy, starting or stopping oral contraceptives, perimenopause)
4. Time of increased severity of symptoms (usually following discontinuation of oral contraceptives, after tubal ligation, following hysterectomy without removal of ovaries, after a pregnancy, after cessation of breastfeeding, or after several months of no menses)
5. History of threatened or actual miscarriage, "toxemia" (pre-eclampsia): 86 percent of women with pre-eclampsia developed PMS in the months following birth
6. History of postpartum depression of sufficient severity to require antidepressant treatment. In one study of 100 women treated for severe PMS, 73 percent had a history of significant postpartum depression
7. Weight fluctuations in adult life greater than twenty-five pounds. Obesity increases the likelihood of PMS for reasons that are still unclear, but may be related to increased estrone production in body fat
8. History of past thyroid problems and/or treatment with thyroid hormone
9. History of painless menstruation (*painful* menses is a different problem called dysmenorrhea and is more often due to endometriosis)
10. Pattern of food or alcohol cravings and/or alcohol intolerance during premenstrual phase of cycle
11. Inability to tolerate high-progestin birth control pills. Women with PMS often experience severe side effects and/or exacerbation of PMS with high progestin oral contraceptives, particularly the triphasic pills with changing hormone content
12. Increased libido. Women with PMS frequently report increased sex drive during the premenstrual phase, compared to women with primary depression who usually report diminished sex drive

II. FAMILY HISTORY

Note presence of similar problems, especially among women in family, such as diabetes; thyroid disease; multiple allergies; autoimmune diseases; disorders such as alcoholism, depression, and/or mania; anxiety disorders; and eating disorders (anorexia, bulimia). All of these have been associated with increased risk of menstrually related mood and physical changes seen in PMS.

III. MEDICAL AND PSYCHOLOGICAL EVALUATION

1. Physical examination (if not recently done by gynecologist or primary care physician), with attention to any signs of hormone imbalance
2. Laboratory tests: blood chemistry panel, complete blood count (CBC), thyroid profile with TSH and thyroid antibodies, prolactin, FSH, LH, progesterone, estradiol, testosterone, other lab tests as medically appropriate and indicated by history and physical findings
3. Psychological assessment of emotional and cognitive function, with rating scales such as Beck, Hamilton, or Zung Depression/Anxiety Scales; Profile of Mood States (POMS), Hopkins SCL-90, PRISM Menstrual Calendar, etc.
4. Daily Symptom Log/Journal through at least one and preferably 2-3 menstrual cycles. Should include:
   a. MENSTRUAL SYMPTOMS, WEIGHT, BODY TEMPERATURE
   b. Dietary intake log relating food intake to time of symptoms
   c. Record of alcohol, caffeine, and tobacco use
   d. Record of over-the-counter and prescription medication use

You and your physician should review this information and discuss the various options available that would be helpful to you. I find that a combination of approaches works best. The section that follows lists options to consider, or you may use others that your physician recommends.

Options for Feeling Better

There are a variety of approaches that will help you recapture your sense of well-being and zest. At the most basic level, you really can't expect *anything* to help a great deal unless you first address constructive lifestyle changes to reduce or eliminate potential triggers and aggravators that make you feel worse if you have PMS. Basic and simple, yet many times not done, are the dietary modifications that have been found to be of help in eliminating many PMS symptoms. Frequently I find that it is difficult to get patients to accept that something as "simple" as changing the way they eat can have a profound impact on the way they feel—their mood, energy level, clarity of thinking—BUT IT DOES! The following suggestions are tried and true. They DO work, but you first have to commit to really giving it your best effort for *long enough* to see a difference. I found that when I paid close attention to these basics, I was able to eliminate just about all of my own PMS problems. I admit I wasn't perfect all the time, but these steps do make a big difference. So, before you ask your doctor for medication or rush out for an herbal fix, make certain you try these.

I. Dietary Changes to Diminish PMS

1. Avoid simple sugars (you know what I am talking about: all those sweets that just seem to stick to your fingers!); reduce salt; cut out alcohol, caffeine, nicotine, and *chocolate—especially just before your period.*
2. Increase intake of complex carbohydrates to 40–50 percent of total daily calorie intake (have a low-fat, low-sugar, high-fiber bran muffin instead of a brownie).
3. Decrease intake of protein to about 20–30 percent of total daily calories, and concentrate on the low-fat protein sources—fish, chicken, low-fat cheese.
4. Space meals properly. Symptoms seen to be worsened by long intervals between food intake, perhaps due to the alterations in glucose tolerance seen in the premenstrual phase. More frequent eating, with smaller portions and less of the simple sugars, also reduces the tendency for women with PMS to crave and binge on sweets.

II. EXERCISE PROGRAM.

I can't say it enough: MOVE THE BODY! Exercise is great medicine! When I do it, I feel like a different person; when I don't, I feel sluggish. Our bodies were designed to be active. I educate women about the physiological and psychological effects of exercise that are of benefit in PMS: increase in beta-endorphin, stimulation of NE, reduction of excess anxiety, stabilization of serum glucose, suppression of appetite, increase in energy, improvement of mood, enhancement of sexual energy. I teach women how to safely begin an aerobic exercise activity and how to monitor pulse rate for optimum effect. You don't have to be a marathon runner to get the benefits of increased physical activity. Walking will do it, especially if you have been inactive. If you have any limitations due to medical problems, talk with your physician and get a referral for a trained physical therapist to help you get started with an appropriate program.

III. STRESS MANAGEMENT

Take a look now at the Vicious Cycle diagrams in chapter 17. Stress plays a direct role in negatively influencing the chemical messengers that are out of balance and contribute to PMS in the first place. Look for ways of reducing avoidable stresses, and look for ways you can minimize the adverse effects of unavoidable stresses. One of the techniques I teach my patients is the relaxation response, popularized by Dr. Herbert Benson but used down through hundreds of years in many cultures. You can elicit the relaxation response using a variety of techniques: visualization, progressive muscle relaxation, self-hypnosis, autogenic conditioning, meditation, and others. There are many good books and tapes available to guide you in using these approaches.

Counseling for stress management techniques may be helpful for some women, especially during times when it feels like life is running you over! Getting an outside perspective on what you can do helps you feel more in control, which then decreases the body's fight-or-flight stress response that intensifies PMS.

Another good stress management technique is having massage therapy during the premenstrual week. Therapeutic massage is an excellent way of improving relaxation, boosting endorphins, improving circulation, and decreasing muscle tension, headaches, and back pain. Look for a registered, certified therapeutic massage therapist in your phone book under American Association of Massage Therapists, or call the A.A.M.T. toll-free number for a member therapist in your area. Acupuncture may also be helpful for some of these stress and PMS symptoms, although this modality does not usually have the more rapid onset of beneficial effect, as do the relaxation techniques and therapeutic massage. Acupuncture, to be most effective, typically requires a series of treatments.

IV. Medication Approaches

VITAMINS

A variety of vitamin combinations have been reported to help alleviate PMS symptoms, but there have not been clear-cut benefits found in controlled studies. I think particularly if you are under a great deal of stress, which depletes the B group and vitamin C, adding a low dose of B complex supplement at least during the premenstrual week can be helpful for some women. Pyridoxine (B6) has been recommended and reported to ease some of the symptoms of PMS if used in conjunction with diet and exercise. We are not sure how pyridoxine achieves these effects, except that it is a cofactor in many chemical reactions, including those involved in making dopamine and serotonin, and it inhibits prolactin metabolism. B6 may modulate the action of dopamine and serotonin in the chain of reactions that regulate production of estrogen and progesterone. It is also involved in the metabolism of estrogen by the liver and in the metabolism of fats and carbohydrates.

The usual starting dose of B6 is 50 mg per day. Although some herbal practitioners and naturopaths say that you cannot overdose or become toxic on the water-soluble B vitamins, it has been well documented that excessive supplementation of the B vitamins (particularly B6) may cause neurological problems. **Do not exceed 50 mg per day because of the risk of peripheral neuropathy (numbness, paresthesias, tingling).**

I have found it is better to supplement the **B complex vitamins as a group** in one supplement rather than taking just vitamin B6, because the B complex needs to be present in the proper balance and ratio in order to work optimally. There are now a number of commercial vitamin formulas that have been theoretically designed for the special needs of women with PMS. Although these are usually more expensive than the general brands sold at the pharmacy, they may provide the balance of vitamins and minerals needed by some women. You may want to consider one of these options.

DIURETICS

Many doctors have used the thiazide diuretics (hydrochlorothiazide (HCTZ), Dyazide, Maxide, and others) to alleviate the fluid retention some women experience in the premenstrual week. The thiazides are *not* the diuretics I recommend, because they further increase potassium loss and may actually aggravate PMS symptoms. They also tend to interfere with normal glucose balance and may increase cholesterol.

If you are someone who clearly experiences documented premenstrual weight gain, bloating, and breast tenderness due to fluid retention, I think the only diuretic that makes *physiological* sense to use is *spironolactone* (brand name: Aldactone). The usual dosage is 50 mg (25 mg twice a day) to 100 mg a day (taken in divided doses as 25 mg four times a day, because it is a shorter-acting medication). Spironolactone acts on the fluid-regulating hormone (aldosterone), which is altered by progesterone in the luteal phase of the cycle, leading to fluid shifts. I do not find that most women with PMS need a diuretic if hormonal balance and diet are improved. If you still have fluid retention, however, I think spironolactone is the better choice than a thiazide diuretic.

ORAL CONTRACEPTIVES (OCS).

I find that the steady-dose (monophasic) OCs can provide a marked degree of symptom relief in a large percentage of women, especially pre- and perimenopausal nonsmoking women who are experiencing diminishing estrogen production and erratic cycles. I have found over the years that the key to using OCs in PMS is to start with a pill formulation with *the least possible progestin* (the culprit for most of the unwanted side effects) and a little better level of estrogen. Many of the ones that are commonly recommended are the pills that are *higher* in progestin, and *lower* in estrogen, which is the *reverse* of what a woman over thirty needs. The three OC pill options on the market in the United States that I have found produce the best results in reducing PMS are: Ovcon-35 (least progestin), Modicon, and Brevicon (next lowest amount of progestin). A new OC Diane-35, available in Canada, has a unique progestin/estrogen combination designed to reduce acne by blocking the androgen receptor. Using the OCs during the perimenopause transition was approved by the FDA for nonsmokers just a few years ago, and the OCs have added *health benefits* of decreasing the risk of ovarian and endometrial cancers, uterine fibroids, and fibrocystic breast changes. Perimenopausal use of monophasic OCs also helps maintain adequate estradiol levels to prevent bone loss. You MUST NOT SMOKE if you take the oral contraceptives, because smoking increases the risk of stroke and blood clots in women who take oral contraceptives.

Conventional teaching has been that women with PMS don't do well on the birth control pills due to the **synthetic progestin,** which can aggravate PMS. I have found that this is true *if the progestin content is higher than 0.5mg norethindrone* (or equivalent progestational activity). If one of my patients decides to try the birth control pill to reduce PMS, I prescribe *only* the low progestin formulas. There are still some women who can't take even the lowest amount of synthetic progestin, but in my experience, this has been a minority. For women who cannot take the synthetic progestins at all, natural progesterone may work, and I talk about this further along in this section.

You might find it helpful to listen to the voices of my patients who have benefited from using oral contraceptives to alleviate the midlife PMS:

A forty-seven-year-old white female described her health as "much better. It's Christmas and I am not sick, and that's different from the past three years. I think the hormones [Ovcon-35] are helping me feel a whole lot better. It was really good to find out that there really is something there, I'm not imagining things. I am feeling really good."

A forty-three-year-old woman who developed severe depression on Loestrin oral contraceptive had these comments several months after changing to a higher estrogen/lower progestin pill, Ovcon-35: "I felt much better, I'm not crying, I don't feel depressed, I have my energy, I don't have those headaches. I really have noticed an incredible difference. I have been able to exercise again, and I wasn't able to do that on the other pill [Loestrin] because I just didn't have the energy. I felt wiped out all the time.

A fifty-year-old woman said: "The birth control pills were heaven sent. Since I started taking them, I have not had any cramps, the bleeding is less, the depression is much better, that black cloud has lifted, and that's been wonderful. I'm as pain free as I have ever been with my periods. The minute I started taking them I could tell a difference. I have had only very mild PMS feelings, but the moods going up and down has gotten better. I am so grateful to you that I feel so good.

A thirty-six-year-old woman, now on the monophasic oral contraceptive, said her physician was against her taking the hormones because of family history of breast cancer in her grandmother, "but I discussed it and felt like this was right for me and I decided to do this. I am much, much better. It's been three weeks on the new pills, I am sleeping through the night, the crying spells are almost completely gone even though I have a reason to cry because a family member almost died of a brain abscess and I flew to another city to take care of him. I handled it really well. I don't have the *crying-for-no-reason* spells like I used to. I'm like a different person, a great decrease in anxiety, I'm not irritable, the GI symptoms have resolved, I have enough energy I'm exercising in the morning going to the gym, my mood's even, my secretary even said I seem a lot happier, I feel more focused, and my memory is somewhat better and I am getting more organized at work. I am ecstatic about my improvement, I can't thank you enough. I'm glad to know I wasn't crazy when I was having all the things I was experiencing.

There are some added benefits, and reduced medical costs, for the last woman who described her experience beginning the oral contraceptives. She has been able to stop taking the sleeping pills and daily Xanax she had been using; she has had no further migraine-type headaches, which had required numerous trips to the ER for injections to treat the severe pain; her moderate incontinence has resolved without her needing the urological consultation her previous physician had recommended; *and* she is enjoying improved quality of life. Pretty good results for about $25.00 a month.

PROGESTERONE.

The use of natural progesterone, as opposed to the synthetic progestational agents found in oral contraceptives, has been recommended by Dr. Dalton in Britain, who has used it successfully for PMS relief in her patients. There are no controlled studies demonstrating its effectiveness. Progesterone has not yet been approved by the FDA for PMS, but then I can't think of *any* of the currently widely used medications for PMS that have been approved by the FDA specifically for use in PMS therapy. The most recently published double-blind, placebo-controlled study of natural progesterone for PMS again showed that progesterone was no better than placebo to reduce symptoms. These results are in contrast to the successes reported by Dr. Dalton; no one seems to be certain of the reasons for the differences. One explanation appears to be that Dr. Dalton's recommended progesterone doses are quite high and therefore exert *pharmacologic* effects beyond the natural *physiologic* effects of this hormone.

Progesterone has been helpful for some women, and the rationale for its use is its effects on the brain pathways involved in producing PMS symptoms. Progesterone inhibits norepinephrine release and reuptake (an antianxiety action), it alters dopamine neurotransmission, and has an anticonvulsant effect at levels in the normal range for the luteal phase. At higher doses, metabolites of progesterone produce an antianxiety effect by also increasing the inhibitory neurotransmitter, GABA, the same way the tranquilizers Valium and Xanax work. Progesterone used for PMS is usually given in the pharmacologic range to exert these antianxiety effects. Such doses produce circulating levels of progesterone much higher than normal for the menstrual cycle. In fact, based on studies in the 1970s, it takes only an oral dose of 300 mg daily to reach blood levels like those seen in the last stage of pregnancy, when progesterone levels are at their highest. At these drug-equivalent doses, progesterone acts on the brain as a **sedative**, and also has anesthetic properties. **If you have a history of major depression, or a family history of depressive illnesses, be cautious about using progesterone for PMS, since it may trigger an episode of major depression in these higher doses.**

In my opinion, progesterone (like estrogen or testosterone) should not be used lightly or without good, knowledgeable medical supervision. Even though it is a natural hormone, if you take more than you need, or you already have certain medical conditions, you may find yourself with multiple unwanted side effects. Progesterone creams and PMS doses can actually be risky for diabetics and women with existing weight gain problems. Current studies have shown that even over-the-counter progesterone creams can give very high blood levels that persist for a number of weeks after stopping use of the cream. I have treated numerous patients who had exaggerated PMS, depressive symptoms, worsening diabetes and allergies, increase in yeast infections, worsening fatigue, and loss of libido from high doses of progesterone. Stopping progesterone abruptly causes a withdrawal syndrome just like stopping Valium, Xanax or alcohol abruptly, because the same brain receptors and pathways are involved.

Women who have declining estradiol but normal progesterone levels may actually become significantly depressed if large doses of progesterone are used for PMS. I have other concerns about long-term progesterone at the high doses used for PMS, since we don't have good data about the potential adverse effects on breast tissue when it is used continuously in supernatural amounts. Remember, in the normal menstrual cycle, progesterone is present for only about *half* the cycle. In addition, using progesterone for a week or ten days and then stopping it with menstruation can cause mood changes that result from the combined endorphin-serotonin drops triggered by estradiol and progesterone dropping sharply at the same time. If you are using natural progesterone and have *more* symptoms of tearfulness, irritability, and anxiety during menses after stopping progesterone, you may have *progesterone withdrawal*. If you have been on higher doses of progesterone for PMS, remember that you need a **slow tapering** to avoid having withdrawal symptoms.

In chapter 15, I have summary charts on the comparative potencies of some of the over-the-counter progesterone creams, so you may want to check this information and think twice before you start using any of these products. Remember, side effects can occur even from *natural* substances.

OTHER HORMONES

Danazol is a potent progestin with androgen properties that has been used in the treatment of PMS and endometriosis. It can be effective, but with a very high price, both in dollars and in very unpleasant side effects: depression, weight gain, acne, increase in facial and body hair. It appears to reduce PMS and endometriosis by suppressing ovarian cycles in hormone production, which eliminates the "triggers" for

PMS and the estrogen stimulation of endometrial growth. I do not use it just for PMS because I think there are just too many severe side effects that are more disruptive of quality of life than the PMS. I have usually been able to help women find another alternative when treating PMS. I have had patients whose gynecologists prescribed Danazol for severe endometriosis not responsive to other treatments, and for these women, the side effects may be worth the decrease in endometriosis pain that itself can be severe and debilitating.

Lupron (leuprolide) is a medication that mimics the gonadotropin-releasing hormones in the brain and results in shutting down the ovaries to eliminate the hormonal cycling that sets off PMS. It has been used to treat severe fibroids, endometriosis, and PMS, but it causes a full menopausal syndrome with hot flashes and even bone loss if it is used for a long period of time, since it shuts off estrogen and progesterone production. To eliminate the hot flashes, sleep problems, and other negative side effects of Lupron, your physician would need to "add-back" a steady amount of estrogen. But if you have heavy bleeding and fibroids, your doctor really couldn't give you the add-back estrogen. Furthermore, you canot take estrogen alone for an extended period of time due to the increase in abnormal bleeding and hyperplasia of the uterine lining. In addition to the careful monitoring needed, and the fact that Lupron has to be given by injection (daily, or as a long-acting shot once a month), Lupron is also quite expensive (approximately $500–$700 per month). If the PMS is so severe and incapacitating that your physician has recommended removal of the ovaries and uterus, it may be worth a two- or three-month trial of Lupron with add-back estrogen to see whether eliminating the ovarian cycling alleviates the severe PMS. This approach helps you feel more confident that a surgical approach would help. I would not recommend such major steps for treating PMS unless the PMS is extremely severe, causing major disruptions in your life, and you have found *nothing else* that worked.

ANXIOLYTICS (ANTIANXIETY AGENTS)

Buspar (buspirone) belongs to a new generation of anxiolytics that act primarily as a serotonin 1A receptor "booster" in the presynaptic neurons and a partial agonist "booster" in the postsynaptic neurons. Buspirone is not an addictive or habit-forming drug, it does not produce withdrawal symptoms if stopped abruptly, and there is no known abuse potential. Buspirone is not a tranquilizer; it does not cause sedation or adverse effects on memory or coordination. Generally, it tends to cause relatively few side effects. In a study of PMS patients at East Carolina University, Dr. Daniel David found that using buspirone in women with *mild* PMS resulted in an 80 percent "helpful" response; women with *moderate* PMS showed a 92 percent "helpful" response; and women with *marked* PMS showed a 100 percent helpful response. I have not personally found such dramatic results, but I have found that Buspar does help a number of women with PMS. It is another option for you to discuss with your own physician. Buspirone is *not* a medication to take "as needed" (or PRN). It takes at least seven days to effect a significant enough level in the brain to produce its beneficial effects and reduce anxiety. A method that works well with this medication is to begin taking it at the end of the menstrual period and take it daily until the next menses starts, then stop for the days of bleeding. What I find interesting about Dr. David's study is that the more severe the PMS was, the better the response to buspirone, which is what I would expect if indeed PMS is triggered by a serotonin deficiency or imbalance. But keep in mind that declining estradiol also causes decreased serotonin activity, so it may be that buspirone effects on serotonin help to offset the effects triggered by decline in estradiol. You may want to check your hormone levels before adding antianxiety medication.

The Benzodiazepines (Xanax, Ativan, Serax, Valium, Klonopin, and others) act on the GABA receptor sites and have multiple effects on the brain: anticonvulsant, sedative, muscle relaxant, and anxiolytic. I find that these medications *may* have limited helpfulness for some patients, but they may also aggravate the dysphoric (or unpleasant) mood states of PMS and may also impair thinking, concentration, and memory in larger doses. I don't recommend these very often because they have an additive adverse effect with alcohol, and produce a dependence syndrome requiring careful tapering off when being stopped. They are also drugs that tend to be frequently abused. If they are used in the management of "crisis" symptoms in PMS, they should be used sparingly, and short term, with the goal being to help you make lifestyle changes that will reduce symptoms in other ways. Of the benzodiazepines listed above, Xanax (alprazolam) is the only one that has been shown in double-blind, placebo-controlled studies to reduce PMS symptoms significantly. It can safely be taken just during the luteal phase when symptoms are present, and then tapered off during your bleeding days. Used this way, in low dose, it usually does not cause any significant withdrawal symptoms.

SEROTONIN-REUPTAKE INHIBITORS (SSRI)

The medications currently available are Prozac, Paxil, Zoloft, Celexa, and Luvox. Another drug, Serzone, has some characteristics that are similar to the SSRIs, but I do not recommend Serzone due to its marked adverse drug interactions that lower estradiol levels and interfere with the effectiveness of birth control pills when given with prescription hormones. Prozac was the first one of these medications that was FDA-approved in 1988 for the treatment of depression. It has now been tested in double-blind studies of PMS patients and found to be significantly effective for the treatment of PMS. A 1995 double-blind, placebo-controlled study of Prozac for PMS, this time in seven centers in Canada with a total of over 400 women, again showed significant reductions in women's symptoms. Current double-blind studies have also shown the effectiveness of Zoloft in reducing PMS symptoms.

I have prescribed Prozac successfully since its release in 1988 to help treat PMS by boosting serotonin in the last two weeks of the cycle. In fact, I had been waiting for Prozac to come on the market so I could use it with my PMS patients. I had already been working with the serotonin connection in PMS for a number of years and thought that a "serotonin-booster" should be helpful for women with this problem. I have found it to be dramatically helpful for many PMS patients *if the hormone approaches I now use* are not enough to alleviate the symptoms. Other PMS specialists report equally good results, with estimates of 70 to 85 percent positive response to SSRIs. When I use an SSRI for PMS, I usually find that these medications can be given just in the luteal phase of the cycle. This is unlike the situation in major depression where the onset of therapeutic effect of these medications may take several *weeks*. With the availability now of Zoloft, Paxil, Luvox, and Celexa, this provides several options for women to try. You may respond well to one but not the others, so don't give up. But remember, I think it is crucial to check the ovary and thyroid hormone levels carefully before assuming that all you need is a serotonin-boosting medication.

All of the SSRIs have far fewer side effects than the older antidepressants: tricyclics (TCA) and the MAO inhibitors. Generally the side effects may be a mild queasiness, anxious feelings, loose bowel movements, and possibly headaches. All of these early side effects tend to diminish over time or with a decrease in dose. Relatively few people have to stop these medications altogether due to unpleasant side effects. SSRIs are also helpful for other disorders due to serotonin abnormalities: chronic pain syndromes, migraines, bulimia, obsessive-compulsive disorders, and others.

The one problem that does tend to make women (and men) want to change to a different medication is that all of the SSRIs can markedly reduce your interest in sex (libido), also make orgasm more difficult to reach (in men this occurs as delayed ejaculation), and diminish the intensity of orgasms when they occur. In some people, SSRIs prevent orgasm altogether. This is especially true with the more potent ones, Paxil and Luvox. If the SSRI medication is important to your well-being, yet you want to counteract the sexual dysfunction side effects, ask your physician about the possibility of taking Wellbutrin, either a low dose daily or possibly 75 to 150 mg about two hours before having sex. For many patients who have found welcome relief of symptoms with SSRIs, Wellbutrin has been helpful to allow normal sexual arousal and orgasm in both men and women. One drawback to Wellbutrin, however, is that it may cause anxiety and insomnia, so you need to let your doctor know if this happens so the dose can be decreased. SSRIs may also cause another strange side effect called *bruxism,* or clenching of the jaw and tooth-grinding that occurs usually during sleep. Nocturnal bruxism can lead to chronic daily headaches, neck and shoulder pain, cracked dental fillings, and wearing down of tooth enamel. This side effect of SSRIs is thought to be due to the fact that SSRIs cause a lowering of the chemical messenger dopamine, which inhibits certain involuntary movements such as jaw-clenching.

"Withdrawal syndromes" are potentially serious problems that occur with abruptly stopping or rapidly decreasing SSRIs like Paxil and Luvox, the ones that are short-acting and more potent. Withdrawal problems are generally not a problem with Prozac, since it longer acting and provides a "smoother" decline in blood level as the dose is decreased. Even so, I recommend tapering Prozac off as well to allow your body time to adjust and regulate the serotonin pathways without the medication. Effexor is another antidepressant with a severe withdrawal syndrome. All of these medications need to be tapered down very slowly.

TCA ANTIDEPRESSANTS
(ELAVIL, PAMELOR, AND OTHERS)

In my opinion, now that the SSRIs are available, I rarely use this group of medications for PMS, since they produce many more side effects, including appetite stimulation, weight gain, significant dry mouth, constipation, racing heart, and, in older patients, problems with blood pressure regulation. A TCA may be indicated if you have a *coexisting mood disorder;* in this case, you should be evaluated by a psychiatrist knowledgeable in psychopharmacology. The TCA group of medications is *highly lethal* if taken in an overdose, accidentally or intentionally (not true of SSRIs, which makes them a safer choice).

MOOD STABILIZERS (ANTICONVULSANTS)

Tegretol (carbamazepine), Depakote (valproate or valproic acid), Neurontin (gabapentin), and others. The mood changes that come with hormone rises and falls can be mistaken for bipolar or cyclo-thymic disorders, which leads some physicians to recommend a "mood stabilizer" medication. While there is certainly a role for these medications if one actually has a rapid-cycling mood disorder, it is unwise to overuse these medications since they all have the potential to cause serious side effects. Depakote, in particular, has been reported to cause a significant increase in polycystic ovarian syndromes. I get concerned when I see these medications being widely used in younger women without any awareness of the potential for adverse effects on ovarian function. Since many of these medications also cause a rise in prolactin, it is common to see such other side effects as weight gain, headaches, and breast enlargement. Remeron is another medicine often used as a mood stabilizer in women and it causes significant weight gain as well as daytime drowsiness. Before you turn to one of these medicines, check to see if your symptoms follow your menstrual cycle hormonal shifts and could possibly be helped with hormonal therapies. I think it is crucial to have reliable testing of follicular and luteal phase ovarian hormone levels prior to starting one of these medications. If your ovarian or thyroid hormones are out of balance, it is important to restore those to optimal levels first, and then see if you still need one of these mood stabilizers.

LITHIUM

Lithium is very effective for bipolar disorder (manic-depressive illness) to stabilize moods, and some physicians have used it to help PMS. I have not found it to be of much use, and since Lithium is a salt in the same family as sodium, it tends to aggravate fluid retention, and it also increases appetite, thereby contributing to weight gain. Lithium has potentially more severe side effects, and tends to cause hypothyroidism, which is already common in women in this age range. I do not recommend lithium as a PMS therapy, although it has well-established beneficial mood-stabilizing effects in unipolar depression and bipolar mood disorders. I think lithium should be given only after you have had a careful evaluation by a knowledgeable psychiatrist to be certain you actually have one of these major affective disorders. Lithium also requires careful monitoring of blood levels, and effects on blood counts, kidney function, and thyroid function.

Summary: Heading Into the Future

PMS. PCOS. Postpartum depression. Premature menopause. Peri-menopause. Depression. All have important implications for your health and well-being. All share common connections in having lower than optimal levels of estradiol, with an imbalance of other important hormones. Each is treatable and each responds to a variety of hormonal therapies and other medications as well as mind-body approaches to rebalance brain chemistry, in addition to the healthy-living lifestyle choices I have described. The midlife years may be a time of "hoppin' hormones" and other changes in the body, but this doesn't mean you should resign yourself to not feeling your best. Midlife is a time to refocus, a time to pay attention to *ourselves* and take care of these wonderful gifts of our mind and body. No one else can do it for you. Ultimately, *you* are your own best physician, and your healing comes from within. The choices you make *now*, whatever your chronological age, have a major bearing on your health for the future. The name of the (health) game is, first and foremost, ***Prevention!***

Chapter 8

Is It Chronic Fatigue, "Yeast," or Perimenopause?

Consider these four symptom clusters, which I have seen in several books recently:

I. fatigue, low energy level, joint pain, impaired reasoning, memory loss, depression, sleep disturbances, anxiety, irritability, muscle weakness, dizziness, balance problems, lethargy, difficulty concentrating, low sex drive, joint aches, insomnia, chronic infections, chronic sinusitis, vision changes, menstrual irregularities, menstrual cramps, vaginal itching, vaginal burning, mood swings, irritability, feeling foggy mentally, difficulty concentrating, short attention span, diarrhea and/or constipation, bloating, indigestion, chemical sensitivities, appetite changes, cravings for certain foods

II. fatigue, low energy level, joint aches and pains, insomnia, bladder irritations and infections, intermittent diarrhea, episodic constipation, bloating, indigestion, allergic reactions, chemical intolerance, skin eruptions, chronic sinusitis, menstrual irregularities, severe menstrual cramps, vaginal discharge, vaginal itching, low sex drive, painful intercourse, rectal itching, vision changes, depression, irritability, angry outbursts, mood swings, migraine headaches, mental fogging, inability to concentrate, loss of memory, loss of alertness, feeling of spaciness, short attention span, restless sleep, appetite changes, alcohol and sweet cravings, dry brittle hair, dry eyes, dry skin

III. menstrual irregularities, severe menstrual cramps, vision changes, dry eyes, chronic sinusitis, joint aches and pains, insomnia, bladder irritations and infections, intermittent diarrhea occurring along with episodic constipation, bloating, indigestion, allergic reactions, chemical intolerance, food cravings—especially sweets—skin eruptions, vaginal discharge, vaginal itching, low sex drive, painful intercourse, rectal itching, fatigue, depression, irritability, angry outbursts, mood swings, migraine headaches, mental fogging, inability to concentrate, loss of memory, loss of alertness, feeling spacey, short attention span, low energy, fragmented sleep

IV. mental fogging, inability to concentrate, loss of memory, loss of alertness, feeling spacey, short attention span, low energy, fatigue, depression, irritability, angry outbursts, mood swings, migraine headaches, bladder irritations and infections, intermittent diarrhea occurring along with episodic constipation, bloating, indigestion, allergic reactions, chemical intolerance, skin eruptions, vaginal discharge, vaginal itching, low sex drive, painful intercourse, rectal itching, menstrual irregularities, severe menstrual cramps, vision changes, dry eyes, chronic sinusitis, joint aches and pains, insomnia

Now, see if you can match the symptom cluster, I through IV, with the proper "diagnosis" from the list below:

    A. Candida albicans ("Candidiasis")
    B. Hypothyroidism
    C. Menopausal syndrome
    D. Chronic fatigue syndrome (also called Epstein-Barr virus syndrome)
    E. Anemia
    F. Major depressive illness
    G. None of these

Did you get them all correct?
The correct answer is: *Any one of the clusters I through IV may occur with any of the illnesses, A through G.*

One of the reasons I wanted you to think about all of these different syndromes and the multiple symptoms that can be produced is that you are seeing the importance of the total picture, instead of just approaching "diagnoses" based upon a list of symptoms. Western-trained M.D. and D.O. physicians, Chinese medicine practitioners, homeopaths, chiropractors, herbalists, naturopaths, and other alternative practitioners all have one practice in common: *They are trained to treat people based on a cluster of symptoms,* whether the treatment used is pharmaceutical medications, herbs, homeopathic remedies, manipulation, acupuncture, or any other modality.

Granted, symptom clusters are extremely important in leading one to a particular type of disorder to decide what treatment options will be helpful. We cannot use just symptoms alone, however, because a wide variety of illnesses and imbalances may produce similar kinds of physical and psychological changes. The problem is that when you are faced with *any* illness or major biological change affecting the brain and body, you will see a wide range of symptoms. This is due to the fact that many body systems are affected by imbalances produced by various stimuli, referred to as *stressors*. In this context, *stressors* can be psychological or physiological (physical). Physical stressors can be due to hundreds of things—these are just a few common ones: hormonal change, illness such as diabetes or arthritis, viruses infecting the body, bacteria overgrowth, "yeast" overgrowth, environmental pollutants, medication side effects, reactions to herbs or excess vitamins. I have had patients with the symptom list above who were toxic from multiple vitamin and herbal supplements. Almost indistinguishable symptoms may occur with hypothyroidism or decline in ovarian hormones or anemia. Another example I have encountered in my practice is chronic insecticide exposure that may lead to a clinical picture of chronic fatigue syndrome (CFS), hypothyroidism, or menopausal syndrome.

Our problem, particularly in women's health, is that both patients and physicians have been taught to look for *one* cause of an illness based on *one* list of symptoms. That's not quite how our body works. The fight-or-flight stress response produces the *same* body reactions ("symptoms") whether you are faced with an oncoming grizzly bear, an oncoming car, fear about financial collapse, a rapid fall in blood sugar, or a rapid fall in estrogen before your period. That's why I think it is crucial for women to have a hormonal evaluation as part of the diagnostic process when they are experiencing a group of diverse symptoms. If you are working with a non-M.D. health practitioner, I think it is important for you to first have a good diagnostic evaluation by an M.D. or D.O. so you know more clearly *what* it is you are treating. I made sure I had my herniated discs treated with what Western medicine had to offer (in my case, surgery) *so I could walk again,* and then I used a whole range of complementary therapies to get well again.

The syndromes I listed at the beginning of this chapter are all examples of ones that are difficult to diagnose with certainty because they produce a variety of symptoms. The best treatment options for you will vary depending upon which condition is the primary one triggering the symptoms. Two that often come up in my work with midlife women are **chronic fatigue syndrome (CFS)** and **Candida albicans (Candida).**

There are a number of good resources to read further about both CFS and candida. There simply isn't room in this book for me to go into all that we know and don't know about these syndromes. However, before you jump to the conclusion—based on just symptoms—that you have one of these syndromes, I strongly encourage you to have a thorough medical checkup to rule out other common problems such as subclinical hypothyroidism and declining ovarian hormone production, which can mimic these other two syndromes. Both of these hormonal factors are *usually* overlooked in both traditional medical settings and in complementary or "integrative" health care settings.

Whether the initial trigger is a viral infection, yeast overgrowth, hormone changes, or other stressors, there is strong evidence that the resulting debilitating syndromes happen primarily due to the accumulation of stressors, which have adversely impacted on the immune system and the neuromodulators that coordinate functions of the brain and body organ systems. A brain-mediated response mechanism, initially triggered by an imbalance in ovarian, thyroid, or adrenal hormones, would contribute to the diversity of clinical symptoms and the overlap in symptoms that we often see in the way these disorders manifest. I do think that if we look for common patterns in all of these, instead of just listing symptoms, it will assist us in developing integrated approaches to helping women feel well again. For example, in addition to more natural hormone options, we are also finding that serotonin-augmenting medications (SSRIs) help reduce the symptoms of many of the disorders I listed above. SSRIs are much broader in their beneficial effects than the old term antidepressant would suggest, so I am sorry that they are still called antidepressants. I prefer to call them "serotonin-boosters." In addition, many different modalities that boost endorphins and serotonin—such as acupuncture, relaxation training, biofeedback, and massage therapy— are also helpful in alleviating some of the symptoms of CFS, candida, perimenopause, and depression. Common threads of positive response to different modalities provide further support to the theory of a brain-mediated mechanism creating a cascade of events triggering multiple effects (or symptoms) in many body systems.

What are Epstein-Barr Syndrome and CFS?

First described by Drs. Paul Cheney and Daniel Peterson of Incline Village, Nevada, in 1984, chronic fatigue syndrome (CFS) was initially dismissed as "yuppie flu." Many physicians are skeptical that it is a "real" disorder, and the condition has been shrouded in controversy because researchers have been unable to identify a cause, predict its course, or find very many effective treatments. It was initially thought to be due to a chronic infection with Epstein-Barr virus, a type of herpes virus that triggers mononucleosis ("the kissing disease") commonly seen in teenagers and young adults. In the past, CFS was thought to be a more chronic form of infectious mononucleosis. Then the medical thinking expanded to attribute CFS to a variety of viral causes—the herpes group (EBV, herpes simplex oral and genital), cytomegalovirus (CMV), rotaviruses, and others, as well as possibly Candida albicans, a yeast. As our laboratory tests have become more sophisticated, recent studies have found elevations in antibodies to a variety of infectious agents, as well as autoimmune antibodies to the adrenal gland, thyroid gland, and possibly the ovaries. These newer findings have weakened the case for any single virus as "the" cause of CFS. Even though the onset of CFS may be *triggered* by a viral illness, the current view is that the *chronic* symptoms are not likely to be caused by an active viral infection. More current views are that CFS is one of a cluster of *neuroendocrine* disorders that includes fibromyalgia (FMS) and multiple chemical sensitivities (MCS). Dr. Riccardo Baschetti, from Italy, has published extensively on the similarities between Addison's disease (adrenal insufficiency) and chronic fatigue syndrome. He has proposed that CFS is a less severe form of Addison's disease, since both physical and neuropsychological symptoms are so astonishingly similar. Although there are many theories about causal factors in these conditions, there has not been any *one* cause that has been clearly demonstrated in the research to date.

There is another connection, however, that is not often discussed in either the medical or the consumer literature. That is the connection all of these conditions may have with women's ovarian hormones. The statistics are simply overwhelming in pointing to the ovarian hormone connection as an issue critically needing more study: CFS is 70–75 percent female in distribution, FMS is over 80 percent female in distribution, and MCS is reportedly variously as 60–80 percent female in distribution. One possible connection with the viral theory that could help to explain the marked female preponderance of cases, is that viral infections like EBV, CMV, herpes, and many others can lead to a viral infiltration of the thyroid gland or ovary itself. Such as infiltration leads to a viral *thyroiditis* and/ or a viral *oophoritis*, with subsequent decline in the optimal functioning of the thyroid or ovary gland. Viral-induced loss of gland function leads to subtle forms of hypothyroidism causing fatigue, or subtle forms of ovarian decline causing infertility and fatigue syndromes. Both of these types of viral syndromes (thyroiditis, oophoritis) are commonly overlooked in most medical settings as potential causes of chronic fatigue. There may also be a viral infiltration of the pancreas, leading to later diabetes from viral damage to the insulin-producing cells of the pancreas. In addition, viral illnesses are known to trigger later development of autoimmune disorders affecting many endocrine organs, so this is another potential link between a viral illness and subsequent appearance of CFS, FMS, or MCS.

Other stressors to the body's immune system have also been implicated in CFS. Persistent low-grade infections such as mycoplasma (a cause of "walking pneumonia") may lead to symptoms of CFS but be hard to detect unless a clinician thinks to do the appropriate tests for mycoplasma. Environmental pollutants ("sick building syndrome"), toxic chemicals ("Persian Gulf" syndrome, insecticide toxicity), and even low-grade toxic effects from chronic use of common household chemicals may lead to immune suppression causing symptoms of CFS. Some of these same chemicals also damage endocrine tissues like the thyroid gland, ovaries in women, and testicles in men, causing disruption in hormone production by these glands. Prolonged stressful life situations also suppress the ovaries and may lead to the neuroendocrine changes associated with CFS, FMS, and MCS. Illnesses like depression and generalized anxiety that stress the immune system have also been considered to play a role in CFS, and we know that declines in both thyroid and ovarian hormones can affect the onset of these mood symptoms. So you see, there are many potential causes for CFS that need to be carefully assessed. Most physicians think to check the adrenal hormones in people with CFS, but the balance of ovarian hormones plays a critical role that must also be investigated, and we need to check for more subtle degrees of thyroid dysfunction that are far more common in women. For example, autoimmune thyroiditis, discussed in chapter 2, will be missed in its early stages if doctors just look at TSH and fail to also check thyroid antibodies in CFS patients.

Our definitions of CFS have been evolving over the last two decades. Initially, this syndrome was given a working definition by the Centers for Disease Control (CDC) as follows: "new onset persistent or relapsing, debilitating fatigue lasting at least six months in a person with no previous history of similar symptoms." Numerous other clinical conditions that could produce similar symptoms *must be excluded* before giving a diagnosis of CFS: malignancy; autoimmune diseases; bacterial, fungal, parasitic, or viral disease; chronic psychiatric disease (depression in particular); chronic inflammatory disease; neuromuscular disease; endocrine disease; drug abuse; side effects of chronic medication or other toxic agent. Simply ruling out all of these can in itself be expensive and exhausting. These are considered the major criteria and must be met for the diagnosis of CFS.

Prior to 1994, a more rigid definition of CFS was used by the CDC and included the following minor criteria for CFS, at least *eight* of which must be present: mild fever, sore throat, painful anterior or posterior cervical (neck) or axillary (underarm) lymph nodes, unexplained generalized muscle weakness, muscle discomfort (myalgia), generalized fatigue for at least twenty-four hours after previously tolerated exercise, generalized headaches unlike any previous pain, migratory arthralgia without joint swelling or redness, sleep disturbance, a main symptom complex arising within hours or days, presence of neuropsychologic symptoms (such as mood changes, forgetfulness, confusion, difficulty concentrating, depressed mood, and others). In 1994, a less restrictive definition for CFS was adopted, since it became more evident that some of the above symptoms actually didn't occur that often in CFS. The diagnosis of CFS now requires severe, persistent fatigue plus *four* of the following eight symptoms: myalgia (muscle pain), arthralgia, sore throat, headache, sleep disruption, malaise following exercise, tender neck, cognitive difficulty (memory, concentration, focus difficulties). Whichever definition is used, there are two factors that I think make it plausible to consider checking women's ovarian hormones as part of a fatigue evaluation: (1) the striking female dominance of the disorder, and (2) the known occurrence of many of these same symptoms as a result of declining ovary hormones in perimenopause.

Hormonal Decline:
An Unrecognized Cause of Fatigue

Seventy percent of patients with CFS are women. I think it is crucial to look at what hormonal changes could be playing a role in this enormous gender difference in incidence of CFS. In all the medical articles I have read on CFS, however, *I have not yet seen one address this issue.* In one recent study of the characteristics of CFS patients, 60 percent were female and the average age was 41.9 years—do you see possible clues here? Premenopause (perimenopause) changes can *begin* about a decade before menopause; shouldn't *this* be considered? The same researchers also studied patients with fibromyalgia: 90 percent were female, and the average age was 44.0 years. Do you see another clue here? Again, nothing mentioned about hormones. The amazing thing to me is that the two investigators for this study were *both female physicians* and there was **not one word about ovarian hormonal factors** mentioned anywhere in this medical article about common disorders in women. In the discussion summarizing these study results, there was not even a comment that checking hormonal factors was important in future research. More recent review articles on this subject share the same deficiency, in spite of our advances in understanding the many metabolic effects of the ovarian hormones on every organ system in the body. We have a **long** way to go.

CFS as a severe form of fatigue may have many causes and contributing factors, with ovarian hormone levels being only part of the picture. But milder forms of fatigue and loss of "vitality" or loss of "zest" are described by a large numbers of women experiencing major ovarian hormone changes, whether they are adolescents with polycystic ovary syndrome, or postpartum women with low ovary hormones as a result of suppression by nursing, or women with infertility due to premature loss of ovarian hormones, or perimenopausal and menopausal women with naturally declining ovary hormone levels. Estradiol and testosterone in particular have significant activating or stimulating effects on energy level. Losing your optimal levels of these key metabolic hormones makes you feel more tired, even if you don't have the full-blown CFS.

An example of severe fatigue developing in the postpartum phase is illustrated by a patient I saw a few weeks ago. Luala, now thirty-seven years old, described the following history:

> I've had a horrible struggle with total exhaustion and hormonal problems since the birth of my daughter 8 years ago. I was never the same after that. I had pre-eclampsia and then a severe hemorrahge after the placenta came out. I was healthy before all that, and afterwards I was totally exhausted all the time and never could get my energy back. My doctors told me I had chronic fatigue but they said there wasn't anything to do about it. I live in a constant brain fog, I have no retention, my memory is terrible. I don't sleep well and I don't have the energy to exercise. I am still having periods, so my doctor said it couldn't be hormonal. I can feel the ovulation twinge most of the time, but not every month. My bleeding varies but my periods have changed in that they aren't as long and the cycles change from short to long. I just know it is connected to my hormones somehow.

Her adrenal and thyroid hormones had been checked numerous times, but none of her physicians had ever checked her ovarian hormone levels. When I did this, her serum estradiol on Day 1 was significantly low at 27 pg/ml, as was her Day 20 (luteal phase) estradiol at 61 pg/ml (it should be about 200 pg/ml or so). Like many younger women I see with this pattern of low estradiol, she still made a healthy luteal-phase ovulatory rise in progesterone to a level of 15.2 (quite normal).

Another finding added support to the observation that her estradiol level was lower than optimal for her body needs: her N-telopeptide (NTx) level was higher than it should be at 55, indicating more rapid bone breakdown already occurring, even though she was only thirty-seven. Her blood pressure was very good at 110/68, so there was no evidence of hypotension as a cause of her fatigue. She was not overweight, her cholesterol profile was very good, and her thyroid tests, including antibodies, were all negative for evidence of thyroid disease. She did not have adrenal insufficiency; in fact, her 8 A.M. cortisol was slightly higher than desirable at 25 as a stress response to her low level of estradiol. Her serum ferritin, a measure of iron stores, was lower than it should be, although not enough to account for her marked fatigue. After eight years of struggle to feel better, she finally had some test results and answers that made sense to her based on what she had observed. Even though she did not have a full-blown Sheehan's syndrome, her ovarian hormone production had not "bounced back" to optimal levels following her pregnancy and the postpartum hemorrhage. Loss of these vital hormones had caused her fatigue and other neuroendocrine symptoms. She was not clinically depressed; she was just missing a critical hormone that affects brain and body function in many ways. I took a fairly simple approach to her treatment and suggested a steady-dose, estrogen-dominant birth control pill. At each of her three-month follow-up appointments, she was feeling more and more "like my old self." At her one-year appointment, her fatigue symptoms had completely resolved, along with the brain fog and other symptoms. It was such a straightforward problem to help, once she and I had reliable hormone levels to clarify what was causing her problems.

In addition to the kinds of difficulties Luala experienced, there is another issue to keep in mind about the ovarian hormone connection with persistent fatigue. There are dramatic and profoundly disruptive effects on sleep caused by declining estrogen levels. I describe these in more detail in chapter 11. Keep in mind that these sleep changes may begin as much as eight to ten years *before* you stop menstruating. Sleep deprivation causes suppression of the immune system and robs you of your normal daytime energy, so it is a major factor in causing persistent *fatigue*. It seems so obvious to me, I don't understand why there aren't a wealth of articles on these connections in the medical literature. Menopause may not explain why CFS occurs in males, but if about 70 percent of the patients with CFS are women, wouldn't it make sense to try and help the majority of sufferers who are female by checking for hormonal factors? In the same vein, what if we looked into what's happening to *male* hormone levels in men with CFS? I haven't seen a formal study of that connection either. I bring this observation to your attention in the hope that you will ask your physician to look into these possible hormonal factors if you think you may have one of these syndromes. It is tragic, in my opinion, that we turn to "heroic measures" to treat these conditions—a recent such heroic measure described in the Wall

Street Journal in late 1999 was neurosurgery costing more than $30,000 to open up the base of the skull—and yet we say testing hormone levels for women is too expensive. This degree of illogical thinking is mind-boggling. We overlook something so obvious as basic ovarian hormone balance that could be helped in some fairly straightforward and low-cost ways.

Progestins in Birth Control Pills: Overlooked Causes of Fatigue

I had a physician colleague call and ask if I would do a consult for his wife. He was very worried about the changes he had seen in her over the previous few months. In his words, "She has always been such a cheerful, outgoing, high energy person. On the go, exercising every day, and normally *very* even in her moods. She's only forty-three and she still has periods. Her gynecologist started her on hormones, but she's continued to get more depressed and talks about feeling so exhausted. She doesn't even have the energy to exercise." He was concerned that she had chronic fatigue syndrome and wanted to be sure that I considered that diagnosis along with checking for possible side effects of the hormonal regimen she was taking.

When I met with his wife in the spring of 1994, she described experiencing severe depressive symptoms, mood swings with a lot of irritability, and sudden tearfulness for no apparent reason. She also reported decreased energy, hot flashes, insomnia, diffuse arthralgias, myalgias, and marked fatigue. "I feel like I've had a long bout with the flu." She also noted difficulty having orgasm, and diminished libido because she was so tired all the time.

I'll give you just the highlights of a comprehensive evaluation, which in her situation did not have to involve extensive laboratory testing for reasons that will become clear as you read on. Her father, to whom she had been very close, had died a year and a half earlier, but she felt she had "come through the grief pretty well." She also had been having times of heavy menstrual bleeding, so her gynecologist had done a D&C in the spring of 1993, and then started her on Loestrin to keep her periods lighter and reduce problems with cramps. Loestrin is an oral contraceptive with a higher progestin content and a lower amount of ethinyl estradiol estrogen (hence the name, "lo-estrin"). This was one reason it was not necessary to check her hormone levels, since oral contraceptives (OCs) suppress the ovaries' hormone production. She said, "I did pretty well at first, and then I noticed that my depressed mood, irritability and low energy became significantly worse about two months before my husband called you."

After her evaluation, I told her I thought that I did not think she had a true CFS syndrome, although I couldn't conclusively eliminate this because there are not any good diagnostic tests for CFS. I explained that an important issue was the timing of her symptoms relative to beginning the particular birth control pill (Loestrin) that was higher in progestin and low in estrogen. Our first step should be to see how she did on a pill with the reverse ratio: higher estrogen and lower progestin. Then, if that didn't lead to improvement, we would consider an antidepressant to improve her sleep, mood, and energy level. I changed her oral contraceptive to Ovcon-35, with much less progestin and slightly more estrogen. I also suggested using estradiol alone for the days between Ovcon pill packs to keep her estrogen from falling abruptly and triggering her migraines. She would still have a normal period at the end of the Ovcon pack when the progestin level dropped, but she wouldn't have to have the estrogen drop causing her migraines. I have to admit, however, at the time her symptoms were so severe, I thought she might also need an antidepressant in addition to the BCP change.

At her first follow-up appointment two weeks later, she said: *"I feel like I've come back from the cellar. I'm not crying, I don't feel depressed, I have my energy, I don't have the headaches, I feel like someone flipped a switch on me. It was remarkable to feel well again in such a short period of time. When I first talked with you, I felt like I knew why people committed suicide, even though suicide isn't an action I would take. This is amazing."* The only thing she had noticed was some breast fullness and tenderness, but said "that's a minor problem compared to how I felt before." A few weeks later, she faxed me a note with a big sunshine face beaming beneath the typing:

Dr. Vliet:
I no longer experience insomnia, swimming in the head, hot flashes, night sweats, joint pain, palpitations at rest, utter fatigue, feelings of absolute hopelessness, nonproductivity, low self esteem, lack of humor and playfulness, terrible witch-like mood swings, short temper, lack of sexual interest, difficulty in reaching orgasm, thoughts of my husband losing interest in me, indecisiveness, inability to concentrate, and not wanting to do anything with anybody for any reason . . . YUK.

Now, I am incredibly back to normal. I feel strong and hopeful . . .

I'm vibrant with color. It is difficult to believe I was viewing the world in black and white. Gray is such a nasty color. I lost all hope for everything.

I'm back to exercising a couple hours a day, and weightlifting is back in my routine. I'm currently contemplating boxercise at home.

Before the change of hormones, life had very little meaning to me. Napping and unexplainable sobbing were two big menu choices for me.

Excitement and thrills of a new day await me now. No person or thing can break my stride, and I am on the move. Thank you Dr. Vliet for your expertise in this area.

D.

This patient ended up having a total of three appointments with me to get back on track with her hormone prescription. I didn't hear from her for several years until she contacted me in 1999 for a medical appointment. She said "I had been doing great and my husband simply continued your prescription for me until this year when we got a divorce. My gynecologist took over prescribing my hormones for me and said '*I don't agree with this concoction and you can take what everybody else takes.*' He switched me to the Mircette pills [Note to reader: Mircette has a lower estrogen and higher progestin content, more like the Loestrin that had caused so many problems for her], and it wasn't long before my body hurt, I had constant headaches again, I felt depressed and bloated again. I lasted for five days on Mircette and I said to myself, screw it, I am going back on the Ovcon, so I called for this appointment."

Her laboratory results, done on the seventh day off her birth control pills, showed lower estradiol and testosterone levels you would expect with her age now at of forty-nine, but her FSH had not yet risen into the menopausal range. This meant that if she didn't want to get pregnant, it would be wise to continue the Ovcon-35 for its contraceptive effects as well as for her perimenopausal hormone balancing. Her laboratory results showed other interesting findings related to the higher progestin content of the Mircette: Her 8 A.M. cortisol was now higher than it had been on Ovcon, which indicated a "stress response" of the body being activated by the low estrogen-high progestin pill, and her *free* T3 and T4 (thyroid hormones) were now lower than they had been, another finding affected by the progestin level of a birth control pill: Her TSH was still in a desirable range, but the *effectiveness* of her thyroid hormones was being negatively affected by the high-progestin pill. These other lab changes are common contributing factors to symptoms of depression, tiredness, and waistline weight gain when women are on birth control pills that are high in progestin content relative to the estrogen balance.

Fortunately for D, she knew right away what the problem was and didn't doubt her own wisdom about the right course for her to take. She got right back on the pills that had been working so well for her. She decided she wasn't going back down that road of seeing a physician who didn't believe her descriptions of how she felt or was unwilling to work with what had helped her so much. She is now in a new marriage, but does not want to get pregnant at age forty-nine. There is still a degree of unpredictability about ovulation and fertility in this phase of life, before the FSH has reached 15 or so, indicating loss of fertility. She doesn't smoke, her cholesterol and bone markers were all really good, and she felt terrific on the Ovcon regimen. Together, she and I agreed that she really wanted to continue taking the birth control pill, and Ovcon-35 was the best choice for her. She left the appointment feeling that her desires had been honored, and her insights validated.

Hormonal balance is certainly not going to be the *only* answer for everyone with fatigue or depression, but for women in their forties, it certainly seems like a good place to start in our evaluations. In addition, whenever the symptom pattern begins in conjunction with starting new medication, I think it is always important to look to the medication as a possible cause of unwanted changes, as well as to evaluate other possibilities. I am constantly amazed at the extensive workups and multiple treatment options (many quite expensive and time consuming) that have been tried in women with fatigue and depressive symptoms without anyone even thinking about trying a different birth control pill or checking the ovarian hormones, the free fraction of the thyroid hormones, or thyroid antibodies. Other physicians, and some women, have said it is too expensive to check the hormone aspects. Now I ask you, which was more "expensive" for the woman above—continuing on the way she was going, or looking for resources to help get answers? What price do you put on *your* good health? What price do we put on women's health collectively? Don't you think these are issues that deserve attention? Ask your physician to check into these aspects of your health if you aren't feeling better with the current treatments for fatigue, yeast, or other problems you may be experiencing.

Hormone Imbalance: A Factor in "Yeast" Infections and Syndromes

Chronic candida has been another of the "women's diseases" that is purported to cause over a hundred different symptoms in multiple body systems. It was popularized by the 1985 book *The Yeast Connection*, based on the work of Drs. Crook and Truss. The mainstream medical community remains skeptical of the existence of a true "chronic yeast syndrome," since there are no well-done studies to document it, and we all have Candida albicans and related organisms throughout the genital and intestinal tracts as part of the normal flora. On the other hand, there are many unanswered questions in women's health. The mainstream medical community has also remained skeptical of hormonal factors in women triggering syndromes like PMS and migraines. You can't find a connection if you don't look for it! Dr. Truss was the originator of the "yeast theory," and Dr. Crook has developed these ideas further. I think there is merit to what they have presented, but I also think many people over diagnose yeast syndromes and fail to properly evaluate women's ovarian (and sometimes thyroid) hormones, with the end result that hormonal aspects triggering similar symptoms, or even making us more susceptible to chronic yeast infections, are rarely addressed. Somewhere between the extremes of overenthusiasm and overskepticism, there lies the reality—we just don't yet fully understand all of the nuances involved.

The advantage of what Dr. Crook is describing in his book is that most of what he recommends is based on dietary change, eliminating use of repeated cycles of antibiotics, and other basic measures that carry little risk and may be very helpful to women with recurrent vaginal yeast problems. I do want you to have information on the basics of hormone factors that you need to investigate if you are having "yeast problems." Once again, since we are dealing with a possible "syndrome" that occurs predominately in women—younger women with hormonal imbalance as well as in midlife or perimenopausal women. Like other disorders more common in women, might this one have a connection with the decreases in female hormones? It turns out that the answer to this question is yes. There are a variety of ways that changing balance in our ovarian hormones will predispose us to having more yeast infections. Let's explore these relationships.

Allergies, herpes outbreaks, yeast infections, sinusitis, and asthma: all of these health problems typically are aggravated premenstrually and have to do with some of the very significant physiological changes that occur with the hormonal shifts each month. Most physicians can tell you that they see a relationship, but there haven't been good studies to try and identify some of the specific reasons for it. Hormonal balance alters immune system function, with *more optimal* immune function in the first half (estrogen-dominant) phase of the menstrual cycle. As progesterone rises in the second half of the cycle, there is more suppression of the immune response. Remember, progesterone is the hormone that has been shown to suppress the mother's immune system during pregnancy to help prevent the mother's immune system from destroying the "foreign tissue" of the fetus. If the progesterone level is high, particularly if estradiol has declined from optimal levels needed to give the normal balance to progesterone, then the increased immune suppression makes us more susceptible to viral and other infections. The changing hormone balance in the second half of the menstrual cycle causes other immune alterations that also contribute to the increased frequency of luteal (premenstrual) phase allergies and herpes outbreaks.

One thing many women don't realize is that during their thirties and forties, the changes in hormone production, particularly declining estradiol levels and progesterone dominance, will further alter the pH balance of the tissue lining the vagina. The vagina is normally more acidic in pH, and this acid environment helps prevent unwanted bacteria and yeast from dominating and causing infections. As estradiol levels decrease (especially if you still have high progesterone levels in the second half of the cycle), there is a rise in vaginal pH to a more alkaline level. The alkaline pH in turn allows *unhealthy* bacteria (such as E. coli from the intestines) and yeast (such as *Candida albicans*) to overgrow in the vagina. The overgrowth of these organisms upsets the healthy balance of the normal vaginal types of bacteria and creates the well-known problems of itchy, burning, smelly discharges.

Another aspect to the potential vicious cycle with candida is that not only does the decrease in estrogen contribute to pH and other changes that make yeast infections more common, but also the presence of excessive candida organisms further *decreases* available estrogen, making the entire problem worse. It has been hypothesized that candida organisms may actually bind the estrogen and prevent it from plugging into the body's estrogen receptor sites, producing an additional estrogen deficit in the body. This is an awful double whammy. It's like adding insult to injury. If you are taking progesterone supplements or using progesterone skin creams that raise blood levels, the higher levels of progesterone help *increase the available blood glucose,* allowing the candida to flourish even more and making the candida problem even worse. Another vicious cycle.

How do you get help for these problems? Certainly dietary changes can help. A simple, gentle approach to help treat vaginal yeast is acidophilus vaginal suppositories, available from compounding pharmacies. Your gynecologist can check the vaginal pH with a simple test and let you know if this is a factor in your continued problems with yeast infections. Some over-the-counter "ovulation predictor" kits are also based on vaginal pH changes. Another simple test, called a maturation index, with tell you whether the vaginal cells have enough estrogen effect to help keep the vaginal lining healthy enough to ward off repeated infections. If not, your gynecologist can prescribe estradiol creams or a estradiol vaginal ring to help restore a healthy estrogen level to the tissues. Estriol is sometimes also used for this purpose, but since it is a less-potent estrogen, estriol isn't generally quite as effective for this purpose as estradiol is. If you are having chronic bacterial or yeast vaginal infections, you want to minimize use of creams or suppositories containing progesterone. You may also ask your doctor to give you a try on birth control pills with *less progestin* if you are currently using one of the high-progestin BCPs, which tend to aggravate vaginal yeast and overall fatigue symptoms.

I have not given you here an exhaustive review of candida syndromes. I just wanted to raise your "index of suspicion" about possible overlooked hormonal connections, and I encourage you to consider these if you have been experiencing repeated vaginal yeast infections, or if you think you may have a broader problem with yeast. I find that the repeated vaginal yeast problems at least *improve,* if not resolve completely, once a more normal hormonal balance is reached. I think it is worth having these hormone issues checked carefully before you take repeated courses of antibiotics or the more potent antifungal drugs. If you are on a menopausal hormone regimen using a synthetic progestin every day, it may help to ask your doctor about (1) reducing the dose, (2) changing to a cycle of only ten or twelve days a month so you don't have the progestin every day, or (3) changing to one of the new FDA-approved natural progesterone products, such as Prometrium. If you are using large amounts of progesterone supplements for PMS treatment, talk with your health professional about trying to achieve a more normal physiological balance with adequate estradiol and keeping the total progesterone dose lower. There are a number of safe and relatively simple hormonal changes that may provide some relief from such an annoying health problem.

**FACTORS CONTRIBUTING TO INCREASED
CANDIDA ("YEAST") INFECTIONS:**

- high-carbohydrate diets, especially if the carbohydrate source is refined sugars
- progesterone excess or high-progestin birth control pills
- chronic or repeated use of antibiotics
- regular use of corticosteroids such as cortisone, prednisone, etc.
- medical illnesses such as diabetes, hypothyroidism, and others
- premature ovarian decline, perimenopause, menopause
- stress: alters levels of many different hormones that affect pH of mucosal linings in the mouth, vagina, and intestinal tract
- excess alcohol consumption
- cigarette smoking (causes earlier loss of ovary hormones)
- stimulant abuse: has effects similar to, *but greater than,* chronic stress (over-the-counter stimulant diet pills, daily use of decongestants containing stimulants, stimulant herbs such as ephedra or Ma Huang, caffeine, cocaine abuse, etc.)

© Elizabeth Lee Vliet, M.D., 1995, revised 2000

Heading Into The Future

As we think about health care reform and what women's health needs must be addressed, clearly heavily female-predominant problems such as CFS will become significant concerns from both *quality of life* and *economic* points of view. In Australia, where the health care system makes it much easier to collect data on cost issues, CFS represents a staggering **$59 million** cost to their society annually. Each individual patient incurs medical costs, on average, of **$9,429.00**. The potential burden on the health care system—both financially and for delivery of health care services—is potentially enormous from CFS alone. Now do you suppose it *might* be cost-effective and make sense to look at the women's hormone levels here?

Chapter 9

Estrogen and Memory: The Words Escape Me

Women's Fears: Am I Losing My Mind?

Words slip out of your mind, suddenly you can't seem to spell simple words, you forget the tasks you wanted to do, you forget where you *put* your To-Do list, you walk into a room and then wonder what you wanted to get, you can't find your keys, you feel scattered in your thinking, and you can't seem to focus like you used to. Does any of this sound familiar? If so, you aren't alone. You aren't imagining it. You may be in the beginning of menopause. What's happening? Why do changes in the ovaries seem to affect your brain so profoundly?

During my residency at Johns Hopkins, one of the specialty rotations was the Dementia Research Program. I remember being very struck upon learning that dementias of all kinds are about *four times more common in elderly women* compared to elderly men of the *same* age. I was bothered by this statistic because, at the time, no one had any explanation for this marked difference in dementia rates between women and men, and researchers were not thinking about studying female hormone effects on the brain.

Based on current projections, a female born in 1994 has a *one in six chance* of developing Alzheimer's, if she lives to an average life expectancy of about eighty years. For women, this lifetime risk is *greater* than the lifetime risk of breast cancer. A male born in 1994, who lives to the average male life expectancy, has a *one in sixteen chance*. It's about time we begin to research the role of decline in estrogen after menopause as a possible factor in women's higher rates of dementia. This crucial research has now been underway for more than two decades, particularly in Canada, Australia, and Japan to determine the effects of estrogen on nerve cells in the brain, memory pathways, and cognitive function. The United States has lagged behind these other countries in paying attention to the importance of ovarian hormone effects on the brain but has recently begun such studies. Let's look at what has unfolded in our knowledge about the many ways estradiol helps preserve our critical thinking and memory abilities. But first some definitions and explanations that will help you understand these complex neuroendocrine connections.

Dementia is a term that means generalized loss of the brain's ability to retain, perceive, integrate, utilize, retrieve, and act appropriately on information, called *cognitive function*. It is a group of brain diseases with a hundred or more different causes. Some types of dementia are treatable and reversible if the cause is caught early. An example is hypothyroidism. Loss of adequate thyroid hormone causes marked decrease of cognitive function and even full-blown dementia if left untreated, but is reversible if treated with thyroid hormone replacement. Alzheimer's disease is another type of dementia that involves progressive, irreversible degeneration of global brain function. At present, we do not have any treatments that completely restore normal brain abilities in Alzheimer's patients, even though some medications may help to delay progression for a while. Estrogen has a significant role in preserving normal nerve cell growth, repair, and function. Studies in Alzheimer patients now suggest that estrogen has the potential to *reduce* our later risk of developing Alzheimer's disease by 40–50 percent.

Milder forms of memory changes that women describe during pre- and perimenopause are generally *not* the more serious dementia syndromes. Dementia is an *illness* that affects about 10 percent of the population on average. Menopause, of course, is a *normal transition* for all women who live long enough, and does not alone cause dementia. But if hormonal decline in women is *one contributing factor* that would help explain the gender differences in the terrible disease of Alzheimers, then we *must* consider this issue in helping women. To make a wise and balanced decision about whether to use supplemental hormones when our ovaries no longer make what we need, we all need solid information to guide us.

As I worked with hormonal effects on many parts of the body and the effects on brain-mediated phenomena, I began to wonder whether hormonal changes in women were more a factor than we had thought. When women talked about memory changes, they typically said these problems were worse, "before my period" or "during my flow." These menstrual-cycle phases are times of declining or low estrogen. Women's descriptions have been so *uniform* in the way they have talked about what they notice with memory related to these menstrual phases that I felt certain it was not all due to life stress or women being oversensitive to body-mind changes. I became convinced that there is an important effect of estrogen on memory.

Fortunately, in the last several years, there are a number of new research studies in animals and humans that show some of the ways estrogen works in the brain to maintain normal memory function. I will describe these later in this chapter. But first, listen to the voices of these women.

In My Office: Women's Stories

I remember the poignant first appointment with Ann, a forty-six year old homemaker and community leader, who sat in my consult room in tears as she admitted her most terrifying fear:

> My mother died of Alzheimer's and it began when she was in her early fifties. I'm beginning to have memory problems, and I'm so embarrassed. I'm afraid someone will notice, and deep inside I'm really afraid it's the beginning of Alzheimer's for me too. I can't seem to focus on my lists like I used to, I forget names, I go to say a word I know and suddenly it's not there and I feel stupid. I can't seem to add like I used to, and my mind wanders a lot. I'm really frightened. I just don't want to end up like my mother. What's happening to me? I do everything right, and I really try to take care of my health, there's just nothing in my lifestyle to cause this memory problem. That's why I'm sure it must be the beginning of Alzheimer's. What can I do?

Her mother had an earlier menopause at about age forty-six, and then was told she had Alzheimer's dementia at age fifty-five. Her sister's menopause was at age forty-seven. Ann had a hysterectomy four years earlier at age forty-three, but had not had her ovaries removed. She was in good health, was not overweight, did not smoke cigarettes, rarely drank alcohol, exercised aerobically four to five days a week, and also followed a weight-training program. She even made sure she took all the vitamins that were supposed to help memory! She really was "doing everything right."

Kay, a fifty-one-year-old writer, was disturbed by her growing awareness of difficulty finding the right words for her articles, as well as having trouble keeping her attention focused on getting a story finished on deadline. She described her observations:

> My thoughts are fragmented, and I get distracted so easily. I never used to be like that. I was always one of the most focused people I know. My husband said I could tune out a freight train coming through the room. Now I feel like the slightest thing distracts me. I feel like my mind is flying in a million directions. What is happening to me? I'm really worried that I'm developing something like Alzheimer's. What

can I do? I don't want to talk with my other doctors about this. They will just think I'm crazy, or tell me I'm under too much stress. But I've always lived with stress, and I used to thrive under the pressure of a deadline. That's when I did my best writing. I just don't understand this, and I'm frightened. This isn't me.

Kay had not yet gone through menopause, although she had noticed her time of bleeding getting shorter each month, and the flow had decreased significantly. She had less bloating and breast tenderness before her periods now but said her irritability and difficulty concentrating were clearly getting worse and seemed to be much more noticeable the few days before her period and the days she was having her menstrual flow. In the past, the week of bleeding had been a week she typically felt better. She had also noticed a marked loss of interest in sex, and said she felt more tired than usual for her. She had not noticed any hot flashes, but said she had "these funny tingly feelings, like something crawling on my arms, and they come and go." She thought she slept "pretty well." She did not smoke and drank wine occasionally when out to dinner. She had no other health problems but did not exercise and was about ten pounds over her desired weight. Her mother went through menopause at fifty-four and never took any hormones. About twelve years later in life, Kay said her mother became "senile," but she did not know any further information about what her mother's memory problems had been. Her mother died at seventy-one of a heart attack.

Both Ann and Kay had a common finding on their evaluations: Each one had high FSH levels and *low* estradiol levels, typical of menopause. Both Ann and Kay had not thought they were menopausal. Kay was still menstruating (although her periods had gotten lighter, a clue that her estrogen was decreasing), and Ann's doctor had told her she was too young to be menopausal. Kay's doctor told her that since she was still menstruating her problems couldn't be due to menopause. And since neither woman had experienced any of the usual symptoms, such as hot flashes, they had not considered the idea of menopause. All of Ann's other laboratory studies were normal, but she did have a significant degree of bone loss for her age, in spite of her excellent health habits and exercise program. Kay's evaluation revealed no other health problems except high cholesterol with a lower-than-desirable level of HDL.

Although it was the memory problems that brought each woman to see me, the bone loss for Ann and the cholesterol changes for Kay, along with the high FSH, were indications that each woman's estrogen had been declining for longer than either one was aware. After reviewing all of their evaluation data and talking in depth about their respective options and their specific desires, both Ann and Kay decided to try estrogen therapy. Ann wanted to be sure she took steps that would help prevent further bone loss, and Kay thought her risk of heart disease was high, given her own cholesterol picture and her mother's death from a heart attack. I talked with each one about what we know about the effects of estradiol on brain centers governing memory. I explained that in my clinical work with women, I had seen noticeable improvements in memory if the estradiol levels were restored to the normal levels of the first half of usual menstrual cycles.

That was two years ago. Ann called a month after starting the estradiol, and in an upbeat voice, said, *"it's better, I feel like I've got my own mind back again!"* By the time she had been on the estradiol for six months, she reported that all of the previous negative changes in her intellectual ability had now resolved. *"I'm back to my normal self. I feel great. I didn't realize just how scared I had been than I might be getting Alzheimer's like my mother. I am so relieved to know that what was happening was just the hormone changes of menopause and it could be helped."*

Kay also had a positive outcome: Her cholesterol profile improved, and she described feeling *"my ability to focus on my writing has dramatically improved. I didn't realize until I felt better just how much I had been slipping in my concentration. I can keep on track, the problem with words has gone, and I seem to do fine with organizing my thoughts again. I had no idea hormone drops at menopause could create such mental changes. Why doesn't anyone talk about this?"*

I think one reason not many physicians address these issues is that, in general, they have not been taught to think about the brain as a target organ of hormone changes. The focus has been on reproductive organs and the breast for the most part, with more recent attention turned to heart and bone health after estrogen declines. Frequently, when women ask health professionals about things like memory symptoms, the explanation is that memory and concentration changes are due to the stresses that women experience in this phase of life. As one woman succinctly put it, however, *"Stress is ubiquitous throughout most women's lives, and the memory changes don't seem to be a problem in earlier years, so why now? It has to have some connection with hormone changes."*

Often, women don't even want to admit to friends that these subtle memory changes are happening. Many are reluctant to talk any more about it, fearing they really are going crazy or developing some type of dementia, so they end up experiencing their uncertainty and fear alone. In health care settings, the questions and connections women think are important all too often get "written off" and go unanswered, leaving the fear and worry to intensify even more.

There was B.J., a fifty-one-year-old woman who wrote me a note after one of my seminars:

I had not been told that memory problems could be related to meno-pause. No one explained about memory problems, libido changes, insomnia, etc. I was mainly told about hot flashes. I really didn't have anyone to talk to. None of my friends said they had these problems. Thanks for a wealth of information. It makes me feel better, I had really thought I was beginning to get Alzheimer's and it had really bothered me. Now I have some ideas to talk with my doctor about.

May was fifty-three when I saw her for a consultation. She had gone through menopause at forty-nine, and had started estrogen therapy shortly thereafter to help her severe hot flashes. She was also concerned about osteoporosis, since her mother had lost two inches in height in the years after menopause and had died of complications following a hip fracture in her late sixties. May had been on conjugated equine estrogens, 0.625 mg for twenty-five days a month, with a progestin added on Days 16 through 25 of the month, since age forty-nine. She felt the estrogen had really helped her hot flashes and energy level, but she was concerned about continuing problems with memory. She talked about having trouble remembering what she had gone into a room to do, frequently forgot a word she was getting ready to say, had to write down telephone numbers as soon as she looked them up, and said she felt her brain "had a cloud pulled down over it. I just feel foggy, and that's not like me, what's happening?"

May's evaluation was normal on all the tests for other possible causes of her memory problems. Significantly, her estradiol was low and her FSH was still in the menopausal high range even though she was on estrogen therapy. She was a tall woman and very physically active. I thought there were potentially two factors to consider in fine-tuning her hormone therapy: First, I thought she needed a different amount of estrogen, given her body build and level of physical activity that increased her metabolism of the hormones: second, I thought she would see a better improvement in the brain-related symptoms if she changed to a natural human form of 17-beta estradiol instead of the conjugated equine estrogens that she had been taking for so long. In my clinical experience, I find that women generally have a better response on brain function using the natural human estradiol since it is the bioidentical hormone the ovary made before menopause, and it fits properly, like a key in a lock, at the specific brain receptor sites that help to regulate memory and information processing.

She took my suggestion and changed to Estrace (17-beta estra-diol) in a better dose for her, and we made sure this was providing what she needed by checking her blood level in about a month and-tracking her symptom improvement. In about a month, she described how she felt: *"My memory is back, I can concentrate and focus well again. They really are greatly improved, I feel like I have my full abilities back. It's hard to explain, but I just feel like my mind is clearer somehow."*

I do not think estrogen is a cure-all for memory problems. But it is, however, one of the most frequently *overlooked* factors affecting memory function for women. There are still many questions to be answered about exactly how estrogen works in the brain and what types of estrogen are needed for these brain pathways. There are many, many types of medical disorders and lifestyle habits that can affect the brain and cause memory changes. Most importantly, if you are having these kinds of symptoms, you need a careful and complete medical evaluation for the various types of problems, hormonal and otherwise, that can result in these mental and physical changes. While I think probably all of us could use more time and practice in *relaxing*, I do not think that's the whole answer. **Body physiology affects brain function, too. It's that basic.**

For those of you reading this who have had memory problems, at least be aware that checking your ovary and thyroid hormones much more carefully and specifically as I have described are critical dimensions of your health measures to address along with other tests and therapeutic approaches you may be taking. You don't have to sit there and be frightened that something terrible is happening to you. There are ways to properly and thoroughly address your questions and ways of arriving at feeling better. Speak up, and be heard!

Meanwhile, here's the latest information on estrogen effects on memory from worldwide research. The brain is truly an exciting frontier of hormone interactions and effects.

You Are Not Imagining It!
Menopause Does Affect Memory.

First some memory basics. To better understand what has been discovered about estrogen effects on memory, you will need to know some of the names of the brain areas involved in memory function, shown in the diagram below. Collectively, these structures make up the area called the *limbic system*, the mood-regulating area of the brain (rich in estradiol receptors, remember?) I described in chapters 3 and 4. Next to each of the memory-regulating structures, I have given an example of a disease process that typically affects that area of the brain and may cause memory disruption. The *temporal lobes* of the brain are major sites of these memory-regulating centers, so you may also see this term in discussions of memory.

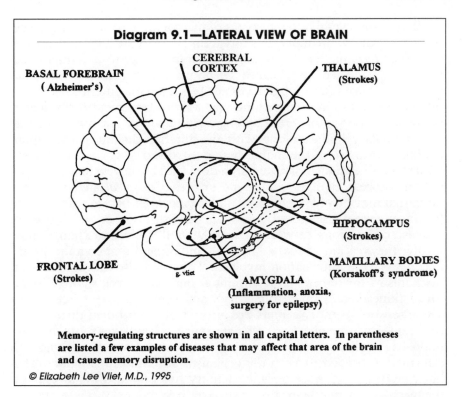

Diagram 9.1—LATERAL VIEW OF BRAIN

BASAL FOREBRAIN
(Alzheimer's)

CEREBRAL
CORTEX

THALAMUS
(Strokes)

HIPPOCAMPUS
(Strokes)

FRONTAL LOBE
(Strokes)

g. vliet

AMYGDALA
(Inflammation, anoxia,
surgery for epilepsy)

MAMILLARY BODIES
(Korsakoff's syndrome)

Memory-regulating structures are shown in all capital letters. In parentheses
are listed a few examples of diseases that may affect that area of the brain
and cause memory disruption.

© Elizabeth Lee Vliet, M.D., 1995

The complex components of our memory system have only
recently been mapped out. It used to be thought that memory traces
were spread throughout the brain and could not be localized to any
particular structures. More recent studies have shown the primary
components of the memory system in the brain are the *hippocampus*, the *mamillary bodies*, the *septal region* of the limbic system,
and part of the *thalamus*. There is a great deal that remains to be
understood about how these various memory processes work in the
human brain, but at present the memory system appears to consist
of "storage centers," which are located symmetrically in both hemispheres of the brain, primarily in the hippocampus and mamillary
bodies. These centers in several parts of the brain provide back-up
systems to prevent memory from being damaged or lost. If one
hemisphere of the brain is damaged, memory will remain intact as
long as the other hemisphere has not been injured. If *both* hemispheres of the brain involving memory centers are injured severely
enough, the person has lost the ability to learn new material and store
it for future retrieval. Memory function, having multiple memory cir-
cuitry centers in various parts of the brain, is thereby different from
other brain functions, which tend to have more specific locations in
one or the other hemisphere.

There are several different types of memory, but to simplify this we can conceptualize memory as short-term memory or long-term memory. *Short-term memory* comes into use in many day-to-day situations, for example, when you hear a telephone number or a name and remember it just long enough to use it. When a name, number or other piece of information is something you wish to remember for a longer period of time, it is converted to *long-term memory*. The hippocampus and mamillary bodies, along with the anterior thalamus and septal region, appear to be the major centers involved in converting short-term to long-term memory. Research does tend to suggest that this conversion process involves some type of actual *physical* change in the brain that may involve creation of *new connections* between nerve cells (estrogen stimulates growth of these new sprouts, or dendrites, to increase connections between neurons). Or this physical change may involve the creation of actual "memory molecules" that contain specific codes for the information involved. The brain also has a variety of mechanisms for remembering specific sound (auditory), sight (visual), touch (kinesthetic), smell (olfactory), and other sensory perceptions. These sensory memory centers are also widely distributed throughout the brain. Since memory is so crucial to survival, it makes sense that the brain has evolved multiple areas for memory storage of all kinds of information needed to keep the organism alive and functioning. The key role of the sex hormones in memory function also fits as part of the mechanisms that help species survive.

New Research on Estrogen and Memory

By now, many of you have seen the headlines in major newspapers about the research on estrogen and Alzheimer's disease, and that estrogen deficiency may play an important role in causing, or worsening, some dementias. At the 1993 meeting of the North American Menopause Society, three researchers agreed that it is a significant, and underrated, factor in some of these aging-related disorders. Dr. Stanley Birge and his associates from Washington University in St. Louis believe that the new research findings support the theory that estrogen loss at menopause contribute to, along with genetic and environmental factors, the deterioration of the central nervous system known as Alzheimer's disease and, potentially, other types of memory changes. Dr. Birge's studies have also found that women over seventy who take estrogen have an improved ability in a balancing exercise, "tandem stance," compared to women not on estrogen. He hypothesized that estrogen deficiency, through effects on postural reflexes and balance, may be a factor contributing to the unusually high rates of falls in elderly women.

Dr. Barbara Sherwin, at McGill University in Canada, has spent a number of years researching estrogen effects on the brain and her studies have shown improvements specifically in *verbal* memory in healthy postmenopausal women on estrogen compared to those who are not. In a separate study, Dr. Sherwin prospectively evaluated surgically menopausal women and found that those treated with estrogen did significantly better on several measures of cognitive function than the women given a placebo. Yet another prospective study of surgically menopausal women showed that taking estradiol specifically enhanced short-term verbal memory. None of these women had any type of dementia; they were all healthy post-menopausal and would not have been considered *impaired* in their memory abilities. Yet, the improved performance in the women on estrogen therapy was statistically significant and also fits with the self-reports I have heard consistently from patients in my practice.

At the Baylor College of Medicine and VA Medical Center in Houston, Dr. Karl Mortel studied postmenopausal women who were either neurologically normal or had mild cerebrovascular disease (CVD), which had manifested as transient ischemic attacks (brief periods of decreased oxygen causing symptoms similar to a mild stroke). He found that among women with CVD, women on estrogen therapy showed improved blood flow to the brain and improved cognitive function compared to the women with CVD who were not on estrogen. He concluded that estrogen therapy may be an effective addition to the treatment of older women with impaired circulation. His work fits with other research that has shown estradiol to have a *relaxing effect* on arteries, leading to more dilation and better blood flow to all organs in the body.

In 1991 and 1992 at the North American Menopause Society meeting, several researchers from Japan presented evidence of estrogen's ability to *improve* cognitive function in elderly women who already had developed Alzheimer's dementia. Dr. N. Hagino found that two-thirds of the fifteen study patients improved significantly in their communication with families, their ability for self-care, and memory for time and daily events. At the time, this research presentation did not get a lot of media attention. Since that meeting, we have seen a marked increase in the interest in, and attention given to, estrogen effects on brain function with additional studies now underway in the United States.

In an ongoing study of 8, 879 female residents of Leisure World, a retirement community in California, researchers at University of Southern California (USC) studied the medical records of those who died during the period from 1982 to 1991, and found 127 women whose death certificates mentioned either Alzheimer's disease or dementia. These cases were then matched with those of the other women the same age who had *not* died of dementia. The resulting 635 cases were assigned to one of two groups: those women who had taken estrogen and those who had not. The researchers found that the estrogen users were 40 percent **less likely** to die of Alzheimer's disease or dementia than women who had not taken estrogen. Another way of looking at it, the women on estrogen ran only about 60 percent of the risk of getting Alzheimer's women had who did not take estrogen. The USC investigators further found that the higher the maximum reported dose of the estrogen, the *lower* the risk of Alzheimer's. The risk of dementia also *decreased* with a longer duration of estrogen therapy. Women who had been on estrogen seven years or more had *only 50 percent of the risk of dementia* seen in women who did not receive ERT. JoAnn McConnell, senior vice president for medical and scientific affairs of the Alzheimer's Association in Chicago, said "I think that these are very interesting results, and stronger than prior hints for an effect of estrogen." These results are preliminary but bring up potentially important additional considerations in weighing the decision about hormone therapy for women who have a family history of dementia.

In 1986, H. Fillit and colleagues in a limited study found that some patients showed significant improvement in attention, mental function, and social interaction when on estrogen therapy. In 1989, another group of investigators using Premarin 1.25 mg daily as the estrogen therapy found that the women showed improvement in memory, orientation, and calculation. In 1994, Ohlura and colleagues did careful psychometric testing and showed objective improvement after ERT on measures of recent memory, distant memory, attention, orientation, personality, mood, and sleeping and feeding behaviors. Serum estradiol was measured in all study participants prior to and during ERT, with ERT resulting in mean serum levels of estradiol up to the values of mid-follicular phase of a healthy menstrual cycle in younger women. These study results suggest that the amount of estradiol given, and the serum levels achieved with therapy, have to reach such a desirable range to have the observed benefits on memory and other cognitive functions. The positive changes seen with ERT disappeared after estrogen was discontinued, thereby strongly suggesting estrogen's major influence on these cognitive functions. An interesting outcome from this study was that the families of all of these patients had also seen the improvement in their relatives and requested that the estrogen therapy be continued long-term at the completion of the study. They didn't need to wait for more controlled studies to be convinced of the positive cognitive effects of estrogen.

Since that time, a number of other studies worldwide have shown improvement in memory function in postmenopausal women given ERT, whether their menopause was a natural one or due to surgical removal of the uterus and ovaries. Ditkoff and colleagues showed an overall improvement in mood and quality of life in post-menopausal women on ERT. In a 1999 randomized double-blind, placebo-controlled clinical trial published in *JAMA*, Yale researchers found that even a three-week course of ERT changed brain activity in postmenopausal women performing memory tasks. This study went a step further in using magnetic resonance imaging (MRI) of the brain to show brain activation patterns both without and with ERT. The cerebral activity changes mimicked brain activation patterns typically seen in younger women. Sally E. Shaywitz, M.D., principal investigator, concluded that, "These alterations suggest a plasticity in the memory systems of mature women and that these neural systems are neither fixed nor immutable." While the full mechanism of estrogen's effects on the brain memory and cognitive pathways has not yet been clarified, there are a number of intriguing hypotheses about how it works, as we shall now see.

How Does Estrogen Work on the Brain?

A number of studies argue for a direct effect of estrogen on memory, specifically on verbal memory, and there appear to be a number of neurochemical and structural ways estrogen exerts its effect. The biochemical and nerve structure studies have been done in animals. While animal studies cannot always be extrapolated to humans, what we have learned about rat brains in other areas of research seems to also apply to human brains at the biochemical level. There is no practical way to measure these types of biochemical and nerve cell structural changes in people, so the animal research provides a working model of what to look for in humans in later clinical trials. Dr. Bruce McEwen, head of Rockefeller University Neuroendocrinology Laboratory, and investigators from other countries, have done extensive research on the effects of estrogen on brain tissue, and have collectively found the many estrogen effects summarized in the chart that follows.

Dr. McEwen and other neuroendocrine researchers have concluded that the brain is an important target organ for estrogens and that effects on the brain functions, such as memory and cognition, must be considered in relation to the decline of estrogens in women after natural or surgical menopause. I agree. I think it's time we looked at the brain as connected to the body and affected by the same kinds of changes that affect other parts of the body. Psychological symptoms, like memory changes, clearly may have *physical causes* as well as stress-related causes.

**ESTROGEN EFFECTS ON
MEMORY AND COGNITIVE PATHWAYS**

- 17-beta estradiol, the primary estrogen produced by the ovary before menopause, has specific receptor binding sites in many different areas of the brain, and these receptor sites appear to be quite *specific* for the native human form of the molecule. (All of my clinical work with patients strongly supports these basic science findings in animal models.)

- Estradiol promotes growth of new dendrites between nerve cells, making *more* synaptic connections, while progesterone breaks down the nerve-cell connections. More synapse connections mean nerve cells can handle more incoming signals.

- When estradiol declines, synapse density in the hippocampus (memory and learning center) decreases as well. (My comment to readers: Denser synapses allow better cell-to-cell information flow.)

- Estradiol enhances nerve cells' ability to take in *nerve growth factor* (NGF). In animals without ovaries, those who did *not* receive estrogen had a marked (56 percent) decline in the number of nerve cells; the animals given estrogen had only a slight decrease in nerve cells.

- Estrogens regulate cholinergic nerve cells in the *basal forebrain* of rodents. (My comment to readers: This is one of the regions of the brain involved in cognitive function and one of the areas that degenerates in humans with Alzheimer's disease.)

- Estrogens increase the production of choline acetyltransferase, an enzyme needed to make acetylcholine (ACh). Estrogen thereby prevents the marked loss of ACh found in patients with Alzheimer's. (My comments to readers: ACh is the brain's most important chemical messenger for storing new memories in the brain, regulating memory retrieval, and cognition. Loss of the cholinergic nerves and chemical messengers is the most marked brain change in Alzheimer's disease.)

© Elizabeth Lee Vliet, M.D., 2000

Listen to the comments of these women who experienced the benefits on memory that came from making appropriate changes in their estrogen therapy:

After a hysterectomy at age fifty-two, I took Premarin for nearly eight years. My memory began to deteriorate. Never one to be particularly concerned about getting old, I made fun of it at first. I reached a point, however, around age fifty-six when my memory loss was downright embarrassing. I felt I was in a mental fog. I couldn't remember common words, stumbled through sentences, lost my train of thought, had

difficulty following complex conversations or instructions, and even skipped words when I wrote. My work suffered and I could tell my family and friends were being kind and patient with me. Loving and generous of them, but humiliating for me. Dr. Vliet suggested I use Estrace for my hormone replacement therapy. In a short time, I began to notice I was no longer constantly apologizing for lapses in speech and memory. The fog had lifted. Of course, my memory isn't what it was when I was twenty, but I have regained my pride and self-confidence. At last, I'm enjoying this stage of my life and all it has to offer.
—A.F., age 62.

I later received the following letter from this patient's mother, who is in her eighties, after she had seen the improvement in her daughter from the change in type of estrogen:

I believe the first thing I noticed after changing from Premarin to Estrace was a cloud lifting from my skull [mind]. Prior to that I seemed to be going around in a perpetual fog, never feeling as though I was thinking clearly. That was such a relief! I seemed to remember things much more clearly, not stumbling over names that I had known for years, once again being able to reconcile my bank accounts and being able to reply to questions that had previously left me with complete blanks. One of the things that had bothered me a lot was the shaking of my hands. There were days when I could hardly make out checks and when I finished, they looked like some person with palsy had written them and were almost illegible. Physically, I feel 100 percent better, and I am so grateful to you for recommending the Estrace to my daughter so I could ask my own doctor to make the change for me.
—F.L., in her eighties

Don't suffer in silence. Know that help is available, and there are a number of such changes in hormone therapy that can improve your memory, improve your clarity of thinking, and give more of that feeling of energy and zest if you are having these problems.

Thyroid Changes and Memory

After about age forty, women have approximately *five to eight times* the incidence of thyroid disorders found in men of similar ages. We do not yet have a clear explanation for this gender difference. Diminished thyroid function becomes more frequent in women as they age, and must be included in the proper evaluation of women in the perimenopause and menopause years. One of the concerns is that brain symptoms of hypothyroidism such as memory loss, decreased concentration, difficulty organizing one's thoughts, and depressed mood are often so subtle that many women are not properly diagnosed until the disorder has progressed to produce the more obvious physical signs of dry skin, hair loss, weight gain, cold intolerance, slowed heart rate, decreased reflexes, high blood pressure, and high cholesterol, to name a few. The subtle brain symptoms *tend to occur first*, and memory loss is among the early changes when thyroid hormones are not adequately produced, or when their effect is blocked by antibody production as occurs in Hashimoto's thyroiditis. Since the changes found in thyroid disorders may overlap the symptoms women experience with menopause, it is particularly important that both hormonal systems be checked fully. If left untreated, hypothyroidism can progress to a dementia syndrome similar to Alzheimer's disease. I have also had quite a few patients who had been *misdiagnosed with Alzheimer's dementia,* but when proper tests were done were found to have a treatable hypothyroidism causing their memory impairment. The evaluation of thyroid function is significantly overlooked in women's health, particularly as women get older.

Of course, it is important not to *overtreat* thyroid disease and take too much thyroid hormone, since excessive amounts of thyroid hormone can cause heart damage and bone loss. These complications occur whether you take "natural" thyroid extracts or the medications made by pharmaceutical companies. Excessive amounts of thyroid cause your body's metabolic engines to be overly "revved up," with increased heart rate, jitteriness, irritability, excessive weight loss, and increased bone breakdown. Thyroid imbalances, either too high or too low, can produce marked effects on brain function, with resulting mood, behavioral, and cognitive changes. Low thyroid causes memory loss, difficulty concentrating, slow mental processes like a "gray cloud of fog" has dropped down over your brain. Excess or "hyper" thyroid states cause scattered thinking, difficulty focusing, memory disruptions (similar to power surges affecting your computer circuits!), and other brain symptoms much like what we call attention deficit disorder. For optimal function of your brain, including memory, *balance* is the key with all of these critical hormones.

Sleep Deprivation and Memory

Tossing and turning, waking up wide-eyed, looking at the clock, going back to sleep, waking up, looking at the clock. This is a common scenario I hear from midlife women. As estrogen levels drop before a period, after ovulation, or decline with menopause, the drop in estradiol triggers a firing of the "alerting" centers in the brain. These centers then discharge a burst of an adrenaline-type chemical messenger, which has an arousing effect and wakes you up. In addition, the burst of adrenaline hits the brain's heat-regulating center and triggers the hot flash or flush, followed by sweating. These episodes of awakening at night may occur only a few times or may be quite frequent, leaving you feeling tired when you get up in the morning. Sleep disruption over an extended period of time is associated with daytime drowsiness, fatigue, feeling "foggy" mentally, and also with disturbances in memory, concentration, focus, and even loss of libido. Prolonged sleep disruption can even be a cause of the biochemical changes that lead to a major (clinical) depressive episode. Getting a good night's sleep is more crucial to our health than most women realize.

I had always been a good sleeper until I hit age thirty-nine. I thought I was much too young to even think about something like premature menopause. I couldn't figure what in the world was happening to me. My doctors just thought it was the stress of medical practice (made sense to me, given how busy I was), and I acquiesced to that idea. A few years later, I realized, as many of my patients have also said, that I had been under a lot of stress at other times in my medical career and did not have the same problems sleeping. So what was this? It turned out that I was actually in premature ovarian decline. The loss of estrogen was causing the frequent waking episodes. Extensive sleep research in recent years has helped us understand the many beneficial functions of sleep to maintain normal body restoration and repair each twenty-four hour-cycle. The role of healthy sleep patterns in optimal memory function has not yet been fully defined, but researchers have identified a strong correlation between failing memory and abnormalities of the sleep cycle. Estrogen balance in women is important for regulation of both sleep and memory.

The normal sleep cycle and sleep stages are adversely affected in significant ways when women lose the active form of estrogen (17-beta estradiol), a process that begins long before you stop menstruating. I described in chapter 5 some of the current studies that have shown estrogen replacement results in improved sleep, even in women with severe forms of sleep disorders like sleep apnea syndrome. Of course, I recognize that there are many factors that cause disruption in sleep (see list), and these must also be addressed. But, the one factor *frequently overlooked* for women is the effect of estrogen change in triggering fragmented sleep. I think women should have their hormone levels properly tested in their medical workups before sleeping pills are prescribed.

SOME COMMON CAUSES OF INSOMNIA

- hormonal changes (ovary, thyroid, adrenal, pituitary, etc.)

- drug and alcohol abuse (acute effects and withdrawal), tobacco use

- excess caffeine, other stimulants (sodas, coffee, tea, chocolate, "metabolic" or "energy" boosters with phenylpropanolamine, herbs with *ephedra*, weight loss and herbal products that contain Gotu kola and other stimulants)

- medical disorders: examples are COPD, congestive heart failure, asthma, diabetes, fibromyalgia, sleep apnea, and many others

- medications: especially allergy and cold medicines with decongestants, some antidepressants, testosterone, or DHEA (if taken at night), many others

- jet lag, shift work that disrupts normal sleep-wake cycles

- clinical depression, generalized anxiety disorders

- life stress, persistent worries, bereavement, posttraumatic stress disorders

- poor sleep habits (making your bed a second home office doesn't help you relax!)

© Elizabeth Lee Vliet, M.D., 1995

Sleep architecture is the term used to describe the normal pattern of sleep stages (shown in the table on facing page). Each of these is characterized by different electrical activity or "brain wave" patterns, measured on electroencephalogram (EEG) tracings, eye movement measures (EOM), and muscle activity (EMG). Non-REM sleep (NREM) are the four stages in which *dreaming does not occur.* REM sleep is the stage in which dreaming occurs, along with other physiological responses like penile erections in men. Sleep problems (apnea, narcolepsy, and others) can be evaluated in sleep laboratories to determine the specific type of disorder, which in turn directs the physician to the proper treatments.

As you sleep each night, you experience seventy- to one-hundred-minute cycles of these stages, with more NREM sleep in the first half of the night, and more REM (dreaming) sleep in the second half toward morning. Sleep quality decreases with age in all of us, even in healthy individuals. The presence of medical problems, obesity, alcohol use, and cigarette smoking may all contribute to even more rapid deterioration in quality of sleep and may disrupt the normal sleep stages. If you become sleep deprived, the brain actively directs restoring the normal sleep patterns by lengthening total sleep time and the amount of slow wave sleep on the first recovery night. On following recovery nights, there is an increase (rebound) of REM

NORMAL SLEEP ARCHITECTURE			
	EEG Patterns	**Eye Movement**	**Muscle Action**
AWAKE	mainly alpha waves, some beta	depends on task	normal tone, voluntary movement
NREM—Stage 1	mixed theta, beta waves; alpha <50 percent	slow, rolling	relaxed, less tone
NREM—Stage 2	theta, bursts of sleep spindles, K complex	slow, rolling	relaxed, less tone
NREM—Stage 3	delta waves, 20–50 percent	slow	relaxed
NREM - Stage 4	delta (slow wave sleep), >50 percent	slow	relaxed
REM (dreaming)	**similar to waking**	symmetrical, rapid; jerky	none (atonia); penile erections occur

© Elizabeth Lee Vliet, M.D., 1995

sleep to compensate for lost REM during sleep deprivation. REM rebound causes *intense* dreaming for several nights or longer.

One of the reasons sleeping pills become a problem with prolonged use is that they interrupt the normal sleep patterns and the balance of the various stages. Stopping sleeping pills abruptly after more than two weeks of use will typically cause REM rebound, making it harder to sleep normally. Eventually, sleeping pill use makes it harder for the body and brain to function normally and will further impair energy, mood, and memory *independent* of the specific medication's effects on memory (more about this in the next section). This is another reason I do not like to see women have prescriptions for sleeping pills without looking carefully for the *underlying causes* of sleep problems, *including* hormone changes, and more serious kinds of sleep disorders (e.g., SAS), which could be dangerous in combination with sleeping pills.

For most women during the menopause transition, sleep disruption does *not* require sleeping pills. Restoring optimal estradiol balance, learning relaxation techniques, having a carbohydrate snack before bedtime to increase brain tryptophan, which will then boost serotonin production (skim milk and cereal is good), or a trial of herbal remedies such as St. John's Wort or 5-hydroxytryptophan or valerian root may all help to restore normal sleep. There is a positive synergistic effect from using a combined approach with all of these options. I have some women who did not want to take a full therapeutic amount of estradiol who reported good results for sleep improvement with a lower dose combined with serotonin boosters. You should talk with your physician about these approaches to see what fits YOU best.

Sleeping Pills, Alcohol, and Other Memory Robbers

All of the sleeping pills on the market today, both prescription and over-the-counter ones, adversely affect your memory. The other "drug" that many people, particularly women, use to help them fall asleep is alcohol. It, too, impairs memory, along with its many other negative effects on health. Alcohol not only causes direct damage to nerve cells, but it also depletes your brain and body of crucial vitamins that are needed for the brain's memory circuits to work properly. For example, the B vitamins are significantly depleted when you drink alcohol on a regular basis, and all of the B vitamins are needed for the brain to make its memory-regulating neurotransmitters. Each class of medication acts by different means to decrease memory, but all of them contribute to memory loss over time. Fortunately, much of the memory loss produced by alcohol, sedative sleeping pills, and over-the-counter sleeping pills can be reversed if you stop using these substances. After prolonged overuse of alcohol, however, the nerve cells are permanently damaged, and memory loss does not return when a person stops drinking. The *progression* of further memory loss may be stopped by eliminating alcohol, but once tissue damage has occurred, normal memory function does not return. This is another reason to limit alcohol to occasional, moderate intake. Let's look at what happens to the brain with each of these "memory robbers" to help you understand why memory changes occur.

Prescription Sedatives ("Sleeping Pills")

These are generally grouped under the term *sedative-hypnotic* medications and include (1) the older *barbiturates* (Meprobamate, Seconal, and others), which are not used as much today due to their toxicity and addictiveness; and (2) the *benzodiazepine group* (Ambien, Dalmane, Restoril, Halcion, Doral, ProSom; other benzodiazepines that are sometimes used for sleep include Klonopin, Valium, Libruim, Xanax, Ativan, or Tranxene). All of the drugs in this category will initially improve sleep by inducing more rapid sleep onset and helping to maintain sleep. After about ten days to two weeks, these medications lose their effectiveness on sleep and also cause a disruption in the normal *stages* of sleep (mainly loss of stage 4 sleep). The sedative-hypnotics as a group *all cause memory loss* if used for an extended period of time, usually longer than two weeks. For some people, the memory impairment can come much more quickly than that. These drugs typically also cause a hangover effect of daytime "brain fog," feelings of tiredness or excessive fatigue, and daytime drowsiness; this problem will be *worse* with long-acting ones (Klonopin, Dalmane, Valium, Librium) and less noticeable with shorter-acting ones such as Ativan, Ambien and Xanax.

The high potency, very short-acting sleep medications, such as Halcion, produce much more memory impairment the next day and also tend to cause rebound anxiety when the drug wears off. I was concerned about the very short action of Halcion and its high potency; even when it first came out, I rarely prescribed it. With the subsequent publicity about the potential adverse reactions, I do not prescribe Halcion at all. I have personally treated many women who have had severe mood changes (anxiety, irritability, memory impairment, and other problems) from Halcion, and I do not recommend its use. The benzodiazepines have an *additive* effect on sedation and potential respiratory depression if you drink alcohol when taking them. All of the drugs in this category produce dependence and cause withdrawal syndromes if stopped abruptly after more than about seven days of use. It can also be dangerous to use sedative-hypnotics if you have sleep apnea, since these medications further suppress respiration. It is uncommon for me to prescribe sedative-hypnotic medications. I much prefer to first see that the sleep problem is properly diagnosed and then to help the individual develop good sleep habits, use nutritional and other natural methods of improving sleep, consider hormonal options if appropriate and desired, and as a last resort use lowdose serotonin-augmenting medications.

Serotonin-Boosters and Antidepressants Used for Sleep

Older sedating antidepressants that boost serotonin, such as Desyrel (trazodone), Elavil (amitriptyline), Sinequan (doxepin), Tofranil (imipramine), as well as newer medications like Zoloft, are often useful in very low doses to help with insomnia. These medications are not addictive, do not disrupt the normal stages of sleep, and if used in low doses, have fewer side effects than typically encountered in the higher doses used to treat depression. These all have mild to moderate antihistamine effects, enhance serotonin activity, and produce drowsiness at low doses. At higher doses used for treating depression, they decrease nocturnal awakenings, increase non-REM sleep, decrease REM sleep, and normalize the disturbed sleep that is characteristic of biological depression.

I think these medications are safe and potentially helpful, but some of the side effects of all except trazodone are particularly bothersome to midlife women (weight gain, dry eyes, constipation, among others), and these medications also have potential for many drug interactions with other medications you are taking. You will need to discuss these options with your physician and see if they might be appropriate for you. The serotonin-boosting antidepressants are especially valuable in improving sleep in people with perimenopausal hormone changes and chronic pain syndromes. You may want to read more in the chapter on fibromyalgia about how these drugs work to reduce pain. The antidepressants are *nonaddictive*, but if stopped abruptly, you may experience "REM rebound," which results in several days to a week of intense dreaming, irritability, and mood swings. If you are taking these medications, even in a low dose, it is best to taper them off gradually.

Another natural serotonin booster is 5-HTP (5-hydroxytryptophan), a building-block molecule used by the brain to make serotonin. Although 5-HTP is widely available without a prescription, there have been FDA reports of contamination in these products similar to that seen with L-tryptophan a number of years ago. As a result of these concerns, I do not recommend that you use an over-the-counter product of 5-HTP. I recommend getting a *pharmaceutical-grade* form of 5-HTP from a compounding pharmacist you trust. The one we use is Belmar Pharmacy in Lakewood, Colorado (800-525-9473), and we have found that their prices for the prescription pharmaceutical grade 5-HTP are *lower* than many of the over-the-counter products.

Over-the-Counter (OTC) Sleep Aids

These include non-prescription products such as Sleep-Eze, Nytol, Sominex, and a variety of others. These products typically contain antihistamine compounds (diphenhydramine is a common one) that are central nervous system depressants and produce drowsiness and sedation. Daytime sleepiness and difficulty with memory and concentration is common. Weight gain and cravings for carbohydrates are other common side effects of antihistamines. You should let your physician know if you use these OTC sleep aids, because they all can potentially interact with other medications you may be taking. This group has an *additive* effect on sedation if you also drink alcohol. I have also found that many of my patients have the *opposite reaction* to antihistamines and become anxious and agitated rather than sleepy. Be cautious if you use these sleep aids, communicate with your physician and do not use them for an extended period of time without having your sleep problems fully evaluated medically.

Herbal Sleep Aids

There are many herbal remedies that have been used to promote sleep. Some of these include valerian root, lemon balm, chamomile, and passionflower. These can be helpful for some people but may trigger allergic reactions in sensitive individuals. If you would like to use these approaches on a short-term basis, I suggest you consult with a knowledgeable herbalist rather than just taking the advice of a salesperson in a health food store. If you are someone with a lot of allergies to trees, grasses, and other plants, remember that these herbal remedies are derived from *plants* and have the potential to aggravate allergies. It is surprising to me how many people usually do not associate their allergies to plants with the possibility of a reaction to an herbal product.

Vitamins and Memory

A number of vitamins are crucial cofactors, or "helpers," for the brain to make important chemical messengers involved in normal memory function. Several of these, especially B12 and folate, have been known for decades to play a role in maintaining normal brain function, in particular memory and mood regulation. More recently, research in a number of countries had continued to identify the role of various vitamins and minerals in memory processes. Iris Bell, M.D., Ph.D., at the University of Arizona, has significant research documenting the effects of vitamins B1, B2, and B6 in improving both depressive symptoms and cognitive function in elderly patients. Dr. Bell has found that thiamine (B1) deficiency impairs brain glucose metabolism and also contributes to high levels of homocysteine, a risk factor for cardiovascular and cerebrovascular disease that can then lead to memory loss. It appears from a number of studies that significant numbers of patients may have laboratory values of these B vitamins that appear to be in the "normal" range, but may not be adequate for optimal nerve cell function in the brain.

Another area of research into factors affecting memory is the role of *antioxidant* vitamins in prevention of plaque formation in arteries, thereby improving blood flow to the brain. Oxidation, or "free-radical damage," is the process of cell damage and death associated with aging, environmental pollutants, poor nutrition, tobacco smoke, radiation, and other causes. What are free radicals? These are "crippled" oxygen atoms that have lost electrons in the chemical reactions of our body's natural metabolic processes, or as a result of trying to make up for poor nutrition, environmental pollution, and other causes. These free radicals roam the body trying to replace their lost electrons by combining with electrons from healthy cells. This causes damage to the membranes and structures inside healthy cells, much like rust damage to your car. What are antioxidants? These are molecules, such as vitamins E, C, beta-carotene, and selenium (*estradiol* has also been found to act as an antioxidant), which have the capability of losing electrons to free radicals without initiating a damaging chain reaction of electron robbing. Antioxidants serve as "scavengers" to clean up these damaging free radicals and help prevent some of the damage to DNA and cell death. Brain neurons and nerve fibers are particularly vulnerable to damage and death from these free radicals. The antioxidants reduce much of this oxidative damage and help keep brain cells working properly. The effect is to produce modest improvements in memory. Antioxidants, as I will describe in chapter 14, also play a role in helping decrease the risk of certain cancers.

Unfortunately, as most of you now know, nutrition has only received brief mention in most medical school curricula. The critical role of vitamins and minerals in brain function is rarely addressed as an important clinical issue. Consequently, most physicians think that a balanced diet is enough and hardly anyone needs vitamin supplements. I must admit that this was my notion, too, when I first started medical practice. Over the years, with more collaborative work with dietitians interested in preventive medicine, and my own study of nutritional factors affecting mood, energy, memory, and a host of other problems, I have come to clearly see that probably *most of us* would benefit from vitamin supplements. That's quite a turnaround from where I was when I graduated from medical school. I am now diligent about taking my own vitamin-mineral supplements daily.

Vitamins: Difficult to Get with Diet Alone

Very few Americans really eat a balanced diet to begin with, and even fewer women have enough caloric intake and food variety on a daily basis to provide even the RDA for many vitamins and minerals. A classic example is magnesium. The average American woman has a daily intake of about 100 mg. The RDA is 400–600 mg a day. Magnesium is critical for nerve and muscle function, mood and memory processes, and bone development among many other roles in the body. Several years ago, I was struck by a nutritional study done by Angelica Cantlon, R.D. She calculated the amount of calories and variety of food that would be required for the average woman to get her RDA of all the basic vitamins and minerals. She found that daily calories needed to be 1400, and the food groups needed were far more diverse than any patient's food diary I have seen in my entire career in medicine! I was shocked, and so were the women in my seminars when I showed them the results of this study. An average woman who is chronically dieting to lose weight, and this is certainly more common in the premenopausal years when *everyone* seems obsessed with losing weight, has a daily calorie intake of 800 to 1000 calories, followed by marked increases on the weekends at social functions! No wonder there seem to be more memory problems in midlife: not only are important estrogen levels changing, but also women are not eating well enough to sustain the brain's activity at optimal function. Fueling the brain with healthy, quality "fuel" is the best way to have sharper memory.

Start with a basic healthy meal plan, but consider that a good multivitamin with additional calcium, magnesium, beta-carotene, and vitamin E and vitamin C will give you added antioxidant insurance. Magnesium and vitamin E in particular are both difficult to obtain in the typical American diet in order to give you the full antioxidant dose. For best absorption, try a liquid formula of the multivitamin you select. *Centrum* is a good one that is available in major drugstores and not very expensive. I don't endorse *mega*vitamin supplements, since I think these are frequently more expensive than necessary and I have seen many of my patients end up having significant side effects and subtle toxicity syndromes.

"Smart Drugs": Marketing Ploy or Real Help?

A variety of these products are being promoted as "brain enhancers." I continue to be surprised at the amount of money patients spend on these supplements and how many they typically take. It is difficult to make any comments about the effectiveness of these products, since it is often difficult to know exactly what is in the product, and there so far is not a great deal of sound research to document positive results with their use. Deprenyl (selegiline) is one drug in this group that has been shown to be of help in reducing the nerve deterioration characteristic of Parkinson's disease. It has been used in Europe as an antiaging drug and a memory enhancer. I have had a few patients who have been on it for preventing the progression of Parkinson symptoms, but I have not seen dramatic changes in memory or other of its purported actions. It has the potential to cause high blood pressure reactions when taken along with the amino acids tyrosine and phenylalanine, as well as tyramine in certain foods. Since these amino acids are also found in foods, persons on Deprenyl have to watch dietary sources as well as supplements. I do not encourage its use simply as a cognitive enhancer, but if you take it, I urge you to notify your physician. I have worked with a number of women experiencing anxiety symptoms, only to find out later that they were taking *ephedra* supplements or Deprenyl, and these were causing the anxiety problems. Please be sure to talk with *all* of your health care professionals about *everything* you take, even if it is an over-the-counter, nonprescription product.

A promising new Alzheimer's drug called galantamine (Reminyl) was recently approved in Sweden and is being evaluated for approval in the United States and several other European countries. Galantamine preserves the memory-enhancing neurotransmitter, acetylcholine, in the brain by blocking the enzyme, acetylcholinesterase, that breaks it down to inactive forms. Increasing the levels of acetylcholine in the brain is thought to lessen the memory loss, cognitive decline, and functional impairments that occur in Alzheimer's disease.

Emerging work on the plant extract, *Gingko biloba* (GBE), is showing promising results to improve brain blood flow, memory, and cognition. Researchers at the Department of Geriatric Medicine at Whittington Hospital in London studied the effects of *Gingko biloba* on thirty-one elderly patients with mild-to-moderate memory impairment and found a statistically significant beneficial effect over placebo. Their study is significant in that it was a double-blind, placebo-controlled protocol over six months, and also included EEG brain wave results. In another European study, seventy-one outpatients with cerebral insufficiency at three test centers were randomized into a double-blind, placebo-controlled protocol for twenty-four weeks. Statistically significant improvements in short-term memory and learning rate were found in the patients taking the gingko extract (EGb 761) but not in the placebo group.

European research over the past thirty years suggests that *Gingko biloba* extract acts as a vasodilator, improves oxygen and glucose uptake, and also acts to help decrease platelet clumping (a factor in arterial plaque formation). At present, there is no regulation of gingko products, and they are proliferating rapidly (along with rising prices) as word spreads about these research findings. Most of the studies have been done on the original extract, EGb 761, and this is the brand *Ginkold*. Other brands may or may not contain the same percentage and compositions of the active compounds. If you chose to try GBE, look for a brand that is approved by the German Commission E, a regulatory body that oversees the quality control for herbal products sold in Germany. Brands that carry this approval generally contain the amount of standardized extracts that were shown in the clinical studies to be effective. Also I encourage you to use some common sense, and observe your body responses before you buy a year's supply.

I do not have the space to go into all the other "smart drugs" currently being touted as wonder agents to prevent changes in brain function with aging. If you are interested in this subject, I encourage you to seek sound information and discuss it with your physician before adding numerous supplements to your daily routine. The best memory enhancers are still the basics I have discussed in this chapter, with particular attention to eliminating alcohol, tobacco, and fatty foods along with taking your vitamins, exercising regularly, and paying attention to optimal hormone balance.

What Can You Do to Improve Memory?

Think of your brain as a "mental muscle" and *exercise it*. Research has shown that stimulating your brain with new learning actually helps increase the number of neuron connections. Take a class in an entirely different field, learn a foreign language, do crossword puzzles, practice solving brainteasers. When you want to remember something new, focus on it, repeat it several times, and perhaps write it down and look at it as well.

Some simple principles of paying attention to *basic health habits* also improve brain function and memory. These are summarized in the chart that follows.

DR. VLIET'S MEMORY-ENHANCING STRATEGIES

- Stop smoking (it deprives your brain of oxygen).

- Stop or reduce use of sleeping pills (talk with your doctor about how to do this safely, since these medications must usually be decreased gradually).

- Eat smaller meals at regular intervals for steady "fuel" to the brain

- Make sure you have healthy nutrition and balance of protein, fat, and carbohydrates.

- Have your thyroid, ovarian, and adrenal hormone levels checked, and consider hormone therapy if your levels are too low and your memory is fading.

- Reduce fat in your diet. It contributes to plaque deposits in the arteries and blocks blood flow to the brain.

- Exercise aerobically several times a week. Doesn't have to be fancy— brisk walking is fine!

- Take a good basic multivitamin along with antioxidants like vitamin C, vitamin E, selenium.

- Eliminate or reduce alcohol.

- Practice relaxation exercises or meditation.

- Get enough sleep.

- USE IT OR LOSE IT—Stimulate your brain with new ideas, and practice!

©Elizabeth Lee Vliet, M.D., 1995, revised 2000

_._-_._-_._-_._-_._-_._-_._-_._-_._-_._-_._-_._-_._-_._-_._-_

Migraines and Hormonal Headaches

MIGRAINE.

Even the name conjures up images of that throbbing, head-splitting pain; nausea that makes you ill just to *think* about moving around; vision problems that make you think you may be going blind; and wanting to crawl off to the darkest room you can find, and tell the world to **"Leave me alone!"**

For all of you migraine sufferers reading this, have you ever asked a physician the question, *"Could it be related to my hormones? The headaches seem to come (or get worse) right before my period"*? And how many of you have been told categorically, "No, there's no connection"?

The following observations have been true down through the centuries of recorded medical observations

- Migraines are three times more common in women than in men.
- The gender difference begins at *puberty* and ends at *menopause*.

With those statistics, it shouldn't take a rocket scientist to figure out that there just *might* be a hormonal connection to the problem in women. Again, most women know that. You have lived it. You have told me over the years of my practice that your migraines (1) almost always come a day or two *before* your period, or the first day or two *of* your period, or (2) come around the ovulatory phase of your cycle, or (3) may have a number of different triggers but are frequently *worse* right around your period. I couldn't accept that all these women who kept saying the same thing were wrong or just neurotic. These are the comments I often hear about women who try to offer a possible explanation or connection for their symptoms.

Like many health problems that affect women in greater numbers than men, migraine was relatively neglected by medical researchers until fairly recently. When studies were done, they were more often *done in men.* I will never forget the article I came across in the *Journal of the American Medical Association* as recently as 1991, a study of using daily aspirin to prevent migraines. In the first two paragraphs, the authors described migraine being more common in women, yet the study they had just done *did not include a single female patient.* They concluded in the article that aspirin on a daily basis could be helpful to reduce migraine frequency *in men,* but *they didn't know whether it would work in women.* How could they if women weren't included in the study?

Since migraine was most commonly a women's disorder, and also included many unusual symptoms, it was all too frequently dismissed and discounted by doctors who thought it was an imagined problem and labeled it hysterical or psychological. Doctors thought women were just "stressed" from taking care of children and from lack of ability to cope. I can remember being taught this stereotype in medical school. Research has finally clarified this issue and clearly defined migraine as a real biological disorder. Yet, you would think *because* migraines occur more often in women and have a relationship to the menstrual cycle in the majority of sufferers, that clinicians and researchers would have regarded hormonal influences as major additional biological clues to study in migraine headaches. It is hard for me to understand why such obvious connections in women's health have been ignored for so long. The ancient Greeks, in the writings of Hippocrates, knew that the menstrual cycle changes influenced the course of such problems as asthma, allergies, epilepsy, and *migraine.* But as an example of the magnitude of the problem of overlooking women's hormonal changes as important variables, I found that a seven-hundred-page textbook devoted solely to the topic of migraine and written by international medical authorities in research and treatment of migraine did not have a *single* index reference to estrogen, even as a subheading under hormones. This text was published in 1987, over twelve years after the pioneering work by Dr. Somerville to identify falling estrogen as a common trigger of migraine headaches in women.

Fortunately, there has been progress in getting attention focused on the menstrual cycle hormonal changes as headache triggers in women. From the pioneering studies of Dr. B. W. Somerville, we now know that a common trigger for the hormonally related migraine headaches is the drop *in estradiol* (remember, that's the primary type of estrogen made by the ovary). Guess when the estradiol level drops the most quickly? You got it, right before your period. The estradiol level (along with progesterone, beta-endorphin, and serotonin levels) begins decreasing rather dramatically about Days 22 to 24 of your cycle and reaches its lowest point of the month on Days 1 to 3 of bleeding. The estradiol level also remains low for the first four–five days of your bleeding, and this is a reason for the increase in migraines during the early days of menstrual flow. Ovulation is another time in the menstrual cycle when estradiol levels drop and may trigger a migraine. So, for some women, there are two times in the menstrual cycle when they are vulnerable to having a migraine headache due to the drop in estrogen production. When might be some other times that women are more likely to be affected by hormonal headache triggers? You're right if you thought of (1) the week women stop birth control pills to have a period, (2) women who take ERT after menopause and stop their estrogen for Days 25 to 30 of the month, (3) the few days after delivery (postpartum phase) when estrogen, progesterone, serotonin, and endorphin levels drop about one-hundred-fold over twenty-four to forty-eight hours.

If you add to the hormone changes the other common migraine triggers—certain foods, alcohol, caffeine, chocolate, barometric pressure weather changes, stress, "rebound" from pain medication, and all the other classic ones—you have a whole host of potential interactions and headache causes. Most doctors, and most migraine sufferers (called "migraineurs" for short), know about and pay attention to the classic triggers I have listed above. *But the overlooked, hidden estrogen trigger is ignored in almost 99 percent of women who have migraines.* Yet, this hormone trigger can be alleviated in some fairly simple ways that I will discuss further in this chapter. Not only does this overlooked connection cause a lot of unnecessary suffering, it also adds dramatically to the cost of caring for patients with migraines. If the hormone trigger isn't addressed, women are often then using far more other medication to control the headaches. These migraine medications are expensive, often costing women (or their health insurance carriers) several hundred dollars a month. In addition, overlooking common menstrual cycle or other hormone triggers also leads to expensive trips to the emergency room for injections of narcotics and other potent pain medications when the other methods fail, and even hospital admissions for managing refractory, difficult-to-control migraines. There *are* hormonal connections, and there are also some *hormonal treatment options* that work extremely well for many patients. Here are some stories from women who have asked that I share their experiences so that others many benefit.

Listening to Women: Dee's Story

"Dee" came to see me several years ago for a consultation with the following concerns: "I have tried every estrogen there is, and they all cause migraines. How do I find something to take so I can feel better? And I'm worried about osteoporosis if I can't take any estrogen." She was forty-seven at the time, and had undergone at age forty-five a total hysterectomy due to severe bleeding and multiple fibroids. She also had her ovaries removed at the same time. This woman described feeling "desperate" to find some relief for the migraines; her loss of energy and libido, the fragmented sleep with nocturnal hot flashes; and the mood changes, which consisted primarily of depressed mood and marked irritability. She did not have a major depressive disorder, although she did see a psychiatrist for psychotherapy dealing with the adjustments to a new marriage. Her psychiatrist had tried several antidepressants that have been useful for treatment of migraines but had been unable to find a regimen that eliminated her headaches. She had not experienced migraine headaches prior to her hysterectomy, although she had experienced occasional milder vascular headaches prior to her menstrual periods off and on during her thirties and early forties.

About a week following her surgery, she was started on her initial estrogen therapy with the standard Premarin 0.625 mg daily. Within the first week of treatment, she developed bloating, breast tenderness, and severe migraine headaches with classic symptoms: prodromal aura, stabbing pain in the right eye with visual scotomata, nausea, and light sensitivity. She was directed to stop the Premarin and was then started on Estraderm patch 0.05 mg twice a week. Her migraines continued to occur several times a week and were so severe that they interfered with her going to work. Estraderm was stopped and she was started on Estrace 2 mg orally at bedtime. Her sleep improved and the nocturnal hot flashes resolved, but she again had severe migraines, which began midday on the third day of treatment and became daily.

Her physician told her to stop Estrace and informed her that she would not be able to take estrogen due to the migraines. She was then treated symptomatically with a variety of medications to decrease the migraine pain when it occurred: beta-blockers, nonsteroidal anti-inflammatory drugs (NSAIDS), dihydroergotamine (DHE), and serotonin-augmenting antidepressants. None of these were completely effective for her migraines, and she also continued to have severe menopausal symptoms. She had remarried about a year before her hysterectomy, and she was particularly upset by her loss of libido and difficulty with sexual arousal. As expected, the sexual problems were much worse when she was taking the beta-blockers and serotonin-boosting medications. She said her husband was "very supportive and concerned, but he's getting at the end of his patience, too. I'm worried this is going to affect my marriage as well as how I feel." Dee initially called for a consultation after a friend had told her of the work I was doing with hormonal connections in migraines. After our initial telephone consultation about her problems, she came to Tucson for a more in-depth evaluation and to have me work with her to find a hormone regimen appropriate for her.

Dee had been in good health and exercised regularly. She did not smoke cigarettes. Before her surgery, she drank wine occasionally with a special dinner but otherwise did not drink alcohol. She had been unable to tolerate even a glass of wine since the onset of her migraine problem, and at the time I saw her, she had not had any alcohol in about two years. Her two pregnancies in her twenties had been uneventful, and she had not had any problems with postpartum depression or migraines. She had her mammograms regularly, and these had always been normal.

Her family history was important, since her mother had lost an inch of height in her later years and was also on medication for elevated cholesterol. Her mother had gone through a natural menopause in her late forties and had never taken hormones. Her father had high blood pressure and angina and was on medication for this. Dee also had a brother in his early forties who had high blood pressure, high cholesterol, and was already on medication.

When I examined her, she was at a healthy body weight for her build, had a blood pressure of 118/78, and had no physical abnormalities. Her blood tests were quite significant in view of her symptoms and helped her to see quite clearly the hormonal connections. Her FSH at 132.7 and LH at 125.5 were very high as expected due to her surgical menopause and no hormone therapy at the time the tests were done. Her testosterone was low at 15 ng/dl and was a factor in her loss of libido; her estradiol was quite low at 32.8 pg/ml, a cause of her menopausal symptoms. Her total cholesterol was high at 274 and her LDL was also too high at 182 which meant she was moving into a higher-risk group for cardiovascular disease. But since her HDL was excellent at 74, she still had a normal risk ratio of 3.7 and I knew this would improve once her estradiol had been improved. Her regular exercise regimen was likely what had helped her keep a higher HDL and lower heart disease risk than her family history would predict. Her thyroid tests, including the TSH of 1.32, were all normal.

Dee's bone density report showed a reason for more concern. In spite of her calcium intake and her exercise, both of which she had been doing for many years, she already had a significant degree of bone loss (osteopenia) at the hip. Her bone density showed a femoral neck density of 0.72 g/cm^2, almost two standard deviations below the normal expected peak bone mass. This was alarming because she was still so young and so physically active. Clearly, her bone density needed to be improved along with finding a way to alleviate her menopausal symptoms and migraines. Dee was worried about whether she would find a way of taking estrogen that did not cause the severe migraines, but she saw from the results of her comprehensive evaluation that she clearly had a number of reasons for being on an optimal estrogen replacement program: (a) the relatively young age of her hysterectomy and removal of the ovaries; (b) her present abnormal degree of bone loss and family history of probable osteoporosis; (c) her present abnormal cholesterol profile and family history of heart disease; (d) her significant insomnia; and (e) her loss of libido and ability to have orgasm, caused by her low hormone levels, not the surgery itself.

From what Dee had told me, I realized that a key part of the problem she had been having with the estrogen causing her migraine headaches had been the fluctuating levels of estradiol with the previous schedules and types of estrogen. The Estraderm patch dose was too low for a younger woman, abruptly menopausal with surgery, and the patch duration is only about forty-eight to fifty hours. This means if she was changing the patch only twice a week, it wore off and the estradiol dropped long before it was changed. If using this brand of patch in women with migraines, I usually recommend changing it three times a week for better stability in estradiol level. Taking Estrace 2 mg once a day gives a rapid rise in blood level with the higher-dose tablet and then a rather sharp drop in about ten–twelve hours as it wears off. This means she had about ten–twelve hours each day when her estradiol levels were too low between the once-a-day doses of Estrace, and this triggered the return of her headaches.

I explained all this to her and said I thought she was sensitive to both a falling *and* a low estradiol level in between doses as the trigger for the migraines. She and I discussed my rationale for a trial on a regimen of smaller doses at more frequent intervals. She said, "You know, that intuitively feels right. I think you are right about what was happening before." I thought she would likely need to reach a dose of estradiol about 1–2 mg a day, but I knew that we could not start at that amount all at once without having her headaches return. I recommended she start with 0.25 mg tablets, taking them three times a day for the first few days. Her headache came back about six hours after the first two doses, and we realized she would need to take it even more frequently. At least this pattern was helping us to confirm the suspicion that the drop in estradiol was the trigger for her migraine. She was headache-free on a schedule of 0.25 mg four times a day, with about six hours in between each dose of estradiol. She still had milder menopausal symptoms with her total daily dose at only 1 mg, so to reach the point where she felt her best, and her symptoms *plus* headaches were gone, she was gradually increased to 2 mg daily. This amount fits with her age, the suddenness of her surgical menopause, and reaching a point where she felt really well and energetic without any unwanted side effects.

Her blood levels of estradiol were now in the desirable range of 100–150 pg/ml, consistent with levels of the first half of the menstrual cycle before menopause. After the first two months on the estradiol, her sexual difficulties had improved significantly, but she still experienced a diminished libido. Since she had a low bone density along with the libido changes, and no longer had the ovaries to produce her own testosterone, I suggested she try a small amount of micronized natural testosterone. She responded well to 2.5 mg micronized natural testosterone daily. I also recommended magnesium 250 mg twice a day as an additional supplement to help improve bone density and help maintain normal vascular tone that would further help reduce the headaches.

At her six-month follow-up, FSH was 30 (now down to the range expected for a woman on the right amount of estradiol replacement), estradiol 145 pg/ml, testosterone 40 ng/dl, fasting total cholesterol 225 with HDL of 78, ratio 2.8. She had no adverse side effects from the testosterone and had remained migraine-free as long as she took her 17-beta estradiol on the regular schedule. She tried to decrease the dose frequency to three times a day but found that she began to have the onset of the migraine prodrome when she increased the interval between doses. She commented that although it was "a nuisance" to have to take the estradiol four times a day, she was so glad to be free of the migraines and feeling better overall, "it's worth it." Her husband was thrilled that she felt so much better and was no longer having migraines and they both described feeling reassured that the sexual problems had been due to the low hormone levels, not a relationship problem. He said "everything's going really well, our sex life is the way we had been when we first got married, it's wonderful to have my wife back."

Listening To Women: Reba's Story

"Reba," now thirty-five, began having migraines in her twenties after she stopped using birth control pills. She had identified a number of triggers for her headaches: red wine, chocolate, certain cheeses, "low-pressure" days when the weather changed and became cloudy and rainy, the onset of her period each month, and the "let-down" days after times of stressful situations at work or with her family. She had tried a number of medications, with varying degrees of success on these types of migraines, and she had also learned how to use biofeedback to help decrease her headaches. Over the years, she had been able to eliminate most of the triggers she had identified, except, she laughingly pointed out,

I haven't been able to control the weather, or eliminate all the stress from my life. For those times, I just have to use the drugs I've found that will work. The Imitrex shots have been a godsend, and that usually breaks the migraine right away. But the thing that really gets me is the *excruciating* migraines I get *right before my period*. The sumatriptan doesn't seem to work as well on those headaches, and sometimes I've ended up in the emergency room for Demerol shots. I have asked every doctor I've ever seen if it could be my hormones, and they all say no. And they all tell me I can't ever take the pill (birth control), but I wonder if that would help? I keep trying to tell my doctors that these headaches started after I stopped the pills, but *no one listens to what I have to say.* I'm convinced that there is some hormonal factor, *and I just want somebody to listen to me and try and help me figure this out.*

I talked with Reba about the connection I thought was a major factor for her: the premenstrual drop in estrogen triggering migraines. We went over her headache diary that clearly showed the relationship between the time of her cycle when estradiol dropped and the onset of her migraine. I pointed out that her calendar showed that she frequently had a migraine at midcycle, corresponding with the estrogen drop at ovulation. She had not realized this pattern, and thought these were "stress-related." She had been using a diaphragm for contraception after several doctors had told her that her headaches would get worse if she used birth control pills. I suggested that we consider trying a low-dose pill with steady hormone levels (*monophasic* pill) and keep the progestin content low since it seems to be the primary culprit in birth control pills that may aggravate headaches. The low progestin pills I use most often in this situation are Ovcon 35 or Modicon because I have found these work best with the fewest unwanted side effects. Modicon has a little more progestin and I use this if a woman has more breakthrough spotting with the lower progestin content of Ovcon 35. These birth control pills have *half (or less)* of the amount of progestin found in other birth control pills.

Newer pills such as Loestrin, Alesse, and Mircette are particularly difficult to use in women with migraine headaches because these pills are so very low in the estrogen and are quite high in progestin content (more than double the amount or potency of progestin that is in Ovcon 35). If you have recently started one of these high-progestin pills and are having more headaches of any kind, talk with your health professional about changing to one of the low-progestin pills I listed.

Another factor in using birth control pills is the *drop in hormones* when the active hormone pills are stopped for seven days (the placebo pill days) each month to trigger the menses. One of the approaches I began using many years ago to help this problem was to suggest stopping the pills for only *three* days at the end of the active pill cycle, instead of stopping for seven days as recommended on the pill package. The shorter time is enough to allow your period to start, but is not so long off the hormones that it causes an estrogen-withdrawal migraine. Reba thought this made a lot of sense with what she had noticed and wanted to try it. Even just three days off the pills was too long for her: The migraine hit again on the afternoon of the third day following the end of her first pill pack. At first she was a little discouraged and thought this meant she would not be able to continue with the pills. I reassured her and told her it just confirmed what we thought: One of her triggers was the drop in estrogen, and the next step would be to shorten the time between packs of active hormone pills to *two* days instead of three. Voila! This worked. If this had not solved the problem, another option would have been to have her use an estradiol patch between pill packs to keep the estrogen steady and prevent estrogen-withdrawal headaches.

It has now been a year and a half since our first consult. Reba is happy on the birth control pills, glad to be free of the diaphragm and even more excited about finding a way to eliminate the trigger for her menstrual migraines. Since birth control pills also suppress ovulation to provide the contraceptive effect, being able to take the Ovcon eliminated the drop in estrogen at ovulation that had also set off Reba's migraines. She still has an occasional migraine when she's overstressed or the barometric pressure drops suddenly, and she has managed those headaches well with the Imitrex (sumatriptan) injections. Added pluses have been having a reliable form of contraception, lighter menstrual flow, no more bad menstrual cramps, and the elimination of her PMS mood swings now that the hormone levels are steady all month.

These are just two of the hundreds of women I have worked with to find creative options to reduce or eliminate the hormonal triggers for their migraines. I can tell you that these approaches work, but it sometimes takes a little time and patience to figure out a particular woman's regimen because each women is different. The challenge is to listen to each woman's wisdom and insights about what she has noticed, track her headache pattern, and put it together with what I know about the hormone options and the pharmacology of the various preparations available. I also have to know the effects and side effects and half-life of the other migraine medications a woman is using, so we can determine whether she is also having "rebound" headaches as those wear off. Yes, it can be complicated, but together, we come up with treatment approaches that make physiological sense. It takes time, patience, and some detective work, but isn't your health worth it? I hope the hormone suggestions I have used will give you some approaches to discuss with your physicians.

New Understandings of Migraine Mechanisms

Migraine headaches occur in two primary patterns: those with an aura (previously called "classic migraine") and those without an aura (previously called "common migraine"). It had been thought that the phenomena that occurred in migraines—visual changes, sensitivity to light and sound, nausea, throbbing head pain—were due mainly to *circulation* changes: blood vessels becoming first constricted (vasoconstriction) and then dilated (vasodilatation). With more research, other aspects of the many biochemical, neural, and vascular changes in migraine are now better understood, and a unified theory has emerged. Migraine is now best described as a state of central nervous system "hyperexcitability" that predisposes a person to episodes of spontaneous depolarization of the neurons, followed by suppression of neuron function, and then changes in regulation of blood flow. A *genetic predisposition* is thought to be *underlying* the development of migraines upon exposure to a precipitating trigger. The majority of migraine sufferers have a family history of siblings or parents with these headaches. A genetically susceptible individual has a *lowered* threshold in response to the external triggers and internal hormonal changes that can set off the migraine sequence. If a susceptible individual is exposed to the headache triggers, the threshold is exceeded and nerve cells in the brain stem are fired off, activating the exaggerated release of serotonin, norepinephrine, dopamine, Substance P, and other chemical messengers. These changes in turn set off reactions in blood vessels, and there you are in the vicious cycle again.

The aura of migraine is usually fifteen to twenty minutes before the headache pain starts and is itself painless. It is caused primarily by sudden vasoconstriction of arteries called the *intracerebral* arteries that serve the brain. When blood supply to brain areas is suddenly reduced, the loss of oxygen causes the varied neurological sensations that commonly occur during the aura: the characteristic visual phenomena—flashing or sparkling lights before the eyes, blurred or distorted vision, tunnel vision, blind spots, or lightening-like flashes; numbness and tingling in the face; weakness in an arm; smelling pungent or unpleasant odors that aren't really there; sudden mood changes with irritability or tearfulness for no apparent reason; and sometimes rhythmic contractions of the abdominal muscles.

The throbbing *pain* of migraine is caused by the distension and vasodilatation of arteries outside the skull, called *extracerebral* arteries. Vasodilatation occurs as a compensatory response to the diminished oxygen supply when the intracerebral arteries become constricted. Pain results from several factors: nerve endings are tugged and "fired off" by distension of arteries, there are decreases in pain-modulating chemical messengers like serotonin and endorphins, as well as the falling estradiol that lowers the pain threshold of nerve endings and makes them more sensitive to pain-inducing stimuli. What sets off the cascade of events leading to vasoconstriction and vasodilatation to produce the migraine attack? Many different *initial* triggers have been identified as culprits (alcohol, tyramine-containing foods, chocolate, nitrites, MSG, histamine, bright flashing lights, loud noises, stress, barometric pressure changes, altitude changes, and others), but the final common pathway in all of these appears to be through alterations in the release of norepinephrine (NE), serotonin (5-HT), and dopamine (DA), along with other chemicals such as endorphins, Substance P, and prostaglandins. A great deal of research has implicated serotonin pathways in migraines, and it now appears that there are very specific serotonin receptors in the blood vessels of cranial circulation that contribute to the pain of migraine headaches.

These important serotonin receptors are called 5-HT_1 receptors, and drugs that *activate* the 5-HT receptor group are called **agonists.** Activation of both 5-HT_{1A} and 5-HT_{1D} subtypes play a role in the relief of acute migraine attacks. The new group of migraine-pain relievers called *triptans* selectively activate the 5-HT receptors to abort an acute migraine. Examples of medications in this group that have been approved by the FDA include sumatriptan (Imitrex), naratriptan (Amerge), rizatriptan (Maxalt-MLT), and zolmitriptan (Zomig). Additional triptans, eletriptan and almotriptan, are being tested for effectiveness and safety but are not yet FDA-approved. All of the triptan drugs have the same mechanism of action and have become first-line treatment for migraine. Studies have shown that these medications do not differ by more than about 5–10 percent in overall effectiveness and safety, but there are small differences in absorption or half-life that may affect your response. Other migraine "abortive" medications are ergotamine and dihydroergotamine (DHE), older 5-HT receptor agonist drugs that have been used for many years to *abort* migraine attacks but have more bothersome side effects than do the triptans.

Other types of serotonin receptors, the 5-HT_2 group, are involved in prevention of migraine headaches. Medications that block (called **antagonists**) the 5-HT_2 receptors seem to help *prevent* migraine. These include the serotonin-reuptake inhibitor antidepressants (such as Prozac, Zoloft, Paxil and others), tricyclic antidepressants (Elavil, Pamelor and others), cyproheptadine (Periactin), and methysergide (Sansert). It is quite interesting to find that **estrogen modulates both the 5-HT_1 and 5-HT_2 receptors,** so it is not surprising that fluctuations in estrogen with the menstrual cycle, postpartum, and at menopause will cause migraines to get worse. Keeping estradiol levels as steady as possible helps keep these serotonin receptor systems from being set off like a fire alarm to cause the migraine cascade.

Excessive production of prostaglandins (PG) by the lining of the uterus, especially $PG-F_2$, is known to trigger both migraines and uterine cramps. Blood plasma taken from menstruating women that contains these prostaglandins will cause migraine headaches and uterine cramping if the blood is given back at another point in the cycle. This suggests that there is a prostaglandin-generating factor in the plasma, which sets off these symptoms associated with menstruation. One hypothesis is that menstrual migraine may be the result of estrogen withdrawal that decreases serotonin activity and also affects levels of $PG-F_2$ and possibly other prostaglandins. Medications that inhibit PG production and action are the well-known pain relievers: aspirin (and the plant willow bark, from which it is derived), Motrin, Anaprox, and many others belonging to the class of NSAIDs. Later in this chapter, I have included a chart of most of the NSAIDs available in the United States. As most of you know, the NSAIDs are used to relieve menstrual cramps, to decrease joint and muscle pain, and to treat acute headaches and help to reduce the frequency of migraines.

Whole textbooks have been devoted to the subject of migraine headache, so I can give you just an overview of important connections in this chapter. I have included a summary chart later in the chapter to illustrate how estrogen affects the steps in the migraine process. I hope that understanding these steps will help you identify ways to think about the medications and hormone strategies available, to eliminate foods or lifestyle triggers of your headaches and to develop healthy eating and stress management approaches to further decrease the headaches.

Estrogen and Progesterone Effects on Headache

The high frequency of migraines occurring around the onset of menses has been observed for several thousand years, but it wasn't until the mid-1970s that Dr. B. W. Somerville did a series of studies, published in 1975, that clearly demonstrated the differing roles of estrogen and progesterone. Dr. Somerville's study showed that the migraine attack was actually triggered by the premenstrual drop in estradiol, not progesterone. He used injections of estradiol in the study subjects to produce a delay in migraine onset, but giving estrogen did not delay onset of menstruation. When the same women were given injections of progesterone, their menses onset was delayed as expected, but the migraine came at the usual expected cycle day, at the same time the estrogen level dropped naturally.

MECHANISMS FOR ESTROGEN EFFECTS ON HEADACHES

- Estrogen increases serotonin production; adding estrogen to serotonin-boosting medications has a *synergistic* effect.

- Falling estrogen decreases the amount of available serotonin, as well as the number of certain 5-HT receptors, that are important in decreasing migraine pain. The drop in serotonin levels causes cranial blood vessels to spasm painfully.

- Falling estrogen causes a decrease in the pain-relieving beta-endorphins in the brain, spinal cord, and body tissues.

- Estrogen withdrawal (either naturally in the cycle or by stopping hormone-containing medication) causes a rebound in dopamine that may intensify pain.

- Estrogen decline causes vasoconstriction by contraction of the muscles in the artery walls, aggravating pain of vascular headaches.

- Falling estrogen causes a burst of norepinephrine release in the brain's locus ceruleus, which increases vasoconstriction and diminishes blood flow to the area of the brain involved in vision, thus producing the aura. NE release further intensifies pain.

- A decrease in estrogen *lowers* the pain threshold, making the individual more sensitive to painful stimuli.

© Elizabeth Lee Vliet, M.D., 1995

In the few articles that address women's reports of their migraine experiences, the observations of *when* women have most of their migraines in the menstrual cycle also support Dr. Somerville's conclusions that estrogen withdrawal was the key trigger. All of the times of increased headache activity across the menstrual cycle are times of falling estrogen levels: ovulation, premenstrual days, postpartum, perimenopause and menopause, or the days of stopping active hormones of birth control pills. This is one of the things I have found frustrating in trying to help patients all these years. If we have known since at least 1975 that estrogen withdrawal is a very common trigger for women with migraines, *why* haven't we taken this into account in our management approaches for relieving headaches? Why haven't physicians listened to women who tell us so eloquently what the pieces of the puzzle may be? *And why haven't more women been validated in their observations that there is a hormonal connection?*

I look at the publication dates of some of these articles and realize that this information was coming out when I was in medical school. Why weren't we taught some of the male-female differences and taught ways to treat patients according to individual approaches suitable for men and for women? And, why is it that women with migraines who have seen a hormonal pattern are *still* "screaming to be heard" about these connections? I think it makes more sense to *consider* a trial of keeping hormone levels steady, and see if this helps an individual woman, instead of insisting there's no connection and having the patient make repeated trips to the emergency room in excruciating pain.

In a woman with a genetic susceptibility to migraine, the headache is the end result of these many biochemical, neuronal, and vascular changes accentuated by the rise and fall in estrogen. If a woman susceptible to migraines is at the vulnerable point in her menstrual cycle, has rebound effects from other pain medications, *and* has environmental triggers (alcohol, weather, foods, etc.) acting on top of the hormonal shifts, it is easy to see how the vicious cycle of headaches is intensified.

The Role of Progesterone and Progestins

In a number of studies on the role of hormones in migraines, a common pattern noted was the increased frequency and severity of migraine, vascular, and muscle-tension headaches in women on synthetic progestins, with progestin-only contraceptives being the *worst* offenders. The higher the progestin content, the more likely the headaches of all types. For this reason, if I use an oral contraceptive in a woman with migraines, I always try to stay with the lowest progestin pill. I also caution against using the long-acting injectable or implant progestin-only contraceptives (Norplant, Depo-Provera) for the same reason: they have a high frequency of aggravating migraines. Even in women who did not have headache problems prior to the use of progestin-only contraceptives, these hormones given without estrogen have a high frequency of causing new-onset daily tension-type headaches as well as vascular headaches like migraines.

The role of natural progesterone in headache syndromes is a little more difficult to determine. In general, progesterone metabolites exert inhibitory effect at the brain's GABA receptors to produce a calming sensation, like the benzodiazepine tranquilizers (Xanax, Valium, Ativan, Klonopin, and others) that also act at the GABA receptors. This same inhibitory effect at the GABA receptors may also produce central nervous system depressant effects in some women (also like the benzodiazepines do) that can lead to depressed mood, tiredness, lethargy, low energy, diminished sex drive (libido), and diminished concentration. If progesterone is given to *males or females*, it produces *slowing* of the heart rate (evident on the electrocardiogram), brain waves (seen on EEG), and respiratory rate. This is the same physiological response on these measures that we see with benzodiazepine medication. In addition, progesterone also acts as an anesthetic when levels are high (as in the last trimester of pregnancy). Also like the benzodiazepines, high doses of progesterone have anticonvulsant and sedative effects at brain centers. When progesterone levels are falling, studies have shown that convulsive activity increases. It is reasonable to think that these effects of progesterone at brain centers would help to decrease headaches, which some women find to be the case. Other women with migraines, however, report that their headaches are much worse during the progesterone-dominant phase of their menstrual cycle or when taking progesterone (even the natural form).

Observations that would help to explain why progesterone may make headaches worse in some women are that (1) progesterone decreases estradiol binding at serotonin (5-HT) receptors, creating a "low-estrogen" headache trigger, and (2) progesterone stimulates the production of prostaglandins that cause spasm of the smooth muscle lining artery walls, another migraine trigger. Another headache-inducing mechanism of progesterone is that when it has been given in therapeutic doses for several days or weeks and then stopped, progesterone produces withdrawal symptoms similar to those we see with benzodiazepines, barbiturates, and alcohol. The progesterone withdrawal syndrome (similar to sedative withdrawal syndrome) includes anxiety, tearfulness, mood swings, fuzzy thinking, insomnia, diarrhea, muscle spasms, and other effects. Progesterone withdrawal can also cause **throbbing headaches** that can be mistaken for migraines. This is one reason it is important to decrease progesterone gradually if you have been taking it for PMS treatment or for hormone therapy at menopause, especially if you are taking more than 200 mg a day (based on oral dose).

At this time, there is no one universal answer to the question about whether progesterone has a positive effect or a negative effect on migraines. I approach the use of progesterone in migraine sufferers like I do other therapies: I pay attention to what the individual woman tells me about her headache pattern relative to hormone cycles and what she has taken in the past. Then we work together to identify the hormone (and other medication) options that best control the headaches. Overall, I have found not found that giving progesterone in high doses helps prevent migraines. In women who still have headaches when taking natural progesterone, I try to use the lowest dose that will protect the uterine lining, and divide the total daily amount into smaller portions given several times a day. I have also found that nonoral forms of progesterone, such as Crinone vaginal cream or injectable progesterone in oil, also help reduce headache frequency when compared to oral progesterone. In my clinical experience, these approaches have worked well to reduce frequency of headaches during the progesterone phase of hormone therapy.

Pregnancy Effects on Migraine

The dramatic hormonal shifts in pregnancy—more than one hundred-fold increase over menstrual cycle levels—affect migraine headache patterns: Some women develop migraines for the first time during pregnancy, others report *relief* of prepregnancy migraines. In fact, up to 70 percent of women who have migraines *without* aura experience relief of their headaches during pregnancy; still others find that pregnancy *intensifies* migraines—a pattern seen more commonly in migraineurs *with* aura. The pattern is highly variable and depends, to some extent, upon the phase of pregnancy.

In women who experience relief of their migraines, the improvement is most often seen after the first trimester, when progesterone levels have dropped and estrogen levels are higher. Worsening of migraines typically occurs in the first trimester when both estrogen and progesterone are rising rapidly as the placenta begins making hormones independent of the ovaries. Migraines are also typically worse again a few hours after delivery, when estrogen, endorphin, and serotonin levels all drop abruptly. Again, it appears to be *rapidly changing* hormone levels that are the culprit in triggering migraines in pregnancy.

Women very commonly describe enhanced feelings of well-being in pregnancy, and this is now thought to be related to the mood-elevating effects of the high estrogen levels in pregnancy. The absence of a cyclic hormonal "up-and-down" pattern and the increased production of endorphins are considered the primary reasons migraines tend to get better in pregnancy. Researchers in England have used the estradiol transdermal gel and patch, with dramatic results, in the immediate postpartum period as a way of keeping estradiol levels from falling so rapidly and precipitating migraines. Since this is the natural human form of the hormone, and a physiologic amount, it has not been considered a problem for nursing mothers to have this postpartum "boost" of estradiol. Keep in mind, the level of estradiol in a patch is still far less than the very high estradiol levels of pregnancy.

Oral Contraceptives (OC) and Migraine: New Findings

Until recently, it had been thought that women with migraine headaches who used birth control pills had a slight increase in risk of stroke at younger ages than we normally see strokes occurring in women. Earlier studies that had found this connection were done in women on the older, high-dose oral contraceptives rather than today's low-dose pills. In addition, earlier studies had not identified *cigarette smoking* as an *independent* risk factor for stroke in these women. The Collaborative Group for the Study of Stroke in Young Women definitively reported that analysis of the data did not confirm earlier reports suggesting that migraine headaches might increase the risk of stroke in young women using oral contraceptives. Although there are still physicians who think that women with migraine headaches should not use oral contraceptives, this caution has not been borne out by recent and more comprehensive evaluations. For women with migraines, *cigarette smoking* is the most significant risk for vascular disease of all types, and this risk may be further increased by taking oral contraceptives.

Another myth physicians were taught is that use of oral contraceptives will automatically aggravate migraines, so women with migraines should never take birth control pills. This teaching turns out to be another incorrect generalization. Current studies, and my extensive clinical experience in this regard, have shown that many women may actually achieve relief of their migraines with the right oral contraceptive to stabilize hormonal fluctuations. Whether headaches are aggravated or relieved with oral contraceptives has a great deal to do with hormone ratios in the pill and *how* the pill is taken. As in many women's health studies, researchers did not take into account normal hormone physiology in interpreting the study data. Earlier studies, which concluded that OC use *increased migraines,* did not look carefully at the issue of *when* in the pill cycle the headaches occurred. For example, researchers often did not ask whether the headache occurred while on the active hormone-containing pills (which would likely mean the pill did worsen the headaches), or whether the headaches occurred in the placebo days of the pill cycle (which would indicate *hormone-withdrawal* as the culprit). About 40–60 percent of women who have migraines while taking the oral contraceptives experience their headaches in the *last seven days* of the pill pack when taking the placebo pills. This pattern supports the role of *falling* estradiol levels in triggering the headache. In four double-blind, placebo-controlled studies, there were no differences in headache frequency in women on the birth control pill compared to women taking placebo, providing further support for the point that OCs do not make migraine headaches worse.

Current investigation of oral contraceptive effects on migraine reveal that headache patterns may change in one of several ways when women take OCs:

1. Headaches may *increase*. This is more often seen with phasic pills that have changing hormone content, such as Tri-Levlen, Ortho Tri-cyclen, Triphasil; increased headaches are also seen with high progestin pills such as ones I mentioned earlier, or with progestin-only contraceptives such as Norplant, Depo-Provera, or pills (Micronor, Nor-QD, Ovrette) if not given with estrogen to balance the progestin.
2. Headaches may be *eliminated* or significantly *decreased*. This is seen more with monophasic, constant-dose pills with lower progestin content, such as Ovcon 35 or Modicon. Some studies have found as much as a 60–70 percent improvement in migraines when women were started on oral contraceptives.
3. New or different types symptoms, such as aura or visual changes, may occur. This type of change is potentially serious and should be discussed immediately with your physician.
4. OC use may contribute to migraine appearing for the first time, usually in women with a significant family history of migraine. This response would suggest to me that such a person would not do well to continue the OC, although occasionally a product can be found with a hormone balance that is tolerated.

I think all of these responses illustrate just how variable the OC effects can be and once again indicates that *individualization* of therapy is crucial, especially since multiple studies have found that in many women, use of the OC pills can *decrease* headaches. There is no one right answer or one approach or pill type that will fit all women. It will take working closely with a physician who is knowledgeable about hormones and migraines to determine the best options for you. Dr. Stephen Silberstein, a well-known migraine specialist, emphasized this approach in an article published in *Neurology*, March 1992: "Estrogens and OCs are not contraindicated in migraine patients. In fact, they may actually be indicated for certain women. One needs to work closely with specialists to make the best use of the various chemical compositions now available."

My advice to physicians is "Listen to the patient, and use the approaches that give positive results with the least adverse effects." My advice to you readers is to keep reminding your physicians that in *women* with migraines, our approaches certainly have to include taking at look at the hormone factor.

Innovative Hormonal Approaches

For women who have a pattern of migraine headaches when hormone levels are changing or *dropping*, there are several options that can help stabilize the estradiol blood levels and help diminish the likelihood of hormone changes triggering migraines. If you want to try one of these options, you will need to work with a physician who will (1) evaluate you and see if hormone approaches could be used for you, (2) prescribe the hormone option that might work best in your particular situation, and (3) monitor your response and make adjustments as needed. If you have difficulty locating someone in your area, you may want to consider a consultation at our *HER Place* offices in Tucson or Dallas-Ft. Worth to help you address these hormone connections.

Step 1: The Headache Diary. A careful history of the migraine pattern and review of a headache diary is crucial to identifying the hormone triggers. I want a woman to keep her headache diary for at least two, and preferably three or more ovarian cycles before I see her. Most women have already seen a number of doctors and have done a detailed headache diary by the time they ask for a consult with me. I think the diary is so crucial that I insist that my patients do one to help us work together effectively as a "detective" team to solve the problem.

Step 2: Smoothing Out the Hormone Fluctuations. If a woman still has ovaries producing the hormone rise and fall (whether or not the uterus is present), my initial goal is to see if we can find a safe and effective way to achieve suppression of ovarian cycling to determine whether this will indeed reduce the migraine frequency and severity. I have found the approaches I used with Reba to be helpful for a large number of women, especially women with new onset hormonally related migraines developing during the "roller-coaster" thirties and forties as ovarian hormones fluctuate greatly. These are examples of options I consider based on an individual woman's medical evaluation and her preferences. You may wish to discuss these approaches with your physician.

1. **Low-dose oral contraceptives** (only if you are a *non smoker* and there are no other risk factors that would preclude using OCs). Taking monophasic (constant dose) OCs will provide hormonal stability. A woman may take the active pills *continuously* for three to six months and observe the effects on her migraines. The estrogen content will protect against bone loss and heart disease risks, as well as reduce or eliminate menopausal-type symptoms. The progestin content will suppress ovarian cycling and ovulation and reduce the hormonal fluctuations that we think are triggering her headaches. Daily progestin in the pill also suppresses the ovaries and reduces later life risk of both ovarian and endometrial cancer, two very important pluses. As I described with Reba, I first try shortening the time off hormone-containing pills each cycle to just two or three days. If headaches occur during the days off active pills, then

I may suggest *continuous treatment with active pills* to eliminate the fall of hormone levels in between pill packs. There aren't any known risks of taking the birth control pills this way, and it does help determine whether it is the *drop* in hormone level or some other factor that sets off the headache.

If a woman has a history of depression *not on* hormone therapy, or a history of feeling depressed on birth control pills, it is important to avoid an OC with more than 0.4 to 0.5 mg of norethindrone or progestin equivalent. The only oral contraceptives on the market in the United States that fit this criteria are **Ovcon 35** (35 mcg ethinyl estradiol and 0.4 mg norethindrone) and **Modicon** (35 mcg ethinyl estradiol and 0.5 mg norethindrone). When I began working with these issues many years ago, I figured out that a better balance of estrogen relative to the progestin would be needed in a birth control pill in order to cause fewer problems with headaches and depression side effects. I had to look up all the various ones sold in the United States and figure out the estrogen:progesterone (E:P) ratios, because everyone I asked about this just said, "Oh, they are all pretty much alike, it doesn't really make much difference which one you use." Well, I knew that wasn't true based on my patients' descriptions about how they felt. I trusted my own instinct and the insights from my patients, ignored the standard teaching that all the pills were similar, and started exploring options I thought might work better.

Over time, it has become increasingly clear that there are marked differences in the way individuals respond to the various pill formulations. Even changing progestin *only 1/10th (0.1) milligram (mg)* can make a difference in side effects, especially headaches and depressive symptoms. Ovcon 35 has the least progestin of any pills available in the United States and, in my experience, is least likely to aggravate headaches or depression. If you try this one and experience headaches or depression as a side effect, it is *not likely* there are any *other* ones in the United States to try, since all of the others have so much more progestin. If the birth control pills don't work, you may want to explore with your physician some of the other options I describe later in the chapter.

Nausea at the beginning of treatment with birth control pills is usually minimized if you take the pills at bedtime. Temporary side effects—nausea, breast fullness, bloating, slight weight gain, lethargy, and depressed mood—are generally related to the amount of progestin and tend to resolve by the second or third pill pack, if they occur at all. Weight gain is a common complaint about the birth control pills, but again, this is usually more of a problem with high progestin pills. Besides, wouldn't it be worth it to weigh two–three pounds more if you got rid of a lot of your headaches with better hormonal stability?

2. **Estradiol transdermal patch** (Alora, Climara, Vivelle, and Vivelle

Dot). If a woman does not want to try the birth control pill, or cannot take it for medical reasons, I have found that it can work well to use the transdermal estradiol patch to help keep estradiol levels steady before menses and at ovulation. This has eliminated the sharp drop in estradiol before bleeding starts, and in many patients, has been quite effective at eliminating the hormone trigger for migraines they have identified. I have suggested that they put the patch on the buttock sometime between Day 24 and 28 of their cycle, change the patch two or three days later, and wear another one until about Day 4 to 6 of the next cycle. This helps offset the body drop in estradiol, keeps blood levels steady and can prevent the menstrual migraine in many women. In women with premenstrual migraine, I see the typical pattern of Day 27–28 or Day 1–2 estradiol levels dropping to lower than normal levels 20–50 pg/ml, corresponding with their headache onset. I aim to keep estradiol levels between 70 and 90 pg/ml during these days, because this range seems to provide the best response in decreasing headache frequency.

Since the patch is being used for only a few days each month, it does not add much additional estrogen, and doesn't interrupt your normal menstrual cycle flow and pattern. This would not be considered taking "unopposed estrogen" because (1) it's just a few days of boosting estradiol levels rather than continuous therapy, and (2) if you are still menstruating and ovulating in a regular pattern with your normal flow, your own body progesterone "opposes" the estradiol.

3. **Use of a GnRH analogue medication for ovarian suppression with estradiol replacement.** This group of medications acts on the brain's releasing hormones that govern the ovary production of estrogen and progesterone. GnRH agonist drugs such as Synarel or Lupron inhibit the brain's production of FSH and LH that stimulate follicle formation and ovulation. As a result, the cyclic ovarian production of estradiol and progesterone is also inhibited. Replacing *only* estradiol, *at a steady daily level,* enables stabilization of this hormonal component and ideally eliminates the estradiol rise and fall as a migraine trigger. Adding back estradiol alone protects against further bone loss, reduces menopausal symptoms caused by these medications, and also reverses any negative changes in cholesterol.

The goal of this therapy is to use a medical means of eliminating ovarian cycling to provide clues to the role of estradiol fluctuations as migraine triggers, and to provide a therapeutic benefit in decreasing migraine activity. This approach is one I have used only as a last resort in migraine sufferers who have been unable to find relief with any other means. There are a number of **significant drawbacks** to the use of GnRH agonists: (a) both medicines cost several hundred dollars a month, (b) Lupron requires daily injections (at least for the first month), (c) it tends to cause irregular bleeding at the outset, (d) they can't be used long-term due to the unopposed estrogen effects on the uterine lining that over time will increase risk of abnormal bleeding and later development of uterine cancer, (e) since both medications induce a sudden menopausal state, the risk of osteoporosis can be increased if GnRH drugs are used for a long period of time without adding back estradiol.

If you have to use this approach, make sure you work with a physician experienced in using GnRH agonist medications and providing hormone replacement, since the procedures can be complicated and require a significant amount of fine-tuning. One woman I saw for a consultation had been on Lupron injections for several months to try and stop her migraines, but her physician had not realized that he had to add back estrogen at a constant level. She experienced severe menopausal symptoms, *worsening* headaches, marked hair loss, bone loss, urinary incontinence, and other serious problems due to the abrupt loss of estrogen. I do not usually recommend this approach except in difficult situations where literally *nothing else* has helped.

Migraine Headaches with ERT after Menopause

I have worked with a number of women who had migraines before menopause that appeared to worsen with hormone therapy, as well as women who *first* developed migraines only after starting on estrogen therapy after menopause. One of the most frequent causes of headaches getting worse with ERT is the regimen that directs women to take the estrogen twenty-five days and then stop abruptly for five days each month. The sudden withdrawal of estrogen on the five days off seems to be the trigger for the biochemical and vascular changes that initiate the headache. A simple solution is to take the estrogen component *every day* to keep blood levels steady. Menopause specialists now recommend taking the estrogen daily instead of the older twenty-five-day schedule. If you are on the twenty-five-day regimen and are having headaches in the five days off, talk with your physician about changing to the daily estrogen schedule.

OPTIONS TO REDUCE MIGRAINES DURING HORMONE THERAPY

If your own physician is skeptical about these hormone connections, you may want to look up the excellent review articles published by Dr. Stephen D. Silberstein, Director of the Comprehensive Headache Center at Germantown Hospital and Medical Center in Philadelphia, and give a copy to your doctor. I wrote a review article for the medical journal *Menopause Management* that was published in 1995; you may write my office for a copy, although most of the material is included in this chapter (please enclose a large self-addressed, stamped envelope with your request). Dr. Lee Kudrow, Director of the California Medical Clinic for Headache in Encino, has also been a strong advocate of paying close attention to subtleties of hormonal changes to alleviate migraines in women on ERT and has published articles on this subject. Perhaps one of these references will help persuade your physician of the validity of these ideas on hormone changes to reduce headache frequency. Here are some of the approaches I have found helpful in minimizing migraines with HRT:

- Changing to a pure 17-beta estradiol (Estrace, Alora, Climara, Vivelle) instead of the mixed conjugated equine estrogens (Premarin) or conjugated plant estrogens (Cenestin, Estratab), or synthetic estrogens (Ogen).
- Dividing your total daily dose into smaller amounts taken morning and evening to keep estrogen levels from fluctuating widely during the twenty-four hours. This is particularly important when using Estrace, since it only lasts about ten–twelve hours in most women. I often find this works when other approaches have not.
- Changing from an oral form of estrogen to a transdermal, vaginal, or sublingual one. Bypassing the liver metabolism may help keep estradiol levels more stable and reduce the swings that can trigger headaches. If you are using a patch, keep in mind that all of the brands may wear off sooner than the manufacturer states, so you may need to talk with your physician about changing the patch more often to keep the estradiol levels steady.
- I do not use estrogen injections in migraine patients because the shots produce *erratic* blood levels (both rapidly rising to high levels, and unpredictably falling to low levels) that tend to aggravate headaches even more.
- Changing from a synthetic progestin (which also aggravates headaches) to natural micronized progesterone (if you have a uterus and need to take a progestin). I find that natural micronized progesterone, particularly in a nonoral form, is less likely to trigger a headache compared to synthetic progestins.
- If natural progesterone causes too many side effects or increased headaches, you may want to try a lower-dose synthetic progestin derived from testosterone (such as Micronor or Aygestin) instead of the progestins derived from progesterone (such as Provera or medroxyprogesterone acetate [MPA]).
- Adding testosterone to a menopause hormone regimen may help decrease headaches in some women. Doses need to be low enough to avoid unwanted side effects such as acne, facial hair, or irritability; testosterone should be given once a day, in the morning, to avoid interfering with sleep.

The Serotonin Boosters: Triptans, SSRIs, and TCAs

Some exciting new developments have occurred in recent years with new medications designed to act selectively on serotonin mechanisms to help both **abort** and **prevent** migraine attacks. The serotonin system is one of the primary pathways that is involved in the cascade of neurochemical-vascular events in a migraine.

Triptans are a new class of medications that act to interrupt the acute migraine attack and decrease pain. Imitrex (sumatriptan) was approved by the FDA in late 1992, and others (Amerge, Maxalt-MLT, Zomig) have been approved since that time. The triptans act specifically on 5-HT_1 receptors in certain cranial arteries as agonists to enhance the serotonin activity at these receptor sites. They are potent vasoconstrictors of the arteries involved in causing pain and they help to rapidly decrease the throbbing vascular pain typical of migraines. All of the triptans are very effective and now are considered the front-line therapy for acute migraine attacks. Use of one of these medications at the first sign of a migraine often enables the sufferer to return to normal activity in a few hours. Each medication has a slightly different pharmacological profile, so they have different rates of onset and varying duration of action. Imitrex nasal spray (20 mg) is the most rapid in onset, and is quick and easy to use. Imitrex injections are also rapid in onset but more involved to use. Both the nasal spray and injection forms have a shorter duration of effect and greater likelihood of causing "rebound" headaches as they wear off. Maxalt-MLT is a triptan medication using an interesting approach with a waferlike tablet that dissolves on the tongue without water, making it a very convenient and rapid onset option for pain relief. Imitrex tablets start to decrease headache pain in about an hour, and the most effective dose has generally been found to be 50 mg. Zomig tablets (2.5 mg) are a little faster in onset than Imitrex, taking effect on pain in about thirty-five minutes. Amerge (2.5 mg) is slower to start acting (about two to four hours), but lasts longer than the other two. Amerge is often recommended for menstrual migraines because it lasts longer, although if you have adequately addressed the hormone triggers with options I described above, you may not need the additional expense of triptan medication.

Typically, the triptans cause relatively few side effects, and these are usually brief flushing or tingling sensations and throat or chest tightness. A potentially serious side effect, usually with the injectable form rather than tablets, is vasospasm of the coronary arteries and high blood pressure in people with cardiovascular disease. So before using the triptans, discuss these issues with your physician if you have angina or other forms of heart disease. These medications are not recommended for use in pregnancy.

Ergotamine (Cafergot and others) and dihydroergotamine (DHE) are two older drugs in this group of abortive migraine medications. Migranal is a nasal spray version of DHE that some migraine sufferers find effective. But overall, the ergotamines have many more side effects than do the triptans because they act at *multiple* 5-HT receptors instead of being selective for 5-HT$_1$. For example, both ergotamine and DHE also affect the 5-HT receptors that inhibit vomiting, so these drugs have the undesirable effect of aggravating the nausea and vomiting that can occur as part of the migraine episode. Triptans, unlike DHE and ergotamine, *only* activate the 5-HT$_1$ receptors and do not typically cause nausea and vomiting. Drugs such as Phenergan or Reglan, are usually given prior to DHE or Cafergot to decrease nausea and vomiting, but they, too, have unpleasant side effects.

Selective serotonin reuptake inhibitor medications (SSRIs) enhance the activity of 5-HT$_2$ receptors to help prevent migraines. Examples in this category are fluoxetine (Prozac), sertraline (Zoloft), and paroxetine (Paxil). At this time, none of these medications are approved by the FDA for use in migraine prophylaxis (medical term for "preventive" therapy), although they are widely used for this purpose by headache specialists and by primary care physicians. Other medications that have been used for migraine prevention include the older tricyclic antidepressants, but the SSRIs generally have fewer bothersome side effects than the tricyclics have. Again, the side-effect profile is due to a difference in specificity at the receptors: Prozac, Zoloft, and Paxil are more specific for the 5-HT$_2$ receptors that reduce migraine activity; the other antidepressants (shown below in the chart), including serotonin, norepinephrine, and acetylcholine, act on many different receptors and thereby produce a wide variety of both desirable and undesirable effects. Typical side effects of the tricyclics are weight gain, constipation, blurred vision, daytime drowsiness, dry mouth, dry eyes, rapid pounding heartbeat, palpitations, low libido, and difficulty urinating normally. Since many of these same problems occur as estradiol declines in perimenopause, it is no wonder that many women don't like to take drugs like Elavil (amitriptyline) or Pamelor (nortriptyline) that aggravate the hormone-induced symptoms. Methysergide (Sansert) and cyproheptadine (Periactin) are 5-HT$_2$ antagonists that have been used for years to help prevent migraines, but both of these older medications have more bothersome, and potentially serious, side effects. I rarely suggest them since I think there are better options available today with the other serotonin-augmenting medications.

One potential pitfall of the SSRI and Tricyclic medications is their tendency to cause withdrawal reactions if stopped abruptly. Withdrawal reactions are more common with the short-acting, high-potency ones like Paxil, Luvox, Effexor and are rarely seen with the long-acting ones such as Prozac. Since withdrawal reactions may occur with all of these medications, it is important that you don't stop them without talking with your physician, and make sure that you *taper down slowly* when you do stop.

SOME SYMPTOMS OF SSRI and TCA WITHDRAWAL

- DIZZINESS, VERTIGO

- LIGHTHEADEDNESS

- HEADACHES

- SENSORY DISTURBANCES, BLURRED VISION

- ANXIETY, AGITATION

- MOOD SWINGS, TEARFULNESS FOR NO REASON

- NAUSEA

- DIARRHEA

- MUSCLE SPASMS, CRAMPS

- PARESTHESIAS (BURNING, TINGLING, ELECTRIC-SHOCK SENSATIONS IN THE HANDS, ARMS, LEGS, AND FEET

- INSOMNIA

- VIVID DREAMS OR NIGHTMARES

- FATIGUE, FLULIKE FEELINGS

TIME COURSE OF ONSET: WITHIN 1-2 DAYS OF DOSE DECREASE OR STOPPING MEDICATION. DELAYED ONSET WITH LONGER-ACTING MEDICATIONS.

© Elizabeth Lee Vliet, M.D., 2000

Additional Medications for Migraine: A Summary of Options

The nonhormonal medications that are most effective for actually aborting an acute migraine attack or preventing recurrent attacks are described above in the section on serotonin boosters. If you have migraines, I encourage you to talk with your physician about some of these approaches instead of relying on narcotic pain medication (such as Percocet, Vicodin, and others). Narcotics blunt the pain but do not actually abort the migraine attack like sumatriptan and DHE do. In addition, if you determine that there is a strong correlation between hormone changes and your headaches, you may want to discuss with your doctor a trial on one or more of the hormonal options I have found effective and that are described above. Fiorinal is a popular medication to help relieve migraine pain, but it is a barbiturate that may lead to depression, memory and concentration problems, rebound headaches as it wears off, as well as loss of libido (again, some of the same problems that occur when estrogen declines). I recommend that you try to avoid regular use of Fiorinal or Fioricet if possible.

Nonsteroidal anti-inflammatory drugs (NSAIDS) are useful to relieve the pain of migraines and are considered *symptomatic* (i.e., reduce the symptom of pain) rather than abortive or prophylactic therapy. NSAIDS act by blocking platelet aggregating and prostaglandin formation and thereby reduce inflammation and pain. All of these drugs can be effective, but individuals respond differently to the various ones in this group. If one doesn't work, you may respond to another. Common errors in using the NSAIDs are not using enough medication *and* not keeping adequate blood levels by taking the NSAIDS regularly throughout the day during headache times. If you use the over-the-counter NSAIDS, remember that these are *only one-third* the dose of the same medication in prescription form, so you should talk with your doctor about the appropriate amount of over-the-counter pain relievers to substitute for prescription-strength ones. The list shows some of the more commonly used ones in the United States, but new NSAIDs are being developed all the time, so this list will not show all of the NSAIDS now available. Remember, lack of response to one *does not* mean another one won't do the trick. It is important to try a variety of different ones to find one that helps reduce headache pain.

Common NSAIDS for Migraine

- celecoxib (Celebrex)
- diclofenac/misoprostol (Arthrotec)
- etodolac (Lodine)
- fenoprofen (Nalfon)
- flurbiprofen (Ansaid)
- ibuprofen (Motrin, Advil)
- indomethacin (Indocin)
- ketoprofen (Orudis)
- ketorolac (Toradol)
- mefenamic acid (Ponstel)
- naproxen (Naprosyn, Anaprox, Aleve)
- oxaprozin (DayPro)
- piroxicam (Feldene)
- rofecoxib (Vioxx)

© Elizabeth Lee Vliet, M.D., 1995

Other classes of medications that act by different mechanisms to prevent migraine attacks are shown in the next table. One problem with the daily use of preventive medication is that you are taking pills every day, and having the potential for side effects, to prevent something that may happen only a few times a month. Most women that I see would prefer to take a pill only when they feel a headache coming on rather than having to take one every day. This is particularly true for women who may be trying to become pregnant and need to minimize the use of daily medications. Preventive medications I find are more effective for migraine sufferers who are having headaches more than twice a week all the time, rather than for women with headaches limited to certain phases of their menstrual cycle or just a few times a month. A bothersome problem with the preventive medications, as is also seen with the abortive medications, is the rebound headaches that occur as the medicine wears off. A common mistake in using these medicines is to use too low a dose for too short a period of time and then conclude it doesn't work. Most of the preventive medications take six–eight weeks to work, and it may also take time to find the right dose for a given person.

Beta blockers, such as propanolol (Inderal and others) have been used extensively for migraine prevention, but they have some very worrisome side effects for midlife women, including blockage of conversion of T4 to the more active form of thyroid hormone, T3. It may be by inhibiting conversion of T4 to T3 that propanolol contributes to depression, fatigue, weight gain, and memory impairment in people taking it regularly. Another cause for concern with beta-blockers is that they interfere with normal glucose and insulin regulatory pathways. A study by researchers at Johns Hopkins Center for Prevention, published in *The New England Journal of Medicine* in 2000, found in a prospective study of 12,550 adults ages forty-five to sixty-four years of age, that those with hypertension who were taking beta blockers had a 28 percent higher risk of developing diabetes than did those people taking other medications for hypertension or those taking no medicine at all. This is a particularly alarming finding, since women already have higher rates of diabetes than do men.

I prefer to avoid beta-blockers if possible because of their potential to produce significant problems with weight gain, insulin resistance, and impaired insulin secretion, depression, lethargy, fatigue, and loss of sexual drive and ability to achieve orgasm. Another concern I have encountered in women on long-term beta-blockers for headaches is finding greater than expected bone loss in women who have no other risk factors. To my knowledge, there has not been any research on the possible connection between beta-blockers and bone loss, so the question of long-term safety *in women* for the beta-blockers, in my opinion, has not been adequately addressed. If you can find other medications to provide reduction in your headache frequency, I think that would be a more prudent course of action. As a group, I think the angiotensin-converting enzymes (ACE) inhibitors are safer and have fewer side effects than the beta-blockers.

The anticonvulsants—Depakote (valproate), Tegretol (carbamazepine), and Topamax (topiramate)—are also used as prophylactic agents to help prevent migraines, but all of these have the potential for significant side effects, including marked weight gain and daytime sleepiness that may interfere with driving and work performance. In addition, Depakote has been found to increase the formation of ovarian cysts and the likelihood of developing polycystic ovarian syndrome (PCOS) due to its effect on the pituitary and production of prolactin, a hormone that suppresses normal ovarian cycles. PCOS is a potentially serious metabolic endocrine disorder associated with marked weight gain, high blood pressure, abnormal development of facial and body hair, infertility, insulin resistance, and increased likelihood of developing diabetes. I do not recommend daily use of Depakote for migraine prevention for these reasons, especially in younger women who may desire pregnancy. In my view, there are now safer options available.

You and your physician may have to experiment to find a choice that will give you the best response, since each person reacts differently. Be sure you keep a diary of how you feel and descriptions of your headache frequency and severity with each medication you try, so that you can better assist your physician in arriving at an optimal solution for you. I have tried to list some of the more common side effects of each class of medication, but keep in mind this is *not* a complete list. Remember that sometimes side effects may be unique to your body chemistry and may not even be listed in the *Physicians Desk Reference*. If something unusual happens when starting a new medication, talk with your physician about it. You must review with your physician the appropriateness of any medication based on your individual health problems and sensitivities.

MEDICINES TO PREVENT MIGRAINES

Name of Drug	Typical Dose	Side Effects	Comments
Beta-blockers			
• Propanolol (Inderal) • Timolol • Atenolol • Nadalol	40–240 mg/day 10–30 mg/day 50–120 mg/day 40–240 mg/day	weight gain, low blood pressure, lethargy, fatigue sexual problems, thyroid dysfunction, depression, and others	Do **not** stop abruptly, may cause rebound high blood pressure
Anticonvulsants			
• Phenytoin (Dilantin) • Valproate (Depakote) • Carbamazepine (Tegretol)	200–400 mg/day 500–3000 mg/day 200–1200 mg/day	rashes, blood cell problems, fatigue, drowsiness weight gain, ovarian dysfunction, many others	Need careful monitoring of blood levels, CBC, liver enzymes, and side effects
Calcium-channel blockers			
• Verapamil (Calan, others) • Nifedipine (Procardia, Adalat) • Diltiazem (Cardizem, Tiazac) • Nimodipine (Nimotop)	160–720 mg/day drowsiness, 30–180 mg/day 120–360 mg/day 30–120 mg/day many others	fatigue, low blood pressure, dizziness, slowed heart rate hair loss, constipation, lethargy, and	Watch for low blood pressure, All in this group may interfere with oral estrogen
Serotonin-enhancing antidepressants			
• Fluoxetine (Prozac) • Paroxetine (Paxil) • Sertraline (Zoloft)	10–80 mg/day 20–80 mg/day	mild nausea, gastrointestinal upset, diarrhea, anxiety, decrease in sexual desire	Do not use with MAO inhibitors; may cause *more agitation in some;* Paxil causes a withdrawal reaction if stopped abruptly
TCA antidepressants			
• Nortriptyline (Pamelor) • Doxepin (Sinequan) • Imipramine (Tofranil) • Amitriptyline (Elavil)	10–100 mg/day 10–200 mg/day 25–150 mg/day 10–250 mg/day	weight gain, constipation, dry mouth, reduced orgasm, blurred vision, dry eyes	May cause rapid heart rate, blood pressure changes, many drug interactions

© Elizabeth Lee Vliet, M.D., 1995, revised 2000

Rebound Headache: Getting Off Painkillers

When I was Associate Medical Director of the Maryview Pain Management Program in Virginia, one of the most common problems I encountered in helping women with headache syndromes (especially migraine) was that of "rebound" headaches due to the multiple analgesics and ergot medications women were taking on a daily basis. Dr. Joel Saper, founder and director of the Michigan Headache and Neurological Institute in Ann Arbor, Michigan, published the first paper about ergot dependency in 1986, which characterized the increasing severity of headaches due to ergot withdrawal. In contrast to typical migraines, patients with ergot withdrawal headaches have more diffuse and severe head pain, more severe vomiting, and are likely to have headaches persisting three to five days during which time they often become dehydrated due to the vomiting. Ergot dependency also contributes to an increased frequency of headaches.

When the headache medicines wear off, the headache pain cycle starts again, so you take more medicine, pain is relieved for awhile, then it comes back, and the cycle continues. It often becomes a problem to even determine which is the migraine and which is the withdrawal headache. We now know that daily use of **all** of the above abortive and preventive medications, as well as **all** of the pain-reliever analgesics, even simple NSAIDs like aspirin and Tylenol, can *cause* rebound headaches. Rebound headaches then contribute to chronic daily headaches that make it difficult to decide what medications to try and use to prevent migraines. When you are caught in this vicious cycle of rebounding, it doesn't matter which medication caused the rebound headaches: opiates, barbiturates (as in Fiorinal, Fioricet, and others), NSAIDS, SSRIs, triptans, or ergotamines . . . all of these medicines can do it. When this happens, practically speaking, *nothing else* works to prevent your migraines. The first step is to be properly tapered off the offending medications causing the withdrawal headaches, and then be started on a suitable *preventive* regimen.

How can you tell if you are having rebound headaches? There are some important clues that help sort this out. Migraines in their usual form occur at most once or twice a week, and more commonly, only once every two or three weeks. If the headaches are happening as often as three to five times a week in a person on daily medication, then it is more likely that the headache is being driven by medication fluctuations, dependency, and withdrawal. There is a typical pattern to withdrawal headaches, regardless of type of medication causing them: (a) headaches show an increasing intensity the longer one is without the medication; (b) there is a crescendo effect not seen in the same pattern with migraines; (c) the headaches are quickly relieved by restarting the offending drug and typically are *not* relieved by any other medications; and (d) the headaches become more frequent, with timing that relates to half-life of the particular drug. If you see yourself described in this pattern, you might consider a comprehensive pain management program for integrated treatment and supervised medication tapering. You may look into resources at one of the headache centers listed in appendix II, or contact the National Headache Foundation (800-843-2256) for the names of specialists in your area.

Alternative Therapies: Acupuncture, Biofeedback, Hypnotherapy, Neuromuscular Massage, Cranio-Sacral Therapy, and Others

Many studies in recent years have shown that biofeedback can be remarkably effective in reducing migraine headache pain. Acupuncture also can be highly effective and appears to work through a number of the neurochemical pathways I discussed earlier in this chapter. Both of these techniques have provided help to women who have side effects with medications or who simply prefer alternative approaches. I often recommend a trial of either or both options, since there are few side effects associated with either one. The primary drawback is that you have to find a skilled therapist to teach you to use biofeedback or to administer acupuncture and both require a series of treatments for optimal effectiveness. You have to be motivated to practice the technique daily in order for biofeedback to be effective. Acupuncture and biofeedback may not have the long-term preventive effects that can be achieved with some of the newer medications, but these modalities certainly can be beneficial to decrease pain and reduce medication use. Acupuncture and biofeedback are helpful as stress-reduction strategies, which can be another way of decreasing headache frequency.

Meditation, deep-breathing exercises, hypnotherapy (hypnosis), and Yoga are also ways of altering the neurochemical pathways that perpetuate the headache cycle. These methods of pain relief require practice to develop the degree of skill needed to help relieve pain during an acute migraine episode, but they can be helpful additions to your other approaches. These techniques are helpful for general stress management as well as headache relief, so I encourage you to look into classes in your area that teach these skills.

Speaking of stress, remember that eating regularly and well helps reduce the stress response that can trigger migraines and also helps prevent low blood sugar (hypoglycemia), another migraine trigger. Watching your alcohol and caffeine intake particularly at vulnerable times of the menstrual cycle helps avoid known headache triggers. Migraines in some women may also be precipitated by milk and other dairy products. If you suffer with migraines, you probably already have a pretty good idea of the triggers that affect you, so pay attention and avoid these at times in your menstrual cycle when you are particularly susceptible to attacks.

Some people feel that Vitamin B6 and diuretics are useful for migraines although I have not found that either of these approaches is effective for severe forms of migraine headaches. Diuretics typically do not improve premenstrual migraine headaches and may actually make them worse by altering electrolyte balance. Vitamin B6 has been reported to help some women with PMS, but it has not been found to help relieve menstrual migraines, and large doses can cause neurological symptoms of numbness, tingling, and sensory abnormalities. One recent study reported that 400 mg of riboflavin daily helped reduce the frequency of migraine headaches, so you may want to try this. The herb feverfew has been helpful for some migraine sufferers and few side effects have been reported with its use.

A number of bodywork modalities help reduce the pain and spasm that occur in neck and jaw muscles and may trigger migraines or cause the chronic tension-type headaches. I have referred patients to physical therapists for myofascial release, to massage therapists for cranio-sacral, shiatsu, and other massage modalities that are very helpful to diminish headaches, and I have also recommended osteopathic manipulation as an effective technique to decrease mechanical factors triggering migraines and other chronic headaches. Scheduling yourself for a massage therapy session at times of your menstrual cycle that you know are vulnerable times for headaches is a great idea for stress reduction, as well as to decrease muscle tension that aggravates headache pain. I think more headache management programs should include these methods since they are beneficial and have few side effects. Many insurance plans will now reimburse for massage therapy if prescribed by a physician for a particular medical problem such as migraine.

And don't forget exercise! Aerobic exercise on a regular basis improves circulation, boosts endorphins, and helps get rid of excess adrenaline that accumulates with our typical stres-s-s-s-filled days. All of these benefits help to further decrease migraine headache frequency. I encourage you to take charge of your headache problems and begin putting all of these pieces together, along with your awareness of the hormonal influences on migraine. Doing this should help give you a better awareness of factors that are within your control and those you need to discuss with your physician. It takes patience, persistence, practice, and partnership with a physician who listens and works with you, but it's worth it in the long run. The debilitating effects of migraines can be minimized with careful attention to integrating all of these approaches.

Chapter 11

Fibromyalgia, Aches and Pains: The Estrogen Factor

If someone told you that there was a medical disorder in which 80 percent of the patients were women, and the average age of onset was thirty to fifty years of age, what connections do you think might be obvious to study? It seems pretty important to look at a factor, or factors, that make women different from men in that age range, wouldn't you agree? As I mentioned in an earlier chapter, I have done a great deal of work with chronic pain patients since my residency at Johns Hopkins in the early 1980s. Over the years, I have been struck by the fact that almost all of the *fibromyalgia* patients I see are women, typically over forty, and frequently with a history of hysterectomy or early menopause. The obvious gender difference in this common medical disorder made me consider two important points: (1) the age range of thirty to fifty is a time of significant hormonal changes for women, but not typically a time of marked hormonal change for men, and (2) women's pain symptoms typically flared up at certain times of their menstrual cycle and subsided at other times in the cycle. I thought there might be a connection with changes in estrogen and progesterone and how these hormones affect brain chemistry in the pain-regulating centers of the nervous system.

The more I began looking into these connections in evaluating patients, the more I was stunned to find marked degrees of hormonal loss, which clearly could be of clinical significance in addressing the chronic pain problems. The information available was so profound, and so overlooked, I have now written a complete book addressing the overlooked hormone connections in fibromyalgia. I realize that with something as complex as fibromyalgia and chronic pain, there are *multiple* causative and contributing factors. It is too simplistic to say that these medical problems are *due to*, or *only* caused by, declining estrogen and other female hormones. My question, however, is why haven't physicians and researchers in the field of chronic pain even considered female hormonal factors when *the majority of patients with fibromyalgia are female?* I continue to be astounded at the collective lack of awareness of women's physiological differences and the failure to include these variables in clinical management and our research models.

Listen to one woman's voice (one of many who has made the connections with her menstrual cycle menopausal hormonal changes):

> I am forty-five, and I've felt for about ten years that there were problems with my hormones. Around the time of my period, the pain seems to increase markedly. As I have been getting closer to menopause, I feel like my fibromyalgia has increased a lot. My doctors say there is absolutely (!) no hormonal connection in fibromyalgia, I've been made to feel I'm stupid for even asking such a dumb question. When I have asked what can help my pain, I have felt talked down to. The only thing offered me was to exercise more. No one is really listening to me.

In addition to overlooking the role of female hormones in fibromyalgia, we have also been too slow in looking at some of the brain hormones and chemical messengers (serotonin, dopamine, epinephrine, substance P, and others) in approaching chronic pain as a problem very different from *acute* pain. It was over twenty years ago during my specialty training at Johns Hopkins that we were using serotonin-modulating medications to help patients with chronic pain. But use of these types of medication in fibromyalgia is just now beginning to gain more widespread use; such approaches are so important that they need wider use. Management options for *chronic* pain are still largely in the dark ages with negative stereotypes of patients (the majority of whom are women, remember?) as "neurotic," "drug-seekers," "addictive personalities," and so on. I hope this chapter will help you see that new hope, help, and treatment approaches are available if you have been struggling with the chronic pain of fibromyalgia.

Fibromyalgia: The Mysterious, Elusive Medical Condition

Fibromyalgia (FMS) is a condition that has been described in the medical writings for several thousand years, going back to the time of Hippocrates and early Chinese physicians. It is also the second most common rheumatological disorder, following osteoarthritis in frequency. The disorder we currently call fibromyalgia has been called a number of different names over the years: *rheumatism, neurasthenia, myofascial pain syndrome, myositis, fibrositis, fibromyositis, myalgia.* FMS is difficult to diagnose on objective physical findings. Although it is far more common in women, I have only once seen a medical article mention checking blood levels of ovary hormones in women with fibromyalgia. Studies have shown low growth hormone (GH) and low serotonin (ST) levels in FMS patients, but these changes are found in other disorders as well, and both GH and ST are decreased by decline in estradiol. One problem is that there are no consistent lab abnormalities in FMS, such as objective measures of inflammation or actual damage to the muscles. In fact, we are now fairly certain that there is no actual *inflammation* of the muscles in FMS. Furthermore, FMS is a disorder of *diffuse* pain throughout major areas of the body; patients do not have a specific, easily identifiable lesion in one area. For all of these reasons, FMS is a particularly frustrating condition, both for patients who suffer with it, and doctors who want to offer their patients some help and relief. Since FMS has been difficult to pin down, this syndrome was long viewed by many medical people with skepticism and disparagement. Doctors saw it as something vague and psychosomatic because its symptoms come and go, the pain is hard to localize, and there are no objective changes in the body when the person is experiencing pain. Add to all this what we already know about the negative stereotypes commonly applied to the female patient, and you can begin to see how a problem that occurs more often in women and is a vague, ill-defined syndrome was often labeled a psychogenic illness.

In 1990, FMS was finally recognized as a legitimate disorder and was given standard diagnostic criteria based upon the presence of both of these findings: (1) persistent pain or achiness at multiple body sites, and (2) the presence of painful trigger points at a minimum of eleven of the eighteen classic sites shown in the diagram below. Current research has shown that individuals with FMS show increased sensitivity to pain throughout the entire body, even areas such as the forehead, rather than just tenderness at the discrete points shown in the diagram as was originally thought. This observation is helpful because it lends support to the concept that the increased sensitivity to pain (or global reduction in pain threshold) is based in the brain (central nervous system, CNS) rather than just in the muscles or nerves of the body (peripheral nervous system, PNS). There are many mechanisms that may affect the CNS pain centers, such as estrogen balance in women, among others. The summary chart below shows some of the characteristic findings of FMS itself, along with *nonmuscular* associated conditions that have been reported in more current research on FMS. It is striking that many of the associated disorders and conditions that are found to be more common in patients with FMS are also ones that are markedly affected by a decline in ovary hormone production, especially estrogen. Associated conditions described in the FMS medical literature are the *same* conditions being described in the *menopause* medical literature about the widespread effects of declining estrogen. We will discuss these hormone aspects in more detail in this chapter, but I want you to begin thinking about this now as it may relate to your own experience.

HALLMARK FEATURES OF FIBROMYALGIA

- generalized stiffness and soreness, often worse in the morning

- increased pain in neck, trunk, and hips

- restless, fragmented sleep

- exquisite tender points where muscles and tendons meet

- numbness, burning, or cold sensations in muscles and/or extremities

- diminished energy, marked fatigue

- commonly associated with mood changes: irritability, lability, depression

- commonly associated with alterations in memory and concentration

- associated with high incidence of recurrent noncardiac chest pain, palpitations

- commonly associated with smooth muscle dysmotility (irritable bowel, esophageal reflux, urinary frequency, interstitial cystitis, dysmenorrhea, TMJ pain)

- higher incidence of CNS-mediated hypotension in FMS patients than in persons without FMS

- may be associated with hearing changes/decreased painful sound tolerance

- altered motility of ocular muscles, and vestibular abnormalities

- may be associated with migraine headaches, multiple chemical sensitivities

© Elizabeth Lee Vliet, M.D., 1995

What is a trigger (tender) point? This is an area where muscle and tendons meet at bone and produce pain that may radiate to other areas as well. A trigger point is defined as positive when pressure of about 4 kg applied to the area during physical examination causes a localized sensation of increased tenderness and pain. It is possible to have other types of chronic myofascial pain syndromes without having all eleven painful trigger points required for the diagnosis of FMS. In this chapter, I have focused on FMS, but I want you to keep in mind that many of the same factors that make FMS worse will also aggravate other myofascial pain syndromes. The use of tender points to confirm a diagnosis of FMS has some problems, and researchers are trying to find better ways of assessing the abnormalities in pain threshold with this disorder. Studies have shown that tenderness is a characteristic that varies a great deal along a continuum in the general population. This means that some patients who do have FMS will be excluded if tenderness is a primary diagnostic feature, and others who have a biological tendency to have more tenderness sensitivity will be overdiagnosed. Tenderness is also influenced by a variety of other factors that may not themselves predispose to developing FMS: getting older, being female, not being very physically fit, poor nutrition. Again, the problem is that the diagnostic criteria may fail to recognize some people who have FMS and include others who don't. At some point, we will need to find a better method of measuring the pain threshold and abnormalities, such as using a *dolorimeter* (a pressure gauge applied against the skin), in order to better define this disorder.

FMS is often confused with arthritis, a group of inflammatory disorders that lead to *joint* deterioration and pain. FMS may occur *along with* osteoarthritis and other types of arthritis. But unlike *arthritis* (inflammation of the joints) and *arthralgias* (soreness, aching of the joints), *fibromyalgia* does not affect the joints directly. It affects the *muscles, tendons, and ligaments.* When you have muscle pain with movement, or the muscles have become tight in spasm, this can then affect the way joints function and thus may give the impression that fibromyalgia is in your joints. FMS does not cause deformities or permanent crippling as may happen with arthritis, but it can certainly interfere with quality of life and ability to function optimally. Many patients describe the pain as "intrusive," "overwhelmingly present," "debilitating," a "robber of my life." These convey how serious this problem is. In addition, there is often a peculiar fuzziness of thinking that sufferers euphemistically call "fibrofog," but the term doesn't convey how devastating the mental cloudiness and confusion can be and the extent to which it can rob you of your ability to carry out even basic daily activities.

Fibromyalgia may also be precipitated by some type of trauma, whether a car accident with whiplash injuries, a severe jarring type of fall, or a surgery followed by prolonged inactivity. The anatomic and biochemical changes that occur with such traumas create severe, wide-ranging effects in the tissues of the body, and then set the foundation for the chronic pain cycle to begin. Hans Selye, M.D., the pioneer in stress research and keen observer of the multiple body effects of *continued, repeated* stressors, coined the term "calciphylaxis" in 1975 to described the complex series of physiological

Diagram 11.1—FIBROMYALGIA:
FRONT AND BACK VIEW OF TRIGGER POINT SITES

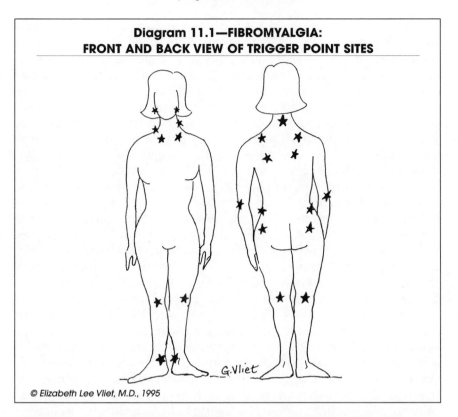

© Elizabeth Lee Vliet, M.D., 1995

changes the body undergoes when responding to stress so that the body is able to fight the stressor or flee from it. Dr. Selye defined calciphylaxis as "an induced hypersensitivity in which tissues respond to various challenging agents with a sudden calcification." He observed that it did not matter whether the stressor was chronic illness, multiple surgeries or injuries, or severe emotional trauma. In all these situations the body tissue changes were the same; the repeated activation of the fight-or-flight response caused adverse changes in the tissues themselves.

Our neuromuscular therapists at ℋℰ𝓡 𝒫𝓁𝒶𝒸𝑒, as well as numerous bodywork therapists I have consulted over the years, all describe the same type of change in the tissues: tight, lumpy bands of muscle, hardened areas of muscle that should feel softer, a doughy feel to the tissues above the muscles, in addition to areas that cause marked pain when pressed. These changes are what Dr. Hans Selye called "calciphylaxis or calcification," and this process causes a tightening and restriction of the tissues in the majority of patients with FMS. The connective tissues around and between muscles, called fascia, become thickened and lose their elasticity, and develop into hard, tight bands. As these bands cause more restriction to the movement of the muscle and fascia, blood flow, lymph flow, and nerve conduction all become impaired. Chemical messengers and nutrients can't get to the muscle adequately, and metabolic breakdown products from cellular actions (often called "toxic wastes" by massage therapists) can't be cleared away and then buildup in the tissue. The accumulation of these irritating metabolic wastes then further causes the "calcification" process, resulting in yet more tightness and pain. Over time this process of "calcification" causes the buildup of bumpy, tender areas and taut bands of muscle fibers we call trigger points because they cause pain at the site and refer pain to other parts of the body.

In addition to interrupting blood and lymph flow and the free movement of muscle and fascia, the fascia that is changed in this way also traps nerves and forms scar tissue and adhesions where the altered tissues stick to each other and don't move freely. When nerves pass through a muscle between taut bands or between taut bands and bone, it causes persistent, unrelenting pressure on the nerve that then causes the nerve to lose its oxygen and nutrients. The nerve then can't conduct signals properly, and this in turn produces numbness, tingling, or areas of hypersensitivity. You know this feeling when you sit on your foot and it goes to sleep—remember the painful prickles as you move your body, the pressure is off the foot, blood flow returns, and nerve sensations return in spades. Your brief episode of the foot falling asleep from pressure is similar to what goes on *continually* in FMS when pressure bands in the muscles compress blood flow and nerve impulse transmission. No *wonder* you hurt all the time. In fact, doctors evaluating FMS patients should ask the question "where *don't* you hurt?" rather than "where *do* you hurt?" If this process continues for prolonged times, and the body is constantly in a state of hyperalertness, the myofascia forms even more of the tight ropy bands around and through the muscle, and these become *contractures* that further restrict movement, and the whole process continues the downward spiral of increasing pain, calcification, and restriction.

It was originally thought that stress and worry, which caused additional muscle tension, caused the symptoms of fibromyalgia. Although recent studies of people with fibromyalgia do not prove that stress itself causes FMS, stress, anxiety, and fatigue can make the pain worse. In fact, chronic pain and fatigue often cause stress and anxiety, which in turn can increase the pain and fatigue. We also know that chronic stress and pain cause suppression of the ovary hormone balance, which in turn causes sleep disruption and suppression of growth hormone and other crucial chemical messengers for pain regulation. Do you see a vicious cycle taking shape? Many times people who are caught in this tension-pain cycle turn to readily available drugs for relief: alcohol, nicotine, caffeine, painkillers, and the like. We are so accustomed to having these substances around that we often do not think of them as the drugs they are. Each one of these substances has many adverse effects on the brain chemical messengers, which collectively result in intensified pain, so again you can see why we must address all of these issues in order to make the journey out of pain. Since there are so many factors involved in aggravating and perpetuating fibromyalgia, it takes a comprehensive and *integrated* approach to achieve optimal reduction in pain and improvement in well-being. Taking painkillers alone will rarely provide for long-term relief and return to normal activity. In order to properly help reduce the pain of FMS, we must look at *all* of these pieces of the puzzle and look at how changes in one group of neurotransmitters or hormones can have a cascade effect on other tissues throughout the body—including the muscles affected by FMS.

There are also crucial hormonal connections in fibromyalgia, as I discuss further in this chapter. To being your thinking about these connections, keep in mind that there is a great deal of overlap in the chemical messengers of the brain and body involved in fibromyalgia and those neurotransmitters affected by the decline in ovary hormones during perimenopause. Stressors (surgical, life situations, or lifestyle habits) that suppress ovary function may also cause decline in ovary hormone levels. I do not find in the medical literature much mention of these *overlapping effects* on pain-modulation pathways and neurotransmitters, and I think there is much to explore in understanding these interconnecting pathways and functions. Although medical researchers and physicians don't know the exact causes of fibromyalgia, they have recognized a number of different conditions and biological changes in the brain and body that are associated with it. The following are some of the basic connections.

Neuroendocrine, Vascular, and Metabolic Changes Associated with FMS

Many people with fibromyalgia have other problems that often confuse their doctors. These include: Raynaud's syndrome (poor circulation to the hands or toes), tension headaches, migraine headaches, dizziness, tingling and numbness, an irritable bowel (abdominal bloating with alternating diarrhea and constipation), muscle tremors, bladder spasms, and blurred vision. Current research has shown that **estrogen loss or decline can result in most of these same symptoms.** Later in this chapter and more in chapter 13, I will talk about the several mechanisms by which estrogen acts to preserve normal muscle and nerve function and normal blood vessel elasticity and to improve circulation. When estrogen decreases, there are subtle effects on blood vessels and blood flow to the tissues that in turn affect muscle tissue's ability to clear metabolic wastes produced by daily activity. There are a number of ways, both direct and indirect, that decline in ovarian hormone can instigate or aggravate FMS, as we shall see. The estrogen factor may have *more* of a role in triggering or aggravating FMS than anyone has realized. Meanwhile, until we have clearer answers from research, if you have FMS you may find it helpful to have a comprehensive neuroendocrine evaluation to see whether hormone factors are part of the problem for you. If an unrecognized decline in your own body estrogen is causing a number of the triggers that will make FMS worse, you may feel better by adding appropriate hormone therapy to your overall FMS treatments.

Immunologic Changes

There's been a great deal of recent interest in the chronic fatigue syndrome (CFS), which had been proposed to have many causes, from a persistent infection with the Epstein-Barr virus (EBV) to abnormalities in the brain centers that regulate blood pressure. EBV as a *causal* link in CFS has not held up under the scrutiny of further research. We have found, however, that many people who had previously been diagnosed as having CFS have been found to have FMS and their fatigue appears to be the result of the chronic sleep deprivation. Fatigue is for some people the most debilitating aspect of fibromyalgia; some women experience it as a lack of muscle endurance, while others describe the fatigue as an overall lack of energy. There are a number of potential links with the immune system that could contribute to FMS patients having a greater tendency to have more frequent infections of all types. Sleep deprivation suppresses immune system function, and so does a decline in estrogen and testosterone. Persistent overstimulation of the fight-or-flight response, for example by ongoing pain stimuli, leads to suppression of the immune system. Chronic pain is a stressor of the body, which also causes excessive production of cortisol, the stress hormone. Increased production of cortisol adds to more suppression of the body's immune system over time. Remember that cortisol production is *also increasing* in response to decline in estrogen. Once again, do you see how the many pieces of the puzzle fit together with women's hormonal changes and the high frequency of FMS in women?

I think it will become clear as you read further in this chapter that our current research findings lend more support to my proposed theory that FMS is triggered by the brain effects of declining ovarian hormones, with multiple brain-body systems, including muscle metabolism and repair, then being affected and leading to the wide variety of symptoms and persistent pain. This integrated model makes more sense to me physiologically, and approaching it from such a gender-specific point of view helps me to develop a more systematic, and physiological, approach to helping women feel better and deal constructively with the menstrual cycle hormonal shifts, and the effects on pain when hormone levels decline following tubal ligation, in the postpartum time frame or in the perimenopause and postmenopausal years. Think of FMS as an "early warning system" of many detrimental metabolic changes, and look at this as your opportunity to grab hold of your health to improve it for many years ahead. This is even truer now that women are living so much longer. The risk of many conditions like FMS increases as we lose our crucial metabolic hormones from the ovary, along with other changes such as thyroid and growth hormone. In 1900, the average age of death for women was forty-eight years. In the year 2000, only one hundred years later, we are fortunate to have average life expectancies of about eighty-eight years. Quite a change, and even more striking if you compare this with the fact that 500 years ago women died, on average, by age thirty-five. I think the most critical point for women to understand is that we want to learn what we need to know about maintaining our long-term health and reducing our long-term individual disease risks so we can live these additional thirty or forty years with the best possible quality of life and good health. Don't just focus on *treating* **or** *bearing with symptoms* NOW; look at your big picture and make decisions based on what is needed for you over the long haul.

Hormonal Changes and Other Conditions Associated with FMS

- FMS more commonly occurs in women at times of significant ovarian hormone change: postpartum, after tubal ligation, after stopping long use of birth control pills, after hysterectomy, and during perimenopause and postmenopause

- Physically unfit muscles and an associated sleep disorder, with disruption in Stage IV sleep in particular

- Metabolic abnormalities: glucose intolerance, insulin resistance, hypoglycemia, elevated or suppressed cortisol

- Immunologic abnormalities such as elevated thyroid antibodies

- Vascular changes, such as Raynaud's syndrome, hypertension

- Neuroendocrine changes: decreased insulin-like growth factor (IGF), decreased growth hormone, low serotonin (all of these are also decreased with decline in estradiol)

- Whiplash and fall-torsion injuries

- Presence of significant situational stressors (affect all of the above)

© Elizabeth Lee Vliet, M.D., 1995, revised 2000

Overlooked Female Hormonal Connections

I have reviewed many books on pain, and nowhere did I find anyone addressing the crucial *ovary* hormonal triggers that can cause and perpetuate pain syndromes far more common in women, such as fibromyalgia, joint pain, back pain, headaches, bladder pain, and other such problems. My own journey into the depths of chronic, debilitating pain has taught me much about these crucial hormone issues and their fundamental role in pain pathways. I know without question that I do not do well with my own muscle and nerve pain problems unless my estradiol is where is should be, and it is in healthy balance with the testosterone the ovaries also produce. But if it were just my own experience with pain, I wouldn't be writing this. I have now treated hundreds of women with a variety of pain syndromes, and this work has shown me time and time again in working with so many women over many years that nothing has fully broken the cycle of pain until their optimal hormonal and nutritional balance is restored. These hormonal connections have been a profoundly important part of the clinical care I have incorporated for my own patients. Obviously, with a subject as complex as PAIN, one approach can't address all the issues or provide all the answers, but I do hope to show you what to look for with the hormone connections, what tests to request from your physicians, and to show you how to begin putting all these pieces of the puzzle together in planning optimal treatment. Then you can begin to benefit from all the other modalities that are recommended in the many books on pain treatment and begin to develop an individualized program for your recovery.

As I noted at the beginning of this chapter, when we look at who gets FMS, some glaring trends pop out: **80 percent are women between the ages of thirty and fifty.** Yes, FMS does occur in men and can begin in adolescence in both males and females, but worldwide statistics show that it is much less common in these groups. When I took careful histories of *when* the onset of FMS symptoms occurred, another glaring trend appeared: For the majority of my patients, the FMS began insidiously following some event that typically is associated with a *significant decrease* in ovarian hormone levels.

I have summarized my hypothesis about the most likely times in women's lives when FMS may insidiously begin due to hormonal shifts. All of these times are when the active form of estrogen, 17-beta estradiol, is low or has fallen sharply. I think this hormonal connection is crucially significant. I am not being sexist. There simply isn't anything else that so *clearly* differentiates male and female bodies. I think many women with FMS find it helpful and hopeful that I discuss these connections. Very commonly, they have already been asking these kinds of questions and have been frustrated with the lack of validation and acceptance of their observations about these connections. *These potential hormonal connections simply have not been explored.*

Dr. Vliet's Hypothesis: HORMONAL CONNECTIONS IN FMS AND COMMON TIMES OF ONSET

- Postpartum (particularly if the pregnancy was after the age of thirty-five)
- Perimenopause, associated with sleep changes
- Postmenopause, particularly if not on ERT or on suboptimal ERT
- Three to five years after tubal ligation
- Two to three years after hysterectomy (even if the ovaries were *not* removed)
- Presence of PCOS (polycystic ovarian syndrome)
- Presence of autoimmune ovarian disorders, especially if results in premature ovarian failure (POF)
- A period of sustained major stresses or illnesses that interrupts menses for several months
- Younger women with chronic anorexia-type dieting that suppresses ovary hormones
- Women who suppress ovarian function with drug or alcohol abuse

© Elizabeth Lee Vliet, M.D., 1995, revised 2000

Scattered in the recent medical literature are other clues to the existence of these ovary hormone connections beyond just my clinical experience. In one study of 100 patients cited by Jon Russell, M.D., Ph.D., of the University of Texas Health Science Center, San Antonio, the average age at which fibromyalgia was diagnosed was forty-eight, a common age of menopausal hormone decline. Dr. Russell described clinical observations that in women who developed FMS between the ages of twenty-five and forty, fully 40–50 percent of them were *menopausal prior to the onset of FMS*—either by surgical menopause or a premature natural menopause.

I think if we actually *measured* blood tests of female hormone levels, we would see an even *higher* percentage of menopausal women in such studies. Instead, the questions about menopause are rarely asked, and most physicians tend to just depend on the patient's chronological age or her own knowledge of whether she is menopausal. This was one of the striking findings I noted when I did the thorough history and medical evaluation of the women admitted to our pain management program. When I actually measured hormone levels in these patients (FSH, estradiol, testosterone, and sometimes progesterone if the woman still had her ovaries), I was quite struck by how low the levels of estradiol and testosterone were compared to the expected normal range for a woman in her twenties through early forties. One of the treatment approaches I used, in combination with the other therapies we incorporated in our overall approach to pain management, was restoring the woman's hormonal balance to normal levels. I was pleasantly surprised to find that the improvements in FMS occurred much more rapidly with optimal hormonal therapy added to the overall therapeutic program.

I must caution that at this time, there is simply no controlled study to determine whether there is a cause-and-effect relationship with female hormones and FMS or whether this observed connection is simply an *association* of the phenomena of *pain/FMS* and *menopausal hormone changes*. Even if there is only an association, it certainly is important enough to at least include in our medical assessments, so that if there are hormonal imbalances, these can be properly addressed in designing an individualized treatment plan. Helping women find an optimal hormonal balance, in my experience, has frequently meant they could reduce the amount of pain medication.

Ria's Story

Ria is an example of the significant improvements that can happen in women with fibromyalgia when hormonal balance is addressed. She is now fifty-three, and had been injured in an automobile accident about eight years ago. Following the accident she developed a severe pain syndrome called reflex sympathetic dystrophy (RSD), which produces a burning, excruciating pain difficult to relieve even with narcotic medication. She underwent extensive evaluation and treatment by physicians very experienced in managing RSD. Two years later, when she went through menopause, she was started on a standard cyclic hormone therapy with conjugated equine estrogen (Premarin), and progestin (Provera). Her menopausal hot flashes stopped, and she was sleeping better. She felt better getting these concerns addressed, even though the RSD continued to cause pain.

Over the past five years, however, she developed a *new and different type of pain*, which she described as clearly distinct from the *burning* pain of RSD. She described the new pain as dull, aching pain in the muscles of her arms, hands, legs, and back associated with intermittent sharper pains along with stiffness in her joints. This pain had gotten so much worse over the last year that she now had difficulty walking and had to begin using a cane. Understandably, she was becoming more and more discouraged about her health. She had observed that this new pain developed after menopause and initiating hormone therapy, so it seemed a reasonable question to ask her doctors if there could be a possible hormonal connection to produce this new type of pain. She did ask several of her doctors whether it was possible to check hormone levels to see if she was taking the right amount. Each time she asked, she was told that it couldn't have anything to do with her hormones. She was told that she had fibromyalgia. She met the criteria I described above for FMS, so this seemed a reasonable diagnosis. She was further told that there was no way to do any tests for hormone levels, and the hormone dose was fine because she wasn't having any more hot flashes. Her doctors recommended physical therapy and anti-inflammatory medication added to the pain medicine she had been taking for the RSD. She continued to have more and more difficulty with both the RSD and this new pain problem.

Ria's friend told her about the work I was doing with women with FMS. Ria scheduled an appointment and had her hormone levels checked along with other important blood tests. In addition to the new pain syndrome, Ria was also having problems with weight gain, loss of energy, diminished libido, restless sleep, and said she just didn't feel "like my old self." Ria and I spent an hour going over all that she had been through, her lab results, and the options I thought could help her. Even though she was taking estrogen, her FSH was still too high in the menopausal range, and her estradiol level was markedly low (less than 30 pg/ml). Her hormone therapy was clearly not giving adequate levels of the estrogen she most needed replenished.

Since she had experienced breast enlargement on the conjugated equine estrogen, as well as the worsening pain symptoms, I did not want to just increase the dose. I suggested she change to the native human form of estradiol, which I thought would give better pain relief. I also recommended that she dissolve the estradiol under her tongue (instead of swallowing the oral tablet) because I knew that would give a better ratio of estradiol (E2) to estrone (E1), which I thought would help reduce the breast enlargement and weight gain she had experienced, and still provide optimal levels of estradiol to help diminish her symptoms. At this time, Estrace is the only commercial tablet form of estradiol that can be dissolved under the tongue and effectively absorbed. (Note: This does not work with other brands or with the generic preparations of 17-beta estradiol.) After I had explained this rationale, she decided to try Estrace. I did not give her any particular suggestions about the change other than to say I thought this estrogen would help her feel better, improve her sleep more effectively, and *perhaps* help with the overall pain she had been experiencing.

At her first follow-up visit about two months later, she said she felt more energetic, was sleeping well again, and had gone down a bra size. She reported that she did not feel as bloated, her joints were not as swollen and painful, and she felt she had a better range of movement. She was surprised to see that over the two months, her overall pain seemed less intense. She asked if I thought that could be related to the hormones, and I told her that this was the response I had seen in most of my patients, and I thought it did have an important hormonal connection. We agreed that she would continue the same amount of Estrace, and she would come back in another two months to be rechecked.

Four months later she returned for follow-up, and I hardly recognized her when she walked in the door. She looked happy and cheerful, walked more quickly and fluidly, did not need her cane to lean on (although she still carried it), and had more normal overall body movements. I commented that I had not seen her in such a long time, I had begun to wonder if she had given up on the hormonal approaches we were trying. She laughed and said,

> No, I was just feeling so much better, I forgot to call and make an appointment! About two weeks after my last appointment, I got up one morning and realized that *my joint and muscle pain was completely gone.* At first, I was afraid to believe it, but after a few more weeks, I realized the resolution of that part of my pain was very real, and it has not come back. The RSD pain is still there, but I can cope with that now that I don't have my joints and muscles hurting so bad all the time. I am even using less pain medicine for the RSD now. Getting off the Premarin and Provera and having my estrogen where it should be made such a difference in my pain, I can't believe how much better I feel now.

The normal premenopausal balance of estradiol in a woman's body has a number of effects on nerves and chemical messengers to reduce pain sensations, particularly chronic pain. Other underlying triggering mechanisms in fibromyalgia can be metabolic, neuroendocrine changes. These chemical changes in the brain and body would then affect the way peripheral nerve fibers function and trigger increases in the painful spasms that set up the vicious cycle of fibromyalgia. An example of this mechanism is the way declining female hormones, particularly estradiol from the ovary, cause *heightened sensitivity of nerve endings to pain* and other stimuli. Decreases in estradiol also cause decreases in serotonin production, so there are several possible ways for hormone change to trigger the variety of pain and aching with FMS. In this way, FMS may be dysfunction of the nerve fibers, with changes or abnormalities occurring in the way nerves to the body transmit pain signals. The stress of chronic pain on the body can also cause *further* decline in ovarian hormone production, so one situation aggravates the other.

The estradiol receptors heavily concentrated in the limbic system areas of the brain provide another connecting link between the chronic pain of FMS and the hormonal changes leading up to menopause. The nerve pathways carrying *chronic pain* stimuli from the body to the brain travel *through* the limbic system centers, which regulate mood and sleep. You can imagine how the *constant* day-to-day presence of pain signals can then disrupt normal sleep regulation and contribute to depressed, irritable moods through effects on the limbic system. Remember that I talked in chapter 5 about the way in which decreases in estradiol can disrupt the limbic system pathways and cause irritable mood and fragmented sleep. Now we see that *both* chronic pain stimuli and decreases in estrogen have similar effects on the same brain centers. *Acute pain* pathways *bypass* the limbic system as they travel from the body to the higher brain centers, so when you experience an *acute* injury producing pain, it is not likely to cause the same types of sleep and mood upsets that we see in people who have a chronic pain syndrome.

What can you do to check these connections for yourself if you have FMS? I suggest asking your physician to check hormone levels, so you can then determine whether adding the hormones might be helpful for you. I discuss these connections with my patients, and then measure FSH, estradiol, and testosterone blood levels. If the results show low estradiol levels, and she wants to try it, I prescribe estradiol alone or possibly with low-dose natural testosterone. If she has a uterus and needs to use a progestin, I try not to use a synthetic progestin (such as Provera, Cyrin, Amen, or Aygestin) unless there is no other choice to control difficult bleeding problems. I have found the synthetic progestins seem to make fibromyalgia pain *worse*. One possible explanation for this observation is that the synthetic progestins actually block estrogen binding at the estradiol receptors in the brain, which will then reduce estrogen's beneficial effects on pain. I have also found that synthetic estrogens (Ogen), the mixed animal-derived estrogens (Premarin, PremPro) or the esterified mixed plant-derived estrogens (Estratab, Cenestin, Menest) also appear to aggravate FMS symptoms. For women with FMS who may benefit from hormone therapy, I *use only the bioidentical human form of 17-beta estradiol* and make certain it reaches optimal estradiol blood levels. If you are having difficulty getting someone to check your hormone levels, you may want to schedule a consultation at a specialty center like our ℋℰℛ 𝒫𝓁𝒶𝒸ℯ programs, where the hormone issues will be addressed as part of a comprehensive evaluation.

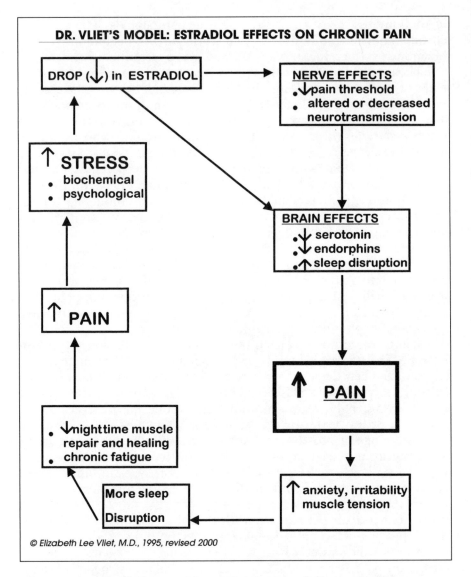

DR. VLIET'S MODEL: ESTRADIOL EFFECTS ON CHRONIC PAIN

© Elizabeth Lee Vliet, M.D., 1995, revised 2000

Serotonin and Other Neurohormonal Connections

There is a great deal of overlap in the chemical messengers of the brain and body involved in fibromyalgia and those neurotransmitters affected by the decline in ovary hormones during perimenopause. Decline in ovary hormone levels may also be caused by stressors (surgical, life situations, or lifestyle habits) that suppress ovary function. I do not find in the medical literature much mention of these *overlapping effects* on pain-modulation pathways and neurotransmitters, and I think there is much to explore in understanding these interconnecting pathways and functions. The list below shows the most important of the known neurotransmitters involved in regulating pain; since there are so many of these, you can begin to see how many different disorders can contribute to making FMS pain worse. I have already mentioned that hypothyroidism is *many times* more common in women than men, and this hormonal disturbance may be another overlooked factor in FMS. Careful and complete evaluation of thyroid function is another crucial hormone system to be checked. In FMS patients, I think it is particularly important to also check antithyroid antibody levels and the levels of the free T3 and free T4 thyroid hormones. Autoimmune thyroid disorders may cause significant muscle pain in the early stages of the disorder, even if TSH is normal. These antibody tests are more sensitive indicators of thyroid dysfunction that may be contributing to FMS pain.

Key Neurotransmitters and Hormones Involved in FMS and Pain

- Serotonin (pain-relieving chemical messenger)
- Tryptophan (building block for serotonin found in many foods)
- Norepinephrine (NE) and Epinephrine (EPI)
- Dopamine
- Substance P (pain-inducing chemical found in higher-than-normal levels in FMS)
- Monoamine oxidase (enzyme that breaks down dopamine, nor-epinephrine, and epinephrine)
- Endorphins
- Thyroid hormone
- Ovarian hormones (some researchers say this is still open to question)
- Adrenal steroids

© Elizabeth Lee Vliet, M.D., 1995

Although medical researchers and physicians don't know the exact causes of fibromyalgia, they have recognized a number of different conditions and biological changes in the brain and body that are associated with it. In order to properly help patients with FMS, we must look at these pieces of the puzzle and look at how changes in one group of neurotransmitters or hormones can have a cascade effect on other tissues throughout the body—including the muscles affected by FMS. I have summarized some of the conditions that are found to be present with fibromyalgia in the table entitled "Hormonal Changes and Other Conditions Associated with FMS" earlier in this chapter.

Unfit Muscles

While it is not yet known whether *unfit muscles* are the cause or the result of FMS, there is increasing evidence that people with fibromyalgia have unfit or poorly developed muscles. Women typically lose muscle mass as they age, so there is less reserve muscle tissue than in earlier years. As the cycle of pain contributes to more inactivity, the muscles become even more unfit and atrophied, which makes them more likely to be injured or damaged with exercise. This is a vicious cycle of more pain causes more inactivity causes more loss of muscle causes more pain causes more inactivity causes more loss of muscle. I think you get the picture. Over time, underuse of your muscles leads to a negative, detraining effect, which results in even more unfit muscles that are more likely to become injured or damaged from exercise. This sort of muscle damage is commonly called microtrauma, and it causes delayed muscle pain and fatigue that may not appear until a day or two after exercising and may last six to seven days. The pain and fatigue make us postpone further physical activity until they are gone and our energy has been restored, thereby again contributing to the vicious cycle.

It is common for anyone to experience the effects of microtrauma after too much physical activity. That's the kind of pain a weekend athlete will experience on Monday or Tuesday. Yet for people who have unfit muscles, these problems may develop after even slight exertion, such as routine day-to-day activities. Microtrauma may also result from other kinds of muscle overuse or injury: poor posture, sitting hunched over at a computer or a desk all day; damage caused by a blow or a fall; or the kind of torsion damage that occurs in a whiplash injury. In the normal person, muscles repair and restore themselves from microtrauma during stage IV sleep each night. But in FMS patients (and in women who have decreasing ovarian estrogen), the deep stages of sleep are disrupted, so normal muscle growth and repair during sleep does not occur.

In addition, there is an important chemical for muscle growth and repair, called Somatomedin-C, released by the liver when the liver is stimulated by growth hormone (GH). Eighty percent of our daily amount of GH is secreted during the deep stages of sleep, which, in FMS patients, are markedly diminished or missing altogether. It may well be, then, that the tendency toward muscle fatigue and weakness may be due to the loss of deep sleep stages, which in turn decreases the normal production of GH. Also keep in mind what I have said about the role of serotonin: This important chemical messenger in the brain is one of the crucial regulators of sleep, and serotonin production is typically also low in FMS patients.

If you think about what I have said about the role of unfit muscles in causing and/or maintaining FMS, you will see why beginning
an exercise program under the supervision of a physical therapist is
one of the cornerstones of effective treatment. It is crucial to break
out of this vicious cycle and retrain your muscles. Patients who diligently follow a graded exercise program have a significantly better,
and more rapid, recovery, because they are rebuilding and strengthening muscle tissue. A gradual increase in aerobic exercise provides
better blood flow to the muscles, which brings new oxygen and fuel
and takes away the waste products (particularly lactic acid), that
otherwise would build up and contribute to more pain.

Sleep Disorders and FMS

Almost all patients with fibromyalgia have a major sleep disturbance as part of the clinical findings. It is not yet known whether
the sleep disorder *causes* FMS or whether the chronic pain produces the
sleep disruption. At the point a person has FMS, sleep is disturbed,
causing a worsening of the FMS and pain. I prefer to view it as an
integrated problem and try to identify ways of constructively breaking the cycle. The clue to the sleep disorder connection in FMS has
been determined from sleep laboratory studies in which patients
sleep in a "bedroom" laboratory, with monitors keeping track of
brain wave patterns, muscle activity, eye movements, heart rate,
breathing rate, oxygen concentration in the blood, and a number of
other objective measures of the quantity and quality of sleep.
Patients with fibromyalgia typically show a marked degree of fragmented sleep, with the deepest or most restful stage of sleep (stage
IV) disturbed or interrupted, and more waking episodes at night.
Physicians refer to this abnormal pattern as "alpha intrusion of
stage IV sleep." Remember that I have also talked about the sleep
disturbances that are caused by declining estrogen levels affecting
the brain centers that regulate sleep. Here we see another hormonal
connection that may aggravate, or help to set up the conditions for,
FMS: **Decreased estrogen makes nerve endings more susceptible to
pain and disrupts sleep; the pain of fibromyalgia disrupts sleep; the
stress to the body of continued sleep loss causes more pain and more
decrease in ovary hormone production.** See how it all fits together?

Sleep disturbances may be a significant reason that women with
FMS describe having such low energy levels and feelings of marked
fatigue. A decline in hormone levels such as estrogen and particularly testosterone may be another reason for the low energy levels.
There is also evidence that **both** sleep problems and decreased ovarian hormones can lead to increased muscle pain. When normal,

healthy volunteers were stressed by artificial disturbance of their stage IV sleep, they developed pain and soreness in their muscles very similar to that seen in FMS. This combination of pain and fatigue then often limits physical activity and endurance. The resulting lack of physical exercise can contribute to the unfit muscles that are more susceptible to further pain, and the FMS symptoms continue to get worse. As I mentioned above, stage IV sleep is important in repairing tissue damage and feeling physically and psychologically rested when you wake up. So if stage IV sleep is reduced, it can contribute to many of the other symptoms of FMS.

If you have trouble going to sleep, you may find yourself turning to alcohol, thinking it will help you sleep better. The problem with using alcohol, especially for FMS patients, is that alcohol contributes to *more* fragmentation in sleep and *more loss* of stage IV sleep. Alcohol used on a regular basis has several other effects that make FMS worse: (1) alcohol depresses the central nervous system and aggravates the biological depression that occurs in about 90 percent of patients with FMS; (2) heavy alcohol use further suppresses ovarian function; (3) alcohol diminishes production of endorphins, the body's natural painkillers; (4) when alcohol is wearing off, it creates an adrenalin rebound that leads to increased muscle tension and pain; (5) alcohol is toxic to muscle fibers. For these reasons, I urge you to avoid drinking alcohol on a regular basis if you have FMS. Nicotine (cigarettes) and caffeine (coffee, tea, soda, etc.) are other common substances that stimulate the adrenaline system, add to muscle tension (and pain), and further aggravate fragmented sleep and reduced stage IV sleep.

I urge my patients with FMS to reduce or eliminate intake not only of alcohol but also other drugs like caffeine, nicotine, over-the-counter DHEA and stimulants found in weight-loss preparations, which may all make chronic pain worse. Take a look at the next diagram, which shows how many different factors are related to one another and create more pain. This may give you some ideas of ways you can begin to make healthy habit changes that will contribute to reducing the chronic pain. At the same time, if you take into account the hormonal factors that are involved in modulating pain sensations, you can begin to see how all these pieces of the puzzle are connected through similar effects on serotonin, endorphins, and other body messenger systems.

Problems with Pain Medications

There are a variety of medications useful in alleviating the symptoms of FMS, including some hormonal therapies. I would like to point out that many of the pain medications we use for *acute* pain treat-

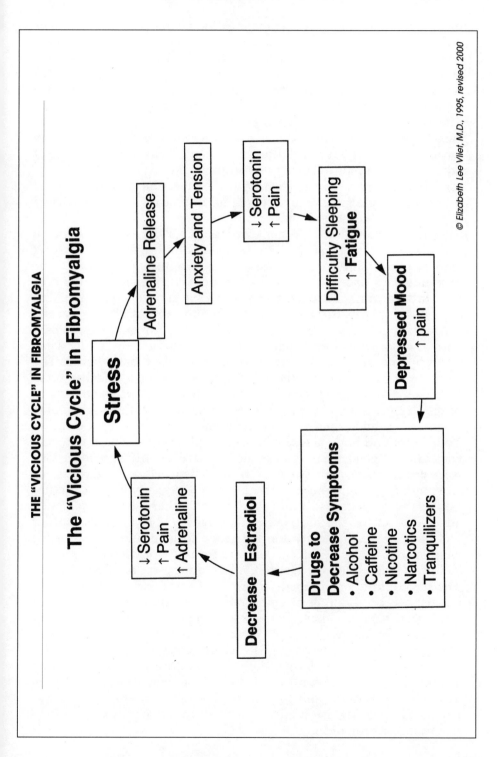

ment could actually be detrimental when working with *chronic* pain. Acute and chronic pain are very different, both in their nerve pathways as I mentioned earlier, and in the biochemical and psychological changes they produce. The best way I can explain the difference between acute and chronic pain is to use the analogy of a loud fire alarm in a building. The fire alarm goes off, gets your attention, and you move out of the building rapidly to avoid harm. Acute pain is the body's alarm that something has gone seriously wrong and needs your attention now. Acute pain triggers bursts of adrenaline, the pain-relieving endorphins, and other chemical messengers to prepare you to deal with the emergency. Narcotics and other potent analgesics are very helpful in relieving acute pain by a number of different mechanisms.

Chronic pain, on the other hand, is like a fire alarm *without* a cutoff switch. The persistent jarring sound of a fire alarm that won't stop is one of the most intrusive and penetrating sounds I have encountered. I once had to handle a patient emergency with the hospital fire alarm ringing persistently in the background. They couldn't get the fire alarm turned off. I thought the sound would literally drive me nuts! This is also very much what your mind-body-spirit goes through with chronic pain: Pain alarms go off continually without stopping and intrude on every dimension of one's being. The spirit feels beaten down, the mind is overwhelmed, and the body feels like it *hurts everywhere*. In chronic pain, the excessive activity of the "alarm system" contributes to an imbalance in the adrenaline system (too much) and the serotonin-endorphin system (too little). Your brain and body actually become depleted of the pain-relieving endorphins, which then *reduces* the effectiveness of the medications we use for acute pain (such as those listed below). Sedatives, or sleeping pills, taken longer than about two weeks will cause disruption in the deep stages III and IV sleep, and alter REM sleep. These adverse effects on the sleep cycle end up making FMS sleep disorder and pain *worse*. If medication is needed to help improve sleep for women with FMS, I prefer to use a *serotonin-boosting* one such as Zoloft, Prozac, Celexa, Desyrel, (trazodone), or possibly Buspar. The serotonin-boosting medications are not sleeping pills. They do not depress the brain as sleeping pills do, so they are safer, do not cause addiction, and have fewer side effects. These medications are more specific for the deficiency of serotonin, which is thought to be a major underlying factor in FMS. While none of these (except trazodone) are *directly* sedating, each works *indirectly* to restore sleep stages back to normal and to also decrease pain by enhancing the activity of serotonin and improving the serotonin-norepinephrine balance. Improving the quality of your sleep is a major part of effective treatment for FMS.

A different class of muscle-relaxant medication, cyclobenzaprine (Flexeril), is also helpful for some patients. It appears to help relax tense muscles and is also significantly sedating, so for many people it also improves sleep. The older tricyclic antidepressants like amitriptyline (Elavil), imipramine (Tofranil), doxepin (Sinequan), and others have been prescribed in the past to promote stage IV sleep. I generally don't recommend using these older tricyclic medications because they have too many side effects, in particular daytime drowsiness and lethargy. One common side effect of *all* the tricyclic antidepressants is that they cause weight gain in a large percentage of patients. Needless to say, this bothers women immensely. Since we now have the more selective serotonin-augmenting options available, I find the SSRIs work better with fewer unwanted side effects. If you are taking one of the tricyclic antidepressants and are having unpleasant side effects, talk with your physician about changing to one of the selective serotonin-boosting medications. Corticosteroids are sometimes used for pain relief in FMS, but they do not seem to be that effective for stiffness and fatigue. In addition, these drugs actually have marked weight gain effects and potentially serious side effects. I do not recommend using corticosteroids in FMS unless you have been carefully evaluated by a rheumatologist, and you have documented low cortisol levels or there is a specific *inflammatory* component that is being treated by the corticosteroids.

Pain Medications to Watch Out For

- narcotics (morphine, Demerol, Vicodin, Tylox, codeine, and others): tend to cause depression, fatigue, decreased memory, and concentration when taken regularly on a daily basis.

- excessive amounts of acetaminophen (Tylenol and generics): taken in large amounts on a regular basis, acetaminophen can lead to liver and kidney toxicity.

- sleeping pills (Restoril, Dalmane, Halcion, Valium, Serax, Ambien, Ativan, Klonopin): alter the normal stages of sleep when taken on a nightly basis for long periods of time. In addition, they are habit-forming, and if you have been taking them for more than a week or two, you will need a gradual tapering when it is time to stop them.

© Elizabeth Lee Vliet, M.D., 1995, revised 2000

Mind-Body Approaches

Fibromyalgia is one of those conditions whose "treatment" is best described as helping people *manage* their symptoms to achieve relief and improved body-mind function. There really isn't a cure for FMS in the sense that physicians could prescribe a medication or other form of treatment that would make all the symptoms and pain go away forever. It can best be compared to a disease like diabetes, in which the symptoms can be controlled and reduced with a "multiple modalities" approach. The destructive effects of FMS pain and progression of muscle deterioration can be dramatically reduced by minimizing lifestyle factors that aggravate pain. There are also *non-addictive* medications that can be used safely for an extended period of time to rebalance body chemistry and help you maintain productivity and pursue fairly normal life activities. It is really important that you plan to work with a team of health professionals over a period of time to decrease the symptoms of FMS. This is not a condition that can be treated quickly in three or four office visits with a physician. It is going to involve *your* active participation in a variety of therapeutic modalities and your commitment to a maintenance program of aerobic, strength, and flexibility exercises on a regular basis. I find that most patients with FMS respond best to a *combined* approach, which ideally would include achieving optimal hormonal balance, appropriate other medication for pain relief and sleep improvement, and these would be supplemented with one or more of the mind-body therapies such as *physical therapy, neuromuscular-massage therapy, cranio-sacral therapy, acupuncture, TENS, biofeedback or relaxation training, vibrational medicine and sound therapy, supportive psychotherapy, stress management, regular exercise, healthy eating habits,* and *vitamin-mineral supplements.* I have successfully used a combination of these approaches for my own recovery following my back surgeries, and I have also prescribed these techniques for my patients who suffer with fibromyalgia and other forms of chronic pain.

Vitamins and Minerals Crucial in Pain Regulation

It is critical to make sure you have adequate intake of certain vitamins and minerals that are important in helping our body make normal muscle tissue and regulate nerve function and pain pathways. I want to mention a few key vitamins and minerals that you will want to include each day, in addition to your multivitamin, calcium, and vitamin D.

Magnesium is especially crucial for nerve cell conduction, muscle contraction, muscle repair, pain regulation, bone building, and it also has a strong independent role in regulating blood pressure. Magnesium's role to decrease blood pressure and prevent seizures is so well known that it is used in an injectable form in the treatment of eclampsia (toxemia) of pregnancy and a variety of heart diseases. It appears to be an important factor in preventing migraine headaches and heart attacks, probably because it helps prevent spasms of the blood vessels throughout the body, but especially in the coronary (heart) arteries.

Magnesium helps maintain normal structure and contraction strength of the heart muscle itself as well as other muscle tissue in the body. In the brain, magnesium is a cofactor in the production of the important pain and mood-regulating chemical messengers such as dopamine. This is one of several reasons magnesium is useful in the treatment of PMS, as well as FMS. Several B vitamins (thiamine, riboflavin, and pyridoxine) require magnesium as a catalyst for the chemical reactions that make these vitamins biologically active in the body. Magnesium also is a cofactor for the chemical reactions for using amino acids to build protein for growth and repair of muscles and other tissues. The pathways for the body to make its energy compounds are also dependent upon magnesium.

In addition to all these, newer research has shown that magnesium plays a key role in helping to block overactivity of the NMDA receptor that is an important player in pain regulation. This receptor complex serves to spread and augment the pain sensations in persistent pain syndromes. Magnesium has been shown to act as a block at this receptor, helping to prevent the calcium channel from opening and causing "hyperexcitable" nerve cells that become overactive and intensify pain signals. Zinc is also important in this blocking process at the NMDA receptor, and the two minerals have slightly different functions to help keep the nerve cells from firing excessively in response to the excitatory amino acids (EAA) like glutamate, aspartate, and glycine. Conditions of low magnesium make the nerve cells more excitable in the presence of EAA, leading to increased pain, increased muscle spasm, and more tissue damage over time. These adverse effects are magnified under conditions when the neurons also have low energy stores of critical nutrients like glucose and oxygen. That's why it's so important in conditions like FMS to eat regularly and keep blood sugar levels steady, maintain optimal intake of magnesium and zinc, as well as practice regular deep breathing to improve oxygen flow to the tissues. Magnesium also is important in preventing free-radical damage to cells. When magnesium is low, not only do we lose this protective effect, but also the low magnesium is itself a trigger that generates *more* free radicals. Again, we have a double whammy that can have a serious cumulative effect in people with FMS.

Since magnesium is involved in so many critical chemical reactions to make energy, use oxygen, maintain "calm" nerve cells, prevent free-radical damage, build muscle, and make the chemical messengers for pain and sleep regulation, it is an absolutely essential mineral to take regularly as part of your supplements, in addition to seeing that you have good dietary sources, such as eggs, legumes, and peanuts. Estrogen enhances magnesium uptake and utilization by the body's soft tissues and by bone, which is another factor helping women have lower rates of heart disease and bone loss if they are estrogen complete. With decline in estrogen, we also lose our ability to absorb and use magnesium optimally, which in turn aggravates the problems that come with loss of estrogen: high blood pressure, greater bone loss, and increased heart disease. But there is a flip side of this coin that you need to keep in mind: If your magnesium intake is too low and you are on supplemental estrogen, the estrogen shifts more of the magnesium into the soft tissues and bone, with a resulting decrease in serum magnesium. This in turn causes a shift in the calcium-to-magnesium ratio, favoring coagulation, and could increase the risk of clot formation. If you are taking calcium and are on estrogen, you need to be certain that you also get enough magnesium each day. But what about getting too much magnesium? Excess magnesium fairly quickly causes diarrhea, so this is a reliable indicator that you are getting more than you need and should cut back on the amount you are taking.

Zinc is a helper for some twenty enzymes and is involved in DNA and protein synthesis, immune reactions, the action of insulin, utilization of vitamin A, the healing of wounds, and it forms part of the structure of bone. It is also a part of the "gatekeeper" minerals at the NMDA receptor involved in pain regulation and serves to help dampen down the activity of this receptor system, thereby helping to decrease the spread of pain sensations. Zinc is as important as protein in the normal processes of growth and maintenance of body tissue. Animal foods are a good source of zinc. Plant sources include whole grains. The recommended intake is 15 mg per day for the average adult. Generally, two small servings of lean animal protein per day are sufficient. Vegetarians should double check that they are getting adequate intake. If you take Zinc supplements, be careful not to take too much, since excess doses cause other problems.

Absorption of zinc depends on adequate dietary intake of tryptophan and B6. A deficiency of either will impair zinc absorption. In the exocrine pancreas the metabolism of tryptophan produces picolinic acid, and this process has a step that requires pyridoxine (B6) as a cofactor for the enzyme to work properly. Picolinic acid is then secreted from the pancreas into the intestinal tract, where it forms a complex with zinc from the foods we eat. This complex of zinc and picolinic acid facilitates the passage of zinc through the mucosa lining the intestinal tract, where it is then taken up into the bloodstream for delivery to the tissues. The quantity of zinc that is carried across the mucosal membranes directly depends on the availability of picolinic acid, which in turn depends on the level of dietary tryptophan along with pyridoxine (B6). A pancreatic extract, Viokase, has been found to contain picolinic acid, as does human breastmilk (but not cow's milk). Studies have shown that picolinic acid added to rat diets promoted growth and increased absorption-retention of dietary zinc. Rats fed diets low in protein sources of tryptophan absorbed significantly less zinc than when dietary tryptophan was adequate. Supplementing with chromium piccolinate can be useful to help keep blood glucose more stable throughout the day and aid in zinc absorption. Current studies have shown that 200 mcg daily is reasonable and has not shown any adverse effects. Higher doses can be toxic, so don't over do it. If you are overweight and have shown clinical symptoms of glucose intolerance, chromium piccolinate with zinc may be helpful as an addition to a properly balanced diet.

Manganese is another mineral needed for the formation of important amine neurotransmitters involved in the regulation of pain and mood. It is essential for normal pituitary function and thereby indirectly regulates is one of the regulatory helpers for hormone production. Another example of its importance in hormone production is that manganese is essential to the process of forming T4 (thyroxine) by the thyroid gland. It also is involved in a number of enzyme pathways needed for the utilization of the B vitamins, vitamin E, and vitamin C, as well as the pathways of energy metabolism, glucose regulation, and immune function. Manganese is also a component of the antioxidant enzyme SOD, or superoxide dismutase, that controls superoxide free radicals formed in the body during cellular metabolism. SOD helps prevent the buildup of excess superoxide radicals that cause cell damage.

Other Tips to Reduce Pain

Aerobic Exercise is another important component of a well-balanced, integrated approach to effective treatment in FMS. Recent studies have shown that regular aerobic exercise can improve energy and decrease chronic pain to provide you with a sustained benefit in many aspects of your health. I find that many women with fibromyalgia are reluctant to exercise because they are afraid it will cause more pain. I suggest having a physical therapist or an exercise physiologist experienced in working with FMS evaluate you and design an exercise program that starts out slowly and gradually becomes more challenging as your strength and endurance increase. If the exercise regimen is gradual, and tailored to your individual needs, there is little risk of increased pain or muscle microtrauma. Your body will eventually be able to accept more vigorous exercise routines. Consult your physician before beginning any aerobic activities, and ask for a referral to a physical therapist to teach you appropriate stretching exercises and help you get started on an exercise program.

I recommend *nonimpact* aerobic exercises for FMS patients to avoid aggravating pain or stiffness. These include brisk walking, swimming, water walking, aqua-aerobics, and using a stationary bicycle or cross-country ski machine. I would suggest that you avoid activities such as jogging, aerobic dancing, "step" aerobics classes, and racquet sports until you have reached a good overall level of physical fitness and your physical therapist feels you are ready to graduate to more strenuous activities. It is especially helpful to do your exercise program in a pool, because this reduces the wear and tear on muscles weakened by FMS. A number of hospitals, YMCAs, Jewish Community Centers (JCC), and fitness clubs now have pool classes available. Remember to gently stretch all your major muscle groups for about five minutes both before and after you exercise. Stretching helps reduce the chance of muscle injury, but make sure that you stay within your body's limits and don't overstretch, since this will cause more injury. Bouncing movements when you stretch also cause more muscle injury and are not recommended. *Stretching* by Bob Anderson is an excellent book I have used for years to provide safe and effective stretching exercises.

Ergonomic Factors. The types of activities you do at home and at work may be additional factors adding to the FMS pain. For example, if you sit slumped over a desk all day, by the end of the day the pain may have gotten worse because of bad posture. I think it can be very helpful to have a posture analysis and recommendations about proper body position for various activities. Your physical therapist is a good resource to help you with these aspects. Many of us are not aware of the abnormal body positions we use daily, which are often the result of compensating for pain. One physical therapist I frequently work with in treating FMS patients does a videotape of the person's posture and movements prior to the session and then again after the treatment. This helps the person to see clearly posture and movement differences and improvements so she is better able to maintain them at home.

Some physical therapists are able to help you assess your home and work environment for body positions that aggravate FMS. It may be helpful to change physical arrangements in your environment to reduce such pain triggers. For example, pain in the arms, neck, or shoulders can be brought on by long hours of typing or working at a computer. If so, you may be able to reduce pain by raising the height of your typewriter or computer table and by learning the acupressure points to use yourself to relieve muscle spasm. Many people are unaware that a wrong mattress for your body needs can put your back into uncomfortable positions overnight, leading to morning stiffness and pain. You may want to have someone take pictures of you lying on your mattress, to check your spinal alignment with your physical therapist. If driving is a problem, try using a backrest or changing the way you sit. I have found that certain makes of cars have seat back angles that I cannot use without aggravating my back problems, so I am particularly careful about which cars I rent when I travel. Being aware of these day-to-day details can help improve FMS pain immensely.

Relieving Stress and Depression. Worries, fears, anger, and other intense emotions may also worsen pain and fatigue. Feelings are sometimes harder to identify than our physical symptoms, yet they may definitely intensify symptoms. Look for appropriate support resources to discuss stresses in your life. I am not saying that FMS is a psychogenic disorder. Everyone has stresses, and everyone reacts to stress in different ways. Always keep in mind what I have been saying throughout this book:

Your mind and brain and body are all connected! More stress causes more muscle tension and more pain!

Thoughts and feelings produce chemical changes in the pain-and mood-regulating chemicals, just like physical pain stimuli produce chemical changes in the body. You may benefit from psychotherapy to help you express uncomfortable or distressing feelings and to help you cope more effectively with situational stresses. Many psychiatrists and psychologists specialize in helping people with chronic pain and may also have experience in teaching self-hypnosis and relaxation skills that reduce stress and tension aggravating pain and fatigue. I typically teach patients techniques such as visual imagery, autogenic conditioning, and progressive muscle relaxation. You may also find it helpful to take a stress management class.

About 80 to 90 percent of patients with chronic pain will develop a biological depression *due to the persistent pain.* Recent studies have shown that chronic pain patients are not typically depressed people who express depression as physical pain; they have ongoing physical pain (even when the cause is unclear), which alters brain-body chemical messengers and produces the depression. In such situations, specific medications, such as the serotonin-boosting ones mentioned in earlier chapters, are needed to alleviate the depression. Psychotherapy can be helpful but is usually not enough to treat a biological depression. A psychiatrist is a physician trained in **both** medication use and psychotherapy, and he/she can be an excellent resource to evaluate your integrated needs for medication and/or psychotherapy. You may then decide to see a psychologist or therapist for ongoing individual or family sessions, but it is better to have your evaluation done by a psychiatrist who knows how to identify and treat biological depression and also understands the physical connections between chronic pain and depression.

In order for any of these treatment approaches to be effective, **you must be an active partner in the process.** This includes becoming knowledgeable about fibromyalgia. You may find it valuable to attend educational lectures on FMS given by doctors and self-help groups in your community. It can be well worth your time and effort to find a physician who is knowledgeable about fibromyalgia and with whom you feel comfortable. Keep in mind that people respond differently to various treatments, so what works for your friend may or may not work for you. It usually takes a trial of several different kinds of treatment before you find an effective combination. If you are working on developing a hormone "recipe" to suit your needs, it may take several months of working with various options to come up with the one that is best for you. Do be prepared to invest the time it takes to find the right combination. I also encourage you to be prepared to modify some aspects of your lifestyle, to expect flare-ups to occur from time to time, and to make time for exercise and practicing relaxation skills. If you invest the time, energy, and effort in carrying out your personalized pain-management program, you will be more likely to achieve positive results.

Fibromyalgia syndrome is now the subject of carefully controlled research studies in many of the leading universities of North America. The leading question facing investigators is whether fibromyalgia represents a true disease process, and what are the metabolic-immune and other abnormalities that cause it. Another major focus of research clearly needs to be on the role of female hormonal decline in triggering and perpetuating the debilitating symptoms of FMS. The results of this research will have a major bearing on whether fibromyalgia can be controlled with new drugs and whether there will need to be more emphasis on assessing and adjusting hormone levels in women who suffer from FMS. Even with use of hormone and medication therapies, I think we will always need to include the complementary approaches I outlined for stress reduction, improved quality of sleep, reduced pain, and maintenance of physical fitness as cornerstone strategies for coping with fibromyalgia. Don't give up hope. There are lots of helpful options available.

Listen to the words of this fibromyalgia sufferer, whose estradiol had been seriously low:

> I am feeling really good now. I think we have hit a good combination, and I feel like I have come such a long way. When I saw you in April and increased the estrogen, that worked really well for me. It seemed like everytime we increased it, I got better. It has helped my sleep

tremendously—within a couple of weeks I was sleeping better. I was taking the Prozac for a while and I decided in August to wean myself off it and see what happened. I didn't feel as tired during the day after I got off it, even though I know that it helped me at first. The fluctuations in the weather and barometric pressure still affect me. One little miracle happened—I took the Micronor for 12 days, and I can actually say I was pain free for that time. When I take it, I got my period about three days after I finished it. The flow was a little heavier and I had a little more cramps, but I did OK on it—not like the problems I had with the other progesterone we had tried. It seemed to actually enhance the effects of the estrogen on the pain. I am really pleased with how much better I feel! The hormones have really made a difference.

Following her own observations that the Micronor seemed to have actually helped decrease her pain, she asked about taking Micronor daily. I told her I thought this would be fine, since she had no medical reasons not to do this. The main reason I had suggested a cyclic regimen was to minimize the progestin use because she had such difficulty taking prior prescriptions of progesterone. But since she was doing so well with the Micronor and the change in estradiol, the daily progestin is a very good solution to preventing cramps, bleeding, and hyperplasia.

So once again, we find that in listening to women's wisdom and working as partners in the healing process, we can find ways to reduce much of the pain and many of the problems that women experience with flares in fibromyalgia pain that occur with hormone imbalance. Fibromyalgia doesn't have to destroy your life. It is possible to recover your zest, energy, and vitality if you focus on addressing *all* these pieces of the pain puzzle.

Chapter 12

Interstitial Cystitis, Vulvodynia, and Leaky Bladders

Odessa's Story

Forty-two years old, Odessa is a typical patient coping with **interstitial cystitis (IC)**. In excruciating pain, up off and on all night long to urinate, exhausted from lack of sleep and the chronic pain, having to urinate *forty to sixty* times a day, and tired of being told "there's nothing wrong, you're just stressed out," she was dismissed by the urologist in her HMO who told her she didn't need any more tests and said, "you just need to stop drinking so much water." Odessa is one of the persistent women who did not give up. She finally found a urologist who knew something about interstitial cystitis, an acutely painful disorder *found almost exclusively in women*. She began getting appropriate help through a combination of medications and lifestyle modifications.

I first saw her two years after her initial diagnosis of IC when she had a consultation to explore the possible hormone connections with IC. She came in with the question "I have interstitial cystitis, could it be estrogen-related? I think I may be starting menopause." I found that she indeed had both *symptoms* of low estrogen and objective *signs*: thinning of the vaginal lining, diminished breast size, decrease in pubic hair, and low blood levels of estradiol. Her bone mineral density had also decreased below normal for her age. She was a good candidate to begin a trial of low-dose estrogen therapy to help improve her health picture as well as to see what improvements could be achieved with her IC.

A year later, her sleep has improved, her energy and concentration are back to normal, her sex drive is back, and she reported that her frequency of urination had decreased by about 50 percent and the intensity of the bladder pain had also decreased. Her IC is certainly not gone, but it is better. Neither she nor I can say whether the improvement was due solely to the addition of estradiol, or to the combination of everything she was doing, but she said "It was encouraging to me to have my questions and insights taken seriously and included in my treatment." Since estrogen has so many direct effects on the bladder lining, nerves, blood vessels, and muscles that govern urinary function, it made a great deal of sense to address this issue in her treatment.

Astoundingly, considering that IC is a *woman's* bladder disorder, there is almost nothing in the scientific literature about the possible effects of hormone change in triggering it, or on the use of hormones as a part of the treatment approach. I was astonished to see a medical review article on current theories of cause and treatment for IC in a 1999 women's health medical journal, written by a *female* urologist, and there was not one mention of ovarian hormone effects on the bladder. When you read further in this chapter and see what is known about the many effects of premenopausal levels of estradiol on the entire urinary system and its function, I am sure you will agree with me that such an omission is staggering. Every single IC patient I have seen has asked me this question "Could it be related to hormone changes?" Seems a pretty logical question, doesn't it, if the problem is pretty much found only in females. I tell women that it makes *physiological* sense that there would be a connection, but there is little definitive research on the question.

What Happens to the Bladder As Estrogen Declines?

Women are frequently embarrassed to tell me that they are having urinary problems, especially if they are experiencing incontinence or urinary "leaks." This is truly a problem no one wants to talk about, yet urogenital problems are estimated to be experienced by as many as one half of women age fifty and up. The Heart and Estrogen/ Progestin Replacement Study (HERS) in the United States found that 56 percent of the 2,763 participants reported weekly incontinence. It is much more common in the years just before menopause and gets gradually worse in the decades after menopause. Is this just due to aging? What is the connection to hormone changes? Another ironic twist: I reviewed many of the current books on menopause to make recommendations to my own patients for reliable resource information, and guess how many had chapters addressing urinary problems—only one. So this appears to be another overlooked, taboo topic even for women's menopause books, even if written by women physicians.

Just like other organs and tissues in the body, the lining of the urinary bladder itself and the urethra have estrogen receptors. These lining cells are sensitive to the effects of rise and fall in estrogen levels during the monthly cycle, in pregnancy, and at menopause. Changes in estrogen cause measurable changes in the characteristics of the cells (cytology), changes in stimuli triggering the urge to void, changes in smooth muscle tone, changes in pain threshold that contribute to the intensity of symptoms experienced, as well as measurable changes in the pressure of the bladder and urethra (urodynamic changes). When estrogen levels decline and remain low, the cells lining the bladder, urethra, and vagina become fewer and thinner (atrophic) as well as more easily torn or damaged with friction ("friable"). The *smooth muscle* of the bladder, urethra, and vagina also contains estrogen receptors. When estrogen declines, the smooth muscle gradually loses its tone and strength. Lack of estrogen contributes to a decrease in the urethral closure pressure, which allows for more leakage. Nerve endings also contain estrogen receptors. With normal estrogen levels, the sensory threshold is raised. When estrogen levels decrease, the sensory threshold is lowered, and the nerve endings become more sensitive, leading to an increase in pain perception that in turn contributes to an increased urge to void.

There are also estrogen receptors in fibroblasts that synthesize collagen, the most abundant structural protein in the connective tissue of the female urogenital tissues. Loss of estradiol at menopause leads to loss of optimal collagen formation that in turn contributes to not only such visable signs as skin wrinkling but also loss of collagen support to help maintain urethral closure and avoid leaks. An interesting study correlating skin collagen with urethral function showed that increased skin collagen was associated with improved function of the urethral sphincter, a muscle circling the opening of the bladder and responsible for urethral closure.

As a result of these hormone-triggered changes in the lining tissues, women are much more susceptible to several problems, as shown in the chart below. When you look at how common all of the various bladder problems are for women, and the increase in such problems just before and after menopause, it is appalling that we still don't have more controlled studies looking at the hormonal effects on these problems. Dr. Vicki Ratner, physician founder of the Interstitial Cystitis Association, acknowledged that women's hormonal changes may play a role in this disorder but also says, "there's just no research on this issue." I have attended a number of medical continuing education meetings on women's health issues, and I have heard presentations on IC, but not one has mentioned possible hormonal factors, even when they describe the disorder as being "epithelial (cells lining the bladder) dysfunction" or "immune dysfunction" (both affected by changes in estrogen).

EFFECTS OF ESTROGEN DECLINE

---

* **vaginal and vulvar dryness, itching, burning, stinging pain** (several disorders: vaginitis, vulvodynia, vestibulitis)

* **pain with intercourse** (dyspareunia)

* **recurrent bladder infections/inflammation** (cystitis)

* **urethral infections** (urethritis)

* **recurrent vaginal infections** (vaginitis)

* **incontinence** (loss of urine—several types)

* **painful urination** (dysuria)

* **urinary frequency**

* **urinary urgency**

©Elizabeth Lee Vliet, M.D., 1995, revised 2000

Interstitial Cystitis: Bladder Pain Doctors Overlook

Interstitial cystitis can be excruciatingly painful, and women often have to see a number of different doctors before being properly diagnosed. There are some staggering statistics with this disorder. Once thought to be relatively rare, current estimates from the National Institutes of Health put the number of sufferers at 500,000 women in the United States. This comes out to 1 in every 260 women. About half of these women are so adversely affected that they cannot hold down a full-time job, and over 75 percent cannot have intercourse due to pain. Fully one-third of women with IC have been abandoned by a husband or lover as a result of their illness. Even more sobering and alarming, *fewer than one out of five sufferers have been properly diagnosed.* Women have seen an average of eight to ten physicians before they are diagnosed. Even if we don't focus on the human suffering involved in such an arduous search for help, what about the financial impact of individuals paying out of pocket and insurance companies paying for multiple doctors' visits, not to mention lost time from work and other responsibilities?

Now some startling additional connections that support my theory that loss of estrogen is an overlooked factor in the development of IC: In a study of 374 IC patients published in 1993, researchers at Scripps Institute found that the mean age of onset for IC is *forty-two years,* and *44 percent* of the patients *had hysterectomies prior to onset of IC.* What else happens in the decade of the forties? You got it, women are often beginning the climacteric time of hormone changes. What else is commonly associated with hysterectomies? You got it, women often begin an earlier ovarian decline of estrogen (even if the ovaries are left in place) due to the effects of surgery on blood flow to the ovaries. Other surveys of IC patients have found that flare-ups tend to occur after ovulation and just before menses. Both are times when estrogen levels are falling. Why aren't these obvious hormonal connections put together and considered? Hormone changes are not the whole story; yet, I think it is a glaring omission to ignore the hormone issues altogether.

Symptoms

Part of the problem with IC is that many women suffer silently until the primary symptom, pain, becomes so severe that it interferes with normal activities. The characteristic symptoms of IC are, unfortunately, *nonspecific* and may occur in other kinds of bladder disorders: increased urination, sudden strong urges to void (urgency), intense pain becoming worse as the bladder fills up and often decreased by voiding (one woman called it "like passing fire"), pain with intercourse, having to urinate multiple times at night (nocturia).

Causes

A variety of possible causes are usually given, but at this time, we simply don't have a definite answer. One of the common findings in women with IC is a history of repeated UTIs and repeated use of antibiotics over an extended period of time (another reason I urge women to avoid indiscriminately taking antibiotics). It has also been suggested that IC is due to a "dysfunctional bladder epithelium" (what about hormone effects here?) or a manifestation of an autoimmune disorder, which are also many times more common in females than males (again, what about hormone effects?). I must sound like a broken record, but it just amazes me that these obvious female connections are overlooked. Other proposed theories are that a toxic substance in the urine, or a chronic persistent infectious agent, damages the bladder lining, leading to the characteristic tiny hemorrhages in the bladder wall.

Nonhormonal Treatments

A large percentage of women are given antibiotics in their primary care or gynecology settings, but most IC specialists agree that antibiotics help this condition very little. Yet many women whose IC has not been properly recognized have been told that they have recurrent bladder infections in the wall of the bladder and need to be on extended courses of antibiotics. In addition to the expense of unnecessary medication, these women often end up with difficult-to-treat yeast infections.

A variety of other **medications** have been tried for IC, with varying degrees of success. An oral medication, (1) Elmiron (pentosan polysulfate or PPS), is a heparinlike compound that provides a protective coating of the bladder lining. The success rate with Elmiron is about 45–50 percent. This drug, given orally, usually 100 mg three times a day on an empty stomach, has few side effects, which are generally reversible when dosage is stopped. Elmiron is somewhat expensive, and it usually takes about three–six months of therapy before symptoms improve. FDA approval for Elmiron in treatment of IC was granted after three U.S. trials indicated that it was more effective than placebo. Other oral medications include: (1) Anti-inflammatory medications (NSAIDS) for pain relief; (2) antihistamines to reduce mast cell activation, such as hydroxyzine, (Atarax, Vistaril) show promising results so far; (3) nalmefene; (4) amitriptyline (Elavil and others), a tricyclic antidepressant that also has good pain-relieving properties. (It is also an antihistamine and its *anticholinergic* properties reduce frequency of bladder emptying.) Amitriptyline has been shown in several trials to be effective, with the usual dose 25–75 mg at bedtime, but there are side effects of sedation, dry mouth, constipation, and significant weight gain.

Intravesical therapy, or bladder distension by filling with fluid, is another approach used for more severe cases of IC. The bladder is distended at 80 cm of water pressure for two to eight minutes, under anesthesia. Some patients report worsening symptoms for a few days, then experience improvement. This relief usually lasts about six–twelve months, and a repeat distention usually again provides a period of pain relief. This form of treatment is one of the oldest known treatments for IC. Until Elmiron, the only FDA-approved medication was DMSO (dimethyl sulfoxide) injected into the bladder (usually 50 ml of 50 percent solution). Symptoms were significantly improved in about 50 percent of the patients. Patients typically receive a treatment on a weekly or monthly basis for six to ten sessions, followed by maintenance treatments less often. One problem is that patients become progressively resistant to it over time. Other drugs inserted directly into the bladder may cause pain and must be done under anesthesia. These include silver nitrate, adriamycin, lidocaine, and chlorpactin WCS-90. Obviously, you should seek out a highly skilled urologist, with experience in treating IC patients, before you undergo these treatments.

Vulvodynia: One Woman's Story

"Robbie" is a forty-three-year-old woman who came for a consult describing "Severe vaginal burning, painful intercourse, lack of lubrication, and diminished orgasm." She said that after reading my book,

> I felt like finally someone was hearing what I was saying. I have been through the mill—I have been to seven or eight different doctors. I went to two different Gynecologists and they said I should see a urologist, who put a scope up my bladder. One Gyn checked an estrogen level but it was a random cycle day. I was told it was normal, but after I read your book I realized it probably wasn't reliable because no one had asked where in my cycle I was. I even had an MRI and they didn't find anything. I went to a specialist at S___ Clinic for vulvodynia and all they did was give me a prescription for citrate and glucosamine. It has helped some but I still had the burning. I am a very bright woman and I wouldn't give up, I felt like they were just treating the symptom not getting at the cause. The doctor at S___ Clinic was even doing surgery on women to remove the damaged tissue. I didn't want to go that route. I then had a reading with a woman who is a medical intuitive, and she said the vulvodynia was due to my having problems with boundaries because I had been in a very stressful relationship for two years. By this point, I didn't know what to think and that's when a friend told me about your book.

I explained to Robbie that there are many biological endocrine factors causing vaginal and bladder problems in women with declining estradiol, and I do not agree with attributing problems like vulvodynia to purely psychological causes and making pronouncements like it is caused by "boundary problems." To my way of thinking, this is again victimizing the woman by blaming her for causing the medical problem, and I do not think this is a very helpful approach.

An interesting fact came to light when I explored with Robbie what her dietary habits had been over the years she was having problems with vulvodynia. She said "I changed to a high soy diet. I started maxing it out, buying tofu and eating it all the time, drinking soy milk—for about two years before the vulvodynia developed. I stopped drinking milk—I heard soy was so good—I changed everything to soy." Otherwise, her diet and lifestyle habits were quite good; she did not use alcohol or tobacco, and exercised regularly. I explained that new studies from three different countries have found that high intake of soy phytoestrogens actually inhibit normal ovarian function in premenopausal women, causing anywhere from 20–50 percent decrease in women's own ovarian hormones, estradiol, and a progesterone. In addition to age, I explained that her high soy intake and low-fat diet were two more factors contributing to her ovaries making less estrogen. It is important to remember that your hormones are made from cholesterol as a basic building block. You must have adequate amounts of cholesterol or your body can't make its steroid hormones (estradiol, progesterone, testosterone, DHEA). Your liver will manufacture cholesterol from food you eat, and from triglycerides, even if you don't eat foods high in cholesterol. Robbie had been on such an extremely low-fat diet for so many years that her body simply didn't have the building blocks it needed to make enough of her ovarian hormones. And then all her soy intake "competed" at the estradiol receptors with what little estradiol her own body did make. Ultimately, the loss of adequate estradiol adversely affected the health of her vulva, bladder, and vaginal tissues.

She also had gone through a lot of infertility treatment and had six months of Clomid, 4 cycles of Pergonal, an in-vitro attempt, and a GIFT (gamete intra-fallopian transfer) procedure. She never became pregnant, but the hyperstimulation of her ovaries meant that more of her follicles were depleted at a younger age than usual. This is another factor adding to her premature loss of estradiol. Her rather marked life stresses added to the premature suppression of her ovaries with diminished hormone production. Remember that stress-induced suppression of the ovaries is part of Mother Nature's protective effects to prevent reproduction when the person (or animal) is not optimally healthy to carry a fetus through a pregnancy. I have to wonder about the possible connection between the last decade of emphasis on very low-fat diets, high soy intake, busier and busier lives with lots of stress . . . and the sharp rise in young women with vulvodynia, infertility, and other hormonal problems I am seeing in my practice.

Checking her hormone levels clearly showed this pattern. Her Day 1 estradiol was 22 pg/ml, when it should have been about 80–90 pg/ml. Her Day 20 estradiol was 156 pg/ml, about half the optimal level for a luteal phase peak in an ovulatory cycle. Her progesterone, in contrast, was at a normal, healthy ovulatory level on Day 20, so she was not progesterone deficient even though her estradiol was too low. Her testosterone was quite low at 10 ng/dl. Her DHEA was really higher than usual, so she did not need this hormone supplemented. All of the rest of her laboratory studies were quite good, including detailed tests of adrenal, thyroid, liver, and kidney function.

It was striking to notice that Robbie's vulvodynia pain flared each month at the time of her cycle when her estradiol was the lowest, at menstruation. The drop in estradiol causes the pain threshold to be lower, so that pain occurs with less stimulation. Low estradiol levels also cause more tissue dryness and burning. In addition, as estradiol declines, stomach pH is altered in such as way that there is less absorption of calcium and magnesium from dietary and supplement sources. If these minerals aren't present in optimal amounts, this is another factor in pain symptoms being worse. I suggested that she try a low-dose hypoallergenic estradiol cream topically to the vulvar area nightly to restore the tissue estradiol more directly, a low-dose estradiol vaginal ring (Estring) inserted inside the vagina near the cervix to reduce the vaginal dryness, and a transdermal estradiol (Vivelle DOT 0.05 mg) patch to bring her serum levels back to the healthy ranges. She had tried Estrace vaginal cream without success, saying that it caused an increase in the burning and vulvar pain. I was not surprised by this report, since all of the FDA-approved commercial estradiol creams contain a chemical (polyethylene glycol, or PEG) that causes a lot of burning when sensitive tissues are damaged by loss of estrogen. I recommended that she use a topical estradiol cream made especially without PEG, and this was compounded at Belmar Pharmacy in Lakewood, Colorado.

When I had a follow-up appointment with Robbie about six weeks later, she said "I had a lot of burning initially with the cream and the Estring, but I stuck it out. Now everything feels much better, the pain is much less. I still have a lot of vaginal dryness but it is slowly getting better. I felt like I had razor blades with the vulvodynia, and that intense pain is gone. I took all your information to my vulvodynia specialist and he said Dr. Vliet is right on. I asked him why he hadn't tested my hormone levels and he said he thought my Gyn had already done them! I told him that he should check hormone levels on everyone who comes through his door!" She was pleased to be feeling so much better so quickly, and could tell she was on the right track. But since her symptoms had not fully resolved and her serum levels of estradiol were still too low, I recommended an increase in her estradiol patch to the 0.1 mg strength and she agreed this made sense to her.

Her next appointment was three months later, and at this time she said "I am coming along really well—the pain with that burning is really low—that burning like razor blades when I urinate is totally gone now. I have some mild pain now at times but nothing incapacitating like it was. It is so much better now with the estrogen! This is just wonders for me." It became time to add natural progesterone because her own ovary production began to decline, and I recommended Prometrium 200 mg a day for twelve days every other month. This produced a normal pattern of bleeding each time, and she tolerated it very well.

I received a follow-up letter from her three months after this second appointment, and she said (in big bold letters): "My pain is still 98% gone for the last 7 months! Thank you truly for your excellent care of me. You have helped me so much. I am doing so much better on the estrogen." She went on to comment that she was really shocked that no one had checked her hormone levels before this, and she planned to talk with her doctors about how important this is for women. She ended her letter with "My health was regained by me listening to my own inner guidance and intuition of what was right for me." Has *your* doctor run thorough tests of your hormone levels?

Unusual Bladder Effects from Dyes, Medications, and Diet

Food Triggers

Certain foods are potent bladder irritants, and some experts recommend that the following culprits be eliminated or reduced: caffeine, alcohol, tobacco (nicotine), chocolate, spices and spicy foods, apples, bananas, acidic foods (citrus fruits, tomatoes), NutraSweet and saccharine, sharp cheeses, coffee, tea, carbonated beverages, chemical preservatives (found in many foods and beverages), lima beans, lentils, and yogurt, to name a few. These foods produce metabolic by-products that may irritate bladder mucosa and increase the urinary urges to void, increase urinary frequency, which in turn end up aggravating incontinence. These foods also cause bladder spasms and pain in some women. Not only are alcohol and tobacco themselves potent bladder irritants, they also significantly interfere with the metabolism and effectiveness of prescription hormone therapies. Diets that are too low in fat reduce absorption of oral ovarian hormones, while diets that are high in fat will increase absorption if taken at mealtime. Thus, bioavailability of any given oral hormone therapy will be affected by when it is taken relative to a meal and the type of meal consumed. When you stop and think about the typical diet of many women "on the run" with busy schedules, you begin to realize just how many of these triggers most people consume every day. Many of my patients obsess over an extra gram of fat, and then drink cola beverages all day that contain a wide variety of irritant chemicals, not to mention all the calories from sugar.

Keeping a dietary diary, correlated with your bladder symptoms, often helps identify the food culprits so you can make the necessary modifications in what you eat and drink. If you are having bladder problems, it really helps to *clean up* your diet.

Dyes

It was during my specialty training at Johns Hopkins that I first became aware of how potentially serious, and bizarre, patients' reactions can be to something as seemingly innocuous as the coloring agents used in medicines (even vitamins and herbal products can have coloring agents that cause these problems). My mother had been researching the role of dyes in atypical allergic reactions at about the same time I had a patient with asthma admitted to our service. In the course of treating the patient's admitting illness (not his asthma), his asthma kept getting worse. We could not figure out what was happening, since his asthma medications were the same and blood levels were therapeutic. Based on the work my mother was doing, I raised the possibility that perhaps it might be the orange-colored tablets we started using to treat his other illness. We changed to a different brand of the medication (one with a *white* tablet), and within a short period of time, the asthma cleared. Since the patient was as curious as we were as to whether the culprit had indeed been the orange dye in the first tablet, he agreed to try taking it one more time. The wheezing returned rapidly. No more orange dye for this person. All of us learned an important lesson.

I started collecting whatever information I could on *tartrazine-based dyes* (a common one is FD&C yellow #5) in medications, foods, and beverages. I was able to find a few articles on allergic reactions to these compounds. The tartrazine-based dyes have a similar chemical effect in the body to that occurring with salicylate, the chemical name for aspirin. Many people who are allergic to aspirin may also react to tartrazine but often don't know it. Since dyes like FD&C yellow #5 are found in so many common products, even including medications used for asthma and allergies, people may be getting a daily dose of a chemical they are allergic to and not realize it. These dyes have metabolic breakdown products that are excreted in urine and are a potent trigger for "irritable bladder," leading to incontinence, that many do not think to check. Over the course of my medical career, I have found this to be a much more common problem than I had ever been taught, and so I have included these cautions in many of the educational programs I do for other physicians. I have seen reactions from rashes to wheezing to severe bladder spasms, all traceable to the dyes in a daily medication.

Janie was an energetic woman in her late forties who came for a consult about her bladder spasms, which had progressed to the point that she had to catheterize herself several times a day to urinate. She had been hospitalized on several occasions with such severe bladder spasms that she had been unable to void at all. She had been healthy, without any history of bladder problems, until about two months after she started estrogen therapy with Premarin. The estrogen effectively relieved her menopausal symptoms of hot flashes and sleeplessness, but she started to develop new symptoms of increased frequency of urination, sudden urges to void, and a burning pain in the area of her bladder. She had seen multiple doctors; had been treated with many courses of antibiotics, pain medications, and tranquilizers; and had been told she was obviously having emotional trouble over her children leaving home, so she should see a therapist. Meanwhile, nothing seemed to help. Janie was having such frequent spasms and difficulty voiding, she had been taught to catheterize herself.

During her visit to our women's health program, she had planned to pursue biofeedback training and acupuncture to help decrease the spasm and pain. In our consultation, she said, "You know, it sounds silly, but I keep wondering if this problem could have any connection to starting the Premarin. Before that, I never had anything like this. I've asked all my doctors this question, but they have all said there's no connection, or it's not possible." I told her that I had seen problems like this, due not so much to the drug or hormone but to the dyes in the tablet. I explained that the simple way to test her idea would be to change her to a completely dye-free form of estrogen and see if it made any difference over the next few months. At that time, there were no commercial estrogens on the market in the United States that were free of dyes. That in itself is amazing and disconcerting to me, given the number of women with allergies, who may need estrogen. So I called the pharmacist in Colorado who had compounded individualized prescriptions of natural hormones for some of my patients and asked him if his tablets had any dyes. They did not, so I ordered the dye-free estradiol tablet for Janie to try.

She was so excited that someone thought she could be on to something that might help, she had it sent overnight mail. I had already told her not to get her hopes up, since this might not be the cause of her bladder problem, but I did think it was worth trying. I also told her that if the dye was an irritant to her bladder, it could still take several weeks for her to see any difference with the change in estrogen tablets. Three days later she called me, and practically yelled over the phone "It's GONE. I have actually been able to urinate on my own without the catheter. This is amazing."

Even I was astonished at the rapid response. I have seen some pretty surprising improvements over the last fifteen years of working with patients, but none this fast. It is now two years later, and at the last follow-up I had with her, her bladder spasms had resolved, and she had remained on the dye-free estrogen. Doctors should be willing to make a simple change like this to a different tablet *without dyes* and see how this affects symptoms.

These same azo-tartrazine dyes are known carcinogens and skin irritants, and some have now been banned due to these effects. My suggestion to you is that if you have bladder sensitivities and an "irritable" bladder (or bowel), it may be wise to watch for these types of chemicals in the foods, beverages, and medicines you consume. Another common irritant for many women is the **propylene glycol** in various vaginal creams, including some of the estrogen vaginal creams that are used to help *treat* vaginal itching and burning. Use of a vaginal 17-beta estradiol cream in a hypoallergenic base without propylene glycol may also help alleviate these problems. Such creams have to be obtained from compounding pharmacies, since all of the commercial estrogen vaginal cream products contain propylene glycol, which may be significantly irritating to tissues.

If you have persistent problems with these symptoms, talk with your physician or pharmacist to see if what you are using contains these dyes and other chemicals. The *Physicians Desk Reference* is now required to list these dyes and other inactive ingredients, so you can always ask your pharmacist if you are in doubt about a particular medicine. Many food manufacturers will send you a complete ingredient list of their products if you write to their consumer information office.

Chronic Bladder "Infections": Is It Really an Infection or My Hormones?

I am very concerned about the trend of women calling doctors' offices for help with "bladder infections" and getting repeated courses of antibiotics. First of all, burning, frequency, and urgency may have many causes. Not all causes are due to infections. Second, repeated use of antibiotics creates problems with resistant bacteria and with chronic yeast infections. So make sure you take the responsible course of action, and go see your doctor for a urinalysis and urine culture before you start on antibiotics. I also think it is important to have your hormone levels checked if you are having problems with burning, frequency, urgency, or leaking of urine. Many people still don't realize the degree to which loss of estrogen plays a role in causing these changes during and after menopause. Rather than continuing to think you have an infection and taking antibiotics, I think it is far more effective to assess the possible hormone causes and address this problem directly, perhaps first with a vaginal estrogen cream or by taking one of the hormone therapy regimens if your doctor feels that is appropriate for you.

If estradiol blood levels are below the 50–60 pg/ml range, it is highly likely that this is a major cause of the urinary problems. Occult diabetes is another very common cause of urinary problems in older women, especially if you are overweight. In its early stages, before the fasting glucose is significantly high, frequent yeast infections, burning on urination, increased frequency, and leaking of urine are common. If you have a family history of diabetes, or have noticed an increase in craving for sweets, you should talk with your doctor about checking more closely for diabetes. In patients I see for consultations, I find that these two endocrine changes are the most frequent *unrecognized* causes of persistent urinary problems.

In addition to the hormone levels, there are some other important tests that you should discuss with your doctor. Not every patient will need all of the tests, but you should at least ask whether any of these are needed to determine the cause of your problem if your doctor doesn't mention them. This is *not an exhaustive list*, since there are many medical problems that can cause urinary problems. But at least this list gives you an idea of some of the newer techniques that are available to aid in the diagnosis of urinary disorders.

What Exactly is Incontinence, or "Leaky Bladder"?

Continence is the ability to control urine flow, and hold urine in the bladder when you feel an urge to urinate. Once we are toilet trained as children, most of us control urination urges unconsciously as we go about our daily activities. Accidental loss of urine, or difficulty controlling the urine flow, is called **incontinence**. A tragic aspect of incontinence problems is the degree to which women do not know it is a *treatable problem*. For example, it is a widespread misconception that urinary incontinence is an inevitable part of normal aging. This is not correct. The Alliance for Aging Research says it best:

> **"You should never think of incontinence as something you have to put up with, or as just a part of growing old."**

And it's not just the issue of comfort that is at stake. Urinary incontinence has a devastating economic impact, individually and collectively, in this country. Americans spend more than *$10 billion* annually on products to either hide the problem of incontinence or to help them cope with it, without looking for ways to treat or eliminate the cause. Medicare cost projections for medical diagnosis and treatment of urinary incontinence are even more staggering: $26 billion annually, more than the costs for dialysis and coronary artery bypass surgery combined. And since this figure includes only the costs for people over sixty-five, the total costs are even greater when one includes the prevalence in younger persons, due to pelvic surgery such as hysterectomy. For older women, the issue carries additional significance: Loss of bladder control is one of the more frequent causes for nursing home admission. Once in a nursing home, patients are even less likely to have a thorough diagnostic evaluation; they are "managed" with catheters and repeated courses of antibiotics, both of which have potential adverse consequences.

With our current knowledge of the causes, and variety of diagnostic and treatment options (and definitely not always just using drugs and surgery), better than 50 percent of incontinence patients can be *cured,* another 35 percent markedly *improved,* and the remaining 15 percent made more *comfortable.* Please do NOT sit home and suffer in silence if you have this problem. See a knowledgeable, caring, and competent physician, or call one of the resources at the end of my book to locate an appropriate professional near you.

There are different types of incontinence, and it helps to understand the characteristics and causes of each.

Stress incontinence is one you hear often, and patients are frequently confused about what it means. I remember one woman in her seventies who came to see me, and when I asked her what was bothering her, she burst into tears and said "My doctor told me I had stress incontinence. I know it's real, and it's not just stress in my life." Her doctor, I am sure, had no idea how upset this lady was by his use of a medical term that she misunderstood to mean something very different, and she was too embarrassed to ask what her doctor had meant. "Stress incontinence" does NOT refer to emotional factors causing loss of urine. It means the *loss of bladder control due to the physical stress of increased pressure in the abdomen* from such activities as laughing, coughing, sneezing, sexual orgasm, jogging, or straining to have a bowel movement.

This type of incontinence is not caused by bladder spasms; it results from weakness or loss of tone in the bladder muscles, which is primarily due to mechanical factors such as damage to the bladder muscles in childbirth, or ligaments and muscles weakened by age or loss of hormone or nutritional components necessary for healthy tissue. Stress incontinence may also be due to hormonal decline contributing to loss of muscle tone. In addition to the effects of estrogen loss seen in postmenopausal women, 35 to 40 percent of women experience postpartum stress incontinence for as long as six to twelve weeks after childbirth due to trauma to the bladder muscles and the sudden drop in hormone levels after delivery. Stress incontinence is usually not associated with urinary frequency and urgency.

Urge (urgency) incontinence is defined as the sudden urge to urinate and the inability to hold your urine long enough to reach the bathroom. It usually results from bladder spasms, and is associated with both increased frequency and urgency. It is common for of urge incontinence to occur without a clear-cut physical cause, but it may also be caused by serious medical conditions such as herniated intervertebral disks, bladder infections, or by gynecological problems such as fibroids exerting pressure on the bladder or loss of normal estrogen effect on urinary and reproductive tissues. Urge incontinence is also aggravated by habits that cause increased urine formation, such as excessive fluid intake, alcohol, use of diuretics ("water pills"), beverages with caffeine, and/or tobacco use. It is important to see a physician for a thorough evaluation, because bladder cancer is also a cause of urge incontinence that has to be ruled out before proper treatment is started. It is not a good idea to keep taking antibiotics for urinary tract infections (UTI), a common cause of urge incontinence, without having a careful medical evaluation to find causes that may need different treatment approaches.

COMMON CAUSES OF URGE INCONTINENCE

- **urinary tract infections**
- **bladder inflammation**
- **estrogen deficiency**
- **spinal nerve-root disorders** (e.g., disc disease)
- **pelvic irritation**
- **chemotherapy**
- **spinal cord injury**
- **pressure from uterine fibroids**
- **emotional stress**

© Elizabeth Lee Vliet, M.D., 1995

Mrs. G. was a seventy-two-year-old professional woman in New York who had a thriving business to run. She came to see me for a variety of health concerns, including bone loss and incontinence. She wanted to discuss the possibility of estrogen replacement therapy. She had been told by her doctor that her incontinence was "to be expected, it's what happens when you get older, just wear pads." Needless to say, this was a difficult idea to accept and a source of embarrassment and anguish for her. Gynecological urology is not my specialty, but I knew that she needed a complete evaluation of her incontinence and this had not been done by her own physician. I referred her to a specialty center in Baltimore, and after the proper diagnostic studies, she was found to have a very treatable type of urge incontinence. She was started on a medication regimen in addition to the hormone therapy I had prescribed. Six months later, her incontinence had dramatically improved to the point where she rarely had any more accidental episodes of urine loss.

Overflow incontinence is the accidental loss of urine from a chronically full bladder. A common cause is a *cystocoele*, which is a vaginal hernia or bulge due to weakened vaginal muscles seen often in postmenopausal women. The bulge from the cystocoele makes a mechanical obstruction and prevents complete emptying of the bladder. A woman can then lose small quantities of urine when she stands, sits, or bends. Another cause of overflow incontinence is damage to the bladder nerves from diabetes, loss of adequate estradiol effects, or from a herniated lumbar disc. This is what happened to me when I was twenty-eight, before I was correctly diagnosed with the lumbar disc. I can certainly relate to the embarrassment caused by episodes of incontinence and the frustration patients experience trying to get help. Overflow incontinence is treated by identifying and resolving the underlying cause. Pessaries, a device inserted into the vagina as a supportive structure, may sometimes be used to lift the bladder away from an obstructed outlet, or bladder surgery may be needed to repair a cystocoele. In my situation, removal of the herniated disc, and getting the pressure off the spinal nerves, allowed normal nerve function to return and the incontinence resolved. As you can see, it is important to distinguish which type of incontinence you have, because the effective treatments are different, for example, stress incontinence is often relieved by bladder surgery, but urge incontinence is not. Loss of urine at night may also occur from a combination of the above types of continence dysfunction.

Some types of incontinence are quite responsive to hormone therapy to restore the estrogen effects on bladder lining, bladder and urethral smooth muscle, connective tissues supporting the bladder, et cetera. There are a few double-blind, placebo-controlled studies that have compared the effectiveness of estrogen therapy in treating urinary urgency, frequency, urge and stress incontinence. These studies have used several types of estrogen: estriol, 17-beta estradiol, and conjugated equine estrogens. To date, the results are mixed. There are several studies from Europe that have shown that *all* of the three types of estrogen above can improve symptoms of burning, urgency, and frequency; but estrogen therapy *alone* has not shown a consistent positive effect on stress incontinence. In the studies I was able to locate, the authors commented that the doses of estriol used may have been too low to achieve optimal benefit. I also thought that the amount of estradiol used was low compared to what we typically recommend for heart and bone benefits. Until we have more definitive scientific data, it is clear that being estrogen-complete for our postmenopausal years does improve and enhance many functions of the urinary bladder, urethra, and vagina, even if estrogen doesn't solve all problems. This is a factor you should explore with your doctor. Don't be afraid to bring it up. Prompt diagnosis is crucial so that a treatable problem can be addressed in time. In my case, if the problem had gone unrecognized another few days, I would have permanently lost the nerve control of my bladder and been left with having to use a catheter the rest of my life.

COMPONENTS OF A DIAGNOSTIC EVALUATION
FOR INCONTINENCE

- **detailed patient history**
- **food/beverage intake diary, and urinary voiding diary**
- **use of prescribed and over-the-counter medications (and herbs, vitamins, minerals, etc.)**
- **physical examination**
- **blood chemistries, hormone levels**
- **urine culture**
- **urine cytology (rule out cancer)**
- **postvoid residual urine volume (measures urine remaining in bladder after voiding, which can contribute to incontinence)**
- **ultrasound (assess kidney size, structure to look for tumors, etc.)**
- **urodynamic studies (check for filling and emptying patterns)**
- **voiding cystourethrogram (checks urethra pressures)**

© Elizabeth Lee Vliet, M.D., 1995, revised 2000

Help Ahead: Hormonal Balance, Biofeedback, Exercise, and Other Options

Hormones

If you are already on ERT or HRT and are still having problems with bladder symptoms like I have described, you may want to ask your doctor to check blood levels of FSH and estradiol to determine whether you are taking the *right amount* of estrogen for your body needs. I continue to find that what we thought was an adequate dose turns out to be less than what's needed for many women. If you are still bothered by symptoms, it is especially important to determine if you are on the right amount of estrogen, because you may not be getting enough for estrogen's *other benefits* either. If serum estradiol levels drawn about twelve hours after a dose of oral medication or on the last day of a transdermal patch are below about 70–80 pg/ml, it is likely that suboptimal estradiol is a factor in the persistence of urinary symptoms. I typically aim for estradiol blood levels of over 100 pg/ml, which is what is typical for the first part of the menstrual cycle. If your ERT/HRT regimen provides estradiol blood levels over 100, the FSH will usually come back down to 35 or less. A residual FSH greater than 20 with estradiol levels below 80 pg/ml confirm the suboptimal estrogen replacement. Vaginal pH may also be a factor. Hypoestrogenic effect and recurrent urinary and vaginal infections are associated with pH levels greater than 4.5 to 5.0. I find these objective measures very helpful in deciding about doses for individual women, especially if they are still having urinary problems.

Another pointer, which I have found helps some women: if you are taking estrogen and continue to have bladder irritation symptoms of burning, frequency, and urgency, you may find it helpful to ask your physician to prescribe an estrogen without dyes in the tablet. Many of the chemical dyes used in medications (and foods and beverages—see earlier section) are irritating to the bladder lining. Looking for dye-free (usually white) tablets for your medications can reduce this source of additional irritation to the bladder. This is a fairly easy step to take, and it may give significant relief. For those of you using a transdermal patch, be aware that some patches actually decline sooner than the manufacturers indicate, which means erratic estrogen levels that can lead to the return of urinary symptoms. A simple strategy to alleviate this problem is to change the patch sooner to give better stability in estrogen replacement.

Another option is to change the *type* of estrogen you are taking. Women have many individual differences in absorption and metabolism of foods, hormones, vitamins, and medications. We have to take this into account. The standard estrogen your doctor uses simply may not be well absorbed in *your* body, and you can ask to change to a different one to see if this helps your symptoms. The equilin or horse-derived estrogens have different binding properties and actions at the estrogen receptors, and these estrogens are also more difficult to metabolize by the human body, since women lack key enzymes in this process. As a result, a number of the equine estrogens remain in the body far longer than does estradiol or estrone. These factors may contribute to incontinence and bladder problems. You may find that a native human 17-beta estradiol works better than the mixed estrogens. In chapters 2, 5, and 15, I have information on the different 17-beta estradiol and the mixed-estrogen preparations available in this country.

Selected pharmacies in the United States will also compound *estriol* tablets and creams, which your physician may consider adding to your ERT/HRT regimen if needed. Estriol has a very short retention time of only one to four hours in cells, making it unlikely that once-a-day doses will provide adequate estrogenic effects when compared to estradiol or estrone. A few studies from Europe have found, however, that intravaginal use of topical estriol cream is of some value in treating vaginal dryness and milder forms of incontinence. Vaginal estriol has been considered by some to be a form of estrogen delivery to urogenital tissue that is safe for breast cancer patients, although long-term clinical trials regarding safety and efficacy have not yet been determined. I *do not recommend* taking estriol without your doctor's knowledge and without adequate monitoring of estrogen effect, since too much estrogen may lead to increased risk of uterine (endometrial) cancer. Phytoestrogens as they naturally occur in foods are too weak to have significant impact on bladder function and incontinence. Although the phytoestrogens are less potent than 17-beta estradiol, it is quite easy with the use of many supplements currently available to produce much higher serum concentrations of the phytoestrogens that competitively inhibit the action of 17-beta estradiol at cellular receptor sites. Dietary and supplement intake of the phytoestrogens are another potential confusing variable in studies of estrogen effects on urogenital measures.

Research

When viewing studies of estrogen effects on bladder function and incontinence, it is important to determine which form of estrogen has been used, since potencies and receptor actions can be quite different. In my clinical experience, optimal effects on bladder are difficult to achieve without having optimal serum levels of the premenopausal estrogen, 17-beta estradiol. Clinical studies that do not measure serum hormone levels, or that use predominately an estrone form of estrogen therapy, may fail to show clinical benefit on incontinence more as a result of suboptimal estradiol replacement than as a result of lack f estrogen effect *per se*. In addition, multiple studies from many menopause research settings worldwide over the last three decades have found that *route of administration* of estrogen makes a significant difference in the therapeutic effect on incontinence. For example, the systemic absorption of low-dose estrogen preparations applied vaginally is dependent on the status of the vaginal mucosa. Absorption is high when the vaginal mucosa is atrophic and gradually decreases to near zero as the vaginal mucosa matures under estrogen influence. Using different routes of estrogen delivery is another issue that makes direct comparison of various studies difficult, since some studies focus on oral delivery, others employ transdermal skin patches, and still others assess intravaginal delivery forms.

Since there is so little written on such an important subject, I am including a summary of the few double-blind, placebo-controlled studies that have compared the effectiveness of estrogen therapy in treating urinary urgency, frequency, urge and stress incontinence. These studies have used several types of estrogen: estriol, 17-beta estradiol, and conjugated equine estrogens. To date, the results are mixed. There are several studies from Europe that have shown that *all* of the three types of estrogen above can improve symptoms of burning, urgency, and frequency; but estrogen therapy alone has not shown a consistent positive effect on stress incontinence. This lack of consistency in the various study results, in my opinion, may be related in part to having suboptimal levels of estradiol due to the type and dose of hormone preparation used. In some studies, authors have commented on this dose effect, and in others, dose-response and type of estrogen issues have not been addressed. Several studies used doses of estriol that were too low to achieve optimal benefit, and this same problem appears to have been the case in some studies using estradiol, since the amount used was low compared to what is typically recommended for cardiovascular and bone benefits.

Yet other authors have found significant clinical benefit on incontinence with various forms of estrogen. The consensus of their studies is that hormonal supplementation with estrogens must be viewed as *critical to the relief* of this impairment in bladder function. A prospective study of continuous combined hormone replacement using 17-beta estradiol and dydrogesterone (a direct progesterone derivative) found that 23.3 percent of the participants reported being cured of their incontinence and nighttime incontinence disappeared in 65.4 percent after six months of oral hormone therapy. At the initiation of the study, urinary incontinence was reported by 44.1 percent of the women, and urinary frequency was reported by 28.4 percent of the women. The authors found that addition of the progesterone derivative did not diminish the effectiveness of estrogen. The results of the above studies correlate with my clinical experience as well.

In spite of such positive findings as those above, a large double-blind placebo-controlled study from England published in 1999 using 2 mg daily of estradiol valerate did not show improvement in urinary stress incontinence when compared to placebo. At least three factors, based on my experience, may contribute to the observed lack of improvement with estrogen in this study: (1) use of the synthetic estradiol valerate in an oral form resulted in conversion to estrone in the liver, inhibiting optimal serum levels of estradiol; (2) the once-a-day dose allows estradiol levels to fall significantly prior to the next dose, which diminishes the estrogen effects on urogenital tissue; and (3) serum estradiol levels were not done to determine whether optimal levels above target thresholds were achieved.

Dose, type of estrogen used, and route of administration have all been found to be significant in determining optimal response on urinary symptoms. Many gynecologists and menopause specialists report that their clinical experience has been that intravaginal delivery has generally been a more effective route of administration of estrogen for the benefit of the urogenital tract rather than oral routes. The estradiol vaginal ring delivery system (Estring), in combination with a 17-beta estradiol transdermal patch for systemic effects, has been particularly effective in my experience. Estring contains 2 mg of

17-beta estradiol in a silicone ring, smaller than a diaphragm, and is intended to remain in place for three months to deliver a low daily dose of the estradiol directly to the urogenital tissues. Some women, however, note a return of symptoms at about two months of having the ring in place, and find it helpful to change the Estring early if this happens. The vaginal ring system has the added benefit of providing mechanical support at the same time it delivers the daily low-dose estradiol. Vaginal creams are also quite helpful to these patients, although somewhat less pleasing esthetically than the vaginal ring system. Vagifem is a vaginal tablet containing 25 micrograms of 17-beta estradiol that has been well-tolerated and effective. In a twelve-week double-blind, randomized, placebo-controlled study, researchers found that treatment with Vagifem significantly improved frequency, urgency, urge, and stress incontinence compared to a placebo. In actual practice, Dr. Boyd, our gynecologist reports that as little as 0.5 to 1.0 gram of 17-beta estradiol cream inserted into the vagina nightly three to seven times a week has provided significant improvement with incontinence in about 50 percent of his patients. Types of incontinence other than stress incontinence have shown the greatest improvement, although modest improvements have been found even in stress incontinence. The vaginal route of administration at these low doses has the added advantage that very little of the estrogen is absorbed systemically (into the whole body). It appears, therefore, that this option may be safe to use in patients for whom systemic estrogen therapy has not been tolerated or is not an option for other medical reasons.

There has not been a great deal of attention yet paid to the urogenital effects of progesterone, synthetic progestins, or testosterone and the role that these hormones may play in causing beneficial or adverse effects on incontinence and other urogenital problems associated with menopause. There is evidence from a wide variety of studies on progestins that these compounds reduce estrogen binding at the estrogen receptor sites in different target tissues and may therefore serve to oppose estrogen effects. I have not been able to locate formal studies of such phenomena with regard to incontinence. My clinical experience, however, has been that women on estrogen replacement therapy have increased problems with urinary infections, frequency, urgency, and all forms of incontinence during progesterone or progestin phase of hormone replacement therapy or with use of progestin-dominant oral contraceptives. My clinical approach has been to slightly increase the amount of estrogen given during the progestin phase of therapy in order to overcome the negative effects of the progestin. This strategy has helped avoid relapse of urinary symptoms in women who had achieved improvement during the estrogen-only phase of their hormone therapy.

Optimizing Hormone Replacement for Bladder Problems

The following are strategies I used for my patients in fine-tuning hormone therapy to give better relief of interstitial cystitis pain, vulvodynia, vestibulitis, and the various types of incontinence. You may want to explore these options with your own physician to help improve urinary system symptoms:

Dr. Vliet's Guide: Optimizing Hormone Therapy to Help Bladder Problems

- Monitor serum levels to ensure that estradiol levels are adequate and are above the known minimum thresholds for estrogen's multiple benefits.

- Intravaginal delivery systems (Estring, Estrace cream, Vagifem) give maximum desired effects on urogenital tissues with less total body absorption (and therefore fewer side effects).

- Change the *type* of estrogen used. Women have many individual differences in absorption and metabolism of foods, hormones, vitamins, and medications. Conjugated equine estrogens (Premarin, Prempro) account for about 75–80 percent of the estrogen prescriptions in the United States, yet these products commonly produce less-than-optimal levels of estradiol, have significant variations in absorption due to the enteric coating, and also contain many different chemicals and dyes in this coating that pose a variety of problems for many women with bladder pain.

- If you are taking estrogen and continue to have bladder symptoms of burning, frequency, and urgency, as well as incontinence, then ask your doctor to change the prescription to a form without dyes in the tablet.

- Minimize the amount of estrone relative to estradiol by using transdermal patches of estradiol or by using oral forms that produce less estrone.

- If you have significant urinary difficulties, particularly interstitial cystitis, stress incontinence, and urge incontinence, try a *natural human 17-beta estradiol:* Estrace or generic estradiol tablets (Alora, Climara, Vivelle and Vivelle DOT) are more effective than the conjugated or esterified estrogens (Premarin, Menest, Estratab, Cenestin) that give you predominately estrone or conjugated estrogens.

- Specialty compounding pharmacies will prepare estriol vaginal creams if you prefer this less-potent form of estrogen, but remember that in general estriol is less effective than estradiol on urinary symptoms. In Europe, low-dose estriol and estradiol vaginal creams have been used successfully for treatment of urogenital problems for women who could not take other types of estrogen. Vaginal forms of these estrogens could theoretically be given without progestin in women who are progestin intolerant.

© Elizabeth Lee Vliet, M.D., 2000

Exercises

You may ask, "How on earth do I exercise my *bladder* muscles?" Dr. Arnold Kegel, in 1951, first described the method of muscle exercise to treat incontinence without the drugs or surgery that were the means used by most physicians at that time. The pubococcygeus, or "PC" muscle for short, is the primary muscle of the pelvic floor that governs control of urinary flow and also contracts the vagina (which may intensify pleasurable sensations during intercourse). The PC muscle also supports the uterus, urethra, and rectum. Dr. Kegel was able to show, by means of a device he invented, that the PC muscle could be trained and strengthened with sets of rhythmic contraction-hold-release actions. When the PC muscle is strengthened, it lifts the organs of the pelvis back into their normal positions and enables a woman to better control her urinary flow. Dr. Kegel monitored the strength of muscle contraction with biofeedback so the woman could objectively see how she was doing and learn how to increase her contraction. By 1956, he reported an 86 percent success rate in 455 women with incontinence who had undergone muscle training exercises at his clinic.

Studies since that time have confirmed the marked effectiveness of these methods. The success rate increases significantly if biofeedback techniques are used at the outset to teach women how to isolate the proper muscles and to contract the muscles more effectively. Patricia Burns, R.N., found dramatic improvement in stress incontinence using biofeedback: She reported 50–99 percent *decrease* in episodes of urine loss. Her research project, conducted at the School of Nursing at the State University of New York at Buffalo, was the first *carefully controlled* study of behavioral treatments for stress incontinence to show their marked effectiveness. In the biofeedback group, women watched a video screen display of the strength of their pelvic muscle contractions while a nurse trained in the techniques measured those contractions using a vaginal sensor probe. A 1999 study led by Dr. Burgio was published in JAMA, with similar very positive results for biofeedback compared to drug therapy. This is certainly an important option for you to explore in your area to find a specialist using biofeedback. Another technique to strengthen pelvic muscles uses low-intensity electrical stimulation to contract the muscles and progressively strengthen them until the patient can learn how to do it herself. Combining the electrical stimulation with biofeedback has been particularly effective for patients who have not responded to Kegels or biofeedback alone.

Once the techniques are learned correctly, these exercises can be practiced anywhere. Not only that, the behavioral techniques are promising because they don't involve the risks of surgery or the possible side effects of medicine. You just need motivation, commitment, and practice. If you are having any of the symptoms I have talked about, bring this up with your doctor to find out what resources are available in your area. And before you rush into "bladder tuck" surgery, make sure you have explored the options for strengthening your pelvic muscles *nonsurgically*. As one woman in her early forties laughingly said, "I practice my Kegels at business meetings, and driving home on the Jersey turnpike, and nobody but me knows what I'm doing. My sex life is great now, and all those embarrassing "leaks" have stopped. And, this way, there's no expense and no side effects." Talk about taking charge of your health and regaining your freedom.

Bladder Training

Another nonsurgical method of relieving urge incontinence is to follow a timed schedule of voiding, with progressive lengthening of the time interval between urinations. For example, if you find that you are not able to go more than three hours without accidental loss of urine, you would be instructed to urinate every two hours, whether the urge to void is there or not. Each week, you would increase the time between voidings by fifteen to thirty minutes until the bladder is trained to reach your goal for time between urinations. This simple method is also dramatically effective, but it does take your commitment to follow the training schedule. Again, it's free and there are no side effects.

Magnetic Field Therapy

A novel approach has been developed using the same principles as magnetic resonance imaging. A few centers in the United States have begun trials of a specially designed chair that is attached to a machine generating various frequencies of magnetic fields. A person sits in the chair for a prescribed period of time, with magnetic field therapy directed to the pelvic floor area. I have participated in a demonstration of this device, and although it certainly feels strange to undergo this therapy, the initial clinical studies are promising. I believe that one resource for this therapy is The Center for Pelvic Floor Disorders in Philadelphia, PA, and it may be worth pursuing before you consider more aggressive options such as surgery.

Medications

In addition to the benefits of estrogen to improve urinary function, there are other medications that help reduce incontinence.

Antispasmodics have been in use for many years and help to reduce bladder muscle spasms that cause urge incontinence. These medications include probanthine, flavoxate, oxybutynin, and imipramine. Alpha-receptor–stimulating medications, such as phenyl-propanolamine, help to improve the bladder sphincter muscle tone. A newer medication, Detrol (tolterodine), acts to reduce urinary leakage and incontinence problems by blocking the muscarinic receptors in the urinary bladder. This enables the bladder to hold more urine and increases detrusor pressure, the muscle that keeps the bladder sphincter closed. Detrol may cause dry mouth and dry eyes due to these muscarinic-blocking properties, but generally its side effects are mild. Imipramine is a tricyclic antidepressant, and shares the same side-effect profile I described in earlier chapters for these medications. Briefly, its most bothersome side effects are increased appetite leading to weight gain, dry eyes, dry mouth, constipation, and palpitations. If you are started on one of these medications, you should be properly monitored by a physician to avoid undesirable side effects. Phenylpropanolamine in particular can cause serious high blood pressure emergencies if taken by someone with hypertension and not supervised carefully.

Surgery

If other methods are not successful, or if there is a specific mechanical repair needed, you may wish to have a consultation with a urologist experienced in the surgical advances for treating incontinence. If you have interstitial cystitis, however, keep in mind that surgical intervention is generally indicated for less than 5 percent of patients. There are a number of new approaches that can be considered, and the specific types of surgery need to be evaluated in the context of your individual needs. Some resources are given in Appendix II to help you locate a specialist in your area. But keep in mind, **get your hormone levels tested reliably to see if this is a factor in your problems.** If you are trying to decide whether to have surgery for incontinence, it is particularly important to know whether you have optimal estrogen effects (since this is a simpler and less-costly option) before you undergo the pain of surgery and long recovery needed, not to mention a more costly procedure with greater overall risks. See the advice at the end of this chapter from one of my patients who had a long struggle with several surgeries.

If surgery is required, local vaginal application of estrogen is vital to prepare the vaginal and pelvic tissues. Use of intravaginal estrogen preoperatively and postoperatively may often be overlooked and has a number of potential benefits to help improve surgical outcome. Improving the estrogen effect gives the surgeon improved tissue quality with which to work and enhances the success rate of the surgical repair. Continued use of vaginal estrogen cream in the post-operative period further improves wound healing, enhances pain relief, improves formation of healthy connective tissue and mucosa, as well as maintains a healthy pH that minimizes infections.

One Woman's Experience

Dear Dr. Vliet,

I really enjoyed reading your article on the bladder especially the part on incontinence. I do agree with your conclusion that estrogen loss affects incontinence. That has certainly been the case with me. **I have lot more leakage when my estrogen level is down.** I only wish I had been given this information years ago . . . My stress incontinence began when I was in my late thirties. I would leak when I laughed, coughed, or sneezed. Ten years later it had become a significant problem. I had started to wear a pad every day. I had to leave the golf course on many occasions because I had not just leaked, but had completely wet through my pad and my clothes were soaked. This also happened several times when I had left a restaurant without going to the restroom first. On the way to the car I would leak through the pad and urine would be running down my legs.

I am sure during this ten-year period my estrogen level had dropped tremendously. This thought had never crossed my mind nor was it ever mentioned to me by my gynecologist. All I was ever told was that my bladder had dropped and needed to be suspended. I finally made the decision to do this and two gynecologists told me it would not be effective unless I also had a hysterectomy. So I had both done. Worst mistake ever made. After the surgery I leaked constantly. I have never been given a good answer as to why. Some doctors have said I had a urethra problem not a bladder one. I feel I must have had some muscle or nerve damage during the surgery . . . Since the first surgery I have had fat injections into the urethra by a doctor in New York. Then I had a sling operation by another surgeon. It did not work so I am now having collagen injections. They have helped, but it is temporary because it tends to break down. The estradiol therapy has helped diminish the leakage, and I will try to find someone here to do the biofeedback you suggested. I hope the information in your book can help other women from having to go through what I have been through. Needless to say, the quality of my life has not been good. It has been a very stressful situation as well as very expensive.

"Annie" [not real name]

Summary

There has been a great deal of progress in understanding estrogen effects on the bladder, yet we have a ways to go in getting this scientific information from research settings better integrated into the general clinical setting where women are seen for their health care. And there are critical areas needing further study, such as: clarifying the differential response to estrogen therapy based upon type of incontinence, identifying a possible role of testosterone on smooth muscle and connective tissue function in the urogenital system of women, and clarifying beneficial or adverse effects of various progestational medications (including natural progesterone) on IC, vulvodynia, incontinence, and overall urogenital health.

Some changes in bladder function certainly do occur with aging, but keep in mind, there are many new treatments, including natural forms of hormones, that may cure, or certainly improve, these problems. For many women, the various estrogen therapies may lead to significant improvement in bladder symptoms without the need for additional medication or surgery. But these estrogen options are often overlooked or not adequately discussed by doctors, particularly in the elderly postmenopausal woman who may never have used hormone therapy. Dietary change and noninvasive behavioral techniques such as biofeedback and pelvic floor exercises can be combined with various forms of estrogen therapy to achieve synergistic benefit. An integrated approach using multiple modalities is often the most effective way to achieve the greatest degree of improvement. Whatever combined strategies are employed, however, it is important for you to talk with your health professional about whether you could benefit from the use of hormone therapy. Since estrogen has the potential for many additional benefits beyond the urogenital tract, including improved balance, cognition, bone preservation, and cardiovascular function, it is crucial that you at least explore this option rather than continuing to suffer in silence. Being estrogen-complete for postmenopausal women is one of several critical factors to improve and enhance the healthy physiological function of the urinary bladder, urethra, and vagina.

Don't let embarrassment keep you from asking for help. I really want to encourage all of you reading this book that there is hope, and help, out there in a variety of organizations, physicians, nurse-specialists, and support groups. I have listed some of these resources in Appendix II. Don't let urinary problems keep you homebound when you have treatment options available.

Chapter 13

Estrogen and Your Heart: Not Just a Menopause Problem

Heart Disease Hits Women, Too

Cardiovascular disease kills approximately 485,000 women per year in the age range of forty to sixty-five, compared to 60,000 deaths annually for *all* reproductive cancers combined: breast, uterine, ovarian, cervical, and vaginal cancers. Over age fifty, *heart disease accounts for 53 percent of the deaths in women. Compare this with the 4 percent of deaths due to breast cancer in women over fifty.* Consider these recent findings:

- Almost 50 percent of women in the United States have had a hysterectomy by age fifty. Even for those women who have *not* had their ovaries removed, about 65 percent will have **menopausal estradiol levels** by **three** years after surgery, regardless of age at which surgery was performed. This means that a woman who has a hysterectomy at age thirty has a better than 60 percent chance of being menopausal by age thirty-three, not the average age of fifty-one for natural menopause. Their heart disease risk more than doubles *when they become menopausal*, not at the older ages we typically associate with heart disease in women.
- Women in their thirties and forties, even though still menstruating, are beginning to show the early effects of declining estrogen that predispose them to higher risk of heart disease after menopause: rising total cholesterol, dropping levels of HDL (the "good" kind), rising levels of LDL (the "bad" kind), and rising blood pressure. Hormonal factors, in particularly estradiol levels, are usually not even considered until *after* menses cease, missing an important window of opportunity for reducing disease risk and preventing serious heart attacks through diet, lifestyle, hormonal and medication approaches.

- A 1999 Yale study of 384,878 hospital patients showed that women *ages thirty to forty-nine* who suffer a heart attack are more than *twice* as likely to die of it in that first hospitalization than are men of the same age. Previous studies had shown that women in general are more likely to die than men following a heart attack but this is the first study to show that this result also applied to such *younger* women. It is particularly alarming that doctors assume this younger age group of women is low risk for serious heart disease, and therefore don't evaluate them as carefully or treat as aggressively as they would men with similar symptoms.
- Women with a serious, but commonly overlooked, metabolic disorder called PCOS, or polycystic ovary syndrome, are at especially high risk of having an early heart attack. PCOS causes waistline weight gain, high blood pressure, high androgen levels, insulin resistance with glucose intolerance, and marked increase in risk of diabetes mellitus.
- Women who present to medical offices and emergency rooms with complaints of palpitations are *far more likely than men* to be given a diagnosis of "anxiety," a prescription for Valium or Xanax, and sent home. Tragic cases abound of women such as this then having a massive heart attack. Some have died as a result of misdiagnosis. I have had many women referred to my practice who had been labeled "anxious," only to find on further evaluation that they had significant early cardiovascular disorders that required *different* medications, or they had perimenopausal decline in estradiol that needed hormonal management.
- Commonly, women in their forties and fifties who describe experiencing palpitations, chest discomfort or pain, and other cardiovascular symptomatology are not given the same degree of comprehensive evaluations and treatment options that are offered men. They are more likely to be given serotonin-boosting antidepressants rather than medications to lower cholesterol or restore estradiol balance.
- Recent studies in the gender differences in health care patterns indicate that women are *less likely* than men to be offered angiography, angioplasty, and cardiac bypass surgery. This is thought to be an additional factor to explain why more women die of their first heart attack compared to men.
- In another 1999 study at Manhattan's St. Luke's Roosevelt Hospital Center, women of all ages were found to have harder-to-diagnose symptoms and more complications of heart disease (internal bleeding, congestive heart failure) than were men. Women need to be especially vigilant about having thorough medical evaluations when they experience less recognizable potential heart attack symptoms such as unexplained sweating, nausea, or shortness of breath.

- Alcohol is known to have specific toxic effects on heart muscle fibers, and excessive alcohol consumption is increasing alarmingly in women. Alcohol is more damaging to women, ounce for ounce, than men because women have less of the enzyme that detoxifies alcohol in the body. Yet women are less likely than men to be identified as alcohol abusers at early, treatable stages of the illness. Women aren't as commonly referred for alcohol treatment until later stages of alcoholism when cardiac and other severe complications have already occurred.

The myth of heart disease as a man's problem, or only affecting older women, appears to be part of the reason that women of all ages with heart disease are sicker when the problems are recognized and have a higher death rate when they have a first heart attack compared to men with first attacks. The myth also helps to explain the overlooked serious heart disease emerging in women in their thirties. Far more women silently, and without much press attention, die of heart disease every year. These alarming trends in heart disease statistics have been present for decades, but women are *still* more aware of and fearful about breast cancer than about heart disease. Perhaps this difference directly results from the greater publicity and media attention given to breast cancer in women. Another reason women view heart disease risk less seriously than breast cancer is that many people have the mistaken belief that heart disease is a "quick and painless" way to die, compared to a prolonged, painful death from breast cancer. Yet, more women than men with heart disease have incapacitating pain, disability, loss of independence, and a prolonged death due to congestive heart failure, angina, or the complications of multiple small strokes. Heart disease may be just as slow, painful, and debilitating as breast cancer is perceived to be.

A significant decline in estradiol will increase your risk of heart disease, whatever your age. When hormone imbalance begins is the best time to evaluate your objective risk factors, not waiting until after problems develop. If you are armed with knowledge, each of you has a unique opportunity *before* actual menopause to identify potential risk factors for cardiovascular disease (CVD) and to implement lifestyle changes at a time when preventive approaches can be the most meaningful for your long-term quality of life. But if you are not aware that heart disease can affect women so dramatically, you may not know to discuss these issues with your physician. And physicians, like all the rest of us, had been taught to think of heart disease as a *man's* disease that did not affect women until sometime after age sixty-five. This misconception still persists, years after the first edition of my book in 1994. You can do something to reduce your risk of these problems, so pay attention to the voices of women in this chapter as they share their stories and comments. Insist on having the proper evaluation by your physician.

Risk Factors Affecting Women and Men

Unfortunately, it has been only in the last few years that women have been included in studies of heart disease risks, as well as clinical studies of new medications to treat heart disease. The information we have shows that women have similar risk factors as men, *except for estrogen*. This seems so blatantly obvious that it is appalling to consider that the role of estrogen in heart disease has been studied only in recent years. Later in this chapter I will talk further about what we have come to understand about estrogen's specific role in reducing risk of heart disease. The general risk factors for heart disease are summarized for your review in Table 1 below. There is a wealth of good books and pamphlets describing each of these risk factors and ways you can modify your lifestyle habits to reduce your risk.

Let me say at the outset: Having a healthy level of estradiol is a critical factor in reducing your risk of serious heart disease. But, before you think of hormones as a "magic bullet" for heart protection, I think it is crucial to make healthy lifestyle changes. These are the *first and most important steps* you can take to help prevent disability or premature death from heart disease. At least **eleven** of the CVD risk factors below are either modifiable or can be eliminated altogether by eliminating the unhealthy lifestyles that are so typical of Americans. Focus on making positive changes, and "JUST DO IT," as the Nike ad says. Your health is your greatest wealth, and you are in control of protecting your investment.

Putting *women's* risk factors in perspective shows the importance of studying gender differences: Total cholesterol levels are better predictors of CVD risk for men, but not for women. High levels of triglycerides are an *independent risk factor* for women, but not for men. *Low* levels of "good" HDL are a greater risk factor for women, while high LDL ("bad" cholesterol) levels are a greater risk factor for men. Among diabetics, high triglyceride levels increase heart disease risk nearly *two-hundred-fold in women,* but only about three-fold in men. A person who has the "lipid triad" of high total cholesterol, low HDL, and high LDL is *thirteen times* more likely to have an acute myocardial infarction (heart attack) in the next four years. What can you to improve your lipid triad? Stop smoking, start exercising, reduce dietary fat and sugars, and for women, consider estrogen therapy. By the mid-1990s, the National Cholesterol Education Program (NCEP) advised that estrogen therapy should be considered for women to lower LDL and raise HDL *before using lipid-lowering drugs,* such as niacin, Mevacor, Pravacol, Lipitor, Zocor, Lescol, or others.

Paying attention to your cholesterol levels, and the ratio of your "good" HDL cholesterol to the total cholesterol is crucial. But

Table I—CARDIOVASCULAR DISEASE RISK FACTORS

- family history of cardiovascular disease
- growing older
- history of chest pain, or prior cardiac problems
- cigarette smoking
- high-fat diets, especially saturated fats
- lack of exercise
- obesity, especially increased abdominal (truncal) body fat (waist-to-hip ratio greater than 0.85); in women, waist over 35 inches
- hypertension (high blood pressure)
- elevated cholesterol and/or low HDL (HDL is a better predictor of CVD risk for women than for men)
- elevated triglycerides (a *greater* risk factor for women than for men)
- diabetes or impaired glucose tolerance
- elevated insulin or exaggerated insulin response to simple carbohydrates
- elevated levels of highly sensitive C-Reactive protein (hs-CRP)
- elevated levels of lipoprotein (a)
- elevated levels of fibrinogen
- elevated levels homocysteine
- low intake or low levels of B vitamins and folate
- clotting abnormalities (coagulopathy)
- premature ovarian failure, or removal of ovaries prior to the average age of natural menopause
- presence of PCOS (polycystic ovary syndrome)
- hypothyroidism (causes high blood pressure and high cholesterol)
- chronic use of prednisone or other corticosteroids
- elevated ferritin (iron stores), whether from ending of menstrual bleeding, excess iron supplementation, or the hereditary iron storage disorder *hemochromatosis*
- emotional stress (causes increased coronary vasospasm, more so in women than men)

© Elizabeth Lee Vliet, M.D., 1995, revised 2000

newer studies have shown that half of all heart attacks occur in people with normal cholesterol levels, so for many years physicians have been looking for additional markers that will help us identify high risk individuals sooner. In a study published in March 2000 in the

New England Journal of Medicine, researchers led by Dr. Paul Ridker in Boston found that C-reactive protein is a powerful predictor of future heart attacks if the highly sensitive form of the blood test is used (hs-CRP). Hs-CRP was an even better predictor of heart attack risk than some other measures we have been looking at in women: lipoprotein (a), homocysteine, and LDL cholesterol. C-reactive protein is a marker of inflammation of blood vessels, an important factor in triggering the damage that leads to heart attacks. Using data on over 28,000 post-menopausal women from the Women's Health Study, women with the highest levels of hs-CRP had more than a four-fold increase risk of heart attack compared with women who had lower levels of this protein. These same researchers have found that even heart patients with normal cholesterol levels who take the medication Pravacol have lower levels of C-RP, and a lower risk of future heart attack, than did the women taking placebo. But if you are concerned about your risk factors for heart attack and want to have some of these tests, be sure and ask your doctor to order the *highly sensitive* C-RP blood test, since not all of the tests for C-RP are as reliable as the newer versions of this test.

Cardiovascular Symptoms and Disease: Many Variations

Symptoms are the changes and sensations you experience, such as headaches, racing heart, clammy skin, pain, flushing, tingling, and a myriad of others. These changes may indicate a normal body response to an environmental stimulus or even to your own thoughts. These sensations may also be a potential warning of *disease.* Not all symptoms indicate disease, and not all diseases (at least in early stages) produce symptoms. Hypertension and osteoporosis are classic examples of diseases that do not produce symptoms until damage has already been done to the body by the disease process. One of my tasks in helping patients is to sort out what the symptoms may indicate, and what diseases could be present that are still silent and not yet producing symptoms.

Palpitations, those fluttering or pounding sensations in the chest that can be quite disturbing and frightening, are quite common as part of the heart response to the brain effects of declining estrogen in the perimenopause and menopause. In numerous studies, palpitations occur in anywhere from 40–60 percent of women in the pre- and perimenopause transition during times of the menstrual cycle when estradiol levels drop (bleeding days and around ovulation). For about 15–20 percent of women, palpitations may be the *only* symptom serving as a clue to the decline in estradiol. But the presence of palpitations does not necessarily mean you have cardiovascular disease. Palpitations may occur as a heart response to the bursts of adrenaline in the brain that occur with drops in estradiol. The increase in heart rate is a normal part of the fight-or-flight reaction; the brain sends a signal to other body organs that something is changing rapidly and is out of balance. Palpitations may also occur in certain types of *benign* heart disease such as mitral valve prolapse or in potentially serious types of heart disease such as *atrial fibrillation*. Such diverse diseases as anemia and hyperthyroidism may also produce palpitations through other mechanisms. Panic disorder is a biological condition of excess, and erratic, production of adrenaline-type compounds in the brain that may produce palpitations as I described for hormone changes. So palpitations as a symptom have *many different* causes. Some causes are just normal responses, but some causes of palpitations indicate more serious conditions. And the best treatment will be different, depending on the specific cause.

Yet, the symptom of palpitations is not often viewed as a possible endocrine-based one that can be caused by falling estradiol or excess thyroid hormone. If women are evaluated medically for the problem of palpitations, they are most often seen by internal medicine or cardiology specialists who check for the possibility of heart disease with cholesterol blood tests, physical exam, electrocardiograms, and exercise (treadmill) electrocardiograms. If nothing abnormal is found on these tests, women are then likely to be told that the cause of their symptoms is stress or anxiety. The average woman is *not told* that her symptoms may be related to menopausal hormone changes, and she typically does not get evaluated with FSH and estradiol blood tests. Listen to CC describe her experience.

CC was thirty-nine years old when she came to see me. She described

> . . . terrible pounding sensations in my chest, and it feels like my heart is going to come right through my chest, it actually hurts it's beating so hard. Then it will go away for awhile, and all of sudden it will come back. It seems to be worse at night, and the funny thing is it doesn't bother me when I'm out jogging. My doctor did an EKG and tells me there's nothing wrong with my heart; he said I'm just too much of a Type A person and I need to relax. But the stress isn't worse now, in fact my life is really pretty good except I want to know what this is because it hurts.

CC had no history of any health problems, did not smoke, seldom had alcohol, did not use any street drugs, and regularly participated in 5K "Fun Run" activities in the community in addition to her daily jogging. Over the past year, she had increased her jogging to between six and ten miles a day, usually six days a week. She reported a lactose intolerance and had cut out dairy products about ten years earlier. With her exercise, she did not think she needed to worry about calcium supplements. She appeared to be healthy and quite fit, and I could not elicit any other problems or symptoms in going through the usual medical "review of systems" checklist.

She was still menstruating, and at her recent gynecological checkup for her annual pelvic and Pap, she said she had been told "Everything's fine, you're normal." When I questioned her more about her menstrual periods, she said her periods had been a lot lighter and less frequent over the past two years that she had been running more. I asked if her heart poundings had any relationship to her menstrual cycle. She said, "Well, now that you ask, I have noticed that it seems to always get *really bad* the day or two before my period starts, and it will last a couple of days and go away. Sometimes it seems to hit again mid-month, then go away again. Other times it will be there occasionally in an erratic way." Her complete medical evaluation, including a thyroid and cholesterol profile along with a Holter monitor of her heart activity for twenty-four hours, were normal. On the first day of her period, when her heart poundings were the worst, her estradiol level was 23 and her FSH 2.0. The low FSH along with the low estradiol is fairly common when women have unwittingly suppressed their ovaries' hormonal function with significant increases in their exercise regimen. I was suspicious from her dietary history and her alterations in menstrual pattern and flow that she may have begun to have early bone loss, and I suggested she consider having a bone density test. She was shocked to find that she had a bone density, at age thirty-nine, one standard deviation *below* the bottom of normal for her age.

When we reviewed all of her information, I explained that the hormone levels were quite low, and I thought the drop in estradiol each month before her period likely triggered the brain burst of adrenaline that increased her heart rate. Since she also had these episodes at midcycle some months, I told her I thought she had the same heart response when her estradiol dropped with ovulation. From her history, I did not think she ovulated every month and this helped her understand why the palpitations did not seem to happen on a regular basis at midcycle. I thought her bone loss had developed gradually with her reduced calcium intake as well as the decline in estrogen when her exercise intensity altered her menstrual pattern and decreased her overall body fat percentage. She did not have any more serious underlying heart disease causing her palpitations.

After we reviewed all of her options and choices, she elected to take the low-dose oral contraceptives (with a lower progestin content) to improve her hormonal balance, maintain her bone mass, and help eliminate the estrogen drop with menses that triggered her palpitations. Needless to say, I also urged her to take calcium and magnesium supplements to help keep from losing further bone. She has done extremely well since then and has not needed further medical visits, since her palpitations have resolved. Her gynecologist agreed with her being on the oral contraceptives and plans to manage that with her as part of her annual checkup. I have seen quite a lot of patients like CC in my practice, and find this rewarding because I feel that together, in a physician-patient partnership, we are arriving at options that *prevent* the progression of disease risks. In my view, this is a great example of "A stitch in time saves nine."

Another difference in the way cardiovascular symptoms appear in men and women is in the pattern of chest pain called *angina*. Men typically experience "crushing" chest pain, with pain that spreads down the left arm and up into the neck area. Women are more likely to have what is called *silent angina,* which does not produce this severe, crushing pain and does not radiate down the left arm and into the neck as we see in men. Women may just experience a "tightness" or "heaviness" in the chest, which can often be mistaken for anxiety if a health professional is not aware of these gender differences in the way angina can present. More often in women than in men, angina may be triggered by spasm of the coronary arteries caused by falling estradiol levels or even emotional stress. So the symptoms of angina as well as the causes tend to be different for women.

The difference in how angina pain is experienced by women compared to men may be due to differences in pain threshold, differences in pain pathways in women, effects of estradiol on the arteries themselves, or other factors we have not yet identified. But it is clear that this difference in the pain symptoms for women is one reason women with angina, or ischemic heart disease, do not get diagnosed early and then have more serious disease by the time it is found. If you are at high risk of heart disease and are experiencing this kind of chest pain, *be assertive* in pursuing an evaluation by your physician. Listen to what this woman went through.

Meg was forty-seven and terrified of having heart disease. **Both** her parents died of CVD. Her mother had a heart attack in her late forties and then died in her early fifties. Meg's cholesterol was 337, triglycerides were elevated at 400, and her CHOL/HDL ratio was 5.5, much too high for a woman her age who had not had any sign of menopause or any menstrual irregularities. She was significantly overweight and had a high fasting glucose. She described physical sensations of angina (ischemia of the heart muscle) with even mild exertion. All of these risks placed her in the highest risk group for her age, yet her HMO physician would not authorize further cardiac testing to evaluate her further, even with her high risk of CVD. Her husband even went in to see the doctor and try and talk with him.

When he came home, he said to his wife, *"Meg, that man doesn't like you!"* They finally talked with the head of customer service at their insurance company, who agreed to reimburse her for the cardiac treadmill stress test she had been requesting and I had prescribed for her due to her many heart disease risk factors. This woman and her husband fought appropriately for what should have been done in her health care. Many patients, however, are more passive than this and simply do not realize that they need to speak up to the health insurance company about such matters. Remember that you are the customer, and you have the right as well as the responsibility to seek appropriate medical evaluation under your health coverage. If you are not being heard, it helps to send a complaint letter to the Insurance Commissioner for your state. Meg and her husband took these steps, and were finally heard. She had her cardiac testing and it showed evidence of blockage of the coronary arteries . . . in time for her to take aggressive steps to prevent a full-blown heart attack. She started estradiol therapy, lipid-lowering medications, a healthy weight-loss program, and a gradual low-intensity walking program. She is doing much better now, with major improvement in all her heart disease risk factors.

Heart Basics—How the System Works

It helps to understand the basics of how the heart and blood vessels work so that when I talk about estradiol effects, you will understand the many ways that this important hormone works to help prevent heart disease. The circulatory system is basically comprised of a **pump** (the heart, a muscular organ about the size of your closed fist) pushing **fluid** (the blood) through a **series of tubes** of different sizes (arteries, capillaries, veins) to provide **nutrients** (e.g., oxygen, glucose) and remove waste products for all the cells, tissues, and organs of the body. This is boiling it down to its most essential aspects. In reality, the massive process of constantly circulating fluids to all parts of the body day and night is incredibly complex, with many different mechanisms for regulating it and keeping the critical balance of the many chemicals the body needs to work properly. It is too complicated to describe further in the short space of this chapter, but at least you have the big picture.

There has to be a **force**, called **blood pressure (BP)**, that moves the blood fluid through the system. BP is measured by two numbers that provide us with information about whether the heart is having to work harder to pump the blood (high blood pressure, hypertension) or whether the pressure is too low to keep blood moving to the necessary organs (low blood pressure, hypotension, can cause fainting spells, lightheadedness, fatigue). The top number is the *systolic pressure;* elevation of this number is usually less serious since it may be briefly elevated by stress, anxiety, and pain as well as by the more serious disorder of hypertension. The bottom number is the *diastolic pressure; sustained* elevation of the diastolic pressure greater than 90 mm Hg indicates hypertension. An average blood pressure is considered to be 120/80 mm Hg, but most women (and many physicians) don't realize this number is based on an average **male.** If we had carefully evaluated gender differences, we would find that the average healthy younger *female* may have normal blood pressures in the range of 110/60 to 110/70. Thus, women who have a blood pressure of 120/80 may actually have a pressure that is *higher* than normal for them.

What happens in the process leading to high blood pressure and arteriosclerosis (cardiovascular disease)? Arteriosclerosis (or atherosclerosis) is basically plaque buildup in the arteries. Plaque is a mixture of cholesterol-containing particles along with platelets and fibrin. These deposits cause a narrowing of the arteries, much like a wad of dirt partially plugging a garden hose. Cholesterol has several forms, and the "good" form (HDL) serves as a scavenger to carry away plaque from the arteries so it can be broken down and excreted by the liver. LDL, or "bad," cholesterol serves to add *more* cholesterol to the plaque deposits lining arteries. When cholesterol levels are abnormally high and levels of the good HDL cholesterol are low, LDL deposits more cholesterol molecules along the artery wall. Since there isn't as much HDL to clean up these deposits and take them back to the liver to be broken down and excreted, plaque builds up on the walls of the arteries. This means it takes more pressure for the blood to get through the arteries, which results in high blood pressure. The narrowing of the arteries due to plaque leads to reduced blood flow to tissues that deprives cells of vital oxygen and nutrients (called ischemia). Loss of oxygen damages or destroys cells (called infarction).

When the damaged cells belong to the heart muscle itself, this is called a myocardial infarction, or MI. When the damaged cells are in the brain, it is called a stroke. The entire process is quite complex, but this is a simple overview of the basics to help you understand the role estrogen plays in reducing risk of both CVD and stroke. Women may be affected by many different types of disorders affecting the circulatory system. These are other common examples and terms, which your physician may use. Make certain to ask for patient education material to read if you are told you have one of these problems.

- **arrhythmias** (heart rate, rhythm disturbances)
- **hypertension** (high blood pressure)
- **hyperlipidemia** (high cholesterol, low HDL, high triglycerides)
- **ischemic heart disease** (angina)

- myocardial infarction, or MI (heart attack)
- strokes, transient ischemic attacks (TIA) (cerebrovascular disease)
- peripheral vascular disease (e.g., thrombophlebitis, or blood clots)
- murmurs, heart valve problems (e.g., mitral valve prolapse)

The Cardiovascular Protection Role of Estrogen: Research Advances

Heart disease rates for women rise dramatically with declining estradiol, regardless of your age when this happens. Heart disease in women rises even more significantly in the years after menopause. Disability, discomfort, and loss of ability to be active every day, as well as premature deaths in postmenopausal women, could be significantly reduced if women were given adequate information about the cardioprotective effects of estrogen replacement therapy and had an *individualized discussion* of their risks of various health problems. Unfortunately, so many women have been frightened by the excessive reporting of the breast cancer risks that they are unwilling to consider taking estrogen after menopause. Even many health professionals are unduly swayed by breast cancer worries and fail to adequately explain to women their much greater risk of being incapacitated or dying from heart disease. Primary care physicians, in particular gynecologists working with menopausal women, can play a major role in correcting the misinformation among consumers. This would help women make informed choices about postmenopausal estrogen therapy based on their own *individual* needs rather than decisions based on fear, or decisions based on what friends may have decided about hormones.

There has been a great deal of exciting research in the last few years that has helped us now understand the many ways that the normal female premenopausal form of estrogen, 17-beta estradiol, exerts its protective effect on heart disease. You may have read about the way that estrogen reduces total cholesterol and increases the body's production of the good type of cholesterol, HDL. But have you seen some of the latest findings?

- *Estrogen decreases LDL, the plaque-forming kind of cholesterol, by increasing liver breakdown of LDL so that it is eliminated from the circulation.* In a 1991 Harvard study of healthy postmenopausal women, oral estrogens reduced LDL an average of 15 percent, and *increased* HDL by 16 percent. Transdermal estradiol did not have the same magnitude of pharmacologic effect on HDL and LDL *initially* but does maintain the natural beneficial effects of estradiol over time to keep HDL and LDL in the premenopausal ranges. In addition, transdermal estradiol *decreases* the triglyceride levels, whereas oral forms of estrogen may *increase* triglycerides.

• *Estrogen stimulates the production of HDL,* the good cholesterol that carries plaque away from the artery wall and back to the liver to be broken down and excreted.

• *Estrogen stimulates the formation of LDL receptors in the liver and possibly the walls of arterial blood vessels.* These receptors bind the LDL so that LDL molecules are removed from the circulation and prevented from forming plaque.

• *17-beta estradiol acts as a calcium-channel blocker to relax artery walls, which helps to dilate the arteries, to improve blood flow throughout the brain and body, and to reduce blood pressure.* Calcium-channel-blocking medications (many are on the market; some examples are Calan, Cardizem, DynaCirc, Isoptin, and Procardia) are used medically to treat a number of disorders such as angina, hypertension, migraine headaches, and bipolar mood disorders. Estradiol has a similar mechanism of action on the blood vessels' calcium channels, so this may be one way estradiol performs its normal function of keeping blood pressure lower in premenopausal women compared to men of the same age. After menopause, as estrogen goes down, we see rises in women's blood pressure more similar to the readings in men.

• *Estradiol given sublingually* (dissolved under the tongue) *improves blood flow in the coronary arteries of the heart as well as women's exercise tolerance on treadmill testing,* an important finding demonstrated by Dr. Philip Sarrel of Yale University in collaboration with cardiologists in London. The women in these studies were postmenopausal women with previously documented coronary artery disease that had caused at least 70 percent occlusion of the arteries. Thus, the improvement seen with estradiol was even more impressive, given that these women had such severe disease.

• *Estrogen stimulates the release of endothelium-derived relaxing factor (EDRF, thought to be nitric oxide) a chemical having an important role in dilating blood vessels to maintain normal pressure and flow.* In a two-year study of twenty-six postmenopausal women, levels of this blood vessel relaxing agent kept *rising in women on estrogen* and continued to increase the longer they took estrogen. Levels of the nitric oxide compound were not changed in women who were not receiving estrogen. Dr. Raghvendra Dubey, of the University of Pittsburgh, who headed this study, said that their results helped to explain another way in which estrogen protects against heart disease before menopause and why it may be important to consider as therapy for postmenopausal women at high risk of CVD.

- *Estrogen maintains the normal balance of prostacycline and thromboxane, two chemicals that regulate clot formation.* Healthy clot formation is a protective mechanism, but excess clot formation leads to heart attacks and strokes. Prostacycline *dilates* blood vessels (improves blood flow and lowers blood pressure) and it also prevents platelets from aggregating or "clumping" and forming plaque to block the arteries. Thromboxane has the opposite effect: It constricts blood vessels and stimulates platelet aggregation as a means of defending the body against hemorrhage. When thromboxane levels are high, blood pressure goes up and more "sticky" platelets aggregate to form plaque along the artery wall. Estrogen *increases* artery production of prostacycline, which *improves* blood flow and *reduces platelet clumping* to form clots and plaque. Estradiol's action is also similar to the way that aspirin works to help prevent clots and reduce the risk of strokes and heart attacks.

- *Estrogen decreases fibrinogen, another clot-forming factor in the blood.* Higher fibrinogen levels are associated with increased clot formation. The Post-menopausal Estrogen and Progestin Intervention Trial (PEPI studies) results released in January 1995 showed that fibrinogen levels rose by 3 percent in women *not* on estrogen. In the Framingham study of heart disease factors, a 3 percent *increase* in fibrinogen *doubled* the risk of heart attack in women. Women who were taking estrogen (Premarin) showed no change in fibrinogen levels in the PEPI study. More recent studies using transdermal 17-beta estradiol have shown that estradiol *decreases* fibrinogen.

- *Estrogen therapy* (to restore estradiol levels to premenopausal ranges) *also improves clot-dissolving ability,* based on recent analysis of the second generation of women in the Framingham Study. Premenopausal and postmenopausal women taking estrogen had significantly *lower* levels of *plasminogen activator inhibitor (PAI-1)* than women not on estrogen therapy. Since PAI-1 is a chemical that *interferes with* natural clot-dissolving ability, lower levels are desirable.

- *Estradiol helps to modulate the various receptors involved in the fight-or-flight response that can lead to stress-induced spasm of the blood vessels to the heart causing angina in women.* Along with this effect, estradiol helps to increase the forcefulness of the heart-muscle pumping action with each heartbeat (positive inotropic effect), and it also increases the "stroke volume" or amount of blood pumped with each heartbeat. Both effects mean improved blood flow to the body.

- *Estradiol also helps to decrease total body vascular resistance, which also means improved blood flow to the entire body.* This beneficial effect was especially enhanced when estradiol was given in the transdermal patch form.

- *Transdermal estradiol has the same beneficial effects on HDL cholesterol as oral estrogen after about six months of transdermal therapy* as shown in studies by Corson (1993) and LaRosa (1994). Corson and LaRosa also showed that *oral* estrogens may sometimes cause an unwanted increase in triglycerides, but *transdermal* estradiol helps *decrease* triglycerides (which lowers CVD risk).

- *Transdermal estradiol significantly decreases both systolic and diastolic blood pressure* as shown in a 1994 study by Cheang and coworkers.

- *Estradiol has several specific effects on the coronary arteries to reduce the buildup of plaque and keep arteries healthy*: Estradiol (E2) inhibits excess growth of arterial smooth muscle (too much smooth muscle makes the artery wall thicker and reduces effective blood flow); E2 inhibits deposits of elastin and collagen that provide a base for plaque formation to clog the artery; and E2 also inhibits lipids (blood fats) from accumulating in plaques in the artery wall. In addition, E2 stimulates up-regulation of vasorelaxin and down-regulation of vasoconstriction, which means lower blood pressure and better blood flow to the body.

- *Estradiol has been found to act as a free-radical scavenger helping to break down plaque in arteries,* demonstrated in a number of studies in recent years. This action is similar to the way other compounds with antioxidant properties (vitamin E, vitamin C) act to help prevent heart disease. In fact, a recent study published in *Menopause: The Journal of the North American Menopause Society* in 2000 (volume 7) found that the 17-beta estradiol made by our ovaries before menopause has an antioxidant potency at least 10-100 times greater than alpha and gamma tocopherol (vitamin E) and melatonin. No wonder younger women don't have heart attacks. In addition to the importance of antioxidants in helping to prevent heart disease, I also talk about their role in cancer prevention (see chapters on nutrition and breast cancer).

All of these exciting developments indicate the depth of the worldwide research on how estrogen in women helps to maintain healthy heart and blood-vessel function throughout the body. Such research helps to better explain why heart diseases increase at menopause when women lose the most active form of estrogen, 17-beta estradiol. The newer research also helps us to understand why heart disease may hit younger women as well if they have conditions like PCOS that cause excess androgens and a relative decrease in the desirable estradiol effects. I am amazed at all the wealth of new information and research just in the five years since I first published this book, as summarized in the following chart.

SUMMARY OF ESTRADIOL (E2) BENEFITS
ON HEART DISEASE RISK

- E2 lowers blood pressure by dilating blood vessels

- E2 increases HDL ("good") cholesterol

- E2 decreases total cholesterol and ("bad") LDL

- E2 improves carbohydrate metabolism, decreasing risk of diabetes

- E2 reduces platelet stickiness and clumping that causes strokes, artery-clogging plaque; increases secretion of prostacycline

- E2 reduces risk of blood clots by several mechanisms

- E2 has antioxidant effects on artery walls

- E2 reverses the impaired vessel response to acetylcholine in atherosclerotic coronary arteries—*Gender specific*

- Estradiol enhances release of endothelium-derived NO (nitric oxide), a potent vasodilator; acts as calcium-channel blocker (vasodilation)

- E2 alters synthesis, release, and response to vasoconstrictive peptides (e.g., endothelin-I and angiotensin-II)

- E2 increases endothelial permeability, transport of blood-derived O2

© Elizabeth Lee Vliet, M.D., 1995, revised 2000

PCOS, Syndrome X, and Your Heart

Millions of women in their twenties and thirties have a hidden disorder that dramatically increases their risk of heart attacks *before* menopause. What is it? It is polycystic ovarian syndrome (PCOS), a commonly overlooked condition affecting about 6–10 percent of premenopausal women, *including teenagers,* that results in wide-spread metabolic changes in the body. PCOS increases the risk of cardiovascular disease as much as eleven-fold by age fifty. Even women from forty to forty-nine years old who have PCOS are estimated to have a risk that is *four times* the risk for women in this age group who do not have PCOS. Syndrome X, a metabolic-endocrine disorder common in women, is another "mysterious" women's disorder seen in premenopausal women and known to be associated with a particularly high risk of having an early heart attack. What are these conditions, and why haven't you heard more about them?

Part of the reason PCOS has been so overlooked is that gyne-cologists have been taught in the past that a woman only had the possibility of PCOS if she had stopped menstruating (called *amen-orrhea)*. In addition, the most common reason women with PCOS see a physician is for infertility. So, if you are not trying to become pregnant, and still have menstrual periods, even though you may have all the *other* metabolic changes that go with PCOS, you are likely to be overlooked in our current fragmented approach to women's health. Endocrinologists is this country haven't focused much on the ovary, since this endocrine organ is the "turf" of gyne-cologists. Gynecologists, on the other hand, haven't worried much about women who were perceived to have "just a cosmetic prob-lem" of waistline weight gain and excess facial hair, or who skipped periods . . . the kinds of changes that occur in both PCOS and Syndrome X. To physicians trained as surgeons, and focused on helping you get pregnant and deliver your baby, these other problems just haven't seemed very important, and they had been taught that PCOS interfered "only" with a woman's ability to get pregnant.

So, what happened? Women who actually had a very serious dis-order (that we now know affects far more than reproduction) were most often discounted and simply told to "not worry, everybody misses periods sometimes" or "just go exercise and lose weight and your periods will come back, and you'll be fine." This happened to a sixteen-year-old young woman I saw recently, who had severe hor-monal imbalance, with a very high level of free testosterone, low estradiol, and a fifty-pound weight gain over six months in spite of a very healthy diet and extensive exercise regimen. She had PCOS, but her gynecologist had not recognized it, because he saw her as simply a teenager obsessed with weight gain. Many physicians don't realize that PCOS has potentially devastating consequences for the rest of a woman's life and could lead to early death from heart attacks or diabetes complications long before menopause. So it isn't "just a cosmetic" issue, it may be your life at stake, as you will see later in this chapter with Susu's story.

First described in 1935, PCOS, or Stein-Leventhal Syndrome, is characterized by excess body hair, lack of ovulation and regular menses, and multiple cysts on the ovaries. Today it is recognized as more than just ovarian cysts and irregular menses; it is a complex endocrine disorder with wide-ranging serious negative effects on fertility, body weight (with marked "middle-body" fat increase), blood pressure, diabetes and cardiovascular disease risks, and later risk of endometrial cancer. Today, we know that these diverse complications of PCOS are caused in large part by the elevated level of androgens, higher-than-normal free testosterone, high estrone-to-estradiol ratio, and insulin resistance with elevated insulin levels causing more vascular damage and abdominal weight gain. With this terrible vicious cycle, young women with PCOS are at especially high risk of developing diabetes, which in turn causes many damaging changes in the heart and blood vessels throughout the body and thereby increases the risk of having a premature heart attack or stroke. Syndrome X, now known to be associated with estrogen deficiency, has a similar picture in terms of causing a marked increase in risk of both heart attack and stroke in younger women. These combined conditions, both affecting normal ovarian hormone balance, affect millions of women, and cause untold pain and suffering, not to mention early death. PCOS and Syndrome X desperately need our careful attention as physicians to get these conditions better recognized and treated when women are younger, *before* they develop permanent problems.

Another cause of concern is that the very treatment of PCOS that is directed toward infertility may itself cause more problems for these young women. International climacteric medicine specialists have published reports that surgical treatments with laparoscopic ovarian diathermy and drugs to stimulate ovulation such as clomiphene citrate (Clomid) may cause premature menopause and a higher risk of ovarian cancer. Using higher-dose content of progestin in a birth control pill to regulate menstrual cycles in these women may lead to further development of lipid and triglyceride abnormalities, which increase risk of plaque buildup in the arteries, particularly if the pills contain higher amounts of the *androgenic* progestins. More on this issue in the next section on progestin effects in heart disease. So women with PCOS have a *double whammy*—they often need specialized treatment if they are going to be able to get pregnant, and some of the treatments themselves may lead to serious problems later.

Newer treatment options for PCOS, and potentially Syndrome X, offer more hope with fewer long-term risks. One promising option is the use of Glucophage (metformin) and other agents that improve glucose intolerance–insulin resistance. Metformin has been shown in a number of recent studies to lower abnormal insulin levels, improve triglyceride and cholesterol abnormalities, improve ovulation (and thereby fertility) and help decrease risk of diabetes and adverse changes in blood vessels. In a 1998 study published in *The New England Journal of Medicine,* 90 percent of the women who took metformin either ovulated spontaneously or with help from the fertility drug Clomid but only 12 percent of the women taking a placebo pill had ovulatory cycles, even if they also took Clomid. More studies are needed on the safety of these medications for the developing fetus, so women trying to get pregnant who want to be treated with metformin should discuss these issues with a fertility specialist.

We have used metformin quite successfully for many PCOS patients that we see at our HER Place offices. Although it is a drug more often used to help young women struggling with infertility, our gynecologist and I have found that it works well to reduce insulin resistance (and its complications) in women who are not necessarily trying to become pregnant. We often use metformin for our patients with PCOS and Syndrome X to help reduce the excess insulin that makes it so hard for these patients to lose weight. In turn, being able to lose weight helps decrease many of the risk factors for both diabetes and heart disease. Because the multiple health risks of PCOS and Syndrome X are so severe, I think metformin has an important role in the treatment of women with suspected PCOS, Syndrome X, or insulin resistance due to weight gain alone, without PCOS. In our experience, bothersome side effects have been relatively uncommon. We usually start metformin at a lower dose than the recommended amount because we find it works well and causes fewer side effects if we start low and increase slowly. Using it this way, side effects tend to be fairly mild (headaches, nausea, diarrhea) and typically disappear with just dietary changes and decreasing the dose.

It is encouraging to me that these newer treatments are so promising, with less reported risks so far than what has been seen with the more aggressive treatments I described earlier. I include all of this information in the heart disease chapter because both PCOS and Syndrome X are conditions that increase heart disease risks in younger women, and the common symptoms of missed menstrual periods, increased body/face hair, and weight gain are often minimized by physicians. If you have these symptoms, or had them when you were younger, keep in mind that PCOS is the culprit about 80–90 percent of the time, and you should be carefully assessed for heart disease risk factors now. The good news is that both disorders are very treatable problems *if they are recognized early* and an *integrated* approach to treatment begun.

Progesterone and Progestin Effects in Cardiovascular Disease

The synthetic progestins have been added to postmenopausal hormone therapy regimens in order to reduce the risk of endometrial cancer of the uterus from taking estrogen alone. The drawback has been that the progestins have tended to offset the estrogen benefits on heart disease risks and to cause significant unwanted side effects such as breast tenderness, bloating, weight gain, loss of sex drive, and depression. These problems were particularly marked when higher doses of Provera (the standard progestin used in the United States) were common. The typical dose of Provera has been 10 mg daily for ten to fifteen days a month. Menopause specialists are now recommending that Provera be decreased to 5 mg daily for a cyclic regimen ten to fourteen days a month, and 2.5 mg if given every day for a continuous regimen. But even at these lower doses, there is still the potential to reduce estrogen benefits on the various heart disease factors I listed above.

To help you understand the concern, keep in mind that all progestins (even natural progesterone) have the potential to **lower the beneficial HDL cholesterol,** and also adversely affect glucose-insulin regulation and increase triglycerides, all of which are other potential heart disease risk factors. It was over a decade ago that we recognized that HDL was more important than total cholesterol in estimating CVD risk, but many physicians still only measure total cholesterol and don't check the HDL. How does this omission affect you? Consider the following examples of two different women and their heart disease risk, and then ask yourself, is it important to know *my* HDL?

- A forty-two-year-old woman, total cholesterol 250
- A forty-nine-year-old woman, total cholesterol 250

Many women and their physicians would be alarmed by the total cholesterol and may rush into taking expensive lipid-lowering medications with the potential for side effects. But, *one* of these women really doesn't need lipid-lowering medication, and *one* of them needs to start it immediately. These two women have very different risks for heart disease. How do you tell which is which? The key lies in their HDL level and calculation of their risk ratios from the total cholesterol number divided by their HDL number.

The forty-nine-year-old has an HDL of 89, giving her a CHOL/HDL *ratio* of only 2.8, about *half* average risk of heart disease. Her excellent HDL is about thirty points above the average for a woman her age. Why is her HDL so high? She is a nonsmoker, takes 17-beta estradiol alone (she had a hysterectomy several years ago so doesn't need a progestin or progesterone), and she exercises regularly. She does not need any cholesterol-lowering medication.

The forty-two-year-old has an HDL of only 25, giving her a CHOL/HDL *ratio* of 10, more than *four times* average risk of heart disease in a woman, and a risk that requires immediate and aggressive intervention to help prevent a sudden heart attack or stroke. Why is this *younger* woman's HDL so low? She is a smoker, doesn't exercise, and has an estradiol level of less than 35, well below the level needed to maintain a healthy HDL level. Her low estradiol is likely a result of cigarette smoking suppressing her ovaries, increasing her risk for early menopause. Obviously, she needs to stop smoking now, but she really does need to be started on lipid-lowering medication right away to quickly bring up her HDL and to help reverse existing damage to the arteries. She is someone who would have even more risk if she were started on the standard menopause "cookbook" approach with Premarin and Provera or PremPro, due to the adverse effects of the synthetic progestin further decreasing her "good" cholesterol.

In addition to decreasing the HDL cholesterol, the adverse effects of progestins on the cholesterol profile are related to several factors:

- *Duration of the dose.* Taking the progestin every day, even at a lower dose, has a more negative effect on HDL, triglycerides, insulin, and glucose than does taking the progestin for only ten to fourteen days a month on a cyclic regimen.
- *Degree of androgen-like properties.* Natural progesterone and the new non-androgenic synthetic progestins (e.g., desogestrel) so far seem not to have as much of the unwanted effect of decreasing HDL, particularly if given transdermally, sublingually, or vaginally and if the doses used are in the therapeutic range for postmenopausal use. (This statement *does not apply* to the much higher pharmacologic doses of natural progesterone often used in treating PMS. I will say more about this issue later).
- *Route of administration.* Transdermal, sublingual, and vaginal types of progesterone bypass the liver and appear not to have as much of the adverse effects on HDL cholesterol, triglycerides, insulin, and glucose that occur when the progestin is taken orally. Oral progestin therapy is standard in the United States. The non-oral routes listed above are more the norm in Europe, where there are also a variety of forms of natural progesterone options as well.

The Postmenopause Estrogen Progestin Intervention (PEPI) studies, a three-year investigation into the benefits and risks of various hormone regimens, was the first major study in the United States to use natural micronized progesterone as one of the therapy regimens and to compare its effectiveness with the standard progestin, Provera. Investigators found that the natural micronized progesterone protected the endometrium (not surprising, since that's what it did for women before menopause!) and did not have the drawback of decreasing HDL to the degree seen with Provera. In fact, micronized progesterone *preserves 60 percent more* of the estrogen-related benefits on cardiovascular measures than does Provera. Another finding of concern in the PEPI study was that the two-hour insulin and two-hour glucose levels were both significantly increased with the MPA (Provera) group, which is another mechanism by which progestins increase risk of both heart disease and diabetes. The results of this study were hailed as a major breakthrough in this country by those of us who have long been advocating the use of natural progesterone for postmenopausal regimens. Hopefully, now that Prometrium and Crinone brands of natural progesterone are available in the United States, we will now see more physicians using progesterone.

Natural progesterone, when given in the low doses currently recommended for menopausal regimens (these are as follows: Prometrium 200 mg orally for ten–fourteen days a month, or 100 mg orally if given every day, or Crinone vaginally 40 mg every other day for six doses a month) has not been found to have the adverse effects on cholesterol, triglycerides, glucose, or insulin that are seen with the synthetic progestins. But there is an important caution to any of you readers who are using natural progesterone in the much higher doses that are being recommended for PMS therapy. Doses in excess of 300 mg a day orally (or creams containing more than 20–40 mg a day) give blood levels of progesterone that are as high as those found in the *third trimester of pregnancy*. These higher doses of progesterone for PMS may cause high blood glucose and worsening glucose control in diabetics or women with insulin resistance, and may also cause high triglycerides, high cholesterol, and higher-than-normal insulin production. These changes are all known to increase risk of heart disease later in life. The problem is that many PMS specialists who recommend such high doses of natural progesterone are not checking serum levels of progesterone or monitoring the cholesterol-triglyceride profile or checking for changes in fasting glucose and insulin, so they miss the fact that these problems are happening.

If you doubt what I am saying about the potential for such problems with high-dose progesterone, simply recall two common pregnancy-related problems most women have heard about: (1) pregnancy-induced ("gestational") diabetes, and (2) toxemia or pre-eclampsia, a very severe form of high blood pressure that can occur in the latter part of pregnancy. These two problems tend to occur in the last stages of pregnancy when progesterone levels are at their highest. So, although I encourage you to consider using natural progesterone instead of synthetic progestins for your HRT in an acceptable dose range (unless you have a medical reason that requires the potency of the synthetic progestins), it is important to be careful about using excess doses or progesterone for other purposes or prolonged use, especially if you are overweight or have diabetes, hypertension, or elevated cholesterol or triglycerides.

Sadly, the PEPI study did not have any groups that were using the natural, bio-identical 17-beta estradiol form of estrogen women have before menopause. Premarin was the only estrogen used throughout all five groups in the PEPI study, so some of the better outcomes on heart disease risk that have been found in other studies since that time (described above in the estrogen section) were not seen in the PEPI study. But even using Premarin as a less desirable form of estrogen, the overall PEPI results showed a 30 percent decrease in heart disease risk, even factoring in the negative effects of the synthetic progestin, MPA. Overall, the PEPI study showed that there was no increase (or decrease) in blood pressure for women on estrogen, whether with or without a progestin. This finding is in contrast to other studies using transdermal 17-beta estradiol that have shown consistent *decreases* in blood pressure in women on estradiol compared to women on no hormone therapy. Since Dr. Whitehead and his group showed many years ago that *increased* blood pressure was a potential side effect of the excess oral estrogen load for the liver when using conjugated horse-derived estrogens, the lack of better effects on blood pressure in the PEPI study is not surprising.

One finding of the PEPI study will be of interest to those of you worried about weight gain with hormone therapy. Even when the women were given the types of hormones *most likely* to cause weight gain (Premarin and Provera), *none of the groups in the PEPI study of women who were taking hormones showed a gain in weight.* The only group that gained weight over the several years of the study was the placebo group on **no** hormones! This also fits with more recent data showing that postmenopausal women on no hormones consistently have higher percentage body fat and more "middle body" obesity than do women taking hormones after menopause. Keeping your healthy *pre*menopausal balance of estradiol, estrone, testosterone, and DHEA is an important part of successfully managing our tendency to get fatter as we get older. I have addressed more on this subject in chapter 17.

The HERS Study: Points to Clarify the Controversy and Confusion

Have you heard the headline saying something like "estrogen therapy shown *not* to help women with heart disease"? Were you confused by this, especially after all the previous positive reports about estrogen therapy *reducing* the risk of heart disease? Most people were. What's the scoop? The Heart, and Estrogen-Progestin Replacement Study (HERS for short) was a large, randomized, prospective study designed to test the effects of a combined daily estrogen-progestin regimen (they used PremPro) in postmenopausal women *who already had coronary heart disease* to see if the hormone therapy would prevent further cardiovascular events, such as heart attack. The HERS trial lasted for just over four years, with half of the women taking a placebo and half of the women taking PremPro containing 0.625 mg of conjugated horse-derived estrogens with 2.5 mg medroxyprogesterone acetate or MPA (the progestin in Provera and Cycrin). None of the women were given estrogen alone to compare estrogen by itself with estrogen plus synthetic progestin. To everyone's surprise, including the researchers themselves, during the first year of the study, women taking the combined HRT had 50 percent *more* heart attacks than women taking placebo, and 3 percent more clotting problems. An interesting pattern emerged later in the study: During the *last* two years of the study, women on the combined HRT had 40 percent *fewer* heart attacks, results that were more in keeping with other studies showing hormone therapy has beneficial effects to reduce heart disease. HERS participants taking combined HRT had an 11 percent reduction in LDL ("bad") cholesterol and a 10 percent increase in HDL ("good") cholesterol. These were positive changes, though not as good as the improvements in cholesterol measures seen with estrogen alone in other studies, particularly when 17-beta estradiol is used. Since it takes on average about 1.5 to 2 years before a reduction in cholesterol will show a decrease in heart disease risk, it may be that the women in the HERS trial were not in the study long enough to see the full benefit of hormone therapy.

But there are other serious problems with the HERS design that I think have been ignored or glossed over by both the consumer and the medical articles on this important subject. Remember the studies I described earlier from Drs. Campbell and Whitehead, published in 1982? They clearly showed that the horse-derived estrogens had the potential to have much worse effects on heart disease risk measures (renin substrate, blood pressure, fibrinogen, elevation of triglycerides, et cetera) than did our own natural 17-beta estradiol. That information has been around almost twenty years, and yet the HERS researchers *still* chose to use only the horse-derived estrogen in the study. The blood-vessel-damaging effects of MPA have also been known for many years: Progestins like MPA *reduce* the beneficial effects of estrogen on a number of heart disease risk factors such as the good cholesterol levels, blood vessel wall elasticity, fibrinogen, and others. Natural progesterone is an available therapeutic option,

and the PEPI studies published in 1995 showed that natural progesterone preserved at least 60 percent of the benefit gained by estrogen. Why wasn't natural progesterone used in the HERS trial?
Again, the HERS researchers *still* chose to use only the synthetic
progestin in the study. No wonder consumers were confused. It is
clear that the news articles didn't give all this additional background. As a consumer, you should be aware that this study was
funded by a grant from the company who makes PremPro. To those
of us who have long advocated use of more natural forms of hormones for women, it was actually encouraging news to see our concerns demonstrated so clearly in the HERS results.

In using PremPro, HERS researchers were giving a potentially
damaging combination hormone product to women *who already
had heart disease*. Progestins are known constrictors of blood vessels, which tends to raise blood pressure and reduce blood flow—
not a good combination in women who already had heart disease.
And then we wonder why the women who participated had *more
heart attacks* the first year. It seems odd that so many medical professionals expressed surprise at the findings. It seems to me that this
result could have been predicted if someone had thought carefully
about information that has been available for quite a few years. I
was appalled that a study like this even passed the pretrial design
review, with what has been published in the past about potential
problems with daily progestins and heart disease, and also what has
been published about potential adverse effects of oral horse-derived
estrogens. I cited other studies earlier in this chapter that had shown
significant cardiovascular benefits from using transdermal 17-beta
estradiol and natural progesterone. Why weren't these options considered, especially since the women being signed up for the study
had *existing heart disease*? It seems that would have been a safer
course of action as a first step.

There has been debate in the medical literature since the HERS
trial results were published about why the early *rise* in heart attacks
occurred, and was followed later in the study by a decline in the
number of women who had heart attacks. My own hypothesis, and
one that I think fits with our current science, is that the women who
had early heart attacks represented the group who were more sensitive to the adverse effects of the constant daily synthetic progestin.
As time went on, this more vulnerable group had been "selected
out" with their heart attacks, and the remaining women may have
simply been less sensitive to the adverse effects of the progestins. I
also think that as time went on in the study, the beneficial effects of
estrogen began to take effect, counterbalancing the negative effects
of MPA, and resulting in a decrease in the number of heart attacks
by the last two years of the study. One OB/GYN from Europe wrote

a letter to *The International Menopause Journal* saying that he thought the dose of the MPA used in the HERS study was too high for women with established heart disease and was higher than he used in his practice.

What's the "take-home" message for you? I think if you already have heart disease, or any of the risk factors I summarized earlier, you would be wise to avoid using a continuous combined horse-derived estrogen and synthetic progestin product like PremPro. If you are already on PremPro and have high blood pressure, high triglycerides, glucose intolerance or diabetes, insulin resistance, high cholesterol, or a history of heart problems, I would urge you to talk with your physician about changing to the bioidentical human forms of estradiol and progesterone to avoid increasing your risk of heart attack or stroke. I think data from a number of other well-done studies over a number of years clearly demonstrate that a nonoral (i.e., transdermal or patch) 17-beta estradiol, alone or with natural progesterone (for women with a uterus), have a much better profile of benefit on multiple cardiovascular risk factors.

Testosterone: Pros and Cons for Heart Disease Risks

I talked in chapter 6 about the role of adding testosterone for some women after menopause, particularly if they have had an abrupt hormone drop from having a surgical menopause with the ovaries removed and are experiencing marked loss of libido. I do think this important hormone has a place in the options we offer women, but it is potentially a problem if a woman has a high risk of heart disease and has abnormal levels of total cholesterol with low HDL. In such a woman, *oral* testosterone, or even transdermal or injections using high doses, may *worsen* the lipid profile by further increasing total cholesterol and *decreasing* the good HDL. For this reason, anyone on testosterone supplements must have regular monitoring of cholesterol, HDL, LDL, and triglyceride levels. I have not found the doses I typically use for women to cause these unwanted changes in cholesterol, but I am using *lower doses* than are often given to women. In controlled studies by Dr. Christopher Longcope, when testosterone was administered continuously in low doses (1.25 and 2.5 mg daily) with estrogen, there were no significant changes in cardiovascular or liver measures, including cholesterol profile.

Testosterone may also increase blood pressure, but this is also related to dose and route of administration and usually only happens at higher doses than I am suggesting. Elevated blood pressure is also more common with the more potent synthetic, chemically different forms than it is with the bio-identical, micronized "natural" testosterone I am suggesting women use. In addition, newer studies, many done in European centers, have shown that when given with the right balance of estradiol, testosterone actually helps maintain the normal mechanisms involved in vasodilatation that serve to help lower blood pressure. If given alone, testosterone and other androgens such as DHEA appear to *promote* buildup artery-clogging plaque (atherosclerosis) and also cause high blood pressure in women. If androgens such as testosterone or DHEA are given *with* estrogen, however, they have the *opposite* effect on the arterial wall and actually help *prevent* buildup of plaque in the arteries. We now have a number of controlled studies showing that *low-dose* testosterone therapy *does not cause increased blood pressure* in most women.

Transdermal patches of natural testosterone would be the most physiologically natural delivery system for restoring optimal testosterone levels for women and would avoid many of the unwanted side effects of oral testosterone, but we do not yet have such a product approved for use in women in the United States. Testosterone patches are available for men, and they work quite well. I have used those extensively in our program **HIS Corner** at **HER Place** for men who are experiencing the hormone decline of "andropause." As a general guideline, for men or women, I think if you are taking testosterone as part of your hormone "enhancement" program, it is a good health practice to have your cholesterol, HDL, LDL, and blood pressure checked at least annually as part of your usual checkup.

In the past, medical practitioners and women have been taught that heart disease does not strike women until after menopause. Recent research, and my own clinical experience with midlife women, has shown that evaluation of ovary hormonal status may be more crucial in premenopausal women than we realized. Keep in mind that women *start* having increased risk for heart disease at whatever age they become *menopausal based on endocrine function, not just chronological age.* A woman who has either natural or surgical menopause at age forty, begins having the cholesterol and other changes that increase risk of heart disease. Those changes don't wait to start until she reaches fifty-five. Testing for the endocrine factor allows us to identify women at risk of cardiovascular disease *at a time when risk factors are reversible* and when lifestyle changes possibly along with hormone therapy can make the most difference.

"Susu" is a woman I first saw for a consult when she was thirty-nine. Her story illustrates many of the points I have made about the role of estradiol and testosterone balance, PCOS, and other issues in younger women related to heart disease risk. Although she was only thirty-nine when I saw her, she had already suffered *three* very serious myocardial infarctions (MI) and almost died during the third one. Her first MI was at age thirty-six. Her story is quite touching, and very meaningful to me. Another patient of mine, along with a friend of Susu's, had taken a copy of my book showing the effects of estrogen on the heart to Susu's husband at the hospital where she was in ICU, in a coma. The doctors had told Susu's family that it was "only a matter of time" before she died, because she wasn't responding to the medications they customarily used for acute MI. Because Susu's friend knew that Susu's heart attacks had always come during her menstrual periods when estrogen is lowest, the two women and Susu's husband shared my chapter on estrogen and the heart with Susu's cardiologist, asking that he consider trying an estradiol patch for Susu. The cardiologist read the material I had summarized about estradiol's many positive effects on heart function and said, "Nothing else is working, we may as well try it." To everyone's amazement, including the doctor's, Susu began recovering. Her "ejection fraction" that had been at critically low values, began increasing within hours of having the Climara patch applied. Slowly she began coming out of the woods and was able to be discharged home.

She had written me about her story at the time she scheduled her first consult, and I was myself overcome with emotion when I read this letter and found that my writing had such a profound impact on a young woman's life. When she was well enough to travel and come to our Texas office, I was amazed at all of the progress she had made since her near-death experience. I was able to review her serum hormone levels with her and show her *why* the estradiol patch had helped so much: Her own menstrual Day 1 estradiol was barely detectable, and her free and total testosterone and DHEA were all quite high, as were her total and LDL cholesterol, triglycerides, and insulin. After a careful evaluation by our gynecologist and me, we were certain she had PCOS as the underlying cause of her cardiovascular disease. It is now three years later, and she is doing well as a more active mom able to be involved with her children and her life again. She is on hormones designed to keep her as steady as possible, lower the androgens, and prevent the falls in estradiol that triggered the severe coronary artery spasms leading to her heart attacks. She has made marked changes in her diet and is following a plan designed to minimize insulin resistance, which has helped her lose the excess weight gradually. And, she is now able to engage in a regular walking program to rebuild her strength and stamina, as well as further improve the insulin resistance. With her involvement in the Internet support groups for PCOS, she has become an avid spokesperson to help other women understand this disorder and get proper evaluation of these hormone issues.

So in summary, I encourage all women, and their physicians, to take into account the *premenopausal* hormone changes, which can be readily checked as part of an overall approach to your health care for women. If you think you are beginning menopause (regardless of how old you are), or if you have a condition like PCOS that causes excess production of androgens and increases your risk of heart disease, and you have a significant family history of heart disease, it is important to ask your physicians to do a simple blood test of FSH and estradiol on Day 1 or 2 of your menstrual bleeding, along with the usual metabolic chemistry panel and cholesterol profile (make sure it includes HDL). This can help identify possible premenopausal changes adding to your cardiovascular disease risk.

If you already have high cholesterol and/or high blood pressure, it is even more important to ask your physician to check your hormone levels so that this can be considered in your therapy. We have good screening and treatment techniques now available for reproductive cancers, so it is crucial that you *also* understand and address the greater risks of disability and premature death from osteoporosis, heart disease, and strokes, which increase as estrogen declines. Today's studies are clear that women *still* seriously *underestimate* their risk of heart disease—most women are off by a factor of *thirty-fold* in their perception of risk of breast cancer compared to their risk of heart disease. If you do not perceive your risk accurately, then you will not take the steps to prevent a problem, so it is crucial for you to have an accurate picture of your individual health risks.

I have found it can be very rewarding as a physician to explain these midlife endocrine changes and their effects on blood pressure, lipid profile, palpitations, and overall risk of heart disease. My women patients have been interested and even excited to learn about these connections and have been even more motivated, by the *knowledge*, to incorporate needed dietary and exercise approaches and to consider whatever hormonal therapy may be desired or appropriate. It also adds to your own sense of taking control of your health by exploring your many options after having a medical assessment that focuses on what makes *your body different* from a man's.

CHAPTER 14

Breast Cancer: Controversies and Risks You Aren't Told, Options to Explore

The Hormone Controversy

Breast cancer is the number one fear expressed by women when discussing hormone therapy, whether referring to birth control pill use or postmenopausal hormone use. A great deal of this fear was fueled by the way that newspapers and magazines headlined (and misinterpreted) findings from the "Swedish Study" in 1989 and the subsequent U.S. Nurses' Health Study a few years later, along with continuing widespread features on breast cancer in newspapers, magazines, and menopause books. Major headlines again occurred across the United States in January 2000 with reports of an observational study suggesting that estrogen-progestin combination therapy had a higher risk of breast cancer than expected (women in this study group were using Premarin and Provera rather than the natural, bio-identical hormones I have recommended throughout my book). What's behind the headlines? Who do you believe? What are your real risks? Let's examine these issues.

It turns out that most of the furor was created *not* by the actual study results, but rather by misinterpretation of preliminary *partial* results by the media and some women's health authors, as I explain later in the chapter. Further confusion has been created by the failure of media articles to list the specific types of hormones being used, since there are many chemical differences among the various products. My desire in this chapter is to help you understand more of the full story behind these headlines and to help you put your individual risk in perspective, as well as to give you options for types of hormone therapies that are less likely to accentuate the known risk factors for breast cancer. I want to help you make some sense of all this and be able to make intelligent decisions for yourself. My goal is that you not feel terrified by all this, but are able to make your decisions based on balanced, up-to-date, solid scientific information.

In women's magazines targeted to all age groups, breast cancer is the number one health topic, leading many women to the mistaken conclusion that this is the only, or at least most important, health concern that we face. This is a classic example of the distortion of health information to generate a sense of fear that in turn sells products (TV ratings, magazine issues, newspapers, books, etc.). Not all women are at the same risk for developing breast cancer, and not all types of breast cancer have the same degree of aggressiveness. Some women have very low risk of developing breast cancer and yet have an extremely high risk of potentially fatal heart problems. The steps to be taken to reduce risk, and the use of hormones, may be quite different, depending on just exactly what the particular health issue or disease may be. When you read articles and books or attend seminars about breast cancer, there are some important aspects of the association with women's hormones that you need to know and that are very often not mentioned.

Let me say right up front: there are two *unchangeable* risks for breast cancer: (1) being female and (2) growing older, whether you take hormones or not.

I, for one, am happy being a woman, and I would like to keep growing older. So, no matter what else you do, and no matter what decision you make about hormones, all of us women have to keep up with our screening mammograms and breast self-exams as we age. Sadly, too many women think that if they don't take hormones, their breast cancer risk goes *down* after menopause. This is not true. Even if you never take hormones, your risk of breast cancer continues to increase as you get older. I will talk more in this chapter about the various risk factors and some of the newest findings that give us all a more hopeful picture than that portrayed in the press.

At the outset, however, I really want to give you some important background on the Swedish study that fueled the fears you have today, and help you understand what happened with publicity in this country for this study. The Swedish study by L. Bergkvist and team was intended to determine the number of cases of breast cancer in women on postmenopausal hormone therapy and compare this with breast cancer incidence in a control group of post-menopausal women who were *not* on hormone therapy. There were several major flaws in the design of the study itself:

- It was a *survey* study based on questionnaires only. It was not a double-blind, clinical *prospective study* that would be the kind of study needed to clarify any *causal* connections.

- The questionnaires were sent out to 23,244 women, but there was *only an 11 percent return* on the questionnaires sent out. Yet, this 11 percent response rate was projected over the *entire 23,244* women in the sample to arrive at their conclusion about relative risk of breast cancer. I am astounded that such a small response rate would have been considered acceptable "science" for the study to be published in a major medical journal.

- The actual number of women in this sample who developed breast cancer was quite small: a total of 253 women, which is too small a study group to provide a causal connection between hormone use and later development of breast cancer.

- **The authors' conclusions on the increased risk of breast cancer with combined estrogen and progestin use was based on** *only ten patients,* another point you won't find in the media articles.

- The type of estrogen used was a *synthetic* estradiol, *estradiol valerate,* not the natural human form of 17-beta estradiol (used in Estrace, Alora, Climara Vivelle, Ortho-Prefest, Combi-Patch, and Activelle). Estradiol valerate is about *one hundred times more potent* than 17-beta estradiol, and even has a different chemical structure from 17-beta estradiol. The two estrogens act somewhat differently in the body, so we cannot make valid comparisons without adjusting for these differences.

- The study's control population had a relative risk for breast cancer of 1.6, not 1.0 as is commonly used for comparison purposes.

- Users of conjugated equine estrogens in this study (the most common estrogen used in the United States) had a relative risk of breast cancer of 1.7, which was not a statistically significant difference from the control group on no hormone therapy. This was another key point not reported in the media.

- In their paper, the authors stated: "whereas a number of the relative risks and associated trends in this investigation were statistically significant, *the number of observations on which they are based was relatively small. Some findings could be due to chance.*" I italicized the last part of the authors' quote to illustrate for you the important statement that was left out of the media reports.

- In a 1992 update publication, Bergkvist reported *corrected* relative risk data for breast cancer in the women in the study. This time, he found a relative risk of 1.0 for both the estradiol valerate group and the conjugated estrogen users. *This is exactly what the relative risk is without estrogen use.* Users of 17-beta estradiol had a relative risk of 0.9, slightly *less than* the control group on no hormones. Tragically for American women, this update was published in a British medical journal, *The Lancet,* so this crucial information, which could help reduce women's fears, did not make it into the American media.

- When Bergkvist published the full results of the initial study in 1989, it was in a more obscure medical journal (*American Journal of Epidemiology*). This time they reported that the relative breast cancer **survival rate** was significantly *higher* in the women who had received estrogen therapy. They found approximately a 40 percent *reduction in deaths from breast cancer* in the women *taking estrogen*. Most women never heard this positive part of the picture. A number of studies since that time have also shown that women on estrogen at the time of diagnosis of breast cancer have less aggressive forms of cancer, better outcomes, and longer survival times.

Why did we get such a distorted picture of the Swedish study in the U.S. press? Could it be that the scare tactics sold more magazines, newspapers, and news shows? Perhaps the authors did not want to point out their earlier incomplete information. Are you feeling angry as you read this? I was, both as a woman and as a physician sincerely trying to help women get accurate and up-to-date information. I remain concerned today that even physicians who counsel women about breast cancer risk are not aware of the above problems with the Swedish study and subsequent studies. This study and the way it was reported did more to terrify women about hormone use than any other single publication I have seen.

Another example of these same distortion tactics emerged a few years later with the release of an analysis of the Harvard Nurses Health Study describing a possible 30 percent increase in risk of breast cancer among the women taking estrogen compared to those who did not. (To put this risk in perspective, instead of seven cancers expected to occur over a ten-year period in two hundred women over age fifty-five, ten such cancers would be found if *all* the postmenopausal women were taking hormones for longer than five years.) Headlines again screamed the alarm and news magazines did sensationalized covers on the subject. And once again, the flaws in the study design was rarely brought out, and the balance of estrogen's benefits on other diseases was not portrayed accurately, if reported at all. Women were again left confused and scared.

When I looked into all this in depth, I found that the Harvard Nurses Health Study had two other important aspects that were omitted from media reports (and many women's health books today, even when written by women physicians). First, the increased breast cancer risk was **only** in the subgroup of women who used estrogen therapy *and also drank alcohol*. The increased risk *was not found* in estrogen users who did not drink alcohol. Did you know that? Most doctors don't even realize this was one of the important findings of the Nurses Health Study. As we shall see later in this chapter, regular alcohol use increases the amount of estrone, the form of estrogen associated with a higher risk of breast and endometrial cancers. You can minimize the "estrone factor" in risk for both breast cancer and endometrial cancer by (a) reducing or eliminating alcohol use, (b) by losing excess body fat, and (c) by using a transdermal form of estradiol that bypasses the liver first-pass metabolism and thereby reduces liver production of estrone. Using a transdermal estradiol instead of Premarin also eliminates the excess estrogen effect of the more potent horse-derived estrogens.

Second, another crucial point was also overlooked in the media reports on the U.S. Nurses Health Study. When I read the original publication in *The New England Journal of Medicine,* I found that the majority of hormone users in the Nurses Health Study were using Premarin for their estrogen. As I described earlier, Premarin gives you much higher levels of estrone and long-lasting horse-derived (equine) estrogens that tend to be strongly bound to breast estrogen receptors and stay in the body longer than our own ovarian estrogen, 17-beta estradiol. I find it alarming that no one seems to be addressing this issue, although I have been asking these questions in medical conferences for a number of years. I think it is imperative for us to conduct research designed to address the potential for *different effects* on breast cancer risk that may occur using *different types of estrogen* therapy (see also chapters 5 and 15). Since we don't have the same enzymes that a horse does to break down the equilin estrogens, what effect does it have on our bodies to have these estrogens remain in the body longer? Do these potent horse-derived estrogens have a greater effect than our own 17-beta estradiol to promote the growth of breast cancers? We *don't know* because leading researchers have simply failed to address these questions and have continued to assume that *all estrogens are alike.* Why hasn't this been considered as a factor in breast cancer risk? Could it be that the company that makes Premarin has so dominated the research and educational programs for physicians that no one will pursue this? If you are concerned about breast cancer risk and choose to use estrogen therapy for all the other health benefits, you can at least choose to eliminate the horse estrogens as a potential risk.

So where DO we stand with our knowledge about ERT/HRT and the risk of breast cancer? **First,** keep in mind that a *causal* connection will show up fairly quickly when there are more women using a given product. For example, in women with a uterus, it became clear within about three years of increased use of unopposed (i.e., no progesterone or progestin) estrogen that endometrial (uterine) cancer rates had risen significantly, to about eight times the previous levels. Uterine cancer rates dropped back to baseline levels as soon as doctors began adding the progestin (or progesterone) to estrogen therapy in women with a uterus. The estrogen–breast cancer issue has not shown this same pattern of significantly increased rates of breast cancer as more women are using estrogen. In fact, if you look at the national cancer data since 1960 (when birth control pills and hormone therapy for menopause first began being widely used), you see that the rates of breast cancer have been "flat," or not increasing. In 1995–96, the graph for breast cancer actually began showing a slight decline. This is not what you would expect to see if use of estrogen or birth control pills actually *caused* breast cancer. During the same period of time (1960–1996), lung cancer in women skyrocketed, as more women began smoking cigarettes, a known cause of lung cancer. Deaths from lung cancer in the United States have exceeded breast cancer deaths since 1996, although you don't hear much about it in the media.

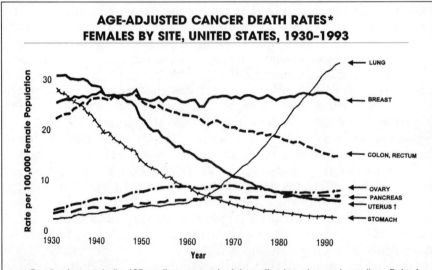

AGE-ADJUSTED CANCER DEATH RATES*
FEMALES BY SITE, UNITED STATES, 1930–1993

NOTE: Due to changes in the ICD coding, numerator information has changed over time. Rates for cancer of the uterus, ovary, lung, and colon and rectum are affected by these coding changes. Denominator date for the years 1930-1959 and 1991-1993 are based on intercensal population estimates, while denominator date for 1960-1989 are based on postcensal recalculation of estimates. Rate estimates for 1968-1989 are most likely of better quality.
* Rates per 100,000 age-adjusted to the 1970 standard United States population.
† Uterine cancer death rates are for cervix and corpus combined.

Data source: Vital Statistics of the United States, 1996.

For about forty years, researchers have been doing studies to answer the estrogen–breast cancer question, and there is still no clear-cut causal connection that has emerged, a fact that bodes well for use of hormone therapy. Analysis of worldwide studies to date by many of our leading menopause specialists, public health experts, epidemiologists, and breast cancer researchers have found that the relative risk of breast cancer in estrogen users is hovering right around 1.0, which means that estrogen is NOT acting as a carcinogen. If estrogen were acting as a carcinogen, the relative risks would be ranging from three to eight or even higher, as was seen with endometrial cancer when estrogen was given alone. If you have a uterus, the relative risk of using estrogen alone is about 8.0, very different from what is seen in the breast cancer studies. *None* of the studies to date have shown that estrogen *causes* breast cancer. What we do know is that estrogen appears to have the potential for *promoting growth* of existing breast cancers that are estrogen-sensitive. This is the end-result message of the few studies that have shown a slightly higher risk of breast cancer in women who have a long duration of hormone use after menopause. But the flip side of this is that when you are taking estrogen and develop breast cancer, the cancer tends to be less aggressive and have a better outcome in terms of survival time than what we see in breast cancers that develop in women not taking hormones. So the news is not *all* bad.

In 1979, for example, Dr. Lila Nachtigall published results of a ten-year double-blind, case-matched controlled study tracking complications that emerged after ten years of hormone replacement therapy. Dr. Nachtigall's study did not show any increased risk of breast cancer in women on estrogen and progestin. All four of the breast cancer patients in this ten-year study were women who were *nonusers* of hormones. There are a number of other studies that have shown similar results. Some studies have shown, however, that there are a few subgroups of women that appear to be at slightly higher risk for developing breast cancer with long-duration use of estrogen: smokers, regular alcohol users, those who are obese, those who have a first-degree relative with breast cancer. Clearly, with the exception of the family connection, women have a choice about whether they continue to engage in lifestyle habits that increase risk. Let's don't be so quick to blame all the risk on hormone use.

In 1999, the results of the Iowa Women's Health Study (over 37,000 women) were published in *JAMA*. The overall news about hormone use and breast cancer was positive. Dr. Trudy Bush, a Johns Hopkins epidemiologist and authority on hormone therapy and breast cancer risk, analyzed the results of the Iowa Women's Health Study and discussed these findings in an editorial. When *all* types of breast cancer were combined and then grouped by duration of use of hormones, estrogen replacement therapy was *not* associated with an increased risk of breast cancer, in either the short term (use five years or less, relative risk 1.07), or the long term (greater than five years, relative risk 1.11). In the Iowa Women's Health Study, only one type of breast cancer—invasive breast cancer with a favorable histology cell type—was found to have a slightly increased risk in women using hormone therapy. Since there is no currently accepted definition of a favorable histology type, Dr. Bush pointed out that it is possible the findings reported occurred as a result of the choice of tumor groupings and not as a result of a true association between hormonal replacement therapy and tumor occurrence. In addition, Drs. Bush and Whiteman emphasized that the study authors elected to focus almost exclusively on those cases of invasive breast cancer with a favorable histology/prognosis even though this specific type of breast cancer was seen in only 5 percent of the study population of over 37,000 women. Drs. Bush and Whiteman emphasized that unlike the association between estrogen replacement therapy and uterine cancer that was convincingly established about twenty-five years ago, the association between estrogen replacement therapy and breast cancer is still being debated because no studies have shown a clear causal connection. After in-depth examination of all the data, Drs. Bush and Whiteman concluded that "any *real* increase in the risk of breast cancer is either too small or too limited to small subgroups of women to be observed consistently in most epidemiological studies" (as was observed in such studies with estrogen therapy and uterine cancer). The overall result of the Iowa Women's Health Study was encouraging with regard to estrogen use, although many women may not have gotten this more positive message from the way the results were reported in the media.

Then in January 2000, a study was published in *JAMA* entitled "Menopausal Estrogen and Estrogen-Progestin Replacement Therapy and Breast Cancer Risk" summarizing the follow-up data on 46,355 postmenopausal women for 1980 through 1995 in the Breast Cancer Detection Demonstration Project, a nationwide breast cancer screening program. This study looked at breast cancers that were found in this group of women correlated with recency, duration, and type of hormone use. Of the 46,355 women followed there were 2,082 cases of breast cancer identified. Of the women who used hormones, the primary type of estrogen used was conjugated equine estrogens (Premarin) and the primary type of progestin used was medroxyprogesterone acetate, a synthetic progestin also known as Provera or Cycrin. The data analysis suggested that women who used a cyclic estrogen-progestin combination had a higher risk of breast cancer than women who used estrogen alone. This finding was also confirmed with a 1999 update analysis of the Swedish study mentioned earlier, in which they also found that combined hormone therapy increased the risk of breast cancer but there was no increase seen for estrogen therapy alone.

The headlines in January 2000 again screamed about hormone use increasing breast cancer risk, but once more, the media did not report the key point that the type of hormones used were ones not natural to the human body. As I have described throughout my book, there are quite significant chemical differences between our natural hormones and Premarin or Provera. It is not appropriate to extrapolate from experiences with Premarin and Provera and then say that all types of hormones, even the ones made by our own body, would have the same effects. This is the message you were not given in the news-papers and magazines. Another surprising finding you weren't told was that this increase in breast cancer risk was seen only in lean women (body mass index less than 24.4 kg/m2 or less), but there was *no increased risk* in heavier women using estrogen alone or the estrogen-progestin combination. So when you are using this infor-mation to help you in your own decisions, keep in mind that the type of hormones being used makes a difference, the type of regimen plays a role (i.e., how many days a month you take a progestin), and your body type and other health risks also have to be considered as part of the total picture.

Many women worry about hormone use if they have had fibro-cystic breasts. Keep in mind this is not considered a disease since it is now known to be a normal variation in over 60 percent of women. Benign fibrocystic changes *do not* give you a higher risk of breast cancer. An increased risk of breast cancer is found in only the subgroup of women who have biopsy-proven atypical or proliferative changes in the breasts. But even for women with atypical hyperplasia kind of fibrocystic changes, many menopause and cancer specialists feel that adding estrogen in the postmenopausal years does not increase their risk further. These women need close scrutiny *with or without* estrogen therapy.

Another way to better understand the estrogen and breast can-cer debate is to look at the pattern of breast cancer in women who *do not take any hormones* after menopause, and compare the pat-tern in breast cancer with the pattern seen in an estrogen-dependent cancer, endometrial (uterine) cancer. Dr. Don Gambrell, a leading menopause and cancer researcher, has summarized these cancer pat-terns in the graph on the following page.

Since so many women are fearful that hormone therapy *causes* cancer, I want to emphasize that this graph shows data from women who are *not* taking hormones after menopause. This chart shows ages twenty to ninety on the horizontal line, and on the vertical line is the incidence of cancer per 100,000 women. Look first at the line for breast cancer. Breast cancer rates continue to increase as we get older, with 80 percent of all breast cancers occurring *after* menopause. A crucial point here is that, **even in women on *no* hor-mone therapy, postmenopausal women are the highest-risk group for breast cancer.** Next look at the line for endometrial (uterine) cancer. Here we know that the risk is directly increased by high estrogen levels over prolonged periods of time. Uterine cancer rates

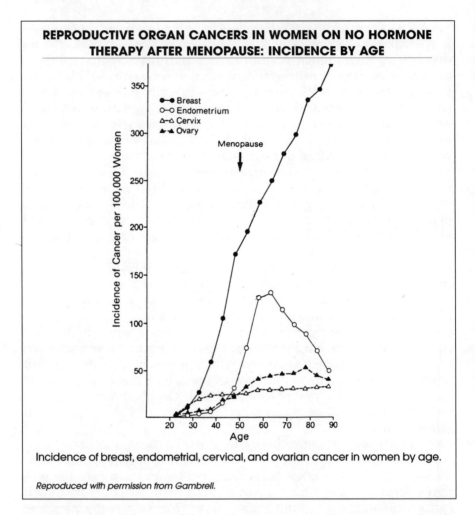

REPRODUCTIVE ORGAN CANCERS IN WOMEN ON NO HORMONE THERAPY AFTER MENOPAUSE: INCIDENCE BY AGE

- ●—● Breast
- ○—○ Endometrium
- △—△ Cervix
- ▲—▲ Ovary

Menopause

Incidence of Cancer per 100,000 Women

Age

Incidence of breast, endometrial, cervical, and ovarian cancer in women by age.

Reproduced with permission from Gambrell.

rise through a woman's life until menopause, when estrogen levels drop. This is what you would expect with an estrogen-dependent cancer: it will decrease in frequency in a woman who is not taking any estrogen after menopause as estrogen levels diminish over the following years. If a woman with a uterus takes estrogen, she also takes a progestin or progesterone in order to protect the uterus, and then there is no increased risk of endometrial cancer.

Now compare the lines for breast cancer and uterine cancer. IF breast cancer were *caused* by estrogen, we would see a pattern like the one for endometrial cancer in women after menopause. As you can see, this is not the case. Clearly the two graph lines are different, and breast cancer has a *rising* rate when the body's *estrogen is decreasing*. This is one of the characteristics of breast cancer that helps us know that estrogen is not the primary causative factor.

What about ovarian and cervical cancers? The evidence is that hormones are not the major risks for these cancers. They are both diseases of aging. In addition to the increase seen with aging, cervical cancer is now known to be a sexually transmitted disease in younger women who have had multiple sexual partners. Cervical cancer is thought to be caused by the human papilloma virus (HPV) and the herpes virus. Regular annual Pap smears help to detect cervical cancer early when it is easily treatable. Death rates from cervical cancer have dropped dramatically as Pap tests have become routine preventive care for women. Ovarian cancer is now understood to have a significant genetic component as well as being related to aging. It is crucial that you know whether you have a family history of ovarian cancer so that you can be more closely monitored. Cigarette smoking and use of infertility drugs have also been associated with an increase in later risk of ovarian cancer. Ovarian cancer is hard to diagnose and tends to spread early in its course, so it is particularly important to know your risk factors. Women at high risk for ovarian cancer may be wise to consider using birth control pills for several years, since this has been shown to decrease risk of ovarian cancer by 40–50 percent.

There is another dimension to this whole issue about hormones and breast cancer that is important for you to consider as you make your own decision about hormone use. *Death rates* from breast cancer have *not increased* in women taking estrogen at the time of diagnosis, a point frequently not mentioned in the media. There are a number of studies that have shown women taking estrogen actually may have a better outlook (prognosis), and longer survival time than women who were not taking estrogen at the time of diagnosis. Something, as yet undetermined, about taking estrogen seems to reduce the likelihood of developing more aggressive forms of breast and endometrial cancer. In addition, even though more women are now using hormones (either as birth control pills or menopausal hormone therapy), death rates from breast cancer in the United States have actually *declined* by 6 percent, a trend that began about 1995. What contributes to the observed decline in death rates? There is now better identification of other risk factors such as alcohol use, lack of exercise, obesity, and high-fat diets; women are becoming better at making lifestyle changes to reduce cancer risk; there is much better technology available for early detection of small, stage I breast cancers; there is better understanding of the different types of breast cancer; and there are more varied and more effective treatment options.

For 1989 through 1994, the above figures show statistically significant improvements in survival for all forms of cancers in white women compared to the 1974–76 time period. For African-American women, there has been improvement in survival for breast

WOMEN'S 5-YEAR SURVIVAL RATES BY CANCER TYPE					
Site	**White**		**African American**		**All Races**
	1974–76	1989–94	1974–76	1989–94	1974–76	1989–94
Breast	75%	87%	63%	71%	75%	85%
Cervix	70%	72%	64%	59%	69%	70%
Uterus	89%	87%	61%	54%	88%	84%
Ovary	37%	50%	41%	46%	37%	50%

Source: National Cancer Institutes, Epidemiology and End Results Program, 1998

and ovarian cancers during this same time period. When looking at all races of women in the United States, we have seen improvements in survival rates for all but uterine cancer. Even though further gains are needed, these are certainly encouraging results. Keep in mind that the *improvements in survival* times with various cancers are happening at a time when more women in this country are choosing to use hormone therapy after menopause, so the picture is certainly not nearly as negative as women are led to believe by the media.

The bottom line? As of this writing, studies throughout the world to date *do not show that estrogen itself is acting as a carcinogen*. Estrogen, whether produced in the body or taken as a hormone supplement, can *enhance growth* of an existing estrogen-sensitive tumor. To date, the majority of medical studies also *do not show* a significant increase in risk of breast cancer in women who use birth control pills or women who take postmenopausal estrogen therapy alone, unless women are also drinking alcohol on a regular daily basis and are using Premarin as the type of estrogen (the only estrogen group in the Nurses Health Study who had an increased risk of breast cancer). Several studies have now shown an increased risk of breast cancer in women using Premarin-Provera type cyclic combination therapy (Nurses Health Study, the Breast Cancer Detection Demonstration Project, and the Swedish cohort study). In these studies, the majority of women used the synthetic progestin for fifteen days or less per month and this is the pattern of use that appears to increase breast cancer risk. It is not yet clear whether using combined estrogen-progestin therapy *every day* causes the same increase in risk. Many physicians are now recommending cycling with progestin less often than once a month, perhaps only three–four times a year, to shed the uterine lining and reduce the risk of endometrial cancer while minimizing the progestin effects on the breast. This approach is logical, and women like having fewer periods, but it will be helpful to see what the long-term studies show with regard to effects on breast cancer risk.

Since breast cancer is a slow-growing form of cancer and may be present for many years before detection, some specialists feel that the estrogen effect to increase growth rate may actually have an indirect benefit: if an existing tumor grows more rapidly, it is likely to be discovered sooner when it can be effectively treated. Also keep in mind the point I made earlier that women who are taking estrogen at the time of diagnosis of breast cancer typically have less aggressive types of cancer and live longer than women who are not taking estrogen when the diagnosis is made.

A very few studies have found that postmenopausal estrogen therapy, used longer than twenty years, may *possibly* contribute to a *slight* increase in breast cancer risk. This slight increase does not translate into a large number of additional cancers, as shown in the summary graph below. There are still far more deaths from heart disease and osteoporosis-related complications than there are from breast cancer, so the picture is certainly more positive than newspapers, magazines, and some menopause books have presented. The bottom line is that we all have an increased risk of disease and death as we get older. The important point is to do what we can to reduce the risks as much as possible, particularly for those that are preventable with lifestyle change and appropriate use of bio-identical natural hormones.

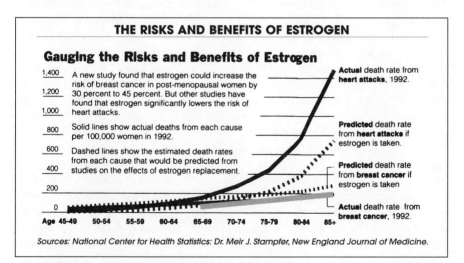

THE RISKS AND BENEFITS OF ESTROGEN

Gauging the Risks and Benefits of Estrogen

A new study found that estrogen could increase the risk of breast cancer in post-menopausal women by 30 percent to 45 percent. But other studies have found that estrogen significantly lowers the risk of heart attacks.

Solid lines show actual deaths from each cause per 100,000 women in 1992.

Dashed lines show the estimated death rates from each cause that would be predicted from studies on the effects of estrogen replacement.

Actual death rate from **heart attacks**, 1992.

Predicted death rate from **heart attacks** if estrogen is taken.

Predicted death rate from **breast cancer** if estrogen is taken

Actual death rate from **breast cancer**, 1992.

Age 45-49   50-54   55-59   60-64   65-69   70-74   75-79   80-84   85+

Sources: National Center for Health Statistics: Dr. Meir J. Stampfer, New England Journal of Medicine.

What is my recommendation? Each of you reading this needs to take the following steps:

1. Determine with your health care professional what your **individual risk** picture is for the various diseases that increase in women after menopause. This assessment will be based on your family

history, your current objective health measures such as bone density, urine bone markers, lipid profile, body mass index, diabetes risk, breast cancer risk, and your lifestyle habits.

2. Weigh the potential benefits of hormone therapy against the risks. This "risk-benefit" analysis should be based on medically sound, up-to-date information, not fear-based on what you read on the Internet or a in consumer health book or heard from a friend.

3. Take your own "values inventory" to determine for yourself what quality-of-life aspects are important to you that may be helped by hormone therapy.

4. Decide what things you worry about the most for your long-term health. Here, each woman will be different. One of my patients, who has severe bone loss, is absolutely terrified of taking estrogen, even though I know it would help prevent further bone loss. I respect her beliefs and I did not push her to take estrogen. I recommended a variety of other medication and lifestyle approaches to preserve bone and she is happy with this choice. Then there was the woman who was more afraid of losing her mind function and developing Alzheimers than of developing breast cancer. She said *"I can be me if I don't have my breast, but I lose everything that is uniquely me if I lose my brain with Alzheimers."* For this second woman, taking estrogen was very important to her feeling of being able to do something positive to reduce the risk of a disease she feared. If you have a family history of colon cancer but no breast cancer, taking estrogen may reduce your risk of colon cancer by as much as 50 percent, quite a significant amount.

Even for women who have had successfully treated breast cancer, there may come a time when an individual woman may want to use estrogen, and I think we as physicians should respect these women's right to choose a course of action they prefer. Two examples came up recently in my own practice. A woman in her fifties who seven years ago had breast cancer and now has severe osteoporosis and back pain, said to me: *"I am terrified of growing older and having even worse osteoporosis and living in such pain. It didn't do me any good to survive the breast cancer if I have to live like this, but my doctors don't listen to me. None of them will prescribe estrogen for me because I have had breast cancer. Will you prescribe it for me?"* Her values and desires for her life are clearly important and I feel I must take this into account in working with her as her professional health care partner. She has decided she wants to restart estrogen therapy, and I have agreed to prescribe the safest form I know, transdermal 17-beta estradiol, rather than one of the mixed or animal-derived estrogen products.

Another woman, now seventy-four and a five-year breast cancer survivor, asked our gynecologist to prescribe estrogen therapy for her because of the way she felt. She had tried various antidepressants and other approaches, without any real improvement and with a lot of problematic side effects. When I saw her for a follow-up appointment two months later, she said: *"I am so much better than I was. I have more energy now, I don't have the dizzy spells I did. The estrogen has been the biggest help. I can concentrate better, my thinking is so much clearer. It has pulled me out of the biggest slump. I was waiting to die . . . I don't have that feeling in my head of being off in another world, off in space. I didn't know hormones were so powerful. Thinking of the alternative, I'd rather have better quality of life—I'd rather have one clear day than live a week longer with that fog. Even though I survived the breast cancer, my life wasn't worth living. I was like a zombie. I didn't care much about anything. That wasn't a good way to live. I knew it wasn't normal to be that way. I'm glad I made this decision."*

At this time, the role of estrogen therapy in breast cancer survivors is unclear. Researchers at MD Anderson Cancer Center in Texas have undertaken a randomized prospective trial of conjugated equine estrogen (0.0625 mg) versus placebo in a selected group of breast cancer survivors to determine the effect of estrogen on breast cancer recurrence. At the 1999 follow-up analysis of outcomes after a median time of forty months, one patient (2.6 percent) taking estrogen developed a new breast cancer and fourteen patients (5.0 percent) *not* taking estrogen developed a new or recurrent breast cancer. All of the women in the study had similar prognostic indicators after the original breast cancer. Other studies are under way in a variety of settings to follow what happens over time when breast cancer survivors elect to take estrogen. For now, such a decision is a highly individual one, based on presence of significantly disruptive symptoms or medical problems due to lack of estrogen that have not responded to other approaches. Certainly with what I know, I would not use a conjugated equine estrogen like Premarin for a woman who had already had breast cancer. I would use only the form of estrogen found in a human woman's body, and then I would recommend using it in a nonoral form (such as patches) to reduce the amount of estrone delivered.

The message is that you and your health professionals need to work together to arrive at a choice that best meets *your* individual needs, not what your friends are doing. I tell my patients, "My job is to give you the best information I know and help you carefully assess your health concerns and risks. I can't tell you what to do. I can help you explore what is right for you, I can help you monitor your health trends, and I can be there to explore other options if you change your mind. The ultimate decision is what YOU want to do." And remember, you should reassess your benefit-risk profile regularly with your physician, perhaps at your annual checkup. No matter what decision you make this year or next year, you always have the option of changing your mind and taking a new approach as your goals and needs and desires may change, or as new information emerges. When you manage your money, you look for the best returns and reevaluate your approaches based on changes and new information rather than doing the same thing year in and year out. You need to approach your health management the same way!

Media Influences

I have been alarmed at the degree of fear and terror I hear from women around the country concerning their risk of breast cancer. I think much of the fear is intensified and exaggerated by the images and headlines used to present the breast cancer story in our magazines and newspapers.

Am I against articles to educate the public? Absolutely not. But I am very much against the degree of sensationalism that is used to sell the product (e.g., a magazine) by excessively dramatizing breast cancer and generating such overwhelming fear among women. I also oppose the portrayal of women as nothing but breasts. A woman is told she has to have a perfect body. If the breast is damaged, she's somehow less of a woman. Many women will say, "I don't want to get a mammogram because I don't want to find anything wrong. Because I don't want a mastectomy. Because that disfigures me. Because that makes me less of a woman." Many of us can relate to this thought process. Yet, today stage I breast cancer is more often treated with lumpectomy and radiation than a mastectomy. Survival rates have been shown to be equally as good with lumpectomy plus radiation compared to mastectomy, if breast cancer is detected early, before it has spread to the lymph nodes. Unfortunately, I find that the majority of women seem to have not gotten this more hopeful message.

Going back to the Swedish study, what happened in the media is alarming as an illustration of how information is manipulated to grab headlines and attention. The first paper from the Swedish group was outlining the study design and preliminary results. This half of the material was published in *The New England Journal of Medicine* (*NEJM*), one of the most prestigious and widely read medical journals in the world. This is also a medical journal that is closely monitored by health and science writers for the newest breakthroughs in medical research and advances of interest to consumers. So, when the Swedish study hit the pages of *NEJM*, the information was immediately picked up by writers on wire services for all the major newspapers. Many of these writers had the information about the latest issue of *NEJM* and the "Swedish breast cancer study" even before most physicians in this country had gotten their copies in the mail. Headlines around the country told *only a piece* of the story before most physicians had even seen the newly published medical article and could digest the information (or lack thereof) from the preliminary study report. Millions of women were alarmed, scared, and confused and stopped hormone therapy without being aware of their individual health risks and without being aware of the inaccuracies, distortions, and limitations in the headlines they had just read.

To compound the problem further, when the *outcome* study results from this *same* breast cancer study were published in the *same* year (1989), they did not appear in *NEJM*, but in the *American Journal of Epidemiology*. Now, you may say, "What's that? I've never heard of that journal." Well, neither have most physicians and certainly most health journalists. It is a medical journal with a much narrower focus than *NEJM*, and a much smaller number of readers. So, why is this important to you? A very key finding emerged in this half of the Swedish study: The women in the Swedish study who were **on** hormone therapy at the time their breast cancer was diagnosed **had a better survival rate** than those women in the study who **were not on** hormone therapy when they were diagnosed with breast cancer.

This crucial information, buried in an obscure medical journal not seen by most practicing physicians and the press, provided an entirely different slant on the issue of hormone therapy and breast cancer risk. It is certainly a piece of information that women deserve to know and to be able to discuss with their physician. But in the world of academic gamesmanship on getting the most "pubs" (publications) from a given piece of research, this highly significant result was *buried* and never reached the headlines where women could see it and use it. As much as I work hard to stay on top of such crucial information in order to responsibly inform patients, consumer groups, and other physicians of new research, it was *over a year* before I was able to find out the full story. The further follow-up came in 1992, when the corrected and more positive data was published, this time in the highly respected British medical journal, *The Lancet*. Of course, that didn't make it to the front pages of our newspapers. I was appalled by the blatant gamesmanship and commercialism that had been demonstrated by this manipulation of both the medical community and consumers. Women ended up being unduly alarmed about their individual risks based on faulty interpretation of statistics, inadequate numbers of patients in the study, and lack of full information on the outcomes.

The point here is not to devalue the role of media articles in providing education and more awareness about breast cancer for women. The point, I think, is to look at the total picture and be aware of imbalances in the information that often distort the true risk for women and frequently portray an overly negative view of progress and treatment options. Read articles with a critical eye on these issues, then talk over your fears and questions with a knowledgeable physician who will help you put your individual risk in perspective.

Dietary Fat and Other Factors

There have been a variety of studies over the last forty to fifty years that have demonstrated a significant connection between high levels of dietary fat, particularly saturated fat derived from animal products, and the subsequent development of breast cancer. The markedly lower dietary fat intake in Japan relative to the United States (as well as differences in soy intake) are thought to be a key factor contributing to the lower risk of breast cancer in Japan compared with the United States. More recent, detailed epidemiological studies of the dietary fat link have failed to *unequivocally* establish quantitative associations between diet and breast cancer, and you may have seen these negative studies in such headlines as "Dietary Fat Not Linked to Breast Cancer." You may find yourself asking, "How can I make sense of such conflicting information? Has there been a 'cover-up' of important dietary factors? What should I do now to protect my health and reduce my risk of getting breast cancer?" I have reviewed about two hundred articles in a Medline search of publications since 1990 and found that the majority of these studies *did* support the link between dietary fat intake and increased risk of breast cancer. These studies have been done in a wide variety of geographic areas, from China and Japan, to Russia, Italy, Australia, Europe, and the United States. The link is stronger for saturated animal fat than for vegetable fat/oils. So, why can't we say definitively that fat intake is a risk factor for breast cancer?

First of all, there are many reasons why *epidemiological* studies, even carefully done ones, may not show a clear, *unequivocal* link between diet and breast cancer:

- Participants' recall of food intake may not be accurate.
- Study of dietary habits needs to be done earlier in women's lives.
- Weak associations are often obscured unless highly accurate dietary measures are used and the number of participants in a study is quite large.
- People may give answers about dietary practices that they think the questioner wants to hear, rather than what they actually eat.
- Dietary factors are more likely to act through *interaction* with other risk variables, rather than as direct (and easier to measure) cause-effect mechanisms.

- Dietary factors may play a more crucial role in cancer promotion at earlier stages in one's life (e.g., adolescence) and may be less important factors in later years (e.g., after menopause), so *when* these factors are studied may be pivotal.

What are some of the data that link dietary fat and breast cancer? The connection was first described in the 1940s, based on higher incidence of breast cancer in rats fed high-fat diets. In addition, observations for many years have confirmed a lower incidence of breast cancer in countries where the fat intake is lower and where the diet is higher in vegetables, whole grains, and fruits. In countries such as the United States, Great Britain, and much of Europe where the fat intake is especially high, and there is more intake of animal fats, we have seen consistently much higher incidences of breast cancer. Following World War II, we have seen a significant rise in breast cancer in Japan, as the typical Japanese diet was "westernized" toward much higher fat intake. Japanese women who emigrated to the United States, and adopted the dietary habits of the American lifestyle, also began to have increasing rates of breast cancer equal to those of American women. There has also been a striking increase in breast cancer rates in the daughters of Japanese immigrant mothers. The daughters have been exposed to higher levels of dietary fat in the United States from earlier ages than were their mothers. Another significant comparison is that of South African Bantu women, who consume about 15 percent of their calories from fat and have a breast cancer death rate of 5 per 100,000 women. Contrast that with African-American women in the United States, who average about 40–45 percent fat in their diet and have a breast cancer death rate of 23 per 100,000 women.

There appears to be from animal studies a *threshold level* at about *20 percent* of total calories coming from fat in the diet that seems to be a key factor. Rats fed diets of 20 percent or less fat had a lower incidence of breast cancer. Rats fed diets *above* 20 percent had a greater incidence of breast cancer; whether it was 30 percent or 40 percent fat didn't seem to make any additional difference in frequency of tumors. An evaluation of the dietary habits of nurses in the Harvard Nurses Health Study did not show a link between dietary fat and breast cancer. The results of this study were headlined across the country: *Harvard study shows no link between breast cancer and dietary fat*. There was a crucial piece of information that *didn't* make it into the headlines: the *lowest dietary fat intake* recorded for the nurses in the Harvard study was above 30 percent fat. *All* of the women in that study had *too much fat* in their diets. It would be like looking at 89,000 women for reductions in lung cancer when all the women in the study are smokers. What the

Harvard study ended up with were *high-fat* eaters and *very high-fat* eaters, so this study was not able to address the potential benefit from a *low-fat diet*. Many doctors didn't know this either. No wonder consumers are confused.

The studies we have now do show a very clear trend toward increased risk of breast cancer in women who consume high-fat diets, particularly if the fat is *saturated (animal) fat*. Another issue, in addition to the *amount* of animal fat in our diet, is *what is in* the fat we eat. Most of the meat and poultry we consume come from animals that have been fed hormones to fatten them up and antibiotics to reduce infections. Pesticides and other toxic compounds become more concentrated in the fatty tissues of our meat sources, so you are also getting more of these toxic chemicals, many of which have been clearly shown to be carcinogenic. In fact, if you look at the data on identified breast cancer risks, and the percent of breast cancer cases *attributable to each risk factor, dietary fat* has the *highest attributable risk*: 27 percent of cases, compared to 12 percent attributable risk for obesity and 17 percent attributable risk if a woman is age thirty or older with first pregnancy. A 1999 Italian study showed a *12 percent* attributable risk due to daily *alcohol* intake. If there is any significant attributable risk due to estrogen use after menopause, it is estimated to be less than 3 percent of total breast cancer risks. So it is important to pursue the "fat factor" as a breast cancer risk, especially in sorting out future health risks for young girls consuming high-fat diets.

In studies showing a positive link with dietary fat, *younger women* in particular appeared at high risk. Dietary fat has been shown to increase the secretion of prolactin and androgens, which can then be used by the body to make types of biologically active estrogens different from estradiol. High prolactin levels are also thought to be a potential risk factor for breast cancer. A 1990 Australian study of 424 women discovered that prolactin levels higher than the average in controls were associated with a more than two-fold increase in risk of breast cancer. Prolactin levels *decrease* with *first pregnancy, low-fat diets, and at menopause,* which fits with the observed decreased risk of breast cancer in women who have first pregnancy before age thirty, and an earlier onset of menopause.

If you should develop breast cancer, it seems wise to clean up your diet by decreasing total fat to about 20 percent, decreasing animal fat and fried foods to the *least* possible, and reduce your intake of meats. Why do I suggest this after cancer has developed? It may have an important bearing on your risk of a *recurrence*. Dietary fat intake is thought to increase both the *growth* and the *spread* of breast tumors, with a greater effect on growth of estrogen-positive tumors. Studies have reported this connection over a number of years. In 1993, two new studies from Sweden and the United States came out showing that women with breast cancer had a lower risk of return of their disease if they changed to a low-fat diet, with about 20 percent calories from fat. So, staying conscious of your intake of animal fat is important both for prevention and for reducing risk of recurrence if you do develop breast cancer.

Keep in mind there is a big difference between seeing a *trend* about a particular risk factor and finding a way to *prove* a cause-and-effect relationship. Are you someone who wants to perk up her ears and take notice at the *early* signs of a problem, or are you someone who waits until a problem hits you over the head before you take action? If you are in the first group of *proactive* types, you will probably want to reduce your dietary fat intake now, based on the last fifty years of *trends* in the clinical data, which show an increase in risk of breast cancer as dietary fat intake increases over time. If you are someone in the second group, who wants to wait until the facts are *proven* before you modify your food intake, stay tuned. We don't have the proof you may want on the breast cancer–fat connection. But since high-fat diets are *unequivocally known* to be a health risk for heart disease, hypertension, diabetes, stroke, and colon cancer, you may want to start reducing the fat in your diet for these other health reasons while we wait for more information on fat's role in breast cancer.

Obesity is another risk factor for breast cancer. Obese women have a two- to four-fold increased risk of getting breast cancer. Excess body fat contributes to higher levels of estrogens (particularly estrone) and a male hormone dehydroandrostenedione (DHA) circulating in the blood. It is *not* known for certain which of these hormones is the culprit in the increased risk of breast cancer in obese women. Two factors imply that it is estrone: (1) 80 percent of breast cancers arise in women *after* menopause, when estrone is the primary estrogen present in the body (produced in the fat tissue and the adrenal glands), and (2) *the location of the fat on the body is important:* there is about a *six-fold increase in risk* of breast cancer in women who have *upper-body* (truncal) fat compared to women whose fat is distributed more around the hips, buttocks, and thighs. A 1991 summary of nutrition and breast cancer risk in Japan revealed that Japanese breast cancer patients were different from matched normal control patients by having *an increase in abdominal (truncal) body fat.* Upper-body fat distribution is associated with *higher* levels of estrone, androgens, and cortisol than with high levels of estradiol.

With most of the evidence pointing to strong links between dietary fat intake and increases in breast cancer, it is tragic that the Women's Health Trial (WHT) in this country was canceled in 1988. The WHT was a landmark project because it was a randomized, prospective ten-year study of the fat hypothesis. Its cancellation is a sad and complex story of political and economic interests put ahead of basic common sense approaches and needs in women's health. A telling point of the attitudes encountered by supporters of this study is found in one of the reasons opponents gave for the WHT cancellation: *Women couldn't be trusted to change their diets and keep good records of their food intake.* Talk about negative stereotypes of women!

Alcohol and Tobacco

The case against alcohol is even stronger than the case against dietary fat. In 1977, the first study to link alcohol consumption with an increase in breast cancer risk was published. Since then, we have many studies from a variety of countries showing similar results: Even moderate alcohol consumption, *three or more drinks per week,* increased breast cancer risk anywhere from 20–70 percent. And drinking more than nine drinks a week increased risk even more. **Alcohol intake is an independent risk factor for breast cancer.** This means that the increased risk is *not* due to other confounding variables, such as total calories, fat, fiber, and vitamins. And *age* at which you begin drinking is an important component of this risk factor. Mothers, take note of this, and talk with your daughters. Drinking alcohol before age thirty increases breast cancer risk, regardless of alcohol consumption patterns later in life. As we are finding with fat in the diet, the main effect of alcohol on breast cancer risk seems to be in the vulnerable time of breast development during puberty. The mechanism for alcohol effect on cancer risk is not yet known with certainty. There is speculation that it may alter hormonal balance by increasing estrone and the androgens in fat tissue. Alcohol also increases body fat deposited in the upper-body areas, which further adds to cancer and heart disease risks. It may act through interference with normal immune function as well.

One more nail in your coffin if you smoke cigarettes: It increases your risk of breast cancer. I cannot think of one single health habit that is more detrimental for women than smoking. If all the other negatives about it haven't gotten your attention, does its role in breast cancer make an impact? The increase in risk of breast cancer due to cigarette smoking is more pronounced for premenopausal women than for postmenopausal women. Tobacco smoke in the body contains many direct carcinogens, adversely affects immune system function, and adversely affects the metabolism of estrogens and other important hormones. Two studies have shown that premenopausal women who have ever smoked daily have approximately a two-fold increased risk of breast cancer, and women who are currently heavy smokers have four times normal risk. It's a "dose-dependent" relationship: the *more you smoke, the higher the risk*. While some studies have not borne out the relationship between smoking and breast cancer, the fact that some *have* is alarming to me in view of all the other terrible effects of smoking on women. Doesn't it just make sense to eliminate this one factor over which you have some control?

Environmental Toxins

Radiation

A known risk factor for many cancers, radiation exposure also causes an increase in breast cancer. The younger a woman is at the time of excessive exposure, the greater her risk of later developing breast cancer. The danger from radiation occurs to the area of the body that receives the radiation. For example, if you had radiation treatment to the cervix for cancer, it does not travel to the breast to increase risk of breast cancer. And the danger also comes from the total *accumulated dose* of radiation. The dose that causes increases in cancer risk is far greater than any you would get having screening mammograms or occasional diagnostic X rays. For example, with modern mammography techniques, you would get about ¼ rad of radiation. The studies that have shown an increased risk of breast cancer after radiation exposure have found that risk increases in a *dose-related manner* from 100 to 500 rads and up.

Terry Tempest Williams, a naturalist and writer from Utah, has written a powerful and poignant book about the human and environmental impact of the aboveground nuclear testing done in Utah and Nevada in the 1950s and 1960s. The "downwinders" (those living down wind from the radioactive fallout at the test sites) have a higher incidence of many types of cancers. The women have a marked increase in breast cancer, and this increase is found in a population dominated by Mormons, who do not drink alcohol or caffeine or smoke tobacco and tend to eat a lower fat diet. In addition, Mormon culture encourages large families, and women typically have their first pregnancy in late teens or early twenties, which normally seems to have a protective effect on later breast cancer development. Traditionally, statistics have shown that Mormon women have a lower-than-average incidence of breast cancer. Ms. Williams's mother was diagnosed with breast cancer at age thirty-eight, fourteen years after she was driving with her husband across the desert not far from an area of atomic bomb testing and saw the fallout dust settling on their car. Listen to the voice of Terry Tempest Williams as she cries out the pain of suffering seen in her family:

I belong to a Clan of One-Breasted Women. My mother, my grand-mothers, and six aunts have all had mastectomies. Seven are dead. The two who survive have just completed rounds of chemotherapy and radiation. I've had my own problems: two biopsies for breast cancer and a small tumor between my ribs diagnosed as a "borderline malig-nancy." This is my family history. Most statistics tell us breast cancer is genetic, hereditary, with rising percentages attached to fatty diets, childlessness or becoming pregnant after thirty. What they don't say is that living in Utah may be the greatest hazard of all.

One by one I have watched the women in my family die common, heroic deaths. We sat in waiting rooms hoping for good news, but always receiving the bad. I cared for them, bathed their scarred bodies, and shot them with morphine when the pain became inhuman. In the end, I witnessed their last peaceful breaths, becoming a midwife to the rebirth of their souls.

When the Atomic Energy Commission described the country north of the Nevada Test Site as "virtually uninhabited desert terrain," my family and the birds at Great Salt Lake were some of the "virtual unin-habitants." I cannot prove that my mother, Diane Dixon Tempest, or my grandmothers along with my aunts developed cancer from nuclear fallout in Utah. But I can't prove they didn't. "

from *Refuge: An Unnatural History of Family and Place* by
Terry Tempest Williams, Vintage Books, 1991, pp. 281-87.

Clearly, there will be more to learn from tragedies such as this, and I hope that all of us will benefit from those like Terry Williams who have had the courage to speak out and identify environmental sources of carcinogens. We are just beginning to understand the degree to which man has polluted and damaged our environment, and the resulting long-term effects on human health.

Pesticides and Pollutants

Environmental Health Perspectives last year published a review article of forty-five different environmental contaminants or classes of chemicals that have been found to cause changes in animal and human reproductive hormone systems. Some of these chemical agents actually mimic estrogen effects in the body even though they are not the same chemical molecules as the native human estrogens. A number of studies already have revealed that women working in the petroleum and chemical industries have significantly increased rates of breast cancer compared to the general public. I, like many others in the health field, have concerns about these *additional* sources of estrogenic compounds in our environment and what effects these substances have on a whole host of health problems, not just cancer development. These chemicals are everywhere in our environment: water supplies, food sources, body fat, breast tissue, and breast-milk. Chemicals in these groups are toxic, tend to be long-lasting in the environment, and tend to be concentrated in fat tissue of fish, animals, and humans. Dr. Mary S. Wolff of the Mt. Sinai School of Medicine in New York City heads a research team that has linked blood levels of DDT to a woman's risk of breast cancer. DDT is the highly toxic pesticide widely used prior to 1972, when its carcinogenic and damaging environmental effects were finally taken seriously. DDT has been banned in the United States since 1972, but due to its long-lasting effects, DDT still pollutes our environment from its use many years ago, and it is still in use in Mexico and other countries today. Those of us born prior to 1972 were exposed to DDT in our diet, because DDT was commonly found in dairy products and meats. Since it is stored in the environment and the body for decades, most Americans alive today carry some DDT residues. In Dr. Wolff's study, women who had the highest levels of DDT is body tissues had *four times* the risk of breast cancer of women with the least amount of DDT residues. The rise in the rate of breast cancer in this country in recent decades followed the increase in use of DDT, suggesting to Dr. Wolff and others that DDT may be linked to breast cancer.

Similar observations and epidemiological date in Israel link breast cancer rates with the pesticides DDT, lindane, and BHC. After twenty-five years of *rising* breast cancer rates in Israel, two researchers noted that Israel was the only one of twenty-eight countries showing a *significant decrease* in breast cancer rates over the ten-year period that ended in 1986. Israel had allowed use of DDT, BHC, and lindane until the mid-1970s, when they were finally banned. Prior to the ban, all three of these pesticides were found in dramatically high concentrations in Israeli milk, dairy products, and human breastmilk. Two years *after* the ban, in studies of human breastmilk from residents of Jerusalem, lindane levels dropped 90 percent, BHC levels decreased 98 percent, and DDT levels showed a 43 percent decrease. Within ten years of the ban on use of DDT, BHC, and lindane, there was a marked drop of 30 percent in breast cancer mortality in women under age forty-four. Researchers could not identify any other significant lifestyle or environmental change to account for these differences except the prohibition against using the three pesticides. To date, the American Cancer Society and other U.S. cancer organizations have done little to explore the critically important evidence of the role of environmental pollutants in breast and other cancers.

Researchers are now looking at the effects on *male* reproductive function, such as lower sperm counts, from these potent estrogen-mimicking pollutants. The noncancer effects of these synthetic compounds may turn out to be far more wide-ranging than we have sus-pected. I bring this up to increase your awareness on these issues and also to help you put in better perspective your decisions about hormone therapy after menopause. After decades of tracking breast cancer patterns in women, therapeutic amounts of *natural human forms of estradiol* have *not* been shown to cause a significant increase in breast cancers. It appears clear, from what studies we do have on these environmental contaminants, that these chemicals activate the body's estrogen receptors in undesirable ways and are more dangerous than previously thought, producing a variety of adverse effects on the body's tissues and immune system.

A Look at Your Real Risks

In addition to the problems I have already talked about in this chap-ter, we have to take a look at what these numbers really mean. Statistics are often misleading and confusing. The one you hear repeatedly about breast cancer is "One in nine women will get breast cancer." How many of you think that one out of nine women right now, regardless of age, are at risk of getting breast cancer? Each time I give a women's health seminar, I find that the majority of the women in the audience raise their hands with a yes response to this question. This statistic has been used in ads and health head-lines for a number of years with the goal of getting women's atten-tion so they will get their mammograms for early detection of breast cancer. The problem is that most women are terrified by it. This fear then keeps women from taking the appropriate preventive and early detection steps available. It's as if many women feel the weight of the statistic saying that there is an *inevitability* about getting breast can-cer, so why bother? I constantly hear women saying "I don't want to get a mammogram, I'm afraid I'll be the one in nine."

What does this statistic really mean? It refers to the *cumulative lifetime risk* of getting breast cancer for Caucasian women. It is *not* a number that can be applied to any one individual woman, since it represents an average risk, taking into account all causes of death over the life expectancy (in this case to age eighty-five). When you see the number change to "one in eight women will get breast cancer," it is actually a revised projection over the longer life expectancy to age ninety-five. It means that one in eight women *by age ninety-five* have a risk of *getting* breast cancer. It does not mean one in eight will die from breast cancer. I have already shown you in the charts above the increases in survival rates with breast cancer. The statistic "one in eight" also does not mean that the incidence of breast cancer is increasing. It means we are expected to live longer and so our risk goes up slightly. These *lifetime* risk estimates give a picture for the whole population, not individual women. Using a lifetime risk estimate will *overestimate* the actual risk for you individually if you have no risk factors for breast cancer and will *underestimate* the risk for you individually if you have risk factors for the disease. I hope this helps put these numbers into a more balanced perspective.

You will see other terms used in articles reporting on breast cancer studies. One, *attributable risk,* refers to the amount of risk for an illness that can be traced directly to one risk factor. For example, with breast cancer, researchers have estimated that dietary fat has an *attributable risk* of 27 percent. This means that 27 percent of breast cancers can be attributed to this risk factor. Obesity is estimated to have a 12 percent attributable risk. I listed other attributable risks earlier in this chapter. Another term, *relative risk,* refers to the relationship between a person's exposure to a risk factor and the likelihood she will then develop the disease. It is determined by the following equation:

$$\text{Relative Risk (RR)} = \frac{\text{Incidence of Disease (exposed persons)}}{\text{Incidence of Disease (nonexposed persons)}}$$

A relative risk (RR) of 1.0 means that the group exposed to the risk has the same incidence of the disease as the nonexposed group. The **higher** the RR, the greater the risk. A relative risk of 1.6 means the exposed group has a 60 percent greater chance of the illness. If the RR is *less* than 1.0, it means that the exposed group has a *lower* risk of the disease. For example, an RR of 0.5 means the exposed group is 50 percent *less* likely to develop the disease.

As I mentioned earlier, most studies to date show a relative risk of about 1.0 for postmenopausal estrogen therapy alone, with the exception of the Nurses Health Study showing a higher relative risk (about 1.3) in the conjugated equine estrogen (Premarin) users *who also drank alcohol regularly.* For postmenopausal women using estrogen, the relative risk of ischemic heart disease is 0.5, based on the most recent research. This means women who are using estrogen have *one-half* the risk of heart disease that nonusers have. Keep in mind that relative risk will change as we age and other risk factors are added.

One problem in applying these various risk statistics to you as an individual is that they don't take into account your specific health profile and the presence (or absence) of more than *one* risk factor (or variable). If you have several of the known risk factors for breast cancer, your individual risk will be higher than the numbers above, and conversely, a woman with none of the risk factors will have a lower risk than the numbers suggest. Your physician will typically review your individual risk and benefit profile with you before recommending a particular therapy. Remember, there are also lifestyle changes you can make now that will help, as well as new medications your physician may suggest. All of this information and these approaches have to be seen as a *total* picture in planning your best health care options.

There is a new computerized risk assessment model, the Gail Model Risk Index, that was developed for assessing risk in the Breast Cancer Prevention Trial. Calculation of the risk number was used in this study to determine which women were at high risk and therefore would qualify for the trial of tamoxifen vs. placebo in preventing breast cancer. The Gail model is a computer algorithm that takes into account five known predictors of risk for breast cancer and calculates your individual risk number based on the number of risk factors you have. The Gail model asks six simple questions related to your current age, age at beginning menstruation, age at first pregnancy with live birth, number of breast biopsies, and number of first-degree relatives with breast cancer. The computer algorithm then estimates the likelihood that you would develop breast cancer in your lifetime if you have certain risk factors. I encourage you to talk with your health professional about doing this risk assessment. A risk index greater than 1.67 percent means you are at high risk and should begin to explore with your physician ways to reduce your risk.

Another problem with our perception of risk is the amount of publicity a given risk gets. All of us are familiar with the shock and fear that happens when we hear about a plane crash, and people rush to cancel flight reservations. Those same people generally don't think twice about getting in a car and driving home. Yet, the chances of dying in a plane crash are estimated at 1 in 11 *million* in the United States and the chance of dying in a car accident are 1 in 5,000! Simply put, because the plane crash generates more publicity, it also creates more impact in the public mind than an automobile crash, and the *perception* of risk from flying appears greater. So the more media attention to breast cancer, and the less the emphasis on heart disease in women, the more you are likely to feel that you are at higher risk of getting breast cancer than heart disease even though the latter is far more common as women age.

CUMULATIVE LIFETIME RISK OF GETTING BREAST CANCER

Age 25:	one in 21,441
Age 30:	one in 2,426
Age 40:	one in 222
Age 45:	one in 96
Age 50:	one in 52
Age 60:	one in 24
Age 75:	one in 10
Age 85:	one in 9
Age 95:	one in 8

Source: National Cancer Institute. All of the statistics are for white women in United States.

We see a similar risk pattern for men with regard to prostate cancer: The two primary risks are being male and growing older. It used to be that most men typically did not live long enough to develop prostate cancer; they more often died at younger ages of heart disease and other causes. And, until recently, we did not have very effective early detection and screening tests for prostate cancer, so many more men had the disease even though they were not diagnosed and died of another cause.

A separate issue is the risk of *dying* of breast cancer. This number is much lower, at all age groups, than the risk of *getting* the disease. The table shows this, again using *averages*. For a given *individual* woman, just how much lower the risk of dying is will depend largely on *how early* the cancer is diagnosed. That's why most physicians are so strongly in favor of regular screening mammograms. In spite of the current debate about whether annual mammograms in women under fifty will reduce total deaths, the mammogram is still the single most effective means of detecting early breast cancers when they are most treatable, are least likely to have spread beyond the breast, and the survival rates are the highest.

Age Range	Risk of Dying of Breast Cancer
Birth to age 110	3.6 percent
Age 20–30	0.00
Age 35–45	0.14 percent
Age 50–60	0.33 percent
Age 65–5	0.43 percent

Source: H. Seidman et al., *CA: A Cancer Journal for Clinicians* 35 (1985); pp. 36–56.

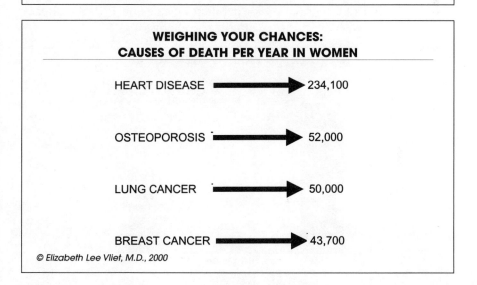

WEIGHING YOUR CHANCES:
CAUSES OF DEATH PER YEAR IN WOMEN

HEART DISEASE   234,100

OSTEOPOROSIS   52,000

LUNG CANCER   50,000

BREAST CANCER   43,700

© Elizabeth Lee Vliet, M.D., 2000

The majority of women who attend my seminars, even though they are generally knowledgeable and interested in health issues, simply do not know the high percentage of deaths in women over age fifty due to cardiovascular disease. Look at the dramatic differences in death rates on the chart below: 4 percent of the deaths in women over fifty are due to breast cancer, but 53 percent of the deaths in women over age fifty are due to cardiovascular disease. *These numbers still hold true today*, as illustrated in the table above. If you have a family history of heart disease, and high cholesterol, then worrying about estrogen increasing risk of breast cancer (and *not* looking at estrogen's 50 percent decrease in heart disease risk) is a little like being worried about getting run over by a donkey cart coming down the road when you are standing on a track ignoring the freight train barreling toward you.

One of the common comments I hear from women is that "I'd rather die quickly of a heart attack than a lingering death from breast cancer." This is another significant misconception. Heart disease doesn't necessarily kill you quickly. Many heart disease victims develop chronic angina and congestive heart failure that rob you of your energy, vitality, and ability to enjoy life and the activities you love. Heart disease can be just as slow and painful in its debilitating effects as breast cancer, perhaps more so since heart conditions are treated with medications that also have energy-sapping side effects but don't necessarily kill you. And remember that osteoporosis is a leading cause of later life pain, disability, inability to engage in daily activities, and premature admission to nursing homes. The 52,000 deaths each year from osteoporosis occur as a result of complications from osteoporosis, such as hip fractures. Contrast these bleak aspects of heart disease and osteoporosis with the fact that the majority of breast cancer survivors today lead completely normal lives once the acute treatments (surgery, radiation, or chemotherapy) are completed, without major debilitating side effects of the disease such as we see with heart disease and osteoporosis.

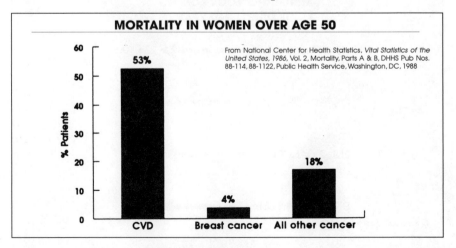

MORTALITY IN WOMEN OVER AGE 50

From National Center for Health Statistics, *Vital Statistics of the United States, 1986*, Vol. 2, Mortality, Parts A & B, DHHS Pub Nos. 88-114, 88-1122, Public Health Service, Washington, DC, 1988

Research Advances: New Findings, Hopeful Outlooks

Talk with a hundred women and ask them what the outlook would likely be for a woman diagnosed with breast cancer, and I am confident that eighty to ninety of those women would list "death" as one of the three first responses. But is this accurate? Is the diagnosis of breast cancer the "kiss of death"? Look at the graph below, and notice that the picture for breast cancer is much more hopeful than for any other cancers that affect women. The **white** bars show the *new cases detected in one year,* while the **black** bars show *the death rates in that year* for each type of cancer common in women. It is striking that we are far better at detecting and treating breast cancer than we are at detecting and successfully treating any of the other cancers shown. I am concerned that most women never get this hopeful message. Media articles on breast cancer, even today, do not adequately convey this encouraging news.

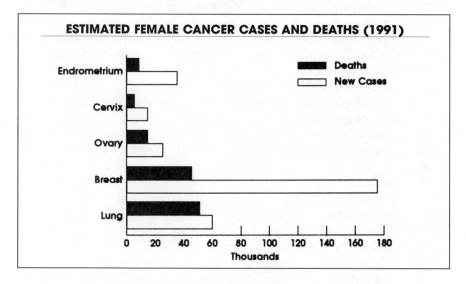

ESTIMATED FEMALE CANCER CASES AND DEATHS (1991)

Survival after breast cancer has improved consistently over the last thirty years: In 1960, the five-year survival rate was only 60 percent overall; today the overall five-year survival rate is better than *80 percent*, and the earlier the stage at diagnosis the better the rate of survival. If diagnosed early on a mammogram, before a lump can even be felt, the *cure rate* for breast cancer is now better than *90 percent*. Notice I said *cure rate*. Breast cancer specialists now talk about cures for Stage I cancers, not just remission. But the most important thing for you to know is that *early detection* is crucial.

So, above all, don't panic. Keep your risk in perspective. If one in eight women by age ninety-five has a risk of developing breast cancer, that means *seven* women out of every eight *escape* having breast cancer. And recall that survival after breast cancer has improved dramatically. Only one in twenty-seven women will die of breast cancer, while *one in two* women over age fifty will die of heart disease. Keep your focus on what health issue is more common in your family, and what your own lifestyle habits are that may be changed to reduce risks.

Mammography Updates

I want to state very clearly: Mammography done in an accredited facility by experienced technicians remains our single most effective method of early detection of breast cancer. No matter what you read in the news about scientists debating whether annual mammograms in women under fifty will save lives, keep in mind that they are debating *statistical correlation*, not what relates to YOU as an individual woman. For you or me, the bottom-line issue is what gives you or me the best means of detecting a breast tumor early, because that's when we have the best opportunity to get it successfully treated and possibly cured. **Period.** Screening mammography has another benefit, based on a 1994 study from the University of Pennsylvania: Detecting a tumor early with mammography *increases* the likelihood that a woman will be able to have a *lumpectomy* instead of a *mastectomy*. As a woman's health advocate, I am incensed by what I see taking place on the mammogram issue and the way headlines screaming at us generate even more fear and confusion for women. And lurking not so far behind the scenes on this subject is the issue of *cost*. Women are being given confusing information about the value of *annual* mammograms during their forties partly because if we move into a national health plan, it will be *more costly* to screen all women in that age group every year. Insurance companies, Medicare policy makers and epidemiologists are looking for trends in death rates to see whether annual mammograms are "necessary" (i.e., translate that to mean "can we save money if we tell women they don't need mammograms every year?"). Don't get caught up in the economic debate on health care general policy when you are making your own individual decision. What these policy makers and insurance payors leave out of the story is that we still know for *an individual* woman, her best chances of survival come from the earliest detection possible. Early detection is greatly increased with mammography. Mammograms can detect tumors several years before they can be felt, and they only miss about 10 percent of tumors overall. It is true that mammograms are not 100 percent accurate, but then nothing else in medicine is either . . . except perhaps a prediction that death occurs for all of us at some point. Looking at it another way, even if you miss 10 percent of breast tumors, it still means that mammograms pick up *90 percent* of tumors. In my view, those are good odds. If there were a device as safe and effective as mammography to screen men for testicular cancer, I doubt seriously that we would have any controversy at all about using the device annually for men.

Another dimension of the controversy is that the National Cancer Institute (NCI) analysis of the mammography data was flawed, according to leading cancer specialists. The American Cancer Society disagreed with the NCI policy change, and requested Dr. Daniel B. Kopans from Harvard to review the studies used by NCI in reaching its conclusions. Dr. Kopans, head of the breast-imaging division at Massachusetts General Hospital, reported that the NCI used studies from ten to thirty years ago, mostly done in countries *outside* the United States. Older mammography equipment frequently produced cloudy, difficult-to-read pictures, and X rays from other countries were often read by technicians who were not as well trained as the radiologists (physicians) who read mammograms in the United States. The average American woman never knew about this crucial information. What you saw were the headlines questioning usefulness of mammography. The combined studies used by NCI had several other crucial flaws: They did not target women in their forties for study, and the sample numbers were too small and followed over too short a period of time. I find all this appalling. Physicians and health activists from many fields have worked too long and hard to help women become aware of the potential life-saving benefits of mammography to have this kind of poor "science" cast doubt on the credibility of years of work and good research. I am outraged at one more example of women being manipulated through misinformation.

Encouraging results were published from a ten-year Swedish clinical study of 24,000 women ages forty to forty-nine. There was a *35 percent decrease in deaths* in the 12,000 women who got regular mammograms compared to the 12,000 who did not have regular breast mammograms. A different type of study of 1000 women, done at Harvard, showed that in women under fifty the tumors detected on mammography were typically *smaller* and had *fewer metastases* at the time of diagnosis. These two tumor characteristics are associated with better survival rates. Remember the key issue for you personally: Getting a mammogram regularly has the *potential* to save your life. Is this important to you? If the answer is yes, then get your mammogram every year and don't worry about the opinions of men debating changes in health policies just for costsavings.

I am also concerned about the significant number of older women who do not get annual mammograms. Only 17–20 percent of women over sixty-five in the United States get their screening mammograms done regularly. Since older, postmenopausal women are the highest-risk group for breast cancer, that means that about 80–83 percent of the high-risk population of women *do not get mammograms* on a regularly scheduled basis. I think one of the reasons for this disturbing trend is that breast cancer is often portrayed in the media as a young woman's disease, so consequently many women over sixty-five simply do not realize that *they are the high-risk group,* not younger women. If only a small percentage of well-informed, health-conscious women know that their breast cancer risk increases with age, what are the implications for other women in our society who may not be as well informed? Add lack of knowledge to the confusion generated in the news, and it's not surprising that we have such a hard time getting more older women to have their mammograms done.

There's a recent ironic twist to all this: At a time when we clearly know that annual mammograms are very effective in reducing breast cancer deaths in older women, Medicare has reduced coverage for mammograms to every *other* year in women over age fifty. It doesn't make much sense from a health standpoint, but it saves money. So what can you do if you are on Medicare and want to get your mammogram annually? I would suggest checking local resources for free or low-cost mammograms offered by hospitals, mobile units, or women's organizations such as the YWCA. Take charge of getting what *you* need.

Promising Advances for Biopsies

There are a number of new approaches that have made mammography even more effective, and I would encourage you to look into what facilities in your area have these latest techniques: use of stereotactic X-ray-guided needle biopsies, injection of radioactive tracers to enhance tumor images, and equipment that can provide more comprehensive views of each breast. University Medical Center and St. Joseph's Hospital in Tucson have introduced an example of such innovative approaches, with a nonsurgical procedure for breast biopsies. For this procedure, a woman lies facedown on a special table with imaging equipment below it. The breast to be biopsied is exposed through an opening in the table, and images are taken and analyzed by computer to give the precise location of a suspicious lump. The radiologist uses a needle to remove a tissue sample from the area, leaving only a quarter-inch scar instead of the usual one- or two-inch incision. Only a local anesthetic is necessary, and typically this procedure requires only cold compresses overnight to prevent swelling. This new approach takes about an hour; results are available in twenty-four hours; and the woman is able to return to usual activity the next day, versus two or three days of rest after a surgical biopsy. Women's satisfaction with this new procedure has been high. I expect we will see even more improvements in the next decade. Even with these advances, you are still in charge of taking the first step: scheduling your appointment.

Options to Explore

Vitamins and Minerals

A number of vitamins and antioxidants have been studied for decades for their possible protective effects in cancer. **Antioxidants,** described further in chapters 9 and 17, include: **vitamin C** (ascorbic acid), **vitamin E** (tocopherol), **beta-carotene** (provitamin A), **selenium,** and **glutathione.** A 1994 study, Diet and Breast Cancer Risk: Results from a Population-Based, Case Control Study in Sweden, had further good news about the role of beta-carotene. The authors found that high dietary beta-carotene intake had a protective effect on the risk of breast cancer development. Their results agreed with findings from several other good studies of the role of diet in breast cancer risk and prevention. There have been a few studies that have not shown the protective effect of beta-carotene, but since the negative studies were ones with small numbers of patients and limitations in the data collection on actual food intake, I think we are on pretty solid ground in suggesting that all of us would do well to increase our beta-carotene intake as part of a total healthy diet to help reduce cancer risk. Eat those sweet potatoes, carrots, and dark green leafy veggies.

Antioxidant compounds have evidence of protective effects on several types of cancer development: lung, breast, colon, pancreas, and larynx, to name a few. There are several good studies that have shown a protective effect of ascorbic acid (vitamin C) on breast cancer, but so far, these studies have primarily shown this protective effect in *post*menopausal women. Of course, this is the group of women at highest risk of getting breast cancer, but we also need more information about the role of vitamins in younger women. Maurice Black, at the New York Medical College Institute of Breast Diseases, found that women with Stage II breast cancer who had weakened immune systems *reduced* their five-year risk of recurrence *from 38 percent to 6 percent* by taking vitamin E. Since the supplement doses generally recommended (400 to 800 I.U. daily) have no known harmful effects, it seems wise to add the antioxidants to your health plan. I typically recommend a good basic multivitamin, along with the combined antioxidants and a calcium-magnesium supplement as part of an overall "health maintenance" program for my patients. For women who have been diagnosed with breast cancer, or who are at high risk due to their family history or environmental exposures, I think it is even more important to add these nutrients to the daily meal plan.

RECOMMENDED GUIDELINES FOR TAKING ANTIOXIDANTS

1. Take them in the recommended doses only—potential toxicity exists at higher doses, particularly with selenium.
2. Take antioxidants from a reputable source. Look for pure USP-grade products, free of additives and contaminants. Make sure you know the complete ingredients in what you take.
3. Be cautious about taking products with a large number of herbal components if you have asthma or allergies, or are taking prescription medications, since the plant components may aggravate these medical conditions or decrease the effectiveness of other medicines.
4. Take the antioxidants as a combination regimen with a good multivitamin as your base. They are more effective when functioning together to provide a positive synergy.

© Elizabeth Lee Vliet, M.D., 1995, revised 2000

Exercise

Dr. Kenneth Cooper, the "father of aerobics" in this country, published in 1990 what I think is a landmark study of the role of physical fitness in reducing cancer deaths. I am very bothered by the fact that this study got so little media attention, when it demonstrated such a significant positive result and is using an intervention (exercise) that has few possible side effects, minimal cost, and a host of additional benefits. Maybe exercise benefits for cancer treatment just aren't "sexy" enough for our media appetite for the "high-tech" approaches? At the Cooper Clinic in Dallas, they followed patients over more than ten years and tracked the correlation between level of physical fitness and cancer deaths. Dr. Cooper's research group found a marked *decrease* in cancer deaths as both men and women increased their level of fitness. Good news for women: his results showed a *greater decrease* in cancer death rates for women who were physically fit compared to males with a comparable level of fitness. There have been other studies that have supported this link between exercise and reduction of cancer, but none with such impressive numbers of participants and dramatic results. Another reason to put on those walkin' shoes and "JUST DO IT"!

Soy Isoflavones and Phytoestrogens

There is preliminary research that suggests increased dietary intake of soy isoflavones such as genistein may contribute to a modest reduction in breast cancer risk. The issues are complex, since soy isoflavones and other phytoestrogens are able to act both as estrogen stimulators and as estrogen antagonists. Which way they act depends in part on the concentration present at estrogen receptor sites, so if you have already had breast cancer, it is important to talk with your physician about whether or not soy and other phytoestrogens are safe for you. If you are worried about breast cancer, and do not have thyroid disease that can be adversely affected by soy supplements, you may want to consider adding 40–80 mg of soy isoflavones to your daily vitamin regimen. I address these issues more in chapter 16, but as always, talk with a physician you trust to guide you in your individual decisions.

Selective Estrogen Receptor Modulator (SERM) Medications

These are synthetically created compounds that selectively stimulate or antagonize the estrogen receptors of different target tissues. For example, some of these medications block estrogen effects at the breast and brain but still stimulate the estrogen receptors in bone and uterus and provide some estrogen-like effects to increase the good HDL cholesterol. Tamoxifen (Nolvadex) was the first such medication developed, initially for the treatment of estrogen-receptor positive breast cancers. In the Breast Cancer Prevention Trial, sponsored by the National Cancer Institute, tamoxifen was tested against placebo for prevention of breast cancer in over 13,000 women older than thirty-five and at high risk for breast cancer (i.e., they had a history of lobular carcinoma in situ or a five-year Gail Model Risk Index of greater than 1.67 percent). In this study, tamoxifen was found to reduce the risk of breast cancer by 44 percent in these high-risk women, although the drug did not increase survival or eliminate breast cancer entirely. Tamoxifen also helps to preserve bone, though not as effectively as does estrogen.

Raloxifene (Evista), another SERM, was approved by the FDA for both prevention and treatment of osteoporosis, although it has only about half of the bone benefit that estrogen does. Studies are under way to assess whether raloxifene will also reduce the risk of breast cancer over the long term. The Study of Tamoxifen and Raloxifene (STAR) trial will randomize 22,000 postmenopausal women to treatment with either tamoxifen or raloxifene to test the hypothesis that raloxifene may reduce the risk of breast cancer as effectively as has been shown for tamoxifene. There are over four hundred centers across the United States, Puerto Rico, and Canada involved in this important study sponsored by the NCI, but results will not be available for several years. Other SERMs are currently being developed, and each one has a different profile of estrogen stimulating and blocking properties, based on the chemical structure of the compound.

Like all SERMs so far, tamoxifen and raloxifene have some significant disadvantages and side effects that make these drugs a problem for many women. Both tamoxifen and raloxifene cause significant hot flashes, insomnia, and memory problems in a majority of users, primarily because they antagonize estrogen effects at brain centers involved in these pathways. Tamoxifen also stimulates estrogen receptors in the lining of the uterus and causes endometrial cancer two to three times the rate seen with placebo. Tamoxifen and raloxifene both cause an increased incidence of potentially fatal pulmonary emboli, deep vein thrombosis (blood clots), stroke, and cataracts, when compared to placebo. Thus, these medications are not replacements for estrogen on all of the cardioprotective benefits estrogen provides. Tamoxifen and raloxifene are not appropriate for all women at high risk for breast cancer, due to their potential for severe side effects. You need to discuss with your physician what the various pros and cons would be for your particular health situation. In a report presented at the 1999 annual meeting of The American Society of Clinical Oncologists (ASCO), the nation's largest group of cancer specialists, the ASCO working group concluded that tamoxifen could be offered to healthy women over thirty-five at high risk for breast cancer, but that "in all circumstances, tamoxifen use should be discussed as part of an informed decision-making process with careful considerations of risk, benefits and alternatives." (*JAMA,* July 14, 1999, vol. 282, no.2, pp. 117–118.)

What about women who are at high risk for breast cancer and are worried about the possibility of increasing their risk by taking hormone therapy at menopause? What are some non-hormonal ways to preserve bone if you also at high risk of breast cancer? What options other than estrogen are there to consider if you have a strong family history of heart disease and are also at high risk for breast cancer? These are important questions that women ask me every day in my medical practice, and these same questions come up frequently in the women's health seminars I conduct around the country. In the chart below, I have summarized some of the options you may explore with your health professional. This is not an exhaustive list of everything available, but it does help you see that you do have new strategies and choices available.

NON-HORMONAL OPTIONS TO EXPLORE IF YOU ARE AT HIGH RISK FOR BREAST CANCER AND HIGH RISK FOR:

ALZHEIMERS

- take antioxidants
- reduce aluminum from dietary and other sources
- consider taking gingko biloba
- exercise regularly to improve blood flow to brain and body
- check ferritin levels to avoid iron overload
- check to be certain thyroid function is optimal (affects brain function)
- control blood glucose
- consider use of newer medications

COLON CANCER

- increase fiber in diet
- reduce animal-fat intake
- reduce nitrates and processed foods
- take antioxidants
- increase dietary intake of magnesium
- use stool softeners such as Metamucil

HEART DISEASE and STROKE

- exercise daily
- reduce intake of simple sugars and animal fats
- stop smoking
- use medication to control blood pressure, cholesterol, and triglycerides if unable to achieve desired targets with diet and exercise alone
- if not allergic to aspirin consider taking 80 mg daily
- take antioxidants daily
- make sure you have appropriate intake of calcium, magnesium, and potassium—all are important in regulating blood pressure and heart function

OSTEOPOROSIS

- perform weight-bearing exercise daily
- reduce intake of alcohol, caffeine, and soft drinks
- avoid excess thyroid or corticosteroids
- make sure you have optimal intake of calcium, magnesium, and vitamin D
- stop smoking cigarettes
- consider use of medication to prevent bone breakdown (resorption): Fosamax, Actonel, Miacalcin, Evista

Integrated Approaches for Healing Body, Mind, and Spirit

For those of you reading this who have already been diagnosed with breast cancer, I understand breast cancer is a disease that profoundly affects us as women at every level: physically, emotionally, sexually, socially, and spiritually. Perhaps more than any other illness, it strikes at the very core of our sense of self as women. This deep fear of breast cancer is in part because we live in a culture that directly and indirectly places value on women related to the perfection of the body, especially the breast. Some women may be more traumatized by this diagnosis than are others, but at some level, we are all profoundly affected by the diagnosis. It strikes too at our sense of mortality, and forces us to think about the meaning of our lives. There have been a number of deeply moving books written by women with breast cancer portraying their journey of dealing with the myriad mixed feelings: from anger to sadness, from denial to despair, from pain to recovery and healing. I encourage you to read one or more of these if you have breast cancer, because I think the encouragement and support will be meaningful and helpful.

At times of pain and struggle in our lives, we all need to know we aren't alone. I also encourage you to take time to reflect on what is important to you, what helps you feel more in control of the disease, what kinds of support you want or need, what gives meaning and purpose to your life, and where you want to put your priorities for time and energy. Go to what I have written about this in the last chapter, and begin to write down the goals that are the most meaningful to you. I find that taking a self-inventory such as this provides focus and a sense of "owning" my life, which helps keep me from feeling overwhelmed when I am faced with a crisis.

Be sensitive to your spiritual needs, too. I think modern medicine too often overlooks the importance of touching the spiritual needs of people as well as serving their physical needs. Modern medicine has also overlooked the power of faith as an important part of the healing process. Seeking support from one's spiritual community is just as important as seeking medical support from a physician or psychological support from a therapist or support group. In working with women who have been faced with breast cancer, I have been constantly impressed by how much better patients do overall when they address their spiritual needs and are also involved in taking an *integrated* approach with a variety of healing modalities they put together for themselves. I encourage women to find ways of *living more fully each moment*. In addition to acknowledging the psychological and spiritual dimensions, I like to help patients focus on improving what they eat and drink; taking vitamins and minerals; keeping up with exercise and physical activity; and incorporating visualization, imagery, and meditation to aid the healing abilities of the body and reduce side effects of chemotherapy or radiation treatments. I have described in chapter 16 a number of options to help alleviate menopausal symptoms when hormone therapy cannot be prescribed. There isn't space in this chapter to elaborate on all of these approaches; I simply want to express my philosophy that **all** of these dimensions are crucial to your emotional and physical health, especially when you are faced with a major illness. I encourage you to explore the many helpful resources—books, audio and video-tapes, support groups, national organizations—that are available to bring knowledge, hope, and encouragement to you. Don't let fear of breast cancer—present or future—rob you of your ability to savor each moment that you are alive.

Chapter 15

Hormone Therapy:
Facts and Fallacies

Taking a Look at The Big Picture:
Symptoms and Health Risks

So often, I hear women saying "I'm confused. There doesn't seem to be **an** answer. Every book I read says something different. Everybody I talk to is *doing something different.* Or, everybody I talk to is on the same thing. Why? What about herbs for hot flashes? What about progesterone cream for osteoporosis? What's the difference with all the estrogens? How do I make sense of all this?" Keep in mind these **two critical points** when reading *any* book on menopause or thinking about hormone therapy:

POINT 1. The *real* issue is not an "either-or" approach: "If I am having symptoms of menopause, do I take hormones *or not*?" "I'm not having symptoms, so I don't need hormones, do I?" Your key question here, and any decision about taking hormones, should not be focused just on whether or not you have symptoms.

You need to look at the big picture of your health and ask questions specific to YOU: "What are my health risks? Which of my health risks will be *helped* by hormones? Which of my health risks could be *made worse* by the type of hormones I use? Which type of hormone therapy, and route of taking hormones, is best suited to my individual needs? What options do I have?"

In my opinion, when women ask the question about taking hormones *just based on presence or absence of symptoms,* they are missing the most important points of all. Hormones are not the only way to manage symptoms. There are *many* other ways to minimize symptoms . . . from acupuncture to herbs to nonhormonal medications to zen meditation. The crucial issue is whether you may be *missing* **silent, subtle changes that may significantly affect your future health,** like bone loss, brain effects, glucose intolerance, or cholesterol changes. For example, both acupuncture and some herbs may reduce hot flashes but may not be providing protection against bone loss that you might not know about for another ten years. How will you feel ten years from now when you have lost two inches in height from vertebral bone loss, you have daily back pain from verte-bral fractures, and your doctor says that you could have prevented this bone loss with good hormone therapy or antiresorptive medica-tion taken earlier? Would you be upset with yourself for not taking more aggressive steps than just herbs in order to prevent bone loss? If the answer to this question is "Yes, I'd do a real guilt trip on myself," then pay attention and check into your options more thoroughly.

When I do a bone density test for my patients, and women discover the bone loss, I hear them say, "Why didn't somebody tell me? I thought the progesterone cream I used for the last three years would prevent bone loss. I thought herbs were all I needed to get rid of the hot flashes. Since I didn't have any more hot flashes, I thought everything was fine." You simply can't assume that all is well inside your body if you don't have any symptoms that you notice. You need the reliable, objective tests at an early stage so that you have this critical informa-tion to guide your decision making for now and the years ahead.

POINT 2. Remember: **Every woman's body is different.** *Any* hor-mone options *must* be designed to provide what *you* need for your body. The amount and type of hormones you take is not likely to be the same as what your friend takes if it is truly individualized to your needs. We cannot continue this crazy "cookbook," "one-prescription-fits-all" approach to women's hormone needs that has been the standard approach in most gynecology settings in the United States for decades. Even now, with all the emphasis on individualizing the prescriptions, and many new natural bioidentical hormone products available, women themselves often say to me, "But my friend is taking Premarin and Provera every day, why are you suggesting something different for me?" Why wouldn't I? Your body is different, your genes are different, your metabolism is different, our health issues are different. Maybe your diet, exercise, and stress level are also different. All of these factors, and more, will determine what type of hormone and what amount you need at any given time. Not to mention that people have different *pref-erences.* Some women say they hate the patch on their skin; other women tell me they hate taking pills. *Vive le difference!* Today, there are many options. Keep in mind also that just because you enjoy trading kitchen recipes does not mean that it's a good idea to trade *hormone* recipes or swap prescriptions when you run out.

Each of us reaches a time when we need to make *our own* deci-sion for our own health. How do you do this in an educated, informed way? In this chapter, and throughout my book, I hope to give you suggestions and guidelines to help in this process. Let's examine some of the issues. First, do I think *all* postmenopausal women need estrogen? No. Many women are healthy and have no symptoms without adding hormones, and they are blessed with good genes and lifestyle habits that give them great bone density, a normal cholesterol profile and great memory as they grow older. But the problem is, how do you determine who does and who doesn't have reasons to use hormones? Is it just postmenopausal women with diagnosed disease who should take hormones? Yes, most women in this category probably should. But by the time diseases like vascular damage and osteoporosis are diagnosed, it may be too late to *reverse the damage*, and all you can hope for is to keep from *getting worse*. What about postmenopausal women with just symptoms? Some may really benefit from hormones, and some may still not need anything more than herbs, healthy diet, and exercise. Some women have *marked symptoms* and *little* disease risk; others have *no* symptoms and *major* disease risk. You really need objective information to determine the best answer for you.

That's what CiCi did when she turned forty-four and came for a preventive medicine consult, saying she wanted to "take charge" of her health and do the "right things" before menopause. She was five feet nine inches tall and had a heavy, sturdy body build. She was still menstruating regularly, and had no symptoms of menopause, not even fragmented sleep. She had continued her walking program three to four times a week after an injury prevented her from running. She did not take calcium, but had been a milk drinker during childhood and continued to have skim milk daily as an adult. She did not smoke, but did drink one glass of wine with dinner on a regular basis. She had been in good health, and said, "I want to stay that way as long as possible!" She asked about having a bone density evaluation done for a baseline, and we did this.

Amazingly, and quite unexpectedly, she was already **two standard deviations below the norm for her age.** She was shocked, and so was I. Neither of us had expected to find *existing bone loss*, since her health picture was so good, and she had not had any menstrual or other changes suggesting she was becoming menopausal. Needless to say, this information changed the picture significantly, and we had to determine what the next steps would be and what her options were. She said later, "I am so glad I looked at this whole picture *now*! What if I had just gone by the risk factors, and hadn't thought I was at risk for osteoporosis? I'm so grateful to find out now when I can do something about it." As CiCi discovered, symptoms frequently do **not** correlate very well with risk of long-term disease.

I was an example of the other situation. I had no disease like bone loss and no heart disease risk, but I was experiencing a great number of really disruptive symptoms beginning about age thirty-eight: fragmented sleep, waking up many times at night and then feeling exhausted the next morning; and what must have been hot flashes but they didn't feel exactly like what I thought hot flashes were like. Also, because I was only thirty-eight, neither my gynecologist nor I recognized these symptoms as the beginning of ovarian decline. Premenstrual mood changes that had not previously been a problem suddenly became noticeable and bothersome. I also started to have frequent ovarian cysts. It turned out that these were all perimenopausal *symptoms*. When I was checked, my bone mineral density was above average, my cholesterol was 130, and I had an HDL of 70. My doctor said he had never seen a cholesterol/HDL ratio that low. I have been exercising most of my adult life, and I also have a heavier body build. Since I did have a lot of symptoms that were interfering with my quality of life, I elected to start a low dose of supplemental 17-beta estradiol, using the estradiol patch. Within a week, it made a world of difference in my sleep and my energy level (from sleeping normally again, I decided); even my clarity of thinking and word recall improved. I had not realized how much I was having these subtle changes until I was given the estrogen patch. At the time, it definitely was not the standard practice to start premenopausal women on even a low dose of additional estrogen. My doctor and I were later vindicated in the validity of our decision as more data became available, and recommendations began changing around 1992 or so. Even before that, however, I felt validated by the rightness of my decision, *for me*, based on my significantly enhanced sense of *feeling well and feeling back to my normal self*.

A letter I received very recently illustrates the same point. This patient, in her early forties, has been struggling with fibromyalgia and persistent insomnia for several years, and our testing revealed her markedly low estradiol even though she was still menstruating, as well as an early phase of low thyroid function. I started her on a 17-beta estradiol, low dose thyroid, cyclic natural progesterone (Prometrium), and natural testosterone, as well as tapered off her amitriptyline which was causing so many side effects. I received this letter four months later, after having only two appointments with her:

> I also want to tell you how good I am feeling. I have a life back. In fact, it is so noticeable that within the past 24 hours, I have been asked by 3 different women about what I have done. One has my book written by Dr. Vliet, one has borrowed a copy and one is looking in the book store for a copy. There is a common thread to their conversations with me. They all have health problems and have all been told by their doctors that it could be hormonal but no tests are offered or a way of addressing that situation. Their doctors have even said that there is not a test for hormones, and all have been given antidepressants, like I was, and told to try to cope. I was not doing well at all on the PremPro. I am so grateful to be feeling so much better and be able to get around, free of pain, and do things again.

Each of us must make our decision based upon knowledge of our whole health picture and our individual needs and desires. Gail Sheehy, in her 1991 book, *The Silent Passage,* referred to osteoporosis, heart disease, and dementia as the "silent thieves" of later life and health because they are ones that typically do *not* announce themselves with many *early* symptoms. I agree with her description, and I am dismayed by the patients I see daily in our practice who have been silently robbed of their quality of life, whether by fear of taking hormones or by failure of doctors to do the proper tests and offer options for individualized prescriptions. The bottom line is that you need to assess the aspects summarized in the table below as you consider your midlife health management and the possibility of taking hormones.

DR. VLIET'S HEALTH CHECK POINTS TO GUIDE DECISION MAKING

1. Check your family history, especially first-degree relatives (parents and siblings) for common problems such as heart disease, high blood pressure, osteoporosis, diabetes, cancers, dementias, thyroid disorders, etc.

2. Evaluate your lifestyle habits (diet, exercise, intake of calcium-magnesium and antioxidants, smoking, alcohol use, forgetting to use seatbelts in your car, etc.) and work now to eliminate or change the unhealthy ones.

3. Examine your own health risks, pattern of illnesses, and diagnosed diseases that might be helped by proper use of hormones (such as high cholesterol, high blood pressure, diabetes, osteoporosis or osteopenia, to mention a few).

4. Work with a physician who will do *objective* tests (in addition to physical exam), such as the following:

   (a) *Measure the serum levels of your ovary hormones.* If you are still menstruating, you need to look at the low point of the cycle, Days 1–3 and the ratio of estradiol to progesterone in the luteal phase or about Days 19–22). If you have stopped menstruating, or have had a hysterectomy, then one time of measuring all the ovarian hormones usually will do.

   (b) *Check your fasting lipid profile* (cholesterol, HDL, LDL, triglycerides).

   (c) *Check your fasting glucose and insulin* to check for diabetes or insulin resistance (both are risk factors for heart disease).

   (d) *Check your bone density of the hip and spine* (DEXA is the most reliabletest) to measure your "bone bank account." Heel and arm tests aren't well correlated with degree of loss at hip and spine.

   (e) *Check the urine or serum test of N-telopeptide* as a measure of the rate of bone building versus bone breakdown. If this number is too high, even if your bone density is still good, it indicates that you are already beginning the process of excessive bone breakdown and are at higher risk for later life fractures. High levels of NTx mean you should be taking more aggressive steps now to preserve bone. Taking calcium and exercising regularly will usually not be enough on their own to reverse this process.

© Elizabeth Lee Vliet, M.D., 2000

If you and your physician decide that you may benefit from hormones, you need to know that the guidelines have changed in the last few years. It used to be that women were told to *wait a year after their last period,* but we now realize that waiting this long allows more bone loss, memory loss, and negative cholesterol-triglyceride changes to occur. Even if you are still menstruating it helps to know your objective measures, such as bone density, to enable you to make a decision that gives you the most benefit. It *may* mean starting hormone therapy *before* menopause for some who have low bone density or other hormone-responsive problems like the women I have described throughout this book. It may mean for other women that your health measures check out fine and you don't need hormones at all. Just reevaluate your picture in a year or two, and keep track of how your body is changing. The key is to intervene with positive action (hormones, other medication, etc.) *before* more serious disease develops.

Current recommendations are that hormones may be started when:

1. symptoms appear and quality of life is diminished (regardless of age);
2. when disease risks are identified;
3. actual disease, such as osteopenia, osteoporosis, high cholesterol is present; or
4. a combination of these issues.

Synthetic Progestins versus Natural Progesterone

There are several terms that many women find confusing, so I will clarify these to help you understand various options.

Progestogen is the broad term used to describe *any substance* that has chemical effects to prepare the body for sustaining a pregnancy, called "progestational" activity.

Progesterone is a biologically natural progestogen produced by the corpus luteum (egg released from the ovary) before menopause, by the placenta during pregnancy, and to a much smaller extent, by the adrenal gland. Progesterone acts by overseeing a number of metabolic effects in the mother's body that will help her carry the baby full term. Progesterone's metabolic effects aren't generally needed after menopause when you are not trying to have a pregnancy. The important exception to this is progesterone opposing the estrogen effect on the uterine lining to prevent hyperplasia and possible development of cancer of the uterine lining.

Progesterone USP is the form of natural progesterone made in a laboratory from building-block molecules (disogenin, diascorea, and others) found in wild yams and soybeans. These plant precursors are chemically different from *progesterone*, and our bodies do not have the enzymes to make progesterone from simply consuming yams and soybeans or using creams with these precursors in them. The yam and soy building-block chemicals have to be changed in the laboratory in a series of steps to make the bioidentical molecule of progesterone that can be biologically active in the body. This synthesized progesterone is then purified to meet FDA standards, and is now called USP (or pharmaceutical grade) progesterone. USP progesterone is used by pharmaceutical companies to make the FDA-approved commercial products: tablets (Prometrium), and vaginal gel (Crinone) used in menopausal hormone therapy and for infertility patients. USP progesterone is also used by compounding pharmacists to make individual prescriptions of tablets, suppositories, and creams for patients. USP progesterone is the active form of the hormone that is commonly added to wild yam creams. When given in the correct dose and schedule for hormone therapy regimens, progesterone generally has far fewer unpleasant side effects than the progestins (like Provera and others).

Progestin is a term that generally refers to chemical compounds made in the laboratory that have properties *similar to* progesterone, but that have a *different* molecular structure and are many times *more potent* than natural progesterone. Progestins are members of the larger group of *progestogens* because they do have progestational ("pro-pregnancy") activity, but they are *not* compounds normally found in the human body. Technically, progesterone itself is a "natural" progestin, but we don't usually mean "natural progesterone" when we use the term *progestin*. Progestins may be made in the laboratory using the natural hormones progesterone or testosterone as basic building blocks. Each of the chemically different progestins has slightly different properties, depending on whether progesterone itself or testosterone is used as a starting point, and depending on what chemical modifications are made. Therefore, each type of progestin has slightly different side effects. Since all of the synthetic progestins are significantly more potent than progesterone itself, they are used in much lower doses than are needed for progesterone. As a result of their potency, and their chemical differences, progestins can produce effects in the body that are at times quite unpleasant and undesirable. Synthetic progestins, whether in birth control pills or given in postmenopause, are the most common cause of unpleasant side effects associated with hormone therapy. I will talk more about this issue in the next section.

As I indicated, the primary reason any progestin (synthetic or natural) is added to a menopausal hormone regimen is to reduce the risk of endometrial cancer in women who have a uterus. Adding a progestogen (synthetic progestin or natural progesterone) causes the uterine lining to become *secretory* instead of *proliferative* (estrogen effect). This change stops the endometrium from growing and allows it to be shed as a "withdrawal bleeding" when the progestogen is stopped. Shedding the uterine lining at regular intervals, whether monthly or every couple of months, protects against the buildup of endometrium that can later lead to cancer. **If you have had a hysterectomy, you no longer have a uterine lining to become cancerous,** so the current consensus of the American College of Obstretricians and Gynecologists (ACOG) and menopause specialists is that *you do not need to take either synthetic progestin or natural progesterone* after menopause. Since all progestins, as well as natural progesterone, may reduce the benefits of estrogen and also have their own side effects, most physicians who understand the metabolic effects of progesterone/progestins don't recommend their routine use if you don't need protection of the uterine lining.

Provera (generic name: medroxyprogesterone acetate, or MPA) is the most commonly used synthetic progestin in the United States for menopause therapy, although it was never actually approved by the FDA for that purpose. Other brand names for MPA include Cyrin, and Amen. MPA was originally approved by the FDA in the 1960s for contraceptive use under the brand name Depo-Provera and has since been used to treat abnormal uterine bleeding and some types of amenorrhea. In more recent years, MPA and other progestins have been used for protection of the uterine lining in menopausal regimens. MPA is derived from progesterone, and is more *progestational* and *less androgenic* than progestins derived from testosterone; other progestins have differing degrees of progestational and androgenic activity to give them varying therapeutic and side effect profiles.

Another group of progestins, such as norethindrone (brand names: Aygestin, Micronor, Nor-QD, Norlutate), are derived from the male hormone 19-nor-testosterone, and as a result they have more *androgenic* effects similar to testosterone in addition to their progestational activity. This group of progestins is often used when women are experiencing a loss of libido since they have less libido-robbing effects than Provera or other progestational progestins. My patients tell me that the androgenic progestins typically cause less bloating, breast tenderness, weight gain, and depression than Provera and other brands of MPA. The more androgenic progestins, however, are not usually recommended (in the standard doses, at least) for women with high cholesterol and low HDL, since the androgenic effects can worsen the risk of cardiovascular disease and decrease the benefits of estrogen. The more androgenic progestins tend to have fewer depression-causing side effects than Provera-type progestins. All of the progestins may cause acne, hair loss, low libido, and weight gain, particularly if used in doses that are too high relative to the amount of estradiol present. The trick is to find the type and dose that works best for you if there is a medical reason, such as suppression of fibroids or endometriosis, that the more potent synthetic progestins are needed. I hope these examples begin to give you an idea how the different progestins ideally should be tailored to a woman's individual health risk profile. I will say it again: We should **not** be using a cookbook approach, giving 80–90 percent of women the same dose and type of hormones!

What about human progesterone? Why even use the synthetic progestins if they tend to cause so many side effects? Why isn't progesterone used as the progestogen for menopause regimens? It is . . . **in Europe,** where it has been widely available and used extensively for several decades. Why wasn't it available in the United States until the FDA approved Prometrium and Crinone in late 1998–early 1999? Primarily for economic, technological, and political reasons: as a natural compound, readily derived from plant precursors found in wild yams and soybeans, progesterone was not itself able to be patented as a unique product, and it was not well-enough absorbed orally to be a reliable way to use it for uterine cancer prevention. Until the process of *micronization* (ability to make the hormone particles smaller) was developed to make the oral forms reliable, and patentable products could be devised, there wasn't a pharmaceutical company in this country willing to invest the millions of dollars needed to gain FDA approval if the company could not recoup their investment with a new patented product.

For many years, Progesterone in oil *was* available in the United States in injectable form made by Upjohn, the company that also makes Provera and Depo-Provera. The injectable form of progesterone USP in oil has been widely used by gynecologists for years to treat bleeding problems, and I was taught to use it more than twenty-five years ago while in medical school. So natural progesterone really isn't an overlooked hormone or a new idea as some progesterone proponents claim. But since most women understandably don't want to have to get an injection on a regular basis, it is not surprising that this form of progesterone has not been widely used for menopause therapy. Compounding pharmacies were the only way to get micronized progesterone in the United States, until 1998–99 when Prometrium was approved by the FDA. These individually made prescriptions tended to cost a lot more than the commercial product Provera, and many doctors were therefore reluctant to recommend them. Other factors limiting the widespread use of the compounded natural progesterone options were: (1) they generally weren't covered by insurance plans, so consumers had to pay out of pocket for them, and (2) each compounding pharmacy had its own formula, making it difficult for gynecologists to feel certain of the reliability of the product. This meant micronized progesterone tended to be used, until now, mainly by physicians who specialized in the treatment of PMS and other hormone-related problems to help women who couldn't tolerate the commercial synthetic progestins.

I have used natural micronized progesterone in my women's health practice since the late 1970s, with a great deal of success. I have learned a lot over the years about the nuances of dose, side effect changes based on how it is given (tablets, suppositories, prescription creams, injectable), and ways of working with progesterone to create individualized regimens and fewer side effects for my patients with all kinds of hormone problems. In fact, the success has been dramatic when compared to the standard cookbook approach using Provera. One of my patients, a woman judge, called me and practically shouted over the phone in a jubilant voice about my changing her to natural progesterone: **"It was 10 million times better than Provera, like night and day. I can live with this, I don't feel crazy and bloated like I did with the Provera. The Provera was really driving me crazy, I couldn't stand it."**

Listen to the voice of this fifty-three-year-old woman, who had been having very bothersome side effects of depression, weight gain, lethargy, and "all that PMS feeling again" with the Provera phase of her HRT, until I changed her to natural progesterone with the Estrace: *"I'm feeling great! I am so pleased with the changes and this combination. I'm floored by all of this. I can't believe the difference in how I feel taking the natural progesterone, it's nothing like what I felt on the Provera. I don't feel so depressed and slowed down like I did. I used to hate those fourteen days on Provera, and sometimes I didn't even take it. I didn't want to tell my doctor, but I just didn't like how I felt on the Provera. I'm thrilled, the natural progesterone worked like clockwork, and my period started within twenty-four hours of stopping the progesterone. It was like a normal period, no pain or any problems."*

Now that we had an FDA-approved commercial product that is standardized in the manufacturing process, has reliable quality control, and is covered by most insurance plans, more and more physicians are now using the oral micronized progesterone for menopause regimens. If the dose or type of oil base (peanut) or dyes in Prometrium cause problems for some women, then we still have the option of micronized progesterone obtained from independent pharmacists who compound the prescription individually for patients based on the physician's prescribed amount. Two independent pharmacies with extensive experience compounding natural progesterone that I have found to be reliable and reputable resources for my patients, are *Belmar Pharmacy* (Charles Hakala, R.Ph.) and *Spence Pharmacy* (Daryl Spence, R.Ph). Phone numbers are listed in appendix II; you may call them for information on their products and services. Both pharmacies will work with your physician to provide doses right for you, and both pharmacies take many of the major health insurance plans.

Even with natural progesterone, there are still some women who simply aren't able to tolerate any progestogen, synthetic or natural. Women who are markedly sensitive to progesterone or progestins may experience intolerable degrees of depression, loss of libido, pain flares, headaches, lethargy, bloating, breast tenderness, and weight gain. For these women, the American College of Obstetricians and Gynecologists published the ACOG Progestin Consensus Statement in 1988 (still valid today), which said: If a woman is intolerant to the progestin, it is acceptable to use unopposed estrogen as long as she is willing to have an annual endometrial biopsy and report immediately any abnormal bleeding. Many physicians are reluctant to use this approach because of the endometrial cancer issue, and because of the erratic and potentially serious bleeding problems that can occur with long use of estrogen only. Going without progestin and having an annual biopsy is an avenue you may explore with your doctor if you have not been able to find any progestin that you can use and natural progesterone doesn't work for you, and if you don't tend to have bleeding problems that could be made worse with this approach. The use of estrogen alone tends to be a greater concern in women who are not getting adequate health care and who have bleeding over a long period of time that is not being properly evaluated. But, for women who have a lot of side effects with the progesterone or progestin, and have severe cardiovascular risks or other problems precluding use of progestogens, then the ACOG position does provide an option for you as long as you take responsibility to see that you are appropriately monitored. There are really not any hard and fast rules in this situation, so it once again comes down to *an individualized approach.*

Progesterone and Wild Yam Over-the-Counter Creams: Caveat Emptor!

The surge of interest in natural hormone options has resulted in a proliferation of over-the-counter products marketed as "natural progesterone" or "extract of wild yam." Many of these products are just scams, since "wild yam" cannot be converted to active progesterone by our bodies, as I explained above. Those creams that do contain USP progesterone often contain amounts that exceed the current recommended doses of progesterone for therapeutic effects. These products are not regulated by the FDA and vary a great deal in the active hormone content and potency. I have found that most manufacturers will not release information about the contents of the products when I have sought this information so I could better advise my patients. I have also been concerned, as a women's health advocate, about yet another spate of misleading and, in many cases, blatantly incorrect advertising for these products. Even though these products are touted as having *no* side effects, if a woman is sensitive to progesterone, there may still be enough hormone content to produce depression, loss of libido, increased appetite, weight gain, worsening of diabetes, increase in yeast problems, acne, bloating, lethargy or tiredness, backaches, flares of fibromyalgia-type pain, and other progesterone-induced body effects. I have had many patients who experienced these problems and had no idea it was the supposedly "safe" wild yam or progesterone cream that was creating these unwanted effects. How do you as a consumer sort out the potential false claims and make an informed decision?

In 1994, I met with researchers from Aeron Laboratories, who have done work in hormone receptor assays for many years, particularly in regard to estrogen and progesterone receptors in breast tissue samples of cancer patients. These scientists had similar questions to the ones I was asking about the over-the-counter creams, and they decided to run *blind* assays of a variety of the commercially available products. They periodically update these assays as new products come on the market, and then publish the current results for consumers and physicians to be able to make informed choices. Aeron gave me permission to publish one of their earlier studies in the following tables. I think this type of technical information provides an important service to women who are being led astray by misleading advertising. Since new products are coming on the market constantly, and manufacturers change their formulas from time to time, it is important to keep up to date on the latest analyses if you want to check out a product. You may be able to find out this information from the manufacturer or check consumer watchdog agencies on the Web.

If you are using one of these products that has a higher progesterone content, you need to let your doctor know. Read the label carefully to see if it says "progesterone" in addition to wild yam extract. If you have been having any of the symptoms I mentioned above since starting one of these products, you may want to stop the product and observe what happens, or change to one from the list that has a lower progesterone activity. In any case, be aware that many of these products have *significant progesterone effects,* even though they are sold as "natural" and/or as "wild yam extract." It is important that you also keep in mind that too much progesterone relative to estrogen can cause heavy bleeding and painful menstruation. This is a point many women don't know, and the makers of these creams don't tell you. We generally hear more about bleeding problems that occur when there is excess estrogen relative to progesterone, but it is also true that constant use of progestins or progesterone *without the right estrogen balance* can cause erratic, heavy bleeding. Your gynecologist needs to know what over-the-counter "hormonally-active" creams or herbs you may be using.

PROGESTERONE CONTENT OF BODY CREAMS

I. MORE THAN 400 MG PROGESTERONE per OUNCE OF CREAM

NAME	Mg prog/oz	Manufacturer
Angel Care	658	Angel Care USA
Balance	408	Vitality Lifechoice
Bio Balance	>400	Elan Vitale
Cumulus	526	Cumulus of Oregon
Derma Gest	510	Broadmoore Labs
EssPro7	502	Young Living
Fair Lady	608	Specialty Living
Femarone 17	536	Wise Essentials
Fem Crème	603	Pure Essence
Fem Gest	522	Bio-Nutritional Formulas
Green Pastures	1,347	Green Pastures
Maxine's Feminique	423	Country Life
Natra Gest	5,506	Broadmoore Labs
OstaDerm	>400	Bezwecken
Pro-Alo	>400	HealthWatchers Sys
Procreme	489	THG Health Products
Procreme Plus	926	THG Health Products
ProDerma	623	Phillips Nutritionals
Pro-Gest	980	Prof & Tech Serv, Inc.
Progesta-Care	484	Life-Flo Health Care
Progonol	>400	Bezwecken
SupraGest	452	Health Alternatives West
Today's Man	501	Specialty Items
Wild Yam Crème	525	Wise Woman Essentials
Woman Wise	523	Jason Natural Products
Yamcon (Pro) Estra	553	Phillips Nutritionals

II. 2-15 MG PROGESTERONE per OUNCE OF CREAM

Endocreme	Wuliton Labs	Palmyra, MO
Femarone	Wise Woman Essentials	Minn, MN
Life Changes	MW Labs	Atlanta, GA
Menopause Form	PMS Relief, Inc	Auburn, CA
Nutri-Gest	NutrSupplies, Inc	West Palm Beach, FL
PhytoGest	Karuna Corp	Novato, CA
PMS Formula	PMS Relief, Inc	Auburn, CA
Pro-Dermex	Gero Vita Int'l	Reno, NV
Wild Yam Ext	Phytopharmica	Green Bay, WI
Yamcon Regular	Phillips Nutr	Laguna Hills, CA

III. LESS THAN 2 MG PROGESTERONE per OUNCE OF CREAM

Progerone	Nature's Nutr., Inc.	Vero Beach, FL
Progestone-HP	Dixie Health, Inc.	Atlanta, GA
Wild Yam Cream	Alvin Last, Inc.	Yonkers, NY

Reference: analysis by RIA at Aeron Laboratories, 5-9-95 and 9-15-98

For comparison, a dose of the FDA-approved, standardized prescription progesterone vaginal cream, Crinone 4 percent, delivers 40 mg per application, and the recommended amount is one applicator every other night for only six doses a month. Using Crinone 4 percent cream would deliver an average of 20 mg a day over twelve days. This is the amount that research to date has shown is sufficient for preventing endometrial hyperplasia. Depending on the amount used, many of the over-the-counter progesterone creams shown above will deliver *far in excess* of the amount delivered by Crinone 4 percent cream. The excess amount of progesterone in many of the over-the-counter creams accounts for such side effects as weight gain, bloating, breast tenderness, headaches, low libido, acne, sweet cravings, depressed mood, lack of energy, fatigue, back aches, and other effects of high levels of progesterone. Just think about the last trimester of pregnancy when progesterone is highest and you have an idea of what may occur with large amounts of progesterone in skin creams.

Myths and Misunderstandings about Hormone Side Effects

One of the common problems I encounter in talking with women about hormone therapy is *which* hormones typically cause what side effects. Most women, and the media, blame estrogen for all the various side effects attributed to the generic terms *estrogen therapy* or *hormone therapy*. This is not the case. As I have described in other chapters, the *type and dose* of estrogen, progestin (or progesterone), and testosterone that you take makes a big difference in what side effects you experience. The *route* by which the hormone is given can also affect the degree of side effects. In addition, each hormone has a typical "profile" of possible side effects. An example I hear a lot is that the "estrogen" causes weight gain, bloating, depression, and breast fullness. These are typical progestin or progesterone side effects. These may be diminished by (1) changing to a different type of progestin, (2) changing to natural micronized progesterone, (3) changing from oral progesterone to nonoral (vaginal or rectal, transdermal, or as a last resort, progesterone injections), and/or (4) decreasing the progestin/progesterone dose.

In many of the newsletters from "alternative" practitioners (usually promoting progesterone skin creams), I have found a consistent pattern of the authors and editors mixing up the side effects of estrogen and progestin: attributing progestin effects to estrogen and giving estrogen a further bum rap. Since many of these people are male and don't live in a female body with our hormonal cycle, they don't realize the major differences between estrogen effects and progesterone. All you have to do is think about how you feel during the first half of your cycle when estrogen is the dominant hormone present (and there is almost no progesterone being produced) and then consider what you typically experience a week or two before your period when progesterone is the dominant hormone to know what I am talking about!

Studies of PMS over many years have consistently found that if women do not ovulate and do not produce progesterone, they don't tend to experience the negative symptoms of PMS that cycle. In addition, very few of the practitioners who proposed the idea that PMS was a "progesterone deficiency" had ever done any actual measurements of hormone levels in the luteal phase of the cycle to see if their theory was correct. I have done these hormone assays in thousands of patients over the last twenty-some years and have consistently demonstrated just the opposite: women with declining estradiol and normal progesterone levels in the luteal phase of the cycle are the ones who report the worst PMS symptoms.

As a simple test of who is "right," go by your own body experience: If you feel the best just before ovulation when estradiol is high and progesterone low, it is unlikely you will benefit from adding a progesterone cream for PMS. If on the other hand, you are someone who has always felt her best the third week of the cycle when progesterone peaks (in an ovulatory cycle), then progesterone may be a therapeutic approach that could work for you. **Just remember, the PMS phase of the cycle is the time *progesterone* is the main hormone and estrogen is lower at that time compared to the first half of a healthy cycle.** This will help you have an easier time remembering which hormone is more often associated with what side effects.

Estrogen may also cause breast tenderness and fullness if the dose is more than usually needed for menopausal therapy. If this occurs, the most appropriate course of action is to decrease the dose and/or change the type of estrogen. I find that the mixed estrogens (esterified or conjugated equine types, as described further in the tables in this chapter) generally cause more breast fullness than do the 17-beta estradiol products. My hypothesis on why this difference occurs is that the conjugated equine estrogens contain such a large amount of long-acting equine estrogens, which appear to be concentrated in the breast and contribute to overstimulation of the tissue. The 17-beta estradiol products are much shorter in their duration of effect and don't accumulate in the body the way the esterified and horse-derived estrogens do. For example, after stopping the conjugated equine estrogens, it may take eight to fourteen weeks for the equilin forms to be cleared from the body; when you stop one of the 17-beta estradiol forms of estrogen, it takes only a day, or perhaps two at most, for the levels to drop back to what they were before you started taking it. All of these differences have a huge impact on the degree of *positive response* as well as the type and severity of *side effects*.

A number of menopause specialists agree that women have different types and degrees of side effects on different hormone preparations. Examples include women on Premarin having more breast tenderness, more problems with atypical elevations in blood pressure, greater increases in triglycerides than patients on 17-beta estradiol as patches or tablets. Drs. Dan Mishell and Rogerio Lobo, both well-respected menopause researchers, have well documented the adverse effects of conjugated equine estrogen (Premarin) on liver parameters, showing that Premarin causes a three-fold increase in angiotensinogen when compared to just estradiol or estrone. Angiotensinogen is a substance in the body that tends to cause increases in blood pressure, so you really don't want anything to increase angiotensinogen too much. The angiotensinogen increase with the equine estrogens was reported by Dr. Malcolm Whitehead, British menopause researcher, **in 1982. Dr. Whitehead's studies have been ignored as a potentially important issue affecting menopausal women in this country.**

The type of tablet formulation is another important issue to consider if you have multiple medication sensitivities and/or allergies to dyes or binders in tablets. According to the advertisement *"Here is what makes Premarin different"* (cited in the table below), this brand of conjugated equine estrogens is prepared by "a unique manufacturing process . . . with more than 63 *coatings"* on the tablet (italics mine). A remarkable number of my patients over the years have experienced complete resolution of such symptoms as skin itching, joint aches, muscle aches, and urinary (bladder and urethra) burning when I switched them from Premarin to estradiol patches or Estrace dye-free tablets. I have hypothesized that many of these symptoms may be triggered by the various dyes and coatings in the Premarin tablet, to which some women are sensitive, even if they do not have an actual allergy. Estrace 0.5 mg tablets are free of dyes and many of the common binders or inert ingredients that tend to cause sensitivity reactions, but the 1 mg and 2 mg tablets have dyes that may be a problem for some women. I raise this issue for you to consider if you have been experiencing any of these symptoms, so that you can talk with your physician about trying another type of estrogen.

When you look at the chart below comparing what is actually in the leading estrogen products, I think it may be clearer to you *why* I find so many more side effects with the conjugated estrogens. Look at how many more different types of estrogens there are in this product and how many more "keys" there are to confuse the "locks" of our body's estradiol receptor sites. The 17-beta estradiol products that are available in the United States provide *only the two types of human estrogen* our bodies are designed to use, estradiol (E2) and smaller amounts of estrone (E1) made in the liver from the E2.

TYPES OF ESTROGEN PRESENT IN VARIOUS PRODUCTS
(Listed in descending order of amount present)

	Cenestin (synthetic plant-derived conjugated estrogens)#	Premarin (conjugated horse-derived estrogens)*	Estratab (esterified estrogens)**	Estrace tablets,* Vivelle DOT, Alora and Climara patches (17-beta estradiol soy/yam derived)
estrone	58%	49.9%	88.8%	
equilin	28%	22.8%	5.9%	
17-α dihydro equilin	15%	13.5%	2.6%	
17-α estradiol		3.6%	1.2%	
δ-8,9-dihydro estrone		3.7%		
equilenin		2.8%	1.1%	
7-β dihydro equilin		1.4%		
17-β estradiol	X	0.5%	—	100%
17-α dihydro equilenin		1.4%	—	
7-β dihydro equilenin	X	?%	—	

* Premarin advertisement, *Journal of the American Medical Assoc.*, February 8, 1995, and manufacturer's prescribing information.
** From manufacturer's prescribing information.
# From manufacturer's prescribing information.

Dose Conversions: Human versus Conjugated Equine Estrogens, Progestins versus Natural Progesterone

As a general guideline, I am including the dose conversions here. Since Premarin (and the other mixed estrogens shown in the table) contain additional types of estrogens, the total estrogen effects from the mixture of compounds is greater so the dose used is smaller than the dose of tablets of oral micronized 17-beta estradiol (Estrace). When you use a patch form of estradiol, there is greater absorption and less hormone lost in the liver "first pass," so the dose for a patch is typically decreased to about 10 percent of an oral dose. For example, 1 mg Estrace tablet is approximately equivalent to a 0.1 mg transdermal estradiol patch. Other approximate comparable amounts are shown in the table. Natural *progesterone* is much *less potent* than the synthetic progestins so the amount you need to provide the protective effect on the uterine lining will be a much larger number of milligrams to give the same effect as the usual dose of Provera, Cyrin, or Aygestin.

DOSE COMPARISIONS	
PROGESTIN DOSE	**PROGESTERONE DOSE**
Provera, Cyrin, Aygestin 10 mg	progesterone 300-350 mg
Provera, Cyrin, Aygestin 5 mg	progesterone 150-200 mg
Provera, Cyrin, Aygestin 2.5 mg	progesterone 75-100 mg
17-BETA ESTRADIOL (Estrace)	**CONJUGATED (or Esterified) ESTROGENS** (Premarin, Cenestin, Estratab)
0.5 mg tablet (white, no dyes)	0.3 mg tablet (Premarin is red)
1.0 mg tablet (lavender)	0.625 mg tablet (Premarin is burgundy)
2.0 mg tablet (aqua-blue)	1.25 mg tablet (Premarin is yellow)

© Elizabeth Lee Vliet, M.D., 1995

Cancer Risks: What's Real, What's Hype

In chapter 14, I talked about the media emphasis on hormone therapy and breast cancer that gives women an exaggerated picture of their risk of this disease. What about the other cancer fears fueled by such articles? What is the real risk of various cancers if you decide to take hormones? How do you determine *your* personal risk? These are aspects to consider in deciding whether or not to take hormones, because the pay-off in benefits is frequently seen in later years. You are making decisions now that will have their full impact a number of years down the road. How do you make sense of the confusing, and sometimes contradictory, information? The cancer concern about using HRT or ERT involves two types of cancers that have been reported to be increased with use of hormone therapy after menopause: breast cancer (see chapter 14) and endometrial cancer. Colon cancer has been shown to be *decreased* by about 40–50 percent in women who use estrogen after menopause, so this is very good news for women with a family history of colon cancer. Lung cancer in women is primarily caused by cigarette smoking and has not been found to have a particular connection with hormone use. Melanoma, a particularly serious type of skin cancer, and cancers of the blood cells (leukemias) are not thought to be increased or decreased by hormone use, based on current studies analyzing cancer patterns in both hormone users and non–hormone users. So let's talk about the two cancers that have an association with hormone use.

Endometrial Cancer

Endometrial cancer is a malignancy affecting the lining (endo-metrium) of the uterus or womb. It tends to be a slow-growing type of cancer, and most often, *erratic heavy bleeding* is an early symptom. Overall, it is a relatively uncommon cancer, particularly today when women are much quicker to seek medical attention for abnormal bleeding. Your risk of getting endometrial cancer is actually quite small: one in one thousand women (0.001 percent) per year. The following chart compares your lifetime *risk of dying* from cardiovascular disease, breast cancer, and endometrial cancer.

LIFETIME MORTALITY RISK FOR WOMEN	
Disease	**Lifetime Risk of Death**
Coronary Heart Disease	31%
Breast Cancer	2.8%
Endometrial Cancer	less than 1%

Source: Cummings, et al., *Arch.Int.Med.* 1989; 149:2445-8

Today, it is even more rare for women to *die* from endometrial cancer for several reasons: (1) it is slow growing, (2) bleeding usually leads to early diagnosis, (3) metastasis, or spread to other organs, typically doesn't occur until later stages in this cancer (unlike ovarian cancer, which typically has already metastasized by the time it is diagnosed), and (4) it is very treatable, usually with hysterectomy, and has a good outcome with treatment. Women with a history of endometrial cancer generally live a normal life expectancy and die of something else. If you have *already had a hysterectomy* for other reasons, then you no longer have the endometrium present and therefore *cannot develop endometrial cancer.*

What are some of the risk factors for endometrial cancer? This is the *only* type of cancer in women that has been clearly demonstrated to be dependent on *sustained high levels* of estrogen for growth. The relationship of estrogen to endometrial cancer is a linear one: The higher the dose of estrogen and the longer the duration of sustained high levels of estrogen, the higher the risk of developing malignant changes in the lining of the uterus. No other cancer affecting women, not even breast cancer, has been found to be estrogen-dependent in this direct way. This connection was discovered in the 1970s, after *estrogen alone* had been the recommendation for postmenopausal women. In women who had been on long-term estrogen *alone*, not taking a progestin, the incidence of endometrial cancer increased about three to eight times normal.

When this increased rate of uterine cancer was noticed, doctors studied the problem and found that *synthetic progestin or* natural *progesterone* needed to be given *with estrogen* to change the uterine lining to a *secretory* stage allowing it to be shed in a periodic bleeding. Progestins keep the uterine lining from overgrowing into the thickened stage of *hyperplasia* that, over a prolonged period of time, could become malignant. Now that standard practice is to prescribe a progestin along with estrogen in women who have a uterus, the incidence of endometrial cancer in women using hormones has dropped back to its usual *low frequency* in women.

If you are on a *cyclic* progesterone or progestin regimen, when you stop the progestin each month, you will have some degree of menstrual-type "withdrawal" bleeding. This is what you **want** to have happen in order to reduce the endometrial cancer risk by getting rid of the lining of the uterus. On the other hand, many women don't like having menstrual-type flow after menopause and may choose to take a progestin every day. The use of any progestin every day suppresses the lining and stops all bleeding in about 80 percent of women after about six months of continuous progestin use. The other 20 percent of women taking progestin daily tend to continue to have annoying, erratic bleeding and spotting. If you fall in this last group, you may want to talk with your doctor about going back to a cycling regimen so that you have more predictable bleeding patterns. Current research has shown that it is medically safe in terms of reducing endometrial cancer risk if you cycle the progesterone or progestin every other month or even every third month. Whether the progestin is given cyclically or daily, the goal is to minimize the amount to the least possible dose that protects the endometrium in order to reduce the likelihood of unpleasant side effects.

Obesity is another key risk factor for endometrial cancer due to the high levels of estrone produced by fat tissue. Obese women *who do not take supplemental hormones* ("exogenous" hormones) are still at higher risk of developing uterine cancer on the basis of sustained high levels of their own body estrogen ("endogenous" estrogen) made in the fat tissue even after menopause. Women who are significantly overweight and have never had children are at even higher risk, because these women have not had the high progesterone levels of pregnancy to help offset the many years of steady estrogen stimulation of the uterine lining. So endometrial cancer is not just related to *taking hormone supplements*; it may also be caused by estrone in your own body after menopause, even if you do not ever take hormones. Excess estrone is also a risk factor for breast cancer in obese women, so these are other reasons we encourage women to reduce body fat and stay within a healthy body-weight range.

Another interesting finding in recent studies, confirmed by researchers in a number of settings around the world, is that the type of endometrial cancer that occurs in women on hormones after menopause has been found to be a *less aggressive* form of this cancer than the one that occurs in postmenopausal women *not* taking hormones. This parallels what has also been discovered with the differences in breast cancer in women on hormones compared to women not taking hormones. Examinations of the cellular patterns of endometrial cancer in women on hormone therapy showed a *well-differentiated* type, which has a *better prognosis* than poorly differentiated or undifferentiated cancer cells. Another positive difference that has emerged is that women *on ERT* who are diagnosed with endometrial cancer have a *95 percent survival rate*, which is significantly better than the survival rate for women who are found to have endometrial cancer and are *not* taking hormones (see graph of survival comparisons).

Dr. Don Gambrell, Jr., a leading cancer and menopause researcher and clinician, published findings from a nine-year study of cancer patterns in women on hormones and not on hormones. He found that the risk of endometrial cancer was significantly reduced in women using combined therapy with estrogen and progestin; in fact, his studies showed that the risk was *even less* in estrogen/progestin users than it was in untreated patients. Findings such as Dr. Gambrell's have been duplicated by other investigators as well. So I think the press reports have given most women an unfairly negative and alarmist view of both breast and uterine cancer risk from taking hormones.

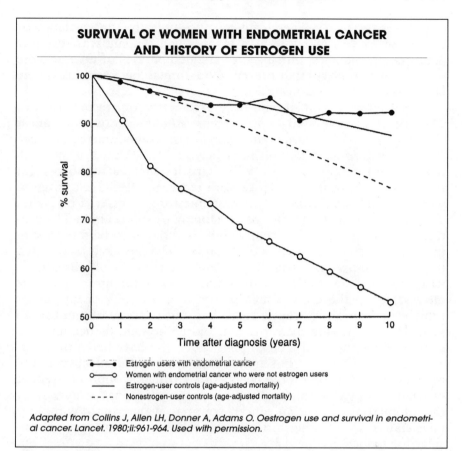

SURVIVAL OF WOMEN WITH ENDOMETRIAL CANCER AND HISTORY OF ESTROGEN USE

% survival

Time after diagnosis (years)

- Estrogen users with endometrial cancer
- Women with endometrial cancer who were not estrogen users
- Estrogen-user controls (age-adjusted mortality)
- - - - Nonestrogen-user controls (age-adjusted mortality)

Adapted from Collins J, Allen LH, Donner A, Adams O. Oestrogen use and survival in endometrial cancer. Lancet. 1980;ii:961-964. Used with permission.

Ovarian Cancer

This type of cancer is the fifth leading cause of cancer death in American women. Even though it is not as common as breast and endometrial cancer, it is more difficult to treat successfully and it tends to spread to other organs earlier in the disease than either breast or uterine cancers. Thus, ovarian cancer strikes a deep chord of fear for women. It occurs in about 4 percent of women in the United States and is primarily a disease of aging, with rates rising dramatically after age fifty. It is also significantly influenced by heredity, which is the reason it is so crucial to know your family history.

Many women have asked "Will hormone therapy increase my risk of ovarian cancer?" There is no direct hormonal association known, but factors that *increase* the number of ovulations a woman has had over her lifetime will increase the risk of ovarian cancer developing later. This is thought to occur as a result of cancer-causing mutations occurring in the rapidly multiplying epithelial cells that cover the ovary. These cells have to multiply after each ovulation in order to repair the area from which the egg was released. Multiple pregnancies, nursing for extended periods of time and use of oral contraceptives that prevent ovulation all help to decrease the later risk of ovarian cancer.

For example, women who have used birth control pills for five years or more have a 40 to 50 percent *reduction* in ovarian cancer risk, and a 60-75 percent *reduction* in risk of endometrial cancer. The longer birth control pills have been used, the lower a woman's risk of both cancers. As of 1999, statistics show a 60-80 percent reduction in ovarian cancer risk with ten years of OC use. Even in women who have the cancer-causing mutation of BRAC 1 or 2, oral contraceptives lower the risk of developing ovarian cancer. The protective effect of the contraceptive pills is thought to be due to suppression of follicle growth and ovulation. The most recent research has found that women who have been on birth control pills continue to also have a **lower risk of ovarian cancer for up to ten years after stopping the OCs.** That's pretty impressive. With my family history of ovarian cancer, if I still had my ovaries, I would in all probability be taking the birth control pills to help reduce my risk. I know of a number of women physicians who have had a tubal ligation for contraception but are taking birth control pills because of this new information on the benefits of birth control pills to reduce ovarian and uterine cancer. If you have a significant family history of endometrial or ovarian cancer, you may want to talk with your physician to see whether birth control pills are an approach to consider for reducing your risk.

CURRENTLY KNOWN RISK FACTORS FOR OVARIAN CANCER

- family history of ovarian and breast cancer
- family history of non-polyposis form of colorectal cancer
- disordered endocrine function (menstrual irregularities, difficulty conceiving), use of fertility drugs for ovarian hyperstimulation
- greater number of ovulations over a lifetime
- previous breast cancer, or breast cancer before age 50
- frequent ovarian cysts
- history of endometriosis
- obesity
- cigarette smoking
- diets high in animal meat/protein/fat
- esidence in heavily industrialized areas (petrochemical pollutants)
- exposure to certain chemicals such as talc-asbestos (hydrous magnesium silicates), which are thought to trigger epithelial cell inflammation around the ovary leading to mutations.

© Elizabeth Lee Vliet, M.D., 1995

One of the difficulties with ovarian cancer is that its early symptoms, such as abdominal distension, bloating, gas/indigestion, chronic stomach pain, fatigue, and unexplained weight loss tend to be very vague, non-specific and are also found in a lot of common benign disorders such as irritable bowel syndrome. Other symptoms may include pelvic pressure or persistent pain, abnormal changes in bladder or bowel function, and severe swelling of the legs. If such problems are present and you have no other explanation for the symptoms, it is helpful to get a blood test for the *ovarian cancer antigen*, CA 125. This protein tumor marker is elevated in about 70 percent of women with ovarian cancer, but routine use of this test for screening purposes is controversial since the CA 125 may be elevated in women who do not have ovarian cancer, and it may be normal in 20 to 30 percent of women who do have cancer. Mild elevations of CA 125 also occur in a number of benign conditions such as fibroids, endometriosis, ovarian cysts, and even early pregnancy.

At this time, there is no definitive way to diagnose ovarian cancer early other than diagnostic laparoscopy or laparotomy. The best available approaches for early detection lie in the combination of (1) careful pelvic examination by your physician, (2) pelvic and transvaginal ultrasound of the ovaries, and (3) the blood test for CA 125. Although the CA 125 is NOT a diagnostic test for ovarian cancer, it is useful in women with a family history of the disease, or women with persistent unexplained symptoms, as *one part* of a complete screening program that also includes the other two tests listed above. The sensitivity of the CA 125 test in picking up ovarian cancer is about 60-70 percent, which means that about 60 to 70 percent of women with ovarian cancer will have significantly elevated levels of CA 125, while 30 to 40 percent of women *with cancer* will have a normal level of CA 125. Since there may be *false* positives AND *false* negatives with the CA 125, it is important that you discuss with your personal physician your particular risk profile and the need for any of these tests.

I use the CA 125 test as part of our preventive medicine evaluations to provide a clue to the presence of possible early ovarian cancer, as well as clues to the presence of the benign conditions listed above, since many of these many not be felt on a routine pelvic exam. This blood test has helped many women find out that they had these conditions when the elevated CA 125 prompted us to order a pelvic ultrasound and the problem was identified. Since the treatment needed can be quite different if one of these conditions is present, I have found it very valuable to include the CA 125 in our preventive medicine health checkups. This helps plan what treatment approaches may be needed, as well as providing the best available test for early detection of possible occult ovarian cancer.

Women with a family history of ovarian, breast, or colorectal (non-polyposis form) cancer may want to have more frequent screening examinations and should consider consulting with a geneticist specializing in oncology to more fully assess risk factors and appropriate testing. Several such programs are available; here are two I think are very good:

1. Hereditary Cancer Institute
   Creighton University School of Medicine
   Department of Preventive Medicine and Public Health
   P.O. Box 3266
   Omaha, Nebraska 68103-9990   1-800-648-8133 or 1-402-280-2942

2. Joann Bodurtha, M.D., MPH; Director, Department of Human Genetics
   Medical College of Virginia-Virginia Commonwealth University
   Clinical Genetics Center
   P.O. Box 33, MCV Station
   Richmond, Virginia 23298-0033   1-804-786-9632

Additional information may be obtained from the Ovary Cancer Resource Center of the American Cancer Society (www.cancer.org) and the National Cancer Institute (www.nci.nih.gov). There are a number of new treatment approaches, and results of new studies are emerging, so if you have concerns about your risk for ovarian cancer, I encourage you to contact one of the above resources.

Hormone Therapy: Options and Choices
To Individualize Your Program

For premenopausal women who are still menstruating but beginning to have either health risks like bone loss or menopausal symptoms such as hot flashes or fragmented sleep, one of the options to help provide hormonal stability is use of the newer low-dose oral contraceptives (OC), or birth control pills (BCP). "The pill," previously not recommended for women over thirty-five, has been found to not only be safe for perimenopausal women, but to actually provide a number of *health benefits*. A June 1999 article in *OB Gyn News* had the following headline: "Prescribe OCs Until Age 52, Expert Advises," and quoted Dr. Patricia J. Sulak of the Scott and White Clinic in Temple, Texas, as saying "OCs are one of the most important preventive health measures in all of medicine. There's no medicine that offers reproductive-age women more benefits; there's nothing out there that even touches OCs." Dr. Sulak went on to say that "Women who don't stay on the pill have heavy periods and irregular periods, premenstrual syndrome, functional ovarian cysts, and they get endometriosis and fibroids. If they start the pill and stay on it except when they want to become pregnant and when breast-feeding, they don't have those problems. . . . The pill was really made for women over 35 . . . once you get over 35 your ovaries start acting up; 90 percent of women will develop irregular bleeding before they get to menopause."

Previous studies that linked BCPs with increased risk of stroke and blood clots (1) did not take into account the independent risk of cigarette smoking on cardiovascular disease, including stroke, and (2) were based on the older, very high dose pill formulations used in the 1960s. None of those high-dose pills are available today. Today's OC formulas are a fraction of the hormone content used when the BCPs first came out. After reanalyzing the past data and evaluating current safety statistics from worldwide studies, the FDA approved the use of oral contraceptives in **nonsmoking** women over age forty because they found that the potential **benefits** for many health problems in women at this age outweighed the slight degree of potential risk. Many women in this age group, even though they may not be ovulating regularly, still need and want contraception. I had one patient, age fifty-one, whose hormone profile confirmed that she had ovulated during her menstrual cycle, and she said (in a tone of shock and disbelief), "You mean I could still get *pregnant*? I thought I stopped ovulating a long time ago. The last thing I need in my life right now is a baby!"

There is other good news about the **protective effects** of the oral contraceptives, and I have summarized this information in the chart below. The percentages given are the **degree of reduction** in that health problem when compared to nonusers of BCPs. In addition to this list, studies from Italy published in 1994, along with other con-firming studies since that time, showed a significant protective effect on maintaining bone density in women who used the OCs during perimenopause. So BCPs help prevent osteoporosis as well as uterine and ovarian cancers, among their many pluses.

If you decide to talk with your physician about using the BCP to help you sail more smoothly over the turbulent waters of peri-menopause, I suggest you ask to try a brand with a better estrogen amount and less progestin to reduce unwanted side effects. These options include Ovcon or Modicon. Pills such as Loestrin, Alesse, Mircette, and others that are *high* in progestin and *low* in estrogen tend to cause more problems and side effects like migraines, tension headaches, loss of libido, weight gain, vuylvodynia flares, increased fibromyalgia pain, depression, bloating, constipation, and a host of other problems (see the women's stories in chapters 8 and 12 in par-ticular). But whatever BCP you use, **do not add St. John's wort** on your own if you have mild depressive side effects. Recent research at the National Institutes of Health has shown that the herb St. John's wort may **decrease** the contraceptive effectiveness of the BCP up to 50 percent. You could be in for a rude surprise with an unexpected pregnancy if you combine St. John's wort with your birth control pill. In addition, since the herb appears to increase the liver's metabolic break-down of the hormones and reduce their effectiveness, you are likely to find yourself back in the cranky, irritable, anxious, "perimenopausal panic" mood roller coaster. Adding herbs on your own may give you more problems than you bargained for!

As one forty-five-year old woman described it to me at a recent follow up appointment: "I felt great on the Ovcon 35 for the first few months. My energy was great, my mind was clearing, my memory was getting better, and I felt so good. I even had my interest in sex back. Then the last two months I felt like I was slipping again. I had more crying spells, I felt on edge all the time, like I was going to fly into a million pieces. And I started having spotting almost every day and that had not been happening before." When I explored with her what had changed in the last two months, she admitted she had added daily St. John's wort and "a few other herbs" recommended by her homeopathic doctor. She said "I didn't think to mention it to you because my homeopathic doctor said herbs are safe and don't have any side effects!" Remember: something as simple as grapefruit juice can interfere with the effectiveness of many medications, so you need to think about drug-herb interactions as very real possibilities. Always go over with your physician *everything* you are taking. Talk with your physician about other types of BCP products to try if you find that you are feeling depressed with one you are taking.

If you use an oral contraceptive in the premenopausal years, you typically do not experience the hot flashes and other symptoms that mark the endocrine transition to actual menopause. That's why I often describe the pills as helping you "sail over the turbulent waters" of perimenopause. But when you are actually menopausal and no longer need contraception, how do you decide when to change over to the usual postmenopausal hormone options? Some women ask me why it is even necessary to make a change to another hormone regimen if the oral contraceptives are working well. The second question is simpler to address: it is important to make the change because even the *low-dose* oral contraceptives contain more estrogen and progestin than is generally needed for *postmenopausal* use. Conversely, keep in mind that **doses of hormones for menopause are *not enough* to provide contraception for the premenopausal women** who still ovulate and could become pregnant. After menopause, since your follicles have been depleted and you no longer ovulate, contraception is no longer an issue, you can use the bioidentical human hormones that are more "natural" and have even fewer side effects than the low-dose BCP.

BENEFICIAL EFFECTS OF ORAL CONTRACEPTIVES

Condition or Disease	Percent Decrease Compared to Non-Pill Users
Menstrual Disorders	
• dysmenorrhea	63%
• menopausal symptoms	72%
• menorrhagia	48%
• irregular menstruation	35%
• intermenstrual bleeding	28%
• premenstrual tension (PMS)	29–80% (degree of reductin in symptoms depends on balance of E:P in pill)
Reproductive Organ Tumors	
• breast: fibrocystic/fibroadenomas	60–75%
• breast biopsies	50%
• benign ovarian cysts	65% (using monophasic pills)
• uterine fibroids (fibroma)	59%
• ovarian cancer	40-80%, based on # of years in use
• endometrial cancer	50-75%, based on # of years in use
Other Reproductive Disorders	
• endometriosis	50%
• pelvic inflammatory disease	10–70%
• toxic shock syndrome	60%
• uterine retroversion	24%
Other Health Problems	
• Rheumatoid arthritis	50%
• iron deficiency anemia	45%
• duodenal ulcer	40%
• sebaceous cysts	24%
• acne	20% (higher reduction with low progestin pills)

Source: Richard P. Dickey, MD, Ph.D. *Managing Contraceptive Pill Patients*, 8th ed., Essential Medical Information Systems, 1994.

Another woman's voice may help you see the some of the potential for feeling better during perimenopause that is possible with the right balance in a birth control pill. RS was 39 when she first consulted me, and these are here words, a year later:

Finding you on the Internet was like a Godsend. I went right out and bought your book. It really helped knowing I wasn't losing my mind. I think every woman should read your book. I had sent up a prayer for help and then found your interview on the Web. I have four children and I am a regional director for a large public relations company and it was getting hard for me to even function. My Gyn said I was too young to be going through menopause, but my intuition was telling me that I was in menopause. He said I just had PMS and all I needed was Xanax. Then I went to my GP and he put me on Elavil. All they wanted to do was give me medicine for depression and anxiety and I really didn't like how I felt on all that. Besides, it really bothered me that they said it was just that I was in a stressful job.

Eleven years ago, I was a single Mom, had just gone through a divorce and my dad died, but I handled all that just fine. But this time, everything in my life was great. I had a husband I loved, a fabulous job and my business was going really well, and I thought to myself why is it that now I have these problems and feel like I can't function? My symptoms were getting so bad I couldn't take business trips and I couldn't think clearly to function well. I was beginning to think I would have to give up my business, but then I realized I didn't want to do that so I kept looking for help. That's when I found about your work and made the appointment with you."

After you started me on the patch, I started sleeping better right away. It was amazing. I could sleep, I didn't have the anxiety attacks or the palpitations – they were gone! Then I started on the birth control pill a couple months later. At first I felt a little nausea with those, but that went away. After being on the pill about 3 or 4 months, I felt 90 percent back to my old self. My mind cleared, I could remember things again, I could focus at work, and I felt like my moods were much more even. It was like a miracle. The only thing that bothers me now is that I'd like a little more of my sex drive back!

The addition of a low dose (1.0 mg) of natural micronized testosterone daily every morning did the trick in helping her achieve just the right balance to restore her usual libido, and she is now quite happy with her overall program. It just takes finding the right combination, so don't give up if it is a little rocky at the outset. It is possible to regain your zest, vitality . . . and even memory!

Making a *smooth* transition to a postmenopausal hormone plan is best done with the assistance of a knowledgeable health professional, so you don't experience any unwanted effects from stopping oral contraceptives abruptly or from differences in potency of the BCPs and the natural hormones. How is this best handled? I recommend that you have an annual blood test to measure FSH, beginning at age fifty-one or fifty-two. The FSH blood test should be done on the fifth to the seventh day *off the active birth control pills, or the "placebo" week when you are menstruating*. If the FSH is checked at the end of the week of placebo pills, you will have been off hormones long enough for FSH to rise into the menopausal range, if you have reached menopause. If you have not yet reached menopause, the FSH will still be low on these days. If you have the FSH done while you are taking the *hormone-containing* pill, it will be suppressed (usually less than 3 or 4) and will not give an accurate determination of your menopausal status. You *do not* have to stop the oral contraceptives for several months in order to check the FSH, as many women have been told. I want you to have this information because your physician may not yet be aware of how and when to check FSH, since it is still relatively new to use oral contraceptives for perimenopausal women into their early fifties. If your FSH is greater than 20 mIU/mL on the days off the hormone-containing BCPs, then you have reached the endocrine stage of menopause and can switch over to the usual postmenopause hormone options. If the FSH is still less than 20, you could *possibly* still become pregnant (although it is uncommon), and you may want to stay on the oral contraceptives until your FSH is higher.

Natural versus Surgical (Induced) Menopause

Many patients ask about the difference between natural menopause and a surgical menopause: Hysterectomy *with removal of the ovaries* is what is generally meant by "surgical menopause," although some people use the term to refer to removal of the uterus alone. If you have had a hysterectomy *without* removal of the ovaries, you will still have ovarian cycles and will be producing your own estrogen, progesterone, and testosterone. Correctly speaking, you are not in the endocrine state of menopause, although you will no longer have menstrual periods because the uterus is removed. If your ovaries are present, you may still have PMS because it is related to *ovarian hormone cycling*, not to the presence of the uterus. Women who have had a hysterectomy without removal of the ovaries do typically, however, have an *earlier* menopause. This is believed to be due to interruption of the blood flow to the ovaries during surgery. Dr. Phillip Sarrel from Yale Menopause Center published a study in the 1990s showing that 25 percent of women will have loss of ovarian function *within three months* of having a hysterectomy even though only the uterus is removed. He also found that by *three years after removal of the uterus*, about *60 percent* of women will have *menopausal levels* of ovarian hormones and show a marked decline in estradiol.

It is crucial for YOU to know this, because *most doctors don't know it.* It is still a common belief that women who have their ovaries after hysterectomy do not become menopausal until about age fifty. Many women today have had a hysterectomy in their early to mid-thirties, and even though they still have their ovaries, may have markedly low estradiol and testosterone levels within two or three years of their surgery. This means they begin suffering from the

many problems associated with loss of these key metabolic hormones: worsening PMS, severe fatigue, weight gain, headaches,
muscle and joint pain, fibromyalgia, disturbed sleep, memory and
concentration problems, loss of libido, incontinence, vulvodynia/
interstitial cystitis, and many others.

Checking Hormone Levels after Hysterectomy

If you begin to have symptoms of menopause following hysterectomy, no matter what your age, I think it is important to check
your hormonal status, and other health risks, to see whether the
ovaries have declined in hormone production to the point that you
may be endocrinologically becoming menopausal and therefore would
benefit from adding estrogen. But if you don't have a uterus, checking remaining ovarian hormonal function becomes a little more difficult because you don't have the external marker of the bleeding
days to know when to perform the blood tests.

What I usually do in this situation is ask the woman to let me
know when she has any body changes like she had the week before
her period (breast tenderness, mood swings, etc.); I draw hormone
levels at that time, and again about a week or so later to get a picture of the most likely low point of the ovarian cycle (the time that
you would have been bleeding, if you still had your uterus). This
helps us determine the relative pattern of residual ovarian hormone
cycles and actual levels that correspond with various symptom patterns. It takes a little more detective work but the effort is worth
it to get the answers we need in order to decide about helpful
approaches to relieve symptoms. I also encourage a woman in this
situation to have a bone density test along with the urinary marker,
NTx, of bone breakdown. Women who have had hysterectomies
at a relatively early age, even if their ovaries are remaining, are still at
higher risk of bone loss than women who have a gradual, natural
decline in hormone production.

If you've had a hysterectomy **with** removal of the ovaries, then
it is even more crucial that you have *adequate* hormone replacement. The younger you are when you have the uterus and ovaries
removed, the more important it is to be sure you are on the proper
replacement hormone amount. In this situation, it truly is *replacement* therapy, because your own ovaries were prematurely removed,
and the body needs the ovarian hormones to function properly. The
sudden loss of estrogen and testosterone can have a profound impact
on all of the health concerns I have been describing throughout this
book. Many times a woman who may have a complete hysterectomy
with removal of the ovaries at thirty-eight or forty may just be given

the lowest dose of estrogen. That often is not enough for a younger woman. Her needs are different and the amount really has to be adjusted to what her body needs. Many women who have had a surgical menopause are also going to need the addition of testosterone. I listen to the patient, and I take my clues from what she describes. A patient may tell me "I've had a hysterectomy, my ovaries were removed and I'm on 0.625 mg of estrogen, but I don't have any energy. I don't have any libido. I'm still having hot flashes. I'm not sleeping well. And I just don't feel quite right." Her description tells me that she's probably not on the right type of estrogen or an adequate amount for her, and that she may need testosterone as well. And yet over and over women are told, "Well you couldn't possibly be having symptoms because you're on 0.625 milligrams of Premarin." The key is not what *dose* you are taking, but what level of estradiol is produced in *your* body from what you are taking. As I described in chapter 5, optimal estradiol levels to help you feel your best are typically the levels produced for most of the time in a healthy menstrual cycle, i.e., somewhere in the range of 90-250 pg/ml.

Remember: *The same dose doesn't fit for everybody.* Also, as you read in earlier chapters, not all estrogens are alike in the way they affect different women. When you are taking a mixture of estrogens or synthetic estrogens you may not get quite the same response at some of the body's estrogen receptors. Even though you may be taking estrogen, if you have not yet had an optimal response, because you are not getting enough of the bio-identical form of 17-beta estradiol that your ovaries made before surgery or before a natural menopause. I would encourage you to talk with your physician about trying one of the many types of 17-beta estradiol options available. Some of the newer ones may be much more effective than what you have been taking. Also keep in mind with the estradiol patches: They all contain the *same type* of 17-beta estradiol. The differences among the patch brands are primarily in the type of adhesives they use, and how long the patch is designed to last. If one causes skin irritation or won't stay on your body well, try another brand.

And be ready to ask your doctor to write your prescription so you can change the patch sooner than the manufacturer says if you find your estrogen-loss symptoms coming back before you are scheduled to change your patch. Brain fog, loss of word recall, hot flashes, restless sleep, night sweats, and/or headaches are some of the common "brain" clues that the patch is wearing off sooner than it is supposed to. If you exercise a lot, you will also metabolize the estradiol faster, which will affect how often you need to change a patch or take a pill. Taking steroids (as for arthritis or asthma) or antibiotics will also increase the metabolism of your ovarian hormones and affect how often you need to change your patch or take the estrogen tablets. These are some of the many issues we deal with every day in my practice trying to help women find the right type and amount of hormone to use.

The old way of prescribing hormones after menopause was 25 days of estrogen (in the United States, this has generally been Premarin). The progestin, usually Provera, was added for Days 16 to 25 of the month. Then women were told to *stop both hormones* for five days a month. I often wondered how this was decided, because the interesting thing is that the ovaries don't **stop** making estrogen five days a month. They just produce *less* for those few days of menses. If you listen to what women say about this schedule, they usually tell you they feel terrible for those five days: hot flashes come back, sleep is interrupted, aches and pains come back, memory isn't as sharp, palpitations hit again. It's miserable to experience both estrogen and progesterone withdrawal symptoms when the hormones are stopped abruptly five days every month. Obviously, it wasn't a woman who came up with that approach. Today, the recommendations are finally more in keeping with what a woman's body normally does: Take the estrogen *every day* and add the progestin or progesterone in a cyclic manner for ten to fourteen days a month. If one progestin bothers you and you don't feel well on it, try changing to natural progesterone or a different progestin at a lower dose. Current recommendations are that you can even take the progesterone or progestin for ten to fourteen days every two or three months rather than the usual fourteen days every month.

As I listen to women, I find they know their bodies so well they tend to get smart after the first cycle or two of that regimen. They quickly realize that it's when they began taking the second pill (i.e., the progestin or progesterone) that they started feeling *really bad*. I can't tell you how many women I have talked with around the country who tell me they just stopped the progesterone or progestin that made them feel so miserable, and kept on taking the estrogen, which made them feel so much better. *But they were too embarrassed or afraid to tell their doctor they had made that change.* What we may have among menopausal women on hormone therapy, and not realize it, is a whole group of women who have taken themselves off the progestin and are taking estrogen alone unaware of the potential problems with doing this. **Physicians simply have to improve communication with patients** and work together to find hormone options that reduce side effects so that women feel well again. On the other side, women need to bring up their concerns more directly to their doctors and *communicate* any medication changes that you may want to make in what you are taking. Keep in mind that there is a lot of fine tuning that can be done in order to come up with an optimal approach that works well for you.

Please, if you have a uterus, **do not** stop your progestin or progesterone unless you discuss this with your doctor. You may cause serious bleeding problems by just stopping the progestin and taking only your estrogen if your body is no longer making progesterone. You and your doctor need to work together to find a solution that works for you, rather than you just stopping on your own. She or he cannot do the best job for you if you don't speak up about your needs and communicate about things you may be doing on your own. If you stop taking a medication of any kind and you don't tell your physician, he or she may not know to see that you get monitored properly for possible consequences. It's so important to your health and well-being for the long run for you to work in an active partnership with the physician you choose.

In the past, the dose of Provera has typically been 10 mg. I find that is too much for most women, and produces an unacceptable degree of bloating, breast tenderness, feelings of lethargy, and depressed mood; or as some women tell me, "I feel like all that awful PMS has come back again." The more common recommendation today is 5 mg of Provera or equivalent amount of another progestin or natural progesterone. At the North American Menopause Society conferences for the past few years, more and more menopause specialists are recognizing the problems with the higher doses of the synthetic progestins and are urging physicians to use lower amounts or change to natural progesterone.

Recent research has shown, whether the progestogen is given monthly or every two or three months, that it is the **duration** of the progestogen phase that is needed to protect the endometrium from hyperplasia. One study of 398 women found that in those who took the progestogen for only seven days, 3.5 percent (fourteen women) developed cystic hyperplasia after several years. When the duration of progestogen was increased to ten days or more, not a single woman developed cystic hyperplasia. If you are supposed to be taking a progestogen, make certain you take it for the **full time** your physician has recommended, even if you should start bleeding earlier, before you have finished your progestin/progesterone cycle. If you continue to start bleeding early each time, talk with your doctor about changing the dose or type of progestin. There is some good news in all this: The longer you are on hormone therapy, what characteristically happens is that the uterine lining does not build up as much as it did earlier in your life so the actual flow is shorter and lighter.

For women who feel strongly that they do not want any more monthly bleeding, another combination or regimen being used is the continuous regimen of giving estrogen and progestin together every day, called continuous-combined therapy. This can be done with various existing tablet or patch options for 17-beta estradiol along with natural progesterone (tablets or vaginal gel) or a low-dose synthetic progestin. In addtion, there are two new *combination* hormone products containing 17-beta estradiol, each with a different type of synthetic progestin, **CombiPatch** (levonorgestrel is the progestin) and **Activelle** (norethisterone is the progestin). **Femhrt** is another new combination product that contains 1 mg of ethinyl estradiol (the estrogen used in many birth control pills) with 5 mcg of norethindrone acetate.

A drawback to all of the combination products is that they are *fixed* dose ratios, and may not provide exactly the balance you need to feel your best. I have been disappointed with CombiPatch and Activelle since these products contain so much progestin relative to the amount of estrogen. So far, only a few of my patients have been able to tolerate them in the fixed dose combinations available. Femhrt is still quite new, but the estrogen–progestin (E:P) ratio in this product appears to be a little better than the others. Since each of these products contains different estrogens and progestins, if you try one and don't like how you feel, it may still be worth trying one of the others since hormone ratios are different and the side effects are slightly different depending on which estrogen and which progestin is used. If the E:P ratio still isn't right for you, and you have too many side effects with the daily progestin, then you may either (1) add an additional estradiol patch along with the combination product, (2) add an oral form of estradiol, or (3) go back to separate prescriptions to be able to individualize the right dose balance you may need.

The advantage of the combined estrogen-progestin approaches is that if you can put up with the spotting and erratic bleeding that is common the first six months, the combined hormones eventually suppress the buildup of the uterine lining, and about 80 percent of women on this regimen do not have any further bleeding. The other 20 percent continue to have erratic and bothersome bleeding, whether from atrophy of the uterine lining due to the constant progestin, or from fibroids or polyps or continued "too-thick" lining of the uterus. These women usually end up changing back to a cycling hormone regimen.

Taking estrogen and progestin every day can work well, unless you are a woman with significant heart disease, diabetes, or elevated blood pressure or triglycerides, or you have a history of headaches or fibromyalgia or depression. The daily progestins tend to make these conditions worse. There are some other problems with the combination regimen taken every day. It has not been studied long enough for us to have a clear idea of its safety and the relationship to later breast cancer. This is one of the reasons I don't recommend continuous estrogen-progestin regimens very frequently. Another reason I don't suggest this form of HRT is that it is not a physiologically normal approach. In our premenopausal years, our ovaries did not make progesterone every day of the month, so I don't feel very comfortable recommending that postmenopausal women take it every day, either. We still have a lot of other unanswered questions about the continuous-combined regimen, including potential negative effects on heart disease risk, more problems with weight gain, interference with optimal estrogen effects on the brain, and others. This regimen still needs further evaluation for its long-term safety. Taking the progestin (or even natural progesterone) every day also tends to cause more weight gain and more side effects in women who are sensitive to the depression-causing effects of the progestin. For women with a family history of heart disease, the progestin every day *may* negate some of the benefits of the estrogen on the heart and the lipid profile. Daily use of the progestin may also contribute to difficulties regulating blood sugar in women with diabetes or insulin resistance. If you are considering this option, you may want to review these pros and cons with your physician. Just keep in mind that this option is one for which we don't have as many studies on long-term effects.

An even newer idea has been incorporated into a product released in the United States in January 2000, **Ortho Prefest** tablets, containing 1.0 mg 17-beta estradiol and 0.09 mg norgestimate. This product has three days of plant-derived 17-beta estradiol followed by three days of combination estradiol and norgestimate in a continuously repeated regimen. This dosing regimen is proposed to capitalize on our emerging understanding of hormone receptor dynamics: (1) delivery of estradiol alone stimulates new hormone-receptor growth, thought to maximize estrogenic benefits, and (2) the combined delivery of progestin with estrogen then down-regulates hormone receptors. Since this product is so new, few of us have much experience with it. It may be a good option for some women who don't have many side effects with progestins and who don't like having monthly bleeding.

The clinical studies prior to release of Ortho Prefest showed that it provides effective relief of vasomotor symptoms and vulvovaginal atrophy, preserves the beneficial effects of estrogen on lipids, and provides skeletal and endometrial protection. The low-dose, intermittent schedule of norgestimate is designed to reduce the unwanted side effects of progestin therapy. In clinical trials for this new product, only 9 percent of women reported bleeding as an adverse event; there was consistent monthly improvement in bleeding and spotting, a low incidence of breast pain (less than 1 percent discontinuation due to breast pain), and a low reported incidence of depression (reported in 5 percent of patients).

I see some potential problems with this regimen for you to consider before asking your doctor about trying it. If you have fibromyalgia, migraines, tension headaches, depression, bladder pain, or struggle with excess weight, even the intermittent progestin may still be more than you can tolerate. The fluctuating progestin levels from starting and stopping the norgestimate every three days may be a particular problem for migraine sufferers and increase the frequency of headaches. If you don't have any of these problems, and don't like having monthly bleeding, you may want to ask your doctor about trying Ortho-Prefest and see how you do.

Another option to explore if you have severe difficulties tolerating progestins of all kinds is the *intrauterine* progestin-delivery system called **Progestasert.** Although this has been on the market for many years in the United States, it has been primarily used as a contraceptive option rather than for progestin therapy in menopausal women. Progestasert releases a small amount of progestin daily directly to the lining of the uterus, and there is very little progestin absorbed into the total body circulation. Because of this, it does not have the usual unwanted side effects of progestin or progesterone taken orally or transdermally. A number of studies have shown that this product delivers enough progestin to effectively suppress the buildup of the uterine lining. If you have a uterus and want to continue estrogen but nothing else has worked to give you a progestin you could take, you may want to ask your doctor about trying Progestasert. There are other intrauterine progesterone/progestin delivery systems soon to be released in the United States, so be on the lookout for these options as well.

Potential Pitfalls and Problems with Hormone Therapy

As new data emerges, there have become fewer and fewer reasons *not* to consider taking hormones after menopause. The primary remaining concerns, or potential "risks," have to do with breast cancer, uterine cancer (addressed earlier in this chapter), headaches, high blood pressure, stroke or blood clots, and risk of gallstones. I have already extensively discussed in chapter 14 the hormone–breast cancer issues, and have tried to give you a balanced view of the data on this complex topic. Headaches with various forms of hormone therapy have been addressed in detail in chapter 10. I find that most of my headache patients actually see *reduction* in headache frequency on hormone therapy, once we have found the right type and dose. Hormone therapy has also been implicated in causing gallstones in some women, particularly *oral* estrogens. This potential pitfall can be avoided by using *transdermal* estradiol that allows bypassing of the liver and, therefore, eliminates most of the unwanted effects on the biliary (gallbladder) system.

Another question that comes up frequently is "What about blood clots and the possibility of stroke?" The newest research from European centers, published since 1990 in the international menopause medical journals, has shown that the current doses and types of estrogen being used for menopause therapy *do not* cause adverse effects on clotting factors. This is particularly true of the transdermal forms of estradiol that bypass the liver "first-pass" metabolism and do not therefore stimulate liver production of clotting factors. The recently reported PEPI trials in the United States further supported the *lack* of adverse effects of estrogen on clotting factors, and also that women on ERT or HRT had *lower levels of fibrinogen* (one of the clot-forming factors) than women not taking hormones. The issue of estrogen-related clotting disorders (thromboembolism, thrombophlebitis) has been more carefully evaluated with modern techniques and was found to be primarily due to use of the older *high-dose* oral contraceptives *in women who were also smokers.*

In addition, the type of estrogen makes an enormous difference in your risk of thrombophlebitis. Dr. Malcolm Whitehead in England published in 1982 his studies showing that the conjugated equine estrogen (Premarin) was more likely to adversely affect clotting factors than is the native human 17-beta estradiol. This is thought to be due to the higher potency and stronger receptor binding of the equilin group of estrogens in Premarin. The same problem is likely to be found with the other "mixed-estrogen" products, Estratab and Cenestin. I definitely would not prescribe the conjugated estrogens, whether derived from plants or horses, to women who have a history of a blood clot or a strong family history of clotting problems. Transdermal 17-beta estradiol is much safer in such situations, and there is a significant amount of data now showing there is no increase in clot formation in women using the estradiol patches. In fact, restoring the estradiol levels to optimal amounts has a number of important effects to *reduce* the likelihood of clots being formed to cause strokes and phlebitis. I have outlined these cardiovascular benefits in more detail in chapter 13, showing the encouraging news from current research that many diseases of the blood vessels—which can lead to stroke, hypertension, ischemia, and heart attacks—are *decreased by estrogen therapy.* In fact, today we know that a woman who is at high risk of stroke is someone who could likely benefit greatly and reduce her risk of future strokes by using 17-beta estradiol to maintain premenopausal estrogen levels.

The following situation is one I commonly encounter, and it illustrates the kinds of side effects that can be reduced or even eliminated by making changes in the specific hormones used. **Rya** is fifty-one, and was referred to me by her psychologist who had been concerned about her mood swings and headaches. He thought they might be related to her hormonal therapy, although she had been told by her gynecologist that this wasn't likely. Her gynecologist thought her mood swings and headaches were due to work stress. (An interesting switch: The psychologist thought the problems were hormonal, and the gynecologist thought they were psychological). When I met with her, this was what she had to say:

> I have terrible mood swings and constant headaches, and I have been so frustrated with this because I have always been so healthy. I just want some answers with my hormones and what I can do to take something more natural and feel better. My psychologist heard you speak and feels you are the person I should see. I started out on Premarin and Provera and I just felt horrible on this. I tried it for three months, and I felt agitated, anxious, depressed, and had headaches almost constantly. Then I was switched to Ogen [a synthetic type of estrone] and Cyrin [the same progestin as in Provera] 5 mg for ten days a month. That's when I have the worst headaches. I've ended up feeling like which do I deal with, my risk of heart attack or feeling lousy every day being on hormones? That's why my psychologist suggested I see you.

Rya was someone who had never had a problem with headaches before starting hormone therapy. She was also experiencing other menopausal symptoms when I saw her, in spite of being on estrogen: marked insomnia, with waking up about 2 or 3 A.M. and then having trouble going back to sleep. She took the Ogen (0.9 mg) in the morning, and I suspected that part of her waking up at night could be either that her estrogen was wearing off or that it wasn't the best type for her. In addition, Rya has a serious family history of heart disease in her mother, father, and her siblings. She expressed a lot of fear about going off the HRT because she's very worried about the heart disease risks, even thought she has made efforts to follow healthy lifestyle habits to minimize her CVD risk. Rya needed, and wanted, the cholesterol-lowering and cardiac protective effects of an oral estrogen, but she had not done well on either of the mixed estrogens she had tried. I told her I thought we could find hormone options that didn't produce so many unwanted side effects, so that she would feel *well* on her hormones and have the benefits she wanted.

I recommended for Rya a change to the oral 17-beta estradiol (Estrace), 0.5 mg in the morning and 1.0 mg in the evening (which is equivalent to her Ogen dose). Spreading out the estradiol provides better stability in blood level throughout the day, more like the physiologic estrogen production by the ovary. I find this works much better for most women than taking estrogen once a day and having a lot of fluctuation in the levels over twenty-four hours. Twice-a-day schedules usually provide much better improvement in sleep as well as reducing headaches triggered by dropping estrogen levels between doses. I also suggested that she try the natural progesterone, 100 mg twice a day, for ten days a month, an amount approximately equivalent to 5 mg of Cyrin or Provera.

At her follow-up appointment she described feeling "like a new person, it's wonderful not to have daily headaches, it's like a miracle. My husband has noticed a big change in my disposition, and said I'm not as irritable and short-tempered as I was. My mood feels more even, I feel a real difference in my ability to let things just run off and not get upset by them. I'm not as tired, and I'm sleeping better. This is a big change!" Where there's a will, there's (usually) a way! I get these comments daily in my practice when women finally get on the right type and amount of hormones they need, and I know it is possible for more physicians to implement these approaches and get similar results.

Target Levels for Optimal Replacement

I regularly use serum hormone levels to monitor need for and response to hormone therapy, and I have consistently found these to be reliable and cost-effective approaches. As I explained in earlier chapters (refer to chapters 3–6 for reasons), the saliva tests just didn't work very well and I stopped using them a number of years ago. The worldwide gold standard for measuring hormone levels remains the use of *serum* assays. I think this type of serum hormone testing will provide you with more reliable and useful information to guide you and your physician in finding the dose and type that is right for you. If you want to request these blood tests from your physician, what should you be looking for as a desirable target range for estradiol?

In my clinical experience, women typically experience their usual energy level, mood, sleep, and memory when serum (blood) **levels of estradiol are** *above* **90–100 pg/ml,** which is the *lower* end of the range for healthy menstrual-cycle levels. It typically takes levels *at least* in this range to achieve remission of the pain in FMS. Levels up to about 200 or so, are the *normal estradiol levels* reached in the first half of the menstrual cycle before women reach menopause. At ovulation, estradiol levels are typically in the range of 300–500 pg/ml, and then in the luteal phase of the cycle (when progesterone is produced), a healthy level of estradiol is generally in the range of 200–300 pg/ml. For restoring hormone function and health benefits after menopause, estradiol levels below about 90 pg/ml are generally too low to provide adequate relief of symptoms from hot flashes to muscle and/or joint pain to disrupted sleep and memory, not to mention maintaining a normal feeling of well-being. Recent research has found that estradiol levels *below* about 80–90 pg/ml result in *increased bone loss after menopause*. Cardiovascular benefits of estradiol have been found to occur at levels *above* about 80 pg/ml as a starting point. Therefore, I suggest you look for a level of about 90 or better and then correlate this with your symptoms.

What should you be looking for as a desirable target range for testosterone? In my clinical experience, women typically experience their optimal normal energy level and libido when serum levels of *total* testosterone are between 40 and 60 ng/dl, with the percentage of free testosterone at about 1–2 percent of the total. Levels below 30 ng/dl are generally too low to maintain your usual libido, intensity of orgasm, energy level, and bone mass. The majority of menopausal women I have evaluated, particularly those who have had surgical removal of the ovaries in their thirties and forties, have had testosterone levels of less than 10 . . . with unmeasureable amounts of free testosterone. No wonder they don't have any sexual desire left! This is also a significant factor in fatigue and low energy. As I described in chapter 6, I usually measure the total, free, and weakly bound forms of testosterone circulating in the bloodstream so I can better help my patients make the best decisions on doses. You may want to go back and read this material again to guide you in what to check.

I have been criticized by other physicians for recommending that women have FSH, estradiol, and testosterone levels checked. They have often told me that it is "too expensive," "unreliable," or "doesn't tell us anything." **I disagree.** Clearly, having this information has made an enormous difference to the women who had been told their symptoms were "all in their head" and who now have a hormone regimen right for them. Many of my patients have also been able to stop the expensive medications for lowering blood pressure and cholesterol, as well as eliminate a variety of pain medications when their estradiol levels were again in the optimal ranges. Furthermore, it is difficult to put a price tag on improving someone's quality of life. I think in the long run it is less expensive to check hormone blood levels than to do all the myriad tests and evaluations that end up being done when hormone problems are *not* recognized, or for women to undergo a long series of psychotherapy sessions, thinking that the mood changes are just stress or an empty nest or a bad relationship. In my opinion, the hormone blood tests are efficient, reliable, cost-effective, and psychologically helpful in identifying a physical cause of disturbing symptoms women frequently experience at midlife and around menopause. I feel strongly that such tests of hormone levels should be available to women, especially those who have had their ovaries removed. There are too many "hidden" medical, psychological, and relationship costs if you don't know your physiological measures. You may find that it is too expensive **not** to have this information as you plan how to best achieve your health goals.

Thyroid Options: "Natural" versus "Synthetic"

The **"natural"** buzzword has also hit the thyroid hormone therapy arena as well as the menopause field. I hear from my patients that there is a lot of debate on the Internet about this one. The question centers around what type of thyroid hormone to give: synthetic pure T4 (Synthroid, Levoxyl, and other generic forms of T4) or a mixed T4-T3 blend that is called natural because it is derived from dessicated (dried) animal thyroid tissue (such as Armour thyroid). There are a number of important aspects of this that I will summarize briefly. Remember, natural can mean "bio-identical" or it can mean coming from a biological source and chemically different from the molecule made by your body. "Synthetic" can simply mean "made in a laboratory" to be identical to what your body makes, or it can also mean "chemically new" and unlike what your body makes. It is crucial for you to know the difference and not get caught up in the marketing ploys.

One concern I have with Armour thyroid is that animal-derived hormones (whether thyroid, insulin, or ovarian, and whether they come from cows, pigs, or horses) have the potential to be antigenic in humans. That means they can cause our bodies to form *antibodies* to the hormones and to our own endocrine glands. This was one of the early problems recognized decades ago with the animal-derived insulins given over long periods of time to diabetics, and also with the allergies to horse serum when this was used as a base for many medicines in the past. Most of these problems have been resolved with the development of synthetic human insulin and medicines not given in a horse-serum base. Similar problems occurred with animal-derived thyroid products when they were all we had and therefore used more widely. Then, scientists created the bioidentical molecule of T4 in the laboratory and were able to produce a bioidentical human form of thyroid hormone that did not cause these problems of stimulating antibody production. I have seen too many women develop high levels of both types of thyroid antibodies when they take animal-derived thyroid products long term, so I prefer not to use these for that reason. This is an especially serious problem for women with fibromyalgia, in whom we need to have optimal thyroid effects on muscle and nerve tissue and avoid triggering antibodies to the thyroid gland.

One of the reasons some practitioners recommend Armour thyroid is that it contains T3 as well as T4. This is not really a valid reason to use the animal-derived product today, when better options are available. For one thing, most people given thyroid medication will be able to take the T4 products and then have the normal conversion in the body to the more active form of thyroid hormone, T3. For those people who can't seem to make this conversion to T3, and still have low T3 levels even on the right amount of T4, I will consider adding a pure, hypoallergenic, sustained-release form of T3 compounded by a specialty pharmacy. I use the compounded product instead of the commercial ones because (1) it isn't animal derived, so it isn't antigenic, (2) I can get it made in a longer-lasting preparation, and (3) I can better individualize the dose of both T4 and T3 if they aren't "fixed" in one tablet. I typically will add T3 *after* I have observed a person's response to T4 replacement, and have checked the lab results for TSH, T3, and T4. I typically start T3 in much lower doses than the commercial products (Thyrolar, Armour, Cytomel) contain. So I really haven't found it necessary to use the animal-derived thyroid products.

Another issue that I hear a great deal about from my patients has to do with when to begin thyroid medication if there is evidence of declining function. TSH values greater than about 5 on most laboratory reference scales indicate hypothyroidism, although many physicians don't treat with thyroid medication until the TSH rises over 8. In my opinion, particularly in women with FMS, PMS, or ovarian problems (including infertility), that is waiting too long and allows symptoms to get worse unnecessarily. In my usual preventive-medicine mindset, "A stitch in time saves nine." I prefer to begin treatment earlier in the process of a failing thyroid gland to avoid having the person get sicker and have more difficulty regaining optimal health. I generally will start medication when TSH is about 3 or 4, occasionally a little sooner if the antibody levels are quite high and/or there are indications that thyroid is needed to help restore normal muscle and nerve function, metabolic regulation, regular ovarian cycles, and/or to improve memory and mood. Current studies also indicate that the *earlier* treatment is begun, the *less likely* the person will have other adverse effects of low thyroid such as hypertension and elevated cholesterol.

If women are given thyroid hormones when they clearly don't need them, however, it can cause more bone loss and possible heart-rhythm disturbances. This is another reason I think it is so important to check both ovarian and thyroid hormones carefully before making treatment decisions. Symptoms of estradiol loss can be almost identical to symptoms of low thyroid function. But if you start thyroid hormone when you don't need it, and your estradiol is low, it will accelerate your rate of bone loss. Obviously, thyroid hormone replacement is a complex topic and I can't give you all the "specifics" in this short space. These are the highlights of some crucial issues I think are important for you to address in talking with your physicians.

Decision Making: Thoughts to Guide You Through the Maze

There is such an explosion of information—some of it very helpful and reliable, some of it terribly out of date, and some of it blatantly wrong. I find that many articles and books still perpetuate old myths about menopause and incorrect myths about hormones. And some of the previous thoughts about reasons not to take estrogen have changed dramatically just in the last several years. I think you have to be very selective about the resources you select in the way of books and articles, as well as the health professionals you choose. Not everyone is interested in, or knowledgeable about, midlife and menopause, as many of you reading this have probably already discovered.

Don't be misled by the word *natural* when looking for remedies for PMS or menopausal changes. Many herbs have been well documented to have toxic effects on the liver and may cause a variety of other symptoms as well. Just because compounds are natural to plants does not necessarily mean they are natural for humans. (Same reasoning I used in talking about the horse-derived estrogens, remember?) In addition, the current research on the human hormone receptor system is revealing incredible complexity of the estradiol, progesterone, and testosterone receptors in various tissues. It is too simplistic to say that herbs with "estrogenic" effects at some receptor sites will do all of the jobs our own hormones are designed to do for us. For example, even though a high-soy diet has been shown to have modest effects to reduce cholesterol, there are also studies now from three different countries that show soy isoflavones compete with our own body hormones at the estradiol and progesterone receptors. This competitive inhibition leads to a 20–50 percent reduction in production of estradiol and progesterone in premenopausal women. That could have a profound impact on your health if you were not aware of this potential adverse consequence of increasing soy intake. For women after menopause, when their own ovarian production of hormones has decreased, it may not be as potentially serious. It really is a complex issue, with no one right answer for everyone. I will discuss these questions in more depth in chapter 16. Herbs have potential downsides, just as taking hormones has potential downsides to consider. For now, I just want you to realize it isn't as simple as we may have thought.

You may not be able to get all of your questions answered in one place, because the specialists in different areas tend to know their own field well but may perpetuate inaccurate information about other areas. For example, I have an area of interest and expertise in the neuroendocrine issues and know a great deal about nuances of hormone therapy as well as how to incorporate a variety of other modalities to maintain good health. But I am not a surgeon and cannot take the place of a gynecologist when my patients need these services. I know about herbal remedies and some basics about their use, but I am not a specialist in the use of herbs, so I don't try to prescribe them extensively. If a patient of mine wants to use just herbal options, I recommend a knowledgeable herbalist. Likewise, you can't expect a non-medically trained herbalist to be as knowledgeable as I am about the current information on hormones. No one of us can know everything about other fields of specialty. If you purchase a book on herbs for menopause, don't expect it to also provide current information on estrogen. In fact, most of these sources I have reviewed are seriously incorrect in the content on both estrogen and progesterone. By the same token, don't expect my book to go into an in-depth discussion about herbs, since that was not my primary focus in writing it. If you are looking for resources, remember to *keep your expectations to the expertise expected for the person's area of specialty*. You will have to do your homework to select a variety of current, reputable, accurate books and other resources to help you develop your health plan. Try to avoid those that are obviously focused on selling products promoted by the author, and look to sources recommended by responsible women's health leaders, such as the Harvard Women's Health Watch Newsletter.

Keep in mind as well that we have different health needs at different stages of our lives. Women's health at midlife and menopause is complex; it requires a variety of integrated approaches and is not likely to fit exactly into any one specialty "box" based on our old models of health care. Just as when our financial goals and needs change, we change financial advisors; as women experiencing changes that have many ramifications on us physically, psychologically, socially, and spiritually, we may need to change our ways of thinking about who may be the best type of health provider to meet our needs and goals. Keep an open mind, and *be prepared to invest time, effort, and money to find someone right for you*, someone who is really interested in midlife and the integration of these important dimensions of your health.

Chapter 16

Complementary Medicine: Making "Holistic" Medicine Whole

In recent years, there has been a dramatic increase in the variety of alternative medicine therapies in use by individuals, hospitals, physicians, and other health professionals in many fields. I am excited to see this changing trend and have been a long-standing advocate for integrating alternative approaches in Western (allopathic) medicine. I am such a proponent for the inclusion of these therapies in our usual medical approaches that I designed an annual continuing medical education course for physicians to learn more about complementary or alternative medicine and use these therapies with their patients. Although *alternative medicine* has been a term in general use, I prefer the term *complementary medicine* because I think these therapies are necessary for many patients and indeed do "complement" the techniques used in Western medicine. I have used many of the complementary medicine modalities for my own healing from various surgeries. I know with certainty that I would not have the mobility and range of motion I have today if I had not incorporated massage therapy, neuromuscular therapy, myofascial release, and hydrotherapy into my own rehabilitation. I have also personally used biofeedback, hypnotherapy, visualization-guided imagery, aromatherapy, therapeutic hot mud packs (prescribed by an Italian physician), physical therapy, chiropractic, acupuncture, and herbal therapies for reducing chronic pain and enhancing relaxation. I have also needed the best of Western medicine, involving complex imaging to diagnose my back and neck problems, precision neurosurgical approaches using high-tech operating microscopes to remove herniated cervical discs, and medications to reduce pain. I know at many levels, intellectually and from personal experience, how important it is for patients to have an *integration* of these therapies in order to get well and become healthy again.

As you read this book and hear me talk about the new scientific advances and hormone therapies in women's health, remember this: First and foremost, my belief system emphasizes wellness and natural options as the foundation, with medical (surgery, medications, etc.) approaches to be added when needed. I know firsthand, however, how important both are to providing complete health care. I am convinced that the key to reducing future health care costs, maximizing patient recovery, and improving well-being will come from the blend of traditional Western and complementary therapeutic approaches.

What Is Wholistic, or Integrative, Medicine?

In the best sense of the word, the blend of traditional Western and complementary therapeutic approaches used together in an integrated approach can be called "wholistic" medicine. The term *holistic (wholistic) medicine* as often used, however, tends to have a different meaning: "holistic" has come to refer primarily to therapies perceived as "natural," and usually ends up meaning any "non-Western medical" approach to healing, such as herbal medicine, homeopathy, naturopathy, chiropractic, Chinese medicine, acupuncture, bodywork, energywork, and others. In this common usage, Western scientific medicine is excluded, making a lopsided approach just like we see when traditional Western physicians ignore the complementary therapies available.

I would like share with you what *wholistic medicine* means to me as a practicing physician: **To make "holistic" medicine truly *whole* or *complete*, it must mean "a *combination* of medical *and* complementary modalities for healing that takes into account the *whole* individual and the individual's physical-emotional-spiritual-social needs in designing a plan for enhancing health, creating an environment for healing, and treating illness."**

Even though we have seen a surge in interest in complementary medicine, the above definition has been my philosophy and approach to health care since *before* I started medical school. I have continued to learn and grow in my own understanding of the many approaches that can help people in "dis-ease." The way I view it, *wholistic* health care is not so much *a technique* as it is *an attitude*. It is an attitude of seeing each individual as a unique blend of physical, psychological, and social needs, then designing a tapestry of techniques and interventions that will best address the particular needs of that person. You may have a definition of wholistic medicine similar to mine and wish it were more available as a model of health care delivery. Consumers who use complementary therapies usually have to pay out of pocket, because these services are not as often covered by health insurance plans. I hope we will see a time in the near future when the benefits of complementary therapies are well established from the point of view of both clinical effectiveness and economically lower cost than is our present fragmented system. As a teacher for physicians and other health professionals, I strongly believe that we are making progress toward an integrated approach. I hear more and more physicians genuinely interested in learning about *complementary therapies* and incorporating these modalities for their patients *and* for themselves.

At the same time, it is distressing that I hear *more condemnation* of Western physicians among the alternative practitioners, who now appear as closed minded to Western approaches as allopathic physicians had previously been to the alternatives. **"Holistic"** medicine cannot be **whole** if its practitioners refuse to accept what allopathic Western medicine has to offer, anymore than we allopathic physicians can be *whole* in our approaches if we fail to include nutrition, exercise, bodywork, biofeedback, acupuncture, chiropractic, and a host of other complementary options. All of us, in the best interests of our patients and clients, need to *stop* the turf battles and *start* collaborating.

Women in particular seek a total approach to their health care, integrating techniques from traditional Western medicine with techniques from traditions of Eastern, Native American, and other ancient healing approaches. Women's wisdom down through the ages provides us with an understanding of the ways women had an intuitive knowledge of the value of all these approaches to healing. In the Greek mythology, the two daughters of Aesculepius (god of healing), Panacea and Hygiea, were the goddesses of different realms of healing: Hygiea's domain was health practices (now known as *hygiene*) and Panacea's role was to apply the "healing balm" of kindness and compassion. The word *panacea* has now come to imply a relatively meaningless cure-all, something of little real value in technological medicine. But in its ancient meaning, you can see how crucial the healing balm of kindness and compassion is whenever there is suffering and a need for healing. In the ancient Greek view, the domains of both Hygiea and Panacea were important to the total healing process. This is the balance we again seek to achieve today.

Such ideas were important to early American women physicians. Elizabeth Blackwell, the first woman in the United States to earn a formal medical (M.D.) degree, had a profound influence on health care delivery for women in the nineteenth century. Dr. Blackwell was a strong proponent of proper use of the medicines available in her time (the late 1800s), along with healthy food, exercise such as walking, fresh air and sunshine, good hygiene, sanitary practices in hospitals and doctors' offices, and other modalities we would today call wellness approaches. At the time she pushed for sanitary practices in hospitals, surgeons still did not know the value of hand washing between surgeries to cut down the infection rate. At Dr. Blackwell's hospital for women, where she insisted upon such procedures of good hygiene and washing, the infection and death rates following childbirth were a minuscule percentage of the rates at the more prestigious New York hospitals run by her male medical colleagues who did not believe hand washing was necessary. Women physicians have often been in the forefront of encouraging the use of traditional therapies and wellness lifestyles, and women patients seem genuinely more responsive to and interested in these complementary approaches.

I have seen an ominous trend in the last several years as I speak to women's groups around the country. I have seen an emerging antagonism toward Western medicine physicians and Western medications (pharmaceuticals). I hear women talk about the "good" alternative therapists and herbal remedies and how "bad" doctors and "drugs" are. Recent medical research has helped to clarify many of the health risks specifically threatening women's well-being and longevity, and to develop effective therapies and medications with fewer side effects compared to those of the past. We have an enormous and exciting body of science to support the rationale and safety of the various medications available today to improve our health. At the same time, however, women are turning away from Western science and medicines in droves. I feel strongly that none of us can afford this "either/or" polarized model of thinking. I recognize all too well, and with sadness, just how much my own profession has failed to address the needs of women, but I believe women around the country are now in danger of throwing out the baby with the bath water when they reject what Western medicine has to offer. Women have rightly asked for more research into the health problems experienced by women. Yet, when that research shows that hormone therapy after menopause reduces the risks of certain diseases, many of the voices who cried out for more research now turn around and accuse physicians of *medicalizing* the natural menopause transition. I have been shocked and saddened by such views, and the anger with which they are spoken.

A mistaken idea often espoused by alternative therapists is that it is only medical drugs that are dangerous and cause unwanted side effects. *Iatrogenic illness*, meaning illness caused or aggravated by treatment procedures or medicines, has been with humankind ever since the first medicine man/woman gave someone an overdose of ground herbs. Curare is a plant-derived nerve toxin causing death by paralysis of the respiratory muscles if given in large enough amounts. You can become toxic on too many vitamin supplements, as well as by taking too much of a particular prescription drug. When I give a seminar, women tell me that herbal medicine is "more natural" and *therefore safer*. Herbs aren't *necessarily* "gentler" or "safer" than pharmaceutical products. For example,

I have seen quite a number of patients, as well as myself, who have had allergic reactions or toxicity symptoms to herbal products, contrary to the reassurances of herbalists who have said herbs are "balanced" and don't cause allergic reactions. I also have patients who have had adverse reactions to Western pharmaceuticals. The street runs both ways. And if you are taking herbs to have a therapeutic effect, isn't it just possible that they can also have *side* effects? Whenever you are taking "medicinals," *no matter what the source,* there is the potential for benefit as well as the possibility of an undesirable reaction.

Yet many times, the same person who objects to taking a purified estrogen because it is made in a laboratory will take an herbal product with *no* ingredient list shown at all, or as a recent patient said to me, "Here is the list of herbs in this tonic, but *I don't have any idea what the words mean or what they do.*" I have a hard time understanding the logic of this. I wouldn't want to put something in my body unless I knew what I was taking, yet I see my patients doing this frequently when it comes to herbs and supplements. I find women often turning to alternative therapists as their primary or only provider of health services, and seek the road to wellness *only* through herbal remedies, vitamin supplements, colonics, and other practices that may or may not have appropriate application for a given person. The potential harm with this approach is that they may miss important and treatable medical problems. A common problem I see is the loss of energy and fatigue that occurs early in the course of thyroid decline, which may be missed if you just take extra vitamins and don't have the appropriate thyroid tests done. Too often, particularly in women's health care, **both** physicians and alternative therapists apply *only their specialty*, regardless of whether this resolves the problem. To put it another way, both groups get too involved with treating a *symptom* rather than the *person* and seeking the underlying cause(s) of the problem.

Keep this in mind as you design your health plan: ***Balance is the key.*** The body is an exquisitely sensitive, precision instrument, and it needs the proper balance in order to function optimally. That balance will be achieved in different ways, and with different techniques, for different individuals, using the tools of modern medicine *along with* the tools of complementary therapeutics. Each one of us is an individual with different needs. The key is to integrate and blend the therapeutic approaches right for you.

Women's Stories: Integrative Medicine at Its Best

Perhaps several case vignettes of actual patients of mine will best illustrate these points and help to explain my philosophy of integrated approaches.

Ms. M. was a young woman in her early thirties who was referred to me by another physician, who said, "She is having significant problems with anxiety and mood swings, and I have her on these various medications, but she doesn't seem to be getting better. She is having a hard time keeping her appointments with me, and I am really not sure what to do to help her. Would you see her and see what you think should be done?"

In doing a systematic medical and psychiatric evaluation of this young woman, I found an unrecognized medical problem (severe changes in her blood sugar levels and abnormally high levels of insulin production) that had a major impact on her mood swings. Her symptoms were much worse just prior to her menses because of the rise in progesterone that also affected her blood sugar regulation, and her symptoms were made worse by the high-dose progesterone suppositories her other physician had been using to treat PMS. She also had an unexpected "anxious agitation" reaction with the tranquilizers she had been receiving from several physicians. An additional factor causing her anxiety and agitation was the "withdrawal syndrome" each month that occurred when she stopped the large doses of natural progesterone she was using. I tapered her off these medications gradually over several months. I later suggested a small dose of a more appropriate anxiety-reducing medicine for her problem of adrenaline overactivity and treated her with a small amount of supplemental estrogen to correct her hormonal imbalance. Her meal plan was designed to increase protein and healthy types of fat to decrease the insulin surge, and I recommended more frequent small meals to stablize the blood glucose highs and lows. She was also started on a basic vitamin program with added calcium and magnesium. As a concert violinist, she had a great deal of stress, muscle tension, and performance anxiety aggravating her headaches and muscle pain. I used techniques of self-hypnosis, with relaxation-visualization training to help her with these problems and also referred her to a massage therapist and a chiropractor for regular bodywork to diminish the muscle tension and spasm. In addition, I recommended she seek training in the Alexander technique of muscle relaxation to improve her concert performance.

This woman also needed more intensive psychotherapy to help resolve problems from her childhood. It was rewarding to see that as she worked through these issues, she did not need the large doses of tranquilizers that had previously been prescribed. She is now doing very well, is taking far less medication, and taking estrogen has greatly improved her bone density as well as mood, sleep, memory, and concentration. She has made enormous strides on her road to well-being by understanding how she needs to eat, using effective relaxation techniques, working with various body therapies to address chronic neck and back problems, and having therapy sessions focused on her particular concerns for psychological health and spiritual growth. She has moved to New York and blossomed as a concert musician and music teacher, confident in her abilities as a soloist, as well as her roles as wife and mother.

What can we learn from this? The message is to *listen carefully*, look for *patterns* of symptoms (such as the premenstrual worsening of her mood changes, blood sugar swings, back and neck pain), and then systematically identify tools to improve overall health, comfort, and sense of control over life's choices. Another lesson reinforced for me as I worked with this woman, is that women often need *much less* medication than the standard doses based on clinical drug studies done primarily on men. If you are not getting better with dose *increases,* talk to your physician about *decreasing* the dose of your medication to see if that will provide relief of troublesome symptoms. The gender differences in response to medication are quite striking and have not been addressed at all adequately in good research. I have addressed a number of these issues in earlier chapters.

Mrs. B. was sent to me by a psychic healer who intuitively "saw" a medical problem that doctors had not been able to diagnose. This woman had a back problem and had seen a chiropractor who recommended adjustment treatments and a long list of vitamin supplements. The manipulation helped ease the muscle spasm, but when this patient began on a lemon juice–maple syrup "cleansing fast" for a week or so (recommended by a naturopathic practitioner), the large doses of vitamins gradually began to create other problems. The imbalanced fasting formula, with such a high level of simple sugar carbohydrate and **no** protein, caused the excessive vitamins and minerals to become even more toxic.

Over the next three months, the patient developed bizarre "burning, electric shock-like sensations up and down my spine and body," along with occasional numbness and tingling, marked mood changes, and generalized muscle weakness. She was seen then by a neurologist, but her unusual emotional expressions and behavior made him think she was "psychotic." Since I worked in both internal medicine and psychiatry, I was asked to see her for a consultation. After getting the history I have just described, I asked her family to bring in *all* of the supplements she had been taking. It turned out to be a *grocery bag full* of various vitamins and herbal products. When I reviewed all of the overlap and duplication among the different products, and put the pieces of the puzzle together, it became clear that she had multiple vitamin and mineral toxicities from excess supplementation. These problems were then made worse by the syrup–lemon juice "cleansing" fasts that further upset body balance. She had not been on any allopathic or Western medications, and yet she clearly had toxicity symptoms. She was also a cigarette smoker, so of course the nicotine only aggravated her other problems. To regain normal nerve and muscle function, along with better mood stability, her body needed to be "detoxified" from these excesses. The situation for this woman was complicated enough that she required hospital admission in order to sort out the problems and do the necessary evaluations. The excessive supplements were stopped, and our dietitian worked with her on a healthy meal plan. Hypnotherapy was used to help with relaxation so she could stop the smoking that she thought was "calming my nerves." Her neurological examination was abnormal, so I ordered a CAT scan of her lumbar spine and found that she had a partially ruptured lumbar disk that had intermittently caused some of the tingling sensations in her legs when she got into certain body positions. I prescribed physical therapy so she could learn good body posture, exercises to strengthen her back, and how to lift correctly. Since this woman's only daughter was about to leave home for college, I felt that some of her mood symptoms were related to feelings of loss and could best be helped with supportive psychotherapy. I referred her to both physical and psychotherapists in her home town to continue this mind-body work.

What can we learn from what happened with this patient? One message is that multiple practitioners can unknowingly create problems by adding therapies that don't blend well with something another therapist has recommended. I see this many times with my patients who may be starting hormone therapy with my guidance and then add herbal supplements from another practitioner at the same time. I also see women that have found a good stability on a hormone regimen and then another physician adds an antibiotic or other medication that alters the hormone metabolism, and the levels go haywire again. When you are seeing several health care providers, make sure that you tell each person what you are doing or taking under the care of someone else. For Mrs. B., the chiropractor had not recognized the toxicity from too much vitamin supplementation, or that his patient needed proper medical diagnosis about the unrecognized lumbar disk problem before she should start on a course of manipulation. Later, when she did see a neurologist, this physician did not take seriously her complaints of back pain because her behavior and emotionality, as well as the multiplicity of her unusual symptoms, made it difficult for him to see a neurological problem; he decided she was "psychotic."

It does often happen that when a *female* patient (compared to a male patient) has symptoms that are unusual or puzzling, the *female* patient much more commonly will be told "there is really nothing wrong," or she is written off as "neurotic" or "psychotic," and the actual medical issues do not get promptly identified and treated appropriately. Neither Mrs. B. nor her family had communicated to anyone information about the juice-syrup fasting or the complete list of supplements she had been taking. Even the best physician cannot put a puzzle together if major pieces are missing. The subsequent integration of medicine, psychiatry, physical therapy, dietary therapy, hypnotherapy, and emotional support was crucial to provide the various modalities she needed for solving the puzzle of interconnected medical and behavioral problems. The point here is that vitamins, although natural, can be toxic in large amounts and can cause changes in mood and behavior along with unusual "nervous" symptoms that could be confused with a medical or psychiatric disorder.

The cases of Ms. M. and Ms. B. illustrate the success of an integrated mind-body comprehensive approach, with traditional medical care an important dimension of their initial assessment and treatment. Even though I am interested in many of the complementary therapies, one physician cannot provide all the therapeutic modalities that are needed to help solve all the problems. It requires the efforts of a team of people, each adding expertise to put together the pieces to create an integrated "whole."These patient cases further illustrate the dangers of taking only one part of the continuum of available treatment approaches. On either end of the continuum, an imbalance may occur, causing the patient to become clinically worse. Modern medicine may take an "overkill" approach at times, but so may chiropractors, advocates of megavitamin supplementation, herbalists, and other alternative therapists who sell people on large numbers of supplements and encourage people to avoid what traditional Western medicine has to offer. At either extreme, such a stance is potentially dangerous. In like manner, physicians must be knowledgeable about and consider the value of complementary therapeutic modalities that may benefit patients, and seek to include these in medical therapeutic regimens.

You must always remember that health problems are *highly individualized*. Similar symptoms in two different people can mean entirely different things. A therapy of any kind that brings rapid relief to one person may be of no help to another and may cause serious side effects in a third. I think it is critically important that all health problems be initially evaluated by a competent, concerned physician, one who you feel listens to you, has your best interests at heart, and who encourages you to add other appropriate and compatible therapeutic approaches to your overall health plan. If you do not now have such a physician, you have every right as a patient to seek one. Such a physician should ideally work *collaboratively* with other therapists and therapeutic options as needed to assist the individual patient reach her optimum level of wellness. It is also important for YOU to tell your physician what supplements you are taking

and what other therapies you are using. I think it is also very helpful when alternative medicine practitioners communicate with you
and your physician when they see something unusual.

I remember one situation that really illustrates this latter point
well. One of the massage therapists working with me in my medical
practice told me she was worried about a woman who had just started bruising excessively during a massage session. I checked on the
patient and discovered she was taking Coumadin (a blood thinner to
help prevent clots); she had misunderstood her directions and was
taking *double* the prescribed dose. She was now bleeding under the
skin, which caused the bruises, and she needed immediate vitamin K
injections as well as to decrease her Coumadin. Even though she did
not know the cause of the bruising, the massage therapist's astute
observations that she promptly communicated to me helped prevent
this patient from having a potentially serious hemorrhage.

This story also illustrates one of the very positive aspects of
modern medicine: the ability, using various laboratory and other
diagnostic means, to determine more precisely what is needed for a
given patient, such as fine-tuning the amount of anticoagulant or
measuring blood sugar levels to determine the amount of insulin to
give a diabetic. This is a valuable aspect of modern health care that
alternative practitioners would do well to recognize and utilize. On
the other hand, there may be many herbal options for common ail-
ments that are safer and more effective than taking repeated courses
of antibiotics. For example, I am very concerned about the overuse
of antibiotics, particularly in women, since this practice increases
recurrent yeast infections and the problem of developing resistant
bacteria, not to mention the enormous cost of these medications.
Using natural approaches, such as acidophilus vaginal suppositories,
helps to prevent both yeast *and* unwanted complications from
antibiotic or antifungal medication overuse.

Issues to Consider with Soy and
Other Alternatives for Menopause Rx

A good example of these principles is the recent surge of interest in
alternative menopause therapies. Aging baby boomers have certainly made an impact. Our market share is being eagerly sought by
makers of everything from acne preparations to portable devices to
induce a state of "Zen." Women have been heavily targeted with the
exponential increase in marketing of "magic bullets" for menopause,
PMS, and perimenopause. These include a wide array of soy supplements, progesterone, and wild yam creams, OTC forms of DHEA
and melatonin. Unbeknownst to the consumer, who has been caught

up with the labeling of all these as natural and therefore safe, all of these products have the potential to cause *harmful* effects if a woman already has a thyroid disorder or a decline in her ovarian hormone production. As one example, we have strong scientific data going back to the 1970s showing the soy isoflavones have marked antithyroid effects, yet that isn't even *mentioned* in the current hype for taking soy supplements or adding soy foods to your diet. Even the ancient Chinese did not routinely eat soybeans until they had developed a fermentation process, hundreds of years after the discovery of soybeans, that eliminated some of these negative effects from eating unfermented soybeans. Fermented soy products include tempeh, miso, soybean paste, and tamari, and these are the forms more commonly eaten in Asian cultures.

There has been a great deal of emphasis on the Japanese high-soy diet being associated with a lower risk of breast cancer, with the result being an intensified sales pitch for soy supplements in pill form and protein powder drinks. But women are not given the balanced message that in Japan, there are many additional factors that also contribute to their lower risk of breast cancer: there is very little alcohol intake, especially among women, and alcohol is a known risk factor for development of breast cancer; Japanese women have far lower fat intake, particularly animal fats; and Japanese women are far more physically active with walking, Tai Chi, and other forms of exercise throughout their lives than are women in the United States. Alcohol, lack of exercise, and high-fat diets are well-known risk factors for breast cancers, as I reviewed in chapter 14. In addition, what you aren't usually told is that the Japanese high-soy diet is comprised predominately of *fermented* soy foods, rather than the soy protein drinks and powders that are marketed in the United States. Why do our women's health newspaper articles and magazines just focus on the *observational,* not causal, connection of high soy intake and lower breast cancer risk in Japan? Could it be related to the advertising dollars that makers of soy supplements spend to advertise their wares in those same magazines? Companies make more money getting us to buy their supplements than by teaching us to go out walking or do Tai Chi every day.

I am well aware of studies that have shown increased soy intake is associated with lower cholesterol, higher HDL cholesterol, and lower blood pressure. All of these factors in turn will help reduce risk of heart disease. But there is also newer research from three different countries that has shown clearly that the phytoestrogens, soy isoflavones, compete with our own body estradiol and progesterone at our body receptor sites. In fact, genistein, a soy isoflavone, even has differential binding affinities depending on *which* estradiol receptor (ER) is considered: It has a six-fold greater affinity for the ER-beta than for ER-alpha. An outgrowth of soy isoflavones binding at the body ERs is that high soy intake has been shown to suppress our own ovary production of estradiol and progesterone by 20–50 percent in several new cross-cultural studies of premenopausal women. If you are already having problems with your ovary hormones, what does the intake of soy do to make matters worse, not better? What about if you are trying to get pregnant, and having problems with infertility, but no one told you that your soy supplements could be interfering with having your ovaries work normally?

What if you have already lost significant bone? What does soy-induced ovarian suppression do to cause further bone loss? What if you are like many younger women I see in their thirties who are having frustrating problems with nightly insomnia, already being triggered by declining estradiol? What effect does soy intake have on your worsening sleep problems if it can further reduce your ovary estrogen production? Do you know the answers to these questions? Is anyone helping you sort this out? See what I mean about the importance of *balanced* information? Is it any wonder that consumers are confused? Could it be this information is left out in the desire to sell more products now that women's economic clout has been "discovered"? If the books and materials you are reading are *not* discussing these issues, then you need to check other sources for your health planning. I am not against soy supplements *per se*, but I do think we should be careful about presenting all the facts, and about how we recommend using these products for different groups of women.

It isn't just consumer magazines that are presenting only part of the picture. Just this summer I received two medical journals, one from the North American Menopause Society (U.S. publication) and one from the International Menopause Society. Coincidentally, they presented exactly the paradox I just described. The U.S. medical journal *Menopause* ran two-page, four-color ads for a red clover isoflavone supplement called Promensil, at the same time the international journal *Climacteric* published the first two placebo-controlled, prospective, randomized, double-blind studies showing that this same supplement had *no effect* greater than placebo on *any* of the menopausal symptoms measured, including objective measures of estrogen effect. *Menopause Management,* another U.S. medical journal that arrived at the same time and is sent to doctors all over the country, went a step further in promoting soy products—they actually packaged an ad and a sample soy protein drink package in the plastic wrap around a recent issue. Personally and professionally, I found this marketing ploy annoying in view of the very mixed results on soy's effectiveness and its known potential problems for women with thyroid disorders and early ovarian decline. I was pleased to see that the editors of *Climacteric* took a higher road than the U.S. journals: their editors wrote a position statement explaining that they will not accept advertising for any health product that has not been proved to be effective on the problems for which it was advertised. And they certainly weren't sending out sample soy products in shrink wrap.

The studies of the phytoestrogen Promensil, published in *Climacteric* in June 1999, were well designed and also had the important dimension of being placebo controlled. These were the first two such carefully done studies in the world. Prior to this, all we had were noncontrolled studies that did not use placebo comparisons. There has consistently been a very high positive response to placebo in studies assessing methods of controlling hot flashes; earlier studies that did not include placebo comparisons therefore tended to overestimate the value of phytoestrogen products such as soy on reducing hot flashes. These two studies were more comprehensive than earlier ones in that they also included several objective measures of estrogen effect as well as effects on standardized menopause symptom-rating scores. Women were defined as menopausal based on having had no periods for at least six months and an FSH greater than 40 IU/l, or based on having had their ovaries removed. Participants were excluded if they had been using any form of hormone therapy for the previous six weeks, if they were vegetarians or regular users of soy products, or were taking medications that induced liver enzymes. Promensil tablets contain 40 mg total isoflavones (genistein, daidzein, biochanin, and formononetin). The three study groups were (1) placebo tablets, (2) one Promensil tablet (40 mg), and (3) four Promensil tablets (160 mg), but all subjects consumed four identically appearing tablets daily. **Pre- and post-trial measures** included daily flushing frequency, Greene Menopause Scale of symptom severity, vaginal maturation index, vaginal pH, FSH, serum level of sex-hormone-binding globulin, complete blood count, liver function profiles, nonfasting lipid profile, and measures of twenty-four-hour urinary excretion of isoflavones.

The two study results were interesting in that the hot flash frequency decreased in all participants, but there was *no difference* in flushing frequency between placebo and isoflavone groups. There were no changes in biological measures of estrogen activity or in subjective symptom scores in isoflavone groups when compared to placebo. As you would expect to see in someone taking isoflavone supplements, there was a measurable dose-dependent increase in the urinary excretion of isoflavone metabolites between baseline and Week 12 in the group on Promensil. An 18.1 percent increase in HDL cholesterol occurred in the 40 mg isoflavone group, but no increase was found between placebo and the 160 mg isoflavone group.

Previous *uncontrolled* studies claiming a therapeutic effect of foods or supplements high in isoflavones appear to have been confounded by a large placebo response. These present studies confirm other studies showing no effect of isoflavones on FSH, SHBG, vaginal epithelium, or pH. Based on these findings in a well-designed, controlled study, my recommendation is that it appears premature to recommend isoflavone products as an appropriate therapy for menopausal symptoms, particularly if patients already have bone loss and/or other more serious consequences of estrogen decline.

In case you may be wondering whether the essentially negative findings might have occurred due to some bias of the physicians conducting the study, I want to point out that funding for both of these studies was provided by Novogen, Ltd., the company that manufactures Promensil, and one of the authors serves as a consultant to this company. So it is unlikely that there was a bias *against* the isoflavone product. The finding of a lack of effect for Promensil in these studies creates an ethical and commercial dilemma for a company that has already successfully marketed its product and has been advertising that use of Promensil leads to significant reduction in hot flashes. I was pleased to see that Novogen undertook proper scientific scrutiny of their product, in spite of the results showing Promensil was no better than placebo in reducing hot flashes.

An interesting finding was the 18 percent increase in HDL cholesterol in the 40 mg isoflavone group, but no increase compared to placebo in the 160 mg isoflavone group. The HDL findings may be confounded by the fact that the lipid specimens were not collected in the fasting state, but the dose-response difference seen here may represent a "therapeutic window" effect of isoflavones. Such a "window" effect has been shown in other studies of genistein effects at estradiol receptors, with one dose range having an agonist effect, and a different dose range having an antagonist effect. Such findings lend further caution to indiscriminate use of isoflavone products until we have a better understanding of the various dose-response relationships.

What does all this mean for you? In my view, it means before we can confidently recommend isoflavone and other dietary supplements for menopausal therapies, we have many issues to clarify in good studies. We need to know more about dose-response relationships for different target tissues, individual therapeutic variation, side-effect profiles based on dose, and effects on long-term disease risks that are known to be strongly linked with estrogen decline. Furthermore, we have to consider potential adverse interactions between dietary supplements and the prescription forms of hormone therapy our patients may also be using. I have been quite concerned by the types of problems I have seen occur in my own patients as a result of such interactions between OTC and prescription medications. For example, I described in chapter 15 the marked decrease in effectiveness of birth control pills when St. John's Wort is added.

If you are using soy and other isoflavone products instead of estrogen in the belief that these plant extracts are more "natural" than estrogen, keep in mind that you may be missing an important window of opportunity to prevent long-term health problems. This is a practical point for you to discuss with your physician when you use OTC supplements instead of prescription medications. It is important to monitor objective measures of bone and lipid markers to be certain that silent disease risks are not going undetected.

Are Herbal Remedies Safe and Effective?

Don't be misled by the word *natural* when looking for remedies for PMS or menopausal changes. While there are many that may help briefly to alleviate minor symptoms, there is a variety of herbs that has been well documented to have toxic effects on the liver, and may cause a variety of other symptoms as well. Just because compounds are *natural* to plants does not necessarily mean they are *natural* for humans. Two recent reports in *Archives of Internal Medicine* and the *Journal of the American Medical Association* reviewed cases of both severe liver and kidney toxicity from herbal products. The patient who had severe liver damage encountered the problem many of us have been worried about: the product had been *adulterated* with chemicals that were not shown on the label, so the woman had no idea what she was getting until she developed serious medical problems and ultimately *required a liver transplant*. Since the FDA does not regulate the manufacture, safety, dosage recommendations, and effectiveness of these substances, you are dealing with two major problems when you use them: (1) the active ingredients simply are not known in many cases, and (2) the bottle may not contain what the label says it does. Even though I am at times frustrated with the slow process of FDA approval for new medications, the advantage is that at least when I prescribe a *pharmaceutical-grade* product, I know that its manufacture and labeling are closely scrutinized for safety, and there are standardized dosage forms and guidelines.

The primary disadvantage to herbal remedies, in my opinion, is that often you are not able to determine the actual amount of the active ingredients you are getting or what is actually in the preparation. Many of the mixed herbal products that are imported from China, for example, are not completely labeled, or have been found to contain adulterants that are not listed. And then there is the problem of determining the correct dose. If, for instance, an herbal prescription says to take six bay leaves every day, how much of the desired ingredient is in that leaf, and what size leaf is used? An advantage of

Western pharmaceuticals is that one knows exactly how much 5 mg of a compound is. The dosage can be adjusted up or down with greater precision and accuracy than a random selection of six leaves or drops of a tincture. On the other hand, physicians may be too heavy handed in the amounts of Western pharmaceuticals they prescribe, especially for women patients. Doses of many medications for women often need to be started at much lower levels than are used for men. I have a number of women who have benefited from Prozac for premenstrual symptoms, but may need only *2 mg* instead of the *20 mg* dose recommended as the usual starting amount. If the differences in women's body size and physiology are not taken into account, there is increased likelihood of adverse side effects. No matter what therapy is being prescribed, all of us involved in the health fields should keep in mind the important premise of all healing traditions: "DO NO HARM."

Another overlooked safety issue with herbs is the problem of significant interactions with prescription medications. While herbs are often marketed as "completely safe, with no side effects," people forget that these plant compounds have to be metabolized by the liver, in the same pathways that the body uses to metabolize prescription medications, foods and vitamins. That means it is possible to have very pronounced *herb-drug-food interactions* that may alter the chemical make-up and effects of each one. You have probably already heard about the serious problems that can occur when taking some medications and drinking grapefruit juice at the same time, or that coffee and fiber in your diet prevent proper absorption of thyroid medication.

Similar problems occur with herbs and prescription medications. One example is the risk of *serious bleeding problems* if you add *Gingko biloba* when you are taking Coumadin, a blood-thinner to prevent formation of blood clots, or if you are taking large doses of aspirin daily for arthritis. Low-dose, baby aspirin daily does not seem to cause bleeding problems when taken with gingko in moderate doses. There are other drug-herb interactions that may cause problems with bleeding, blood pressure regulation and sedation during surgery if you take the herbs too close to the time you are having a surgical or dental procedure. Some of these potentially dangerous interactions, in addition to gingko, include feverfew, garlic, ginseng and vitamin E. All of these decrease the effectiveness of platelets forming blood clots, so you may be more likely to have excessive bleeding if you take these within two weeks before your surgery. Kava, valerian, and St. John's wort interact with sedative medications and anesthetics to intensify the effects of these drugs, possibly leading to prolonged sedation. Ginseng, black cohosh, and St. John's wort can also adversely affect blood pressure, making it difficult to control during a surgery. To be safe, you should plan to stop taking any of the above herbs or supplements at least *two weeks prior* to your surgery. And be sure that you always let your physicians know what herbs, vitamins and supplements you are taking.

Another serious interaction between medications and herbs was reported recently based on studies at the National Institutes of Health. The commonly used herb, St. Johns' wort, has been found to *decrease* the contraceptive effectiveness of the birth control pill *up to 50 percent*. With today's low dose pills, there is no such margin for error if you want your pills to work to prevent pregnancy. **Do not add St. John's wort** for depressive symptoms if you are taking birth control pills, or you could be in for a rude surprise with an unexpected pregnancy, no matter how many people may have found it helpful for relieving depression. In addition, since the herb appears to increase the liver's metabolic break-down of the hormones and reduce their effectiveness, you are likely to find yourself back in the cranky, irritable, anxious, "perimenopausal panic" mood roller coaster. At this time, there is no such known drug interaction between birth control pills and antidepressants such as Prozac, Zoloft, Paxil, Celexa, Luvox, or Wellbutrin. Serzone, however, does diminish the effectiveness of oral estrogen or birth control pills. Both St. Johns' wort and Serzone should be avoided as medications for depression if you are also taking prescription hormones. If you feel depressed on your current birth control pill, first talk with your physician about other types of birth control pill products to try that may have less progestin before you add other medicines or herbs for depression. Adding herbs on your own may give you more problems than you bargained for!

Another concern for menopausal women is that the *amount of hormone effect* may not be enough to provide levels needed to maintain bone density and to avoid increased heart disease risk if you are just using oral phytoestrogen and herbal supplements or from skin creams purportedly containing hormone-like substances. Although a number of natural remedies like black cohosh, evening primrose oil, red clover isoflavones, and soy isoflavones may alleviate milder symptoms such as hot flashes, the important question for you to evaluate is whether these remedies are having other desired effects in the body, such as bone preservation. So, deciding whether or not to use herbs depends upon your individual health needs and goals. If you *know* from testing that your bones and cholesterol levels are in desirable ranges, then you may decide to use an herbal remedy for reducing hot flashes. On the other hand, if your bone density is low, you really need to be sure that you are getting a reliable source of the right amount of estradiol to prevent further bone loss. I hope this approach provides a rational, commonsense way of deciding what is right for you. The following is a brief list of some commonly available herbs with potential for severe adverse effects. This is not a complete list. I encourage you to contact a reputable source (several listed in Appendix II) for additional information.

SOME POTENTIALLY DANGEROUS HERBS TO AVOID

- KNOWN TO CAUSE ACUTE LIVER INJURY, CHRONIC HEPATITIS, CIRRHOSIS, AND/OR LIVER FAILURE: chaparral, comfrey, coltsfoot, germander, margosa oil, mate tea, mistletoe and skullcap, Gordolobo yerba tea, pennyroyal (squawmint) oil, pyrrolizidine alkaloids, aflatoxins, *Amanita phalloides*, Jin Bu Huan (a Chinese herbal product), and others.
- KNOWN TO INCREASE HEART RATE, BLOOD PRESSURE (DANGEROUS IN PEOPLE WITH CVD): ephedra (Chinese name: mahuang), excessive amounts of caffeine (not generally shown on labels, but a common adulterant in tonics), and others.
- KNOWN TO CAUSE LIVER OR KIDNEY DAMAGE (ACUTE INTERSTITIAL NEPHRITIS AND/OR RENAL FAILURE): *Tung Shueh* pills (the culprit for the woman who developed liver failure) found to be adulterated with an anti-inflammatory agent, **mefanamic acid,** not shown on the label; aristolochic acid; products adulterated with phenylbutazone.

Always let your doctor know if you are taking any herbs or other supplements, so that if you develop problems, he or she has more information to use to help you prevent potentially serious interactions with prescription medications.

Summary

I think two overall keys to providing the best health care for women are the recognition of *gender* hormonal differences, and the recognition that *each individual* will have *different needs* and will benefit from a different blend of approaches. I think allopathic, osteopathic, homeopathic, and naturopathic physicians each have much to teach and to learn from the others. To provide optimal care for women of today, health professionals must use a variety of options, integrating the best of prescription hormones and medications when needed, along with healthy intake of vitamins, rational use of supplements, use of complementary herbs when appropriate, counseling and psychotherapy, stress management techniques such as hypnotherapy or biofeedback, as well as incorporating acupuncture, exercise prescriptions and the various types of body work and physical therapy. All of us in the health professions must also remember that prayer and ways of nourishing the soul are crucial elements of the healing process. As Ambrose Pare, a 16th century surgeon said, "God heals the wound, I merely dress it."

There is a great deal of valuable, reliable, scientific information available today about safe and effective ways to blend these approaches and therapeutic options. I encourage you to always work with health professionals who are willing to help you find useful information and to sort out the "product sales" hype from the reputable scientific information now available. Our goal as health professionals should be to find the unique blend of physical, medical, herbal, psychological, and spiritual approaches for each of you as an individual to help you best regain your wellness balance and achieve harmony and good health.

We also need to take better advantage of developing a *health partnership* between the health professional and YOU, the patient, with your own capacity for *self-healing*. If we CHOOSE to use it, engaging our minds to activate the healing ability *within* us, is the most powerful medicine that exists for all of us. When we combine our *internal* healing power with the appropriate *external* modalities available to us, the integration enhances our ability to achieve the best state of health we can. Even if we have a disease, such as diabetes, we may still move to a greater state of *wellness* by eating healthy meals, exercising regularly, practicing relaxation skills, having massage therapy to improve circulation, and maintaining a positive outlook on life. It's a different way of looking at things: Someone who has no disease or illness may still be *unwell* in mind, body or spirit, living a life full of unhealthy habits and feeling a sense of *dis-ease*. Another person who, having a serious disease, yet practices the integration of internal and external healing options, may feel an inner calm, balance, and wellness even with significant disease still present. You choose which way you will live.

As a physician who is formally trained in medicine, I give you the best of my knowledge and wisdom, but *you* choose to use it or not. You are in control of your choices and options. Without YOU having an active commitment to and involvement in YOUR own health care, there can be no true healing process. YOU are the most crucial member of any health care team. My desire is to help you learn the information and skills to TAKE CHARGE of your own well-being, and then help you find the necessary resources to reach your goals. You have the power to *be a well, educated woman.*

Chapter 17

Fat To Fit: Healthy Lifestyle Changes For All Ages

"Women are not frail. By widespread consumer education, early lifestyle behavior modification, and the productive use of modern technology, the image of the shrunken little old lady we hope will be condemned to history and replaced by women imbued with vitality and a zest for an active and productive old age."
—MORRIS NOTOLOVITZ, M.D., Ph.D.

VR's Story

I'm the third girl in a family of four girls. My sisters and my mother had serious medical problems (mostly cardiovascular) while they were alive and they have all died too young. I enjoy life, I want to be physically and mentally active. I don't want to be sickly or to die young. This is the reason for my story.

In 1984 I was fifty-four years old, a widow for a year, and the mother of four adult children. I was enjoying my work with young people, my family and friends, and life in general; however, I sensed something was wrong with my physical condition. I had been diagnosed as having essential hypertension when I was *twenty-nine* years old. Over the years, physicians had prescribed a variety of medications, which usually kept my blood pressure below the 150/90 threshold. I was taking four different medicines for five or six years and my blood pressure was staying within normal limits. But I knew something was wrong. My body just didn't feel like me. Everything was taking more effort than it usually did. I felt like I had to push myself to swim and play golf, my two favorite sports. I would go to aerobics class and really be working out well and never could get my heart rate into the target range. Very frustrating for someone who likes to follow directions and achieve my goals!

When I mentioned this to friends, they made the usual comments, "Remember you're older now, VR!" I knew too many active people much older than I was, so I didn't buy into my friends' excuses. I went to my doctor, whom I'd been going to for seven years. I told him how I felt and suggested that I needed a reevaluation with an up-to-date cardiac stress test (remembering my sisters and their heart problems, it seemed like a reasonable request to me) and then a review of my medications. He looked over my record and said "No, there is no sign that you need a cardiac stress test. Your blood pressure is well-controlled and you seem fine to me." I believe he thought this was true, but I think he was also influenced by the fact that I was on an HMO insurance plan and this would add to his medical expenses. He had indicated there would be problems justifying the cardiac stress test.

At this point I did some serious soul searching. *I felt something was wrong with me physically.* I knew I couldn't prove it, but I wasn't going to let a doctor keep me from getting a correct diagnosis! I thought about my mother and sisters. Mother started having heart attacks in her fifties, had two operations on her carotid arteries in her sixties, had strokes in her seventies and eighties, and died in a nursing home at eighty-five, out-of-touch with reality. My sister Rae, who was seven years older than I, started having heart attacks in her forties and died at fifty-one. My older sister Anne, who is ten years older than I am, started having heart attacks in her fifties, and at sixty-four had a quadruple bypass. She lived an invalid's life until she died at age sixty-nine. With this kind of family history, I knew I needed help immediately.

I shared my story with Dr. Vliet. She asked many questions and then ordered a cardiopulmonary exercise test plus some labwork. My own primary care physician refused to order the test, saying I didn't need it. I had never had such a comprehensive stress test. It was stopped suddenly because my condition rapidly declined. The test report stated I was heavily overmedicated, my heart was blocked so much by the beta-blockers that it couldn't get to a higher heart rate even though the monitors showed that I had already passed the aerobic threshold! The cardiologist's report said I was in danger of sudden death if I participated in physical activities. And here I had been pushing myself in aerobics classes three times a week. I knew my body had been trying to tell me something, I just didn't realize how serious it was. Dr. Vliet urged me not to go on my planned wilderness hiking trip, but to take that time to get my medication changed and my body in better shape. After the abnormal results, my primary care physician then said, "Oh, well, I guess this did need to be done. I'll send the prescription to the insurance company."

I believe Dr. Vliet saved my life. She *listened* to my concerns and accepted the possible validity of them. She ordered the tests that would give her the factual information she needed to confirm or deny my subjective feelings about my body. Dr. Vliet did a complete re-evaluation and, with her colleague, provided me with a new regimen of preventive medicine and appropriate medications.

Now, eleven years later, I follow the basic tenets of preventive medicine: low-fat foods, regular physical activity, relaxation techniques, caring relationships, required medications, and periodic medical check-ups. I have lost weight, yes, but more importantly I have *gained* good health. My blood pressure is controlled; I exercise four times a week. I take only two medications now, instead of *five*, and I am off the beta-blockers. I work full time in a high-pressure job I love, I go jet-skiing and swimming with my grandchildren, and have just taken up scuba diving. Good living for a sixty-five-year-old woman!

Update, 2000: VR is still active and energetic, still scuba-diving, exercising regularly, is taking even less medication, loves how good she feels on her estrogen patches, and has *not* had a heart attack like her sisters and mother. She is now over seventy but has the energy and vitality of someone twenty years younger.

VR wrote her story herself when she learned I was writing a book, because she wanted her voice to be heard by other women who may not be listened to, and wanted to encourage other women to *listen to their own body wisdom*. I feel gratified by her words and inspired by all that she has done to take charge of her life in spite of the "bad genes" she's inherited! She has truly made the efforts that are within her control to change her lifestyle, move from FAT to FIT and healthy. Which will you be? You choose. There is a great deal that is indeed within your control.

VR's story illustrates the many integrated issues I have raised throughout this book and encapsulates what has been wrong in women's health care. She is an articulate, educated, health-conscious professional woman. She knew her body and trusted her instincts. She had appropriately consulted her physician with her concerns. She was not listened to, not taken seriously, not evaluated properly for her health history and risks. She was overly medicated **and then told she was fine,** there was nothing wrong. If someone this knowledgeable and assertive was dismissed and discounted, it makes it even more alarming to think about all the women out there who do not have VR's knowledge and ability to speak out, and then quietly become more debilitated or die from not being listened to and taken seriously.

VR's story is critical in illustrating another problem for women. Weight loss is key to reducing hypertension and heart disease risk. Doctors know that, but too often don't refer patients for nutritional consultations to help with healthy weight loss plans. Instead they tend to prescribe pills to control blood pressure. It's faster, it's what they are taught, and many patients expect and want a "magic bullet." But VR was different. She had been actively involved in a regular exercise program for a number of years, and she had worked hard to decrease her body fat, cut out added salt, reduce alcohol, and stop smoking. What she did not know, and what was potentially lethal, was that the very medications given to decrease her blood pressure were also directly interfering with her ability to lose weight and her ability to accomplish the benefits of her aerobic exercise. She had never been checked for hormonal changes, nor had any physician talked to her about the potential cardioprotective benefits of estrogen therapy so she could consider that option. She was on *five* different antihypertensive medications and cholesterol-lowering drugs when she came to see me, creating problems with drug interactions and side effects that were making it even harder for her to lose weight and have the normal body responses to exercise. Yet, her physician had never looked at the estrogen factor, which is so crucial to preventing heart disease in a woman with all these risk factors and strong family history. For the "bottom-line" folks out there, *if* you ignore all the quality-of-life issues for VR, and *if* you ignore the risk of premature death she was facing, and just look at the dollar cost of her care (over $500 per month on medications alone, in 1995 dollars), isn't it far more cost effective to provide a woman-centered evaluation with appropriate testing of hormone levels, decrease her expensive medications, help her with lifestyle changes, and prescribe hormone therapy than to continue multiple medications and treat the complications, and heart attack, when these occur? Put in this context, a hormone blood test doesn't seem so expensive, does it?

As I indicated above, beta-blockers (like Inderal, Corgard, Atenolol, Tenormin, and other newer ones as well) have several *unwanted* effects: (1) they slow down metabolism; (2) they decrease insulin release from the pancreas, which then impairs glucose regulation and increases the tendency to gain weight; (3) they block the normal heart rate response to exercise, which impaired VR's ability to safely exercise and monitor her heart rate; (4) they decrease one's energy level and tolerance for physical activity; and (5) they interfere with normal thyroid hormone function. Here was a well-motivated and disciplined patient who was being thwarted in her efforts to achieve her health goals due to ignorance of the *unappreciated* side effects of the medication she was taking.

Let's look at some other gender-specific issues and needs for women who are making the transformation from being overfat to being more fit and more lean—notice I didn't say skinny, I said **fit** and **lean.**

Research on Men Doesn't Necessarily Apply to Women

Since estrogen and progesterone are both involved in regulating metabolism, blood glucose, and body-fat storage, you'd think that researchers would have paid more attention to the "female factor" in obesity research. If you and your husband or boyfriend have ever gone on a diet at the same time, you have experienced firsthand that weight loss is very different in men and women. A few years ago, when my husband and I went on a spa vacation, I watched him peel off the pounds, while I struggled to get a *quarter* pound lower on the scale. He even got to eat more calories than I did. Not fair! From an evolutionary perspective, it makes sense that females would be more efficient at storing (and keeping) body fat, to carry pregnancies. Now we live in a culture that *esteems thinness* and at the same time makes *eating* a dominant social activity, rewards good behavior with ice cream or candy, and puts fast-food options on every street corner. What insanity. Our bodies have not had several million years to adapt to the sudden availability of excess food, and we pay the price with an obesity epidemic in the United States.

Sugar and fat are two examples. I lived in Williamsburg, Virginia, for many years, and I was surprised to learn that in colonial American homes, sugar was such a rare and very expensive delicacy that it was often kept under lock and key. Today, we truly live "la dolce vita" (the sweet life) when we put sugar in practically everything, even ketchup. Pounds of it, in fact. Today the average American consumes on average 125 pounds of sugar per person per year. That's incredible. Much of the sugar we eat is hidden. It appears in processed foods of all kinds, including soups, condiments, salad dressings, frozen dinners, and the obvious sources: desserts and soft drinks. It's been calculated that the average American eats *24 percent* of *daily* calories from sugars in various forms, mainly refined sugar (sucrose). Then comes the FAT. Americans consume, on average, *40–43 percent* of daily calories from fat, instead of recommended amounts of 20–30 percent. That means *64 percent* of the calories you eat every day come from *fat* and *sugar.* No wonder Americans have more obesity and obesity-related diseases than any other country in the world. Since simple sugars have no nutritional value except providing energy, that means that most Americans have to get the essential nutrients from only 35 percent of their food intake. It is clear that sugar and fat calories are crowding out more nutritious food groups from our diet. And for women, sugars especially pack a double whammy: eating them tends to create a vicious cycle of craving them, and our hormonal changes each month affect not only how our bodies metabolize both sugars and fats but our cravings for them as well. I will talk more about these vicious cycles further along in this chapter. But first, some metabolism basics as related to women's bodies.

Fat storage is one of our adaptations to the scarcity and unpredictability of food supplies before food was cultivated on a steady basis. Humans who were more efficient at storing body fat were better able to survive the periods of famine. Pima Indians in the southwestern United States are an illustration of the consequences that occur when people have evolved in environments of scarce food, and are genetically more efficient at storing fat. Now that foods, and the wrong types of food, are so plentiful, Pima Indians have the highest incidence of diabetes (and all its complications) of any group in the United States.

Females in particular needed to be able to effectively store fat in order to survive and to also provide the nourishment to sustain a growing fetus for nine months. Estradiol helps to regulate blood sugar to keep glucose levels steady, and it also functions to enhance storage of fat around the hips, thighs, and buttocks, which provides "fuel" able to sustain a pregnancy. Progesterone causes increases in appetite and metabolic rate and also causes lowered sensitivity to insulin that *increases* fat storage and leads to glucose *intolerance,* and further *increased cravings* for sweets. This effect of progesterone encourages a pregnant woman to eat more, which results in better nourishment for the fetus; but alas, more body fat for the mother.

Recent research has confirmed what women have always suspected: We get hungrier the week before our periods, due to the rise in progesterone. Appetite increases about 12 to 15 percent in the second half of the menstrual cycle. If you ignore this increase in appetite because you are dieting, you may find that the sweet cravings become uncontrollable, leading to the binge-on-sweets-feel-guilty-starve-again-then-binge-again cycle. If you eat fruit and whole grain breads high in complex carbohydrates, balanced with more fat and protein, during the progesterone-dominant second half of the menstrual cycle, you provide the fuel needed to sustain blood glucose during this time of increased appetite and metabolism. The result is you are less likely to give in to the craving for sweets that lead you to overeat, the main culprit in adding excess pounds.

Compared to men, women also have more of the *lipogenic* enzymes that help the body *store* fat instead of the *lipolytic* enzymes that *break down* fat so it can be used as fuel. Many of our female tendencies to gain weight and to crave sweets (instead of meats, which men tend to want) have strong hormonal influences that have an adaptive advantage for our species. Unfortunately, our biochemical makeup just doesn't fit well with our current cultural obsession with women having to be rail thin to be considered sexy and attractive. It helps to understand these basics so you don't fall into the psychological trap of beating yourself up mentally because of your body size. You can help improve the ratio of lean muscle mass to fat mass by exercising regularly and eating healthy. As you read further, I will explain ways of achieving a better balance in what and when you eat, the difference between body *weight* and body *composition,* as well as the ways female hormones interact with appetite regulation.

Eating for "Wellness of Being"

I am not perfect. I have been FIT. I have been FAT. I have probably in my lifetime tried almost every diet that came out. Finally I learned some years ago that most diets don't work. What works, plain and simple, is healthy eating with the optimal balance of protein (about 25–30 percent), fat (about 25–30 percent, focusing mainly on unsaturated fats), complex carbohydrates (40–50 percent), along with increased activity and regular exercise. Do I always do it? Not always. I'm just like most of you: too many things to do and too little time to do them. Until 1989 and the last round of surgeries on my neck, followed the next year by my hysterectomy, I had been really diligent about keeping up with exercise and maintaining my healthy body composition. I have to admit, since then it has been much harder. The many months of recovery from surgery got me out of my exercise routine so long, and contributed to enough weight gain, that I have had a very difficult time reestablishing a consistent exercise program that works as well as what I was doing in the past. I got bored with a basic walking program, and about a year ago, took up roller-blading. I loved the exhilaration and it was great exercise, but I forgot I was no longer the limber twelve-year-old who could fall with impunity. I also learned that roller blades are *very* difficult to control. After a spectacular crash (landing of course on all the places that did not have the protective pads) that messed up my shoulder, hip, and neck, I am now back to a more sane exercise regimen of either walking on the treadmill or swimming laps five to six days a week. Walking and swimming are not as exhilarating for me as jogging or roller-blading, but they are a lot safer! And this amount of exercise does help keep excess weight in check. I also make an effort at work to walk up stairs instead of taking elevators a few floors, and I look for ways to walk more during daily activities. Every little bit helps. I really do understand the frustrations and difficulties my patients describe in reaching their goals, since I'm right in there fighting the same battles.

But I will say this: over the last twenty years, in an effort to better practice what I preach and to be healthier myself, I have made some significant changes in the way I eat. I have much less saturated fats. I make sure to have a good balance of protein at each meal and snack to help decrease the insulin surge and blood-sugar drop that come with high-carb snacks. I rarely use butter or margarine, or even much vegetable oil. I used to make homemade mayonnaise, I enjoyed it so much. Now I prefer using nonfat yogurt or low-fat mayonnaise. I have red meat only a few times a month. I cut out colas (even diet ones) and other soft drinks with phosphates. I rarely have any alcohol, maybe a glass or two of wine every several months. I have cut out added salt and pick low-salt options when I eat out or buy a prepared frozen dinner. I don't snack on sweets like I used to. I eat more fresh fruit. I eat whole grain bread. I eat only *plain* popcorn, no butter and no salt. I don't go to work without a good breakfast anymore. I make sure I keep up with my skim milk for calcium without the fat of whole milk. I pay attention to taking magnesium supplements and a multivitamin every day. Taking this inventory really helped me to affirm the positive changes I have made. You might do the same.

Take an honest look at what you eat every day. **Can you find some healthy changes you have already made?** Good. **Make a list of those, and add three or four new ones.** Think of changes to add that you are ready to make *NOW*.

Sorting Out the Fads

As we baby boomers age, one thing is clear: We are getting fatter. Entrepreneurial types have quickly figured out that there is a huge market here and lots of money to be made with diet products of all types. The hype is everywhere, and there are figures to show we are buying into the hype: Americans spend close to $40 billion annually on diet and diet-related products. The sad part is, 95 percent of people who are buying into all these diets will regain the weight. This creates the marketing opportunity of the millennium: selling the same product to the same people over and over again. Fads in food abound. Fads in diets crop up faster than the weather changes. New diets sell products: books, tapes, flash cards, videos, cookbooks, supplements, special foods, prepared meals—you name it and there will be a product designed to go with the newest "diet of the day." There's a diet to suit every taste and every food craving. High fiber, low fat. High fat, low fiber (good if you like being constipated). High protein, low carbohydrate is in. No, it's out. High carbohydrate, low protein is the way to go. Don't mix protein and carbs at the same meal. Don't mix fruits and vegetables at the same meal. Don't mix protein and fat at the same meal. Don't mix protein and fruits and vegetables at the same meal. Eat grapefruit at each meal to burn fat. Don't eat grapefruit, it will cause stomach acid. It would be less confusing to just not eat. 1980: Margarine is OK, butter's bad. 1990: Margarine's bad, butter's better. 2000: Flaxseed oil and Benecol are the way to go.

How do you make sense of all this? (My suggestion: Don't try. It doesn't make sense, *it just sells*.) How do you sort out fads from facts and find something that works for you? I will hit the highlights here, and I have to admit this section on food balance has changed significantly since I first wrote *Screaming to Be Heard* in 1994. At that time, I was still heavily influenced by the emphasis on low-fat, high-carb meal plans based on programs such as those of Drs. Ornish and Pritiken. As time has gone on, and I have done more clinical work with women's hormone changes and their effects of "apple-shaped" weight gain leading to insulin resistance and further weight gain, I have had to modify my original emphasis on the low-fat, high-carb approaches. One crucial factor I had not fully realized at that time was that the positive findings of Pritiken and Ornish with regard to low-fat, high-fiber, lower-protein diets were based mainly on studies of their *male* patients. As we women all know, there are a lot of differences between men and women in terms of fat storage, and loss/gain of fat and body weight, particularly those of us who are in the midlife years or those with abnormal ovarian function such as PCOS.

The emerging data on insulin resistance in women, and the impact of our midlife decline in estradiol, with normal progesterone and relatively more androgen effect, has led me to modify my earlier recommendations of a diet consisting of 60 percent carbohydrates, 20 percent proteins, and 20 percent fats. I now recommend for my patients (and for me, too) a meal plan higher in protein along with healthier fat sources. The earlier emphasis on very low fat (20 percent or less) and high (60 percent or more) carbohydrates works well for men, but not as well for women with the hormonal changes of PMS, PCOS, perimenopause, and menopause. For a while, until periods actually stop, women going through the premenopausal ovarian decline are losing estradiol (E2) first, but progesterone (P) is typically still in the ovulatory range. This means a higher P to E2 ratio, which along with the "unmasking" of male hormones (androgens) due to decline in E2, tends to put weight gain around our waist and upper abdomen. This change in fat distribution makes us tend to be less sensitive to insulin, a condition called *insulin resistance,* which promotes fat *storage*.

There is also another whole dimension to the way hormonal changes in women affect insulin regulation, which makes the syndrome of **insulin resistance** much more common in women, especially as they grow older. *Insulin resistance* refers to the phenomenon of having high levels of both circulating insulin *and glucose* in the bloodstream, but the insulin molecules can't bind properly to the insulin receptor sites on the surface of the cell to allow glucose to enter the cell and be used for energy. This occurs when women (and men) gain weight; the fat cells become distorted in shape with increased fat storage, and the "lock" or receptor site for insulin is "warped" out of proper alignment, so the insulin molecule "key" no longer fits in the receptor. Insulin resistance makes it harder to lose weight, since the cells are not getting enough "fuel," you continually perceive you are hungry even though there is plenty of fuel circulating in the bloodstream. It also causes rising blood pressure and problems with "reactive hypoglycemia" (low blood sugar) when the excess insulin suddenly works, glucose rushes into the cells, and your blood glucose plummets. This sequence creates intense sweet cravings, and the whole cycle starts over; you get fatter, become more insulin resistant, and so on. Such marked glucose swings contribute to feeling lethargic, sleepy, and having trouble concentrating when the glucose levels are rising, and then feeling sweaty, anxious, irritable, or weepy when the glucose levels are falling quickly. You may notice significant changes in how you feel and function relative to the time since your last meal or the types of food you eat. Insulin resistance is one of the "deadly four" that increase the risk of heart disease and diabetes, along with truncal obesity (waist area instead of hips), high blood pressure, and high cholesterol/triglycerides.

It is now known that there are also insulin receptors in ovary tissue, and insulin appears to change the enzymes in the ovary to shift hormone production toward the *androgens* rather than the normal estrogen balance. This type of problem occurs in young women with PCOS, and in perimenopausal woman who are losing estradiol. The imbalance of androgens to estradiol causes deposits of body fat around the middle of the body (similar to males), as well as all the other unwanted effects I just listed. Low-fat, high-carbohydrate diets make this problem *worse* by stimulating more insulin production by the pancreas, and more insulin production in turn tends to push the body toward storing more fat. More body fat then makes more insulin resistance, so it is another of those terrible vicious cycles. Some of you may see yourself and your own struggles in this description. This is why I have revised my earlier recommendations on the balance of carbohydrates, fat, and protein to help reduce this trend toward increased insulin resistance.

I suggest that you read the book *40-30-30 Fat Burning Nutrition* by Joyce and Gene Daoust, for more information on insulin resistance that occurs for us as we gain weight and experience the midlife hormonal changes. This excellent book will also provide suggestions on meal plans for you that are quick, simple, and easy to follow. Another good book on this subject is *The Protein Power Plan,* but my patients have told me that it is harder to follow than the *40-30-30* book. In order to *decrease* the stimulation of insulin with meals, I recommend that you aim for a blend of 40–50 percent complex carbohydrates, 25–30 percent protein, and 25–30 percent unsaturated fat with each meal.

It is also important to focus more on foods with a *lower*

glycemic index to help avoid overstimulating insulin production that in turn triggers more food stored as body fat instead of being burned for energy. What does *glycemic index* mean? Food that are quickly converted to glucose, such as bananas or white flour pastas and breads, cookies, crackers, and sweets, have a *high* glycemic index. Food that take longer to be converted to glucose, such as fat and protein foods or fibrous vegetables, have a *low* glycemic index, and do not overstimulate insulin production. Lower insulin levels help you lose the unwanted body fat, as well as reduce your risk of heart disease and diabetes.

I also recommend smaller meals at more frequent intervals to help maintain your energy level on an even keel throughout the day, increase metabolic rate, and reduce food cravings later in the day. Mood, anxiety, and cognitive changes are quite characteristic of the brain effects of marked glucose fluctuations due to elevated insulin and falling estradiol. These are the same symptoms women with FMS describe as "fibro-fog," which can actually have many hormonal and nutritional causes. In addition, the symptoms we use to diagnose panic disorder are the *same* symptoms that are triggered when the brain's "alarm center" senses a rapidly falling glucose or estradiol. It *feels* the same, even though the cause may be quite different. The more you can achieve stable glucose and estrogen levels with diet, exercise, healthy hormonal balance, and, when appropriate, use medication options such as metformin (Glucophage), the less you will need antidepressant or antianxiety medicines to improve mood and decrease anxiety symptoms. Low-to-moderate-intensity exercise, such as walking, acts as an "invisible insulin" that serves to facilitate delivery of glucose to the muscles and lower the tendency to have *high* glucose levels in the bloodstream. It also decreases the problem of insulin resistance and helps burn fat for fuel as well as improving muscle function.

Food as Fuel for Energy and Zest

Let's take a closer look at these food types, or "macronutrients"— carbohydrates, proteins, and fats. **Carbohydrates** are one of our key nutrient groups. You've heard the term a lot. It used to be that all the magazines talked about cutting out the "fattening" carbohydrates. Then for a while, all we heard was "carbs are good, it's the excess fat we put on them that is bad." This idea focused on all the sour cream, butter, oils, and mayonnaise that were added to foods like baked potatoes or pasta or salads. For example, a baked potato with sour cream and bacon bits and butter could run 500–600 calories, while a plain baked potato has only about one hundred calories yet is loaded with fiber, vitamin C, minerals, and lots of energy. But, now we are coming full-circle to having more books recommending lower carbs and a little more fat (of the healthy kind) again.

Carbohydrates are the body's primary "quick-start" fuel, providing four calories of energy per gram. Carbs are readily converted into glucose, the only fuel the brain can use. Proteins are a little slower to undergo this conversion to glucose, but, they, too end up in the bloodstream as glucose that gives our brain and body the steady fuel it needs to operate. If you aren't getting enough carbohydrates and protein at regular intervals throughout the day, your blood sugar falls, and you feel tired, irritable, and foggy-brained. Both protein and carbohydrates are crucial elements of your "eating well" plan to maintain energy, concentration, memory, stable mood, and a normal metabolic rate throughout the day.

Complex carbohydrates, such as whole grains, whole vegetables, and whole fruits, are your best source but should make up only about 40–50 percent of your daily food intake. Choosing complex carbohydrates over simple carbs such as white-flour pasta, white bread, or crackers will provide more fiber, better stability in your blood glucose, and a healthy feeling of fullness so you won't have the desire to overeat. Complex carbs also don't tend to overstimulate insulin production as much as simple carbohydrates do. In addition, bringing in more of a balance of proteins and fats at each meal, provides better feeling of fullness (satiety), and sustains your energy levels more evenly and longer.

Proteins also provide four calories per gram as energy for the body. Proteins are slower to digest than carbohydrates, so they help keep blood sugar (glucose) levels steady over about three to four hours, compared to the shorter length of time, about one–two hours, that blood glucose is sustained by complex carbohydrates. The role protein plays in our food is to supply the amino acids from which the body can make its own proteins. The protein in food and the resulting amino acids help keep blood-sugar levels steady over several hours, compared to the shorter interval sustained by complex carbohydrates. This is why a healthy balance of protein—about 25–30 percent of your food intake—is important at every meal. Protein is needed for building healthy muscle and bone and for body-repair processes, such as daily muscle repair, particularly as you increase your exercise. Proteins also provide the building blocks to immune globulins and the brain's chemical messengers.

Amino acids are classified into two categories: those the body can make and do not have to be included in the diet, called *nonessential,* and those the body cannot make itself and must get in the diet, called *essential.* There are eight essential amino acids that the body is not able to make, or can only make in very small amounts not fast enough to meet energy demands. One essential amino acid of special interest to women with pain syndromes is DL-phenylalanine (DLPA), an amino acid with mild pain-relieving properties. It is found naturally in foods such as nuts, cheese, avocados, bananas, sesame and pumpkin seeds; it is also available as a supplement sold in pharmacies and health food stores. However, if you are taking MAO inhibitors or have migraines, hypertension, palpitations, or tachycardia, you should not use DLPA supplements. Another essential amino acid is lysine which the body uses to manufacture L-carnitine, a chemical that helps muscle cells to more efficiently use oxygen. Tyrosine is a nonessential amino acid that your body is capable of synthesizing on its own and is used to make both adrenal and thyroid hormones. Are you beginning to see how your diet plays a role in your hormone balance and well-being?

Complete proteins are those that contain all of the essential amino acids and are found in animal sources, foods such as meat, fish, chicken, eggs, and cheese. But these foods contain higher amounts of fat, so you need to select those protein foods that are lower in fat: lean meats, low-fat cheeses, poultry without the skin, egg whites without the yolks, et cetera. If you do not eat animal protein, you need to combine your vegetables in such as way that you get complete proteins, since vegetable sources are lacking in some of the essential amino acids. The combination of beans and rice to make a complete protein source is an excellent example.

Fats are the most concentrated energy source in our macronutrient group, with nine calories of energy per gram. Some fat in the diet is crucial to provide the essential and other fatty acids that are used to make a variety of hormones, including those of the ovaries, as well as to absorb fat-soluble vitamins. I don't think the extremely low-fat diets are as desirable for women, but neither am I giving you license here to throw away all concerns about eating fat, especially the unhealthy saturated or "trans" fats. Actually, I find that if I use just the fat content of my protein sources and don't add much fat to what I eat, I'm generally pretty well on target with the 25–30 percent percent fat goal. As you can see from various calorie tables, you certainly don't need butter or margarine on your grilled cheese sandwich, since the cheese has more than adequate fat content on its own. Most Americans certainly exceed my recommendation of 25–30 percent fat intake.

If you want to maintain health, lose weight successfully, and maintain a healthy body weight, the "secret" is to cut out the *excess* fat in your diet and get your body moving more. Nothing new, I know, but the good news is that cutting out the *excess* or *added fat* is also one of the easiest ways to reduce your total caloric intake. Most people don't realize that **all fats** (whether vegetable oils, olive oil, butter, margarine, or lard) have twice as many calories per gram as carbohydrates and protein (9 cal/gm compared to 4 cal/gm each for protein and carbs). Fat is the most calorie-dense type of food we eat, but high-fat foods don't take up space in the intestinal tract like high-fiber foods do, so we often don't realize how much fat (and calories) we have eaten. It is dramatic how much more dietary fat Americans eat now than we did at the turn of the century: **45 percent now versus 28 percent in 1900.**

A primary source of dietary fat for most Americans is the *hidden fats* in foods that often sabotage our best efforts. The new food labeling will help you detect these hidden fats, such as the salad dressing on your salad, the cream sauce on your pasta (remember that marinara sauce is lower in fat), the olive oil for dipping your bread, fish cooked in butter, donuts at the morning coffee break, pizza dripping with cheese and pepperoni, French fries, those big yummy-looking "bran" muffins (there's probably a day's worth of sugar and fat in each one and not much bran!), the sauce glistening on your steamed vegetables, the list goes on and on. It helps to learn where the fats are hidden in various foods and gradually cut back every day. You may find it helpful to buy a small paperback guide to counting fat grams, since there are now several good ones available. Consider it as "lite" reading. As you make these changes, tell yourself all the wonderful things you are doing for your body, now and down the road. You'll also notice you don't feel as sluggish. Diets that are too high in fat and are not balanced with proper amounts of carbohydrates and proteins slow down the gastrointestinal tract motility, contributing to more constipation, distention of the tummy, and feeling generally fat and miserable, especially the second half of the menstrual cycle.

The real key for women going through hormone changes, such as PMS or PCOS or perimenopause, to help maintain steady energy levels, improved brain clarity, and less pain is to achieve a balance of carbohydrates, protein, and fat at each meal and each of the "snack breaks" of the day. For example, this is why I recommend having a healthy snack in the late afternoon, about 4 PM, when blood sugar normally hits the "afternoon slump." This snack should also have the balanced ratios (40:30:30 or 50:25:25). Making sure you do have this late afternoon snack each day helps your mental sharpness and also helps keep you from coming home from work ravenous and eating everything in sight. Depending on what time you get your breakfast in, I also suggest a mid-morning snack to keep things level.

While I am on the subject of dietary fat, I want to comment about another disturbing trend I have seen in women's health habits. I encounter more and more women who tell me they have *cut out dairy products*, especially milk, *for fear of the fat*. What do they replace milk with? Typically, it's soft drinks, whether regular or sugar-and-caffeine free. Either type poses unique problems for women who want to be healthy and maintain optimal body composition and bone density. All soft drinks contain high levels of phosphates, which attach to the calcium and magnesium ions in the digestive tract and increase the loss of both minerals from the body. Calcium and magnesium then move from the bones to maintain adequate blood levels that are needed for normal nerve and muscle function. So the more soft drinks you consume, the more calcium and magnesium you lose. Regular soft drinks not only leach these minerals from your bones, they are also loaded with sugar. A twelve-ounce nondiet soft drink contains about seven to eight teaspoons of sugar. This becomes a real problem when you drink five or six sugared sodas a day, because you end up with almost *half* your total daily calories coming from a source *without any nutritional value*! If you drink the sugar-free ones, you are still getting artificial sweeteners whose sweet taste contributes to excess stimulation of insulin, a hormone that stimulates fat storage. Think about it. Low-fat milk has about the same *calorie* content as a regular soda, and rather than leaching calcium from your bones, it provides both calcium and protein. I have been drinking skim milk for so long that 2 percent milk now tastes too rich.

Another *gimmick* to watch out for is all of the low-fat and fat-free food items now filling the shelves. The fat may have been removed, but it has been replaced by simple sugars and excess calories with little nutritional value. These play havoc with blood-sugar levels that in turn affect energy levels. Plus, what I find is that because the box of cookies is "fat free," we feel psychologically it is *okay* to eat more. How many of us have come close to finishing a whole box of these in one sitting . . . or just deciding that there are not enough left to bother with putting them back in the pantry? That is not a balanced snack . . . and it is a sure way to increase insulin production and promote more storage of body fat.

Body Weight versus Body Composition

Most women I talk with are absolutely obsessed with the scale and what they *weigh*. Body weight has become the number one statistic women talk about, certainly in large part due to the cultural brainwashing that to be thin is to be desirable and acceptable as a woman. I want to emphasize that we really should be looking at body **composition** rather than body **weight**. Body weight can vary immensely depending upon how much muscle mass you have built up and what your body build is. Someone who has a heavier bone density, for example, and more lean body mass may weigh twenty-five pounds more than a smaller-boned person who has not been exercising, and yet both could have the same percentage of body fat. One patient of mine is a young petite, thin woman (size 4) who is sedentary. Her body-fat anaylsis showed that she has *34 percent body fat*. Healthy ranges for women over 30 are about 25-30 percent body fat, so this woman is in an unhealthy "at risk" range, although she *looks* terrific by society standards. Another patient, who is stockier in appearance and wears a size 14, actually has *25 percent body fat* because she exercises regularly and does weight training three times a week. The second patient, who wears a larger size, is actually healthier overall than the smaller size woman. Fit doesn't mean skinny.

I recently went to my husband's class reunion, and someone remarked that though she wore the same size dress that she had in her twenties, the form inside was much different. One of the things that changes with age is body composition—the relative proportion of fat to muscle, bone, and other lean tissue. In the ongoing Fels Longitudinal study on aging, researchers looked into this. A brief summary shows that both women and men in the study had age-related increases in weight, total body fat, and percentage of body fat during the period from 1976 to 1996. Those who had the higher levels of physical activity predictably had lower percentages of body fat. Women generally experienced a change in body composition rather than a loss of weight or reduction in body mass. Menopause also made a difference. The longer a woman had been postmenopausal, the higher the proportion of body fat to lean body mass; however, those who took estrogen lost less lean body mass, and had a lower body-fat percentage. For postmenopausal women wishing to maintain healthy body composition, the equation then seems to be **Ex + E2 = a healthy body**. That is, **exercise** helps a lot, plus the **right type of estrogen** helps exercise be more effective in building bone and muscle.

The way to really determine an optimal weight for you is to have a body composition test done to measure your percentage of body fat. For women the optimal ranges are 22–30 percent body fat. If you are over thirty, you are more likely to preserve bone if your body fat is closer to 25 percent. The "at risk" range is greater than 33 percent. If you're over age thirty and you're trying to get down below 20 percent body fat, you really do increase your risk of osteoporosis. This is because you're losing enough body fat to lose some of the natural estrogen that's present in body fat tissue, and you begin to actually have some negative effect on your overall health.

Research at the Cooper Clinic, from the National College of Sports Medicine, and other investigators studying optimal healthy ranges, has found that when women get too low on percent body fat, they stop menstruating normally, have declining hormonal production, and begin to lose bone more rapidly. I really strongly encourage women not to go below the 20 percent body-fat level. Actually, if you get down *below* about 15 percent, you lose menses and that's when women become even *more at risk for osteoporosis*. Those of you on a weight-loss regimen, and who are exercising several times a week, should focus on body measurements once a month and not be obsessed with body *weight*. Your weight is not going to be an accurate indicator of the loss of fat tissue (which weighs about ⅙ as much as does muscle tissue). It is much more accurate, and helpful, to focus on how your body is changing in the way of inches. This gives you a much better picture of the amount of *fat loss*. As you exercise you *increase* the *lean body mass*, so by only using scale weight measurement you won't realize that you're losing "light weight" body *fat* as you build up *heavier* muscle mass. I usually recommend to women that they take their body measurements about once a month, and try not to weigh on the scale any more than once every other week. You can go tomorrow to your local health club and have your body-fat percentage measured. Then throw your scale away, and buy a tape measure. Focus on what's happening to the health of your body, not on the number of pounds!

Vicious Cycles: Food Cravings and the Menstrual Cycle

Over my years of clinical practice, I would say that about 75–85 percent of women patients have described cyclic food cravings that are clearly related to the second half of the menstrual cycle. And these cravings are the kind of intense urges that override rational awareness that junk foods aren't healthy! Women have often described going out late in the evening just to buy chocolate (or something salty or whatever) because the craving was so strong. I have to admit, I did that myself on occasion when the premenstrual "have-to-have-chocolate" urges hit! Why is this? And why is it that I have **never** had a **male** patient describe cravings for **chocolate** the way women do. Yes, I have had male (and female) patients who were alcoholic describe cravings for alcohol, but I see that as a different physiological issue and mechanism.

I think there is a key *hormonal* factor that affects women and contributes to these cravings: *the rise and fall in* **progesterone** *during the second half of the menstrual cycle*. How does this work? Progesterone alters the normal insulin response, which regulates blood glucose ("sugar" levels in the blood). Women then experience a greater tendency to have lower blood glucose levels, and more episodes of "reactive" drop in blood glucose following food intake, especially if the food intake is primarily sweets or other simple sugars. This tends to set up the vicious cycles that I have drawn in the diagrams below. Take a look at "The Vicious Cycle" and "Another Vicious Cycle" and see if you recognize yourself! Then read on about what is happening as your body cycles hormonally each month.

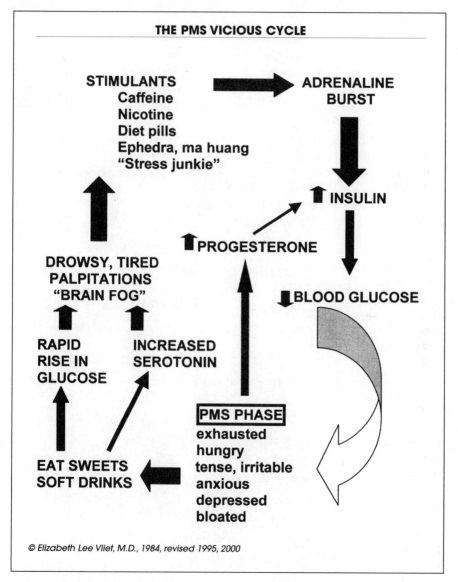

THE PMS VICIOUS CYCLE

STIMULANTS
Caffeine
Nicotine
Diet pills
Ephedra, ma huang
"Stress junkie"

ADRENALINE BURST

↑ INSULIN

↑PROGESTERONE

DROWSY, TIRED
PALPITATIONS
"BRAIN FOG"

⬇BLOOD GLUCOSE

RAPID
RISE IN
GLUCOSE

INCREASED
SEROTONIN

EAT SWEETS
SOFT DRINKS

PMS PHASE
exhausted
hungry
tense, irritable
anxious
depressed
bloated

© Elizabeth Lee Vliet, M.D., 1984, revised 1995, 2000

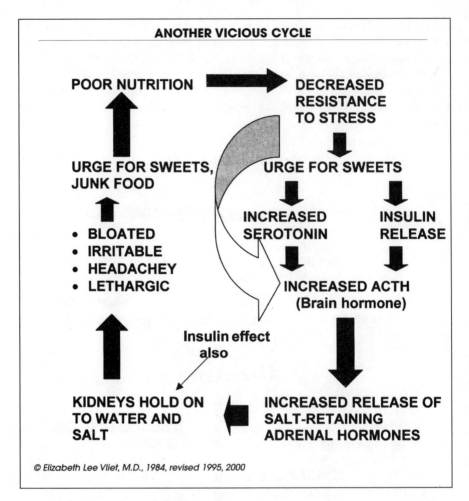

ANOTHER VICIOUS CYCLE

POOR NUTRITION → DECREASED RESISTANCE TO STRESS

URGE FOR SWEETS, JUNK FOOD

URGE FOR SWEETS

• BLOATED
• IRRITABLE
• HEADACHEY
• LETHARGIC

INCREASED SEROTONIN

INSULIN RELEASE

INCREASED ACTH (Brain hormone)

Insulin effect also

KIDNEYS HOLD ON TO WATER AND SALT

INCREASED RELEASE OF SALT-RETAINING ADRENAL HORMONES

© Elizabeth Lee Vliet, M.D., 1984, revised 1995, 2000

Not too long ago, I came across a newspaper notice in bold letters, like this:

THE NUMBER ONE CAUSE OF KITCHEN DEATHS IS EATING AN ENTIRE TUBE OF CHOCOLATE CHIP COOKIE DOUGH . . . RAW!

I howled with laughter at this. And so do audiences of women when I give a talk and show this slide. Most of us who have ever craved chocolate can relate to this, especially premenstrually.

Do any of you have cravings for chocolate? It turns out that the premenstrual rise in progesterone with its benzodiazepine-like effects on the brain may make you feel a little more slowed down, and several compounds in chocolate have mood-lifting, "feel-good" properties: the stimulants phenylethylamine (PEA) and theobromine (like caffeine), and magnesium. Newer research has shown that chocolate also contains calcium and antioxidants. Dark chocolate contains more antioxidants than green or black tea, while milk chocolate contains about the same amount of antioxidants in black tea. Brain levels of serotonin are also boosted by the sugar added to chocolate to make it taste good, so it's no wonder that chocolate makes you feel good when you eat it.

I know I certainly lived with those chocolate cravings for a lot of years. Loss of the ovary cycles (and that progesterone rise), stable optimal estradiol levels, and good magnesium intake all combined to solve that awful cyclic craving problem for me. I know how it is: When you are feeling exhausted, hungry, tense, and irritable, *sweets and chocolate* are quick and easy to turn to. Alcohol, too, is digested to a simple sugar, causing a rapid rise in blood glucose, so women who have premenstrual alcohol cravings are also experiencing a physiological effect of the hormone shifts. Eating sweets in turn causes an increase in serotonin in the brain. If there is too rapid a rise in brain serotonin, it causes drowsiness, palpitations, and nervous/anxious feelings. A more *gradual* rise in serotonin can cause a sense of calming, much like a tranquilizing medication. Actually, sweets are nature's original "tranquilizing drugs." I've had patients say to me, "Well I don't want to take an antianxiety medicine or antidepressant. I don't want to take any drugs." So I'll turn this around and observe, "Did you realize you're using *food* as a drug? Let's look at a way to help you achieve your desired ends more constructively." When you're feeling drowsy and you're trying to get through the afternoon, you often turn to what's quick and readily available: caffeine, sweets, or maybe the nicotine in cigarettes. These all trigger release of the chemical messengers that affect insulin, which in turn drops the blood sugar, and there goes the cycle again. Sound familiar?

In summary, the **vicious cycles** you've experienced premenstrually are *physiologically* based in the hormone shifts, *aggravated* by external stressors, and *intensified* by the wrong food choices and lack of exercise. Then we get into the vicious cycle of poor nutrition, which in turn affects our body's resistance to stress, which increases our craving for sweets, which affects the serotonin and insulin levels, which affects one of the brain hormones that regulates fluid balance. So there's more fluid retention, which is also an effect of insulin; the kidney holds onto water and salt, and you feel bloated, headachy, and irritable. Sound familiar?

Perhaps you are now seeing some places in the "vicious cycle" where you can make a *choice* for types of food or exercise that will *break the cycle*, not intensify it. But, if you *don't know* the vicious cycle is there, and how it works, then you can't deal with it constructively. That's my fundamental message: knowledge of what is happening gives you the power to make new and healthy choices. Be aware that when you're feeling bloated, irritable, and headachy, you don't feel like going out to exercise, yet *that's the very time you need it the most*. You also don't feel like fixing or eating a nice balanced meal with lots of steamed vegetables, but again, that's exactly what you need. **You have the power to perpetuate the vicious cycle or break it!**

It has been described since the 1930s, and perhaps even earlier, that women have altered glucose regulation in the luteal (progesterone-dominant) phase of the menstrual cycle. There are many complex metabolic effects of the hormonal shifts and complicated interactions of the various neuroendocrine "regulator messengers" that control body weight, fluid balance, appetite, food cravings, and other functions. In this discussion, I have presented a *very simplified* overview of some of the key factors. There are a number of good books (see appendix II for ones I recommend) that go into more detail on these metabolic influences for women.

I have for many years been interested in the connections between physiological changes such as blood glucose, and hormones, and so on, and the kinds of physical and behavioral responses that such physiological fluctuations can trigger. I have done five-hour (and sometimes six-hour) glucose tolerance tests (GTT) on many women with PMS during the past twelve years, and have found a strikingly consistent pattern of an abnormal response to glucose *if this testing is done in the mid to late phase of the second half (luteal phase) of the menstrual cycle*. Many doctors have said to my patients "You don't need to do glucose tolerance tests, we don't do those anymore to diagnose diabetes," or "It doesn't matter when in your cycle you do a glucose tolerance test, it's all the same."

Well, I disagree with both aspects. First of all, I am not simply looking for diabetes, I am looking for objective laboratory data to show changes in glucose levels that correlate with my patients' mood swings and physical symptoms and that could help explain the pattern of food cravings. Second, it is clear from *listening* to the patients that there is a definite *cycle-specific* characteristic to these cravings, and if I don't do the testing at the time when the women have the cravings, then how will I discover potential physical and hormonal factors involved in triggering these cravings? Physiologically, the luteal phase of the cycle is when the hormone shifts have the most dramatic impact on the insulin-glucose regulations. If a glucose tolerance test is going to be done *in a female patient*, it is crucial to do it at the right time of her menstrual cycle to get the right information. The GTT should be done three to five days before the period is due. Timing of the GTT with the late luteal phase allows the best opportunity to pick up the way in which the hormonal shifts affect blood glucose regulation. This in turn helps me to individualize a dietary approach for that person, specifically *when* food is eaten and the *balance* of carbohydrate, fat, and protein that will best help that person.

If any of you have ever had a GTT to test for either diabetes or hypoglycemia, you know that patients usually go to the laboratory for the testing. No one except the laboratory technician observes the patient, and then the results (as numbers) are sent to the physician. Typically the physician looks at the individual numbers for each hour of the test, and if the numbers fall into the "normal" range, the patient is told "everything's normal" regardless of how the patient may have felt during the test. Most patients are never asked if they had any symptoms during the GTT. It seemed to me that this process over-looked the most crucial information: what the patient had to say!

I developed a different way of studying this in 1983 and have been using this method in evaluation of women with hormone-relat-ed problems. I have the person come to our office for the GTT, and she (or occasionally, he) is shown how to keep a timed symptom log of everything experienced throughout the test. My staff also makes written observations of the patient during the test and frequently also does a short cognitive assessment (to check memory, attention, concentration, etc.) at each blood draw. These combined objective and subjective observations are kept in the medical record and are reviewed and discussed in detail at the follow-up appointment in conjunction with the lab results. This integration allows us to cor-relate the pattern of body changes with the actual fluctuations in blood glucose and insulin levels. It has been remarkable what has emerged from this approach, both in terms of hidden problems being properly identified, and in terms of helping someone learn how her body responds, what's contributing to the sensations she experiences, and what to do to with eating plans designed to con-structively correct the problem. Nine times out of ten, this process leads us to the insights needed to turn things around. It gives the per-son herself, and the nutritionist, important data to take into account in meal/snack planning. Once again, my approach is fairly basic in concept: observe the person, listen to what she says, pay attention to body physiology and hormonal effects, and figure out how to put it together into a cohesive, integrated, individualized plan of action.

When doing a GTT it is a simple matter to test for insulin resistance by checking insulin levels each time a glucose level is drawn. The GTT is more expensive when the insulin levels are added; yet, if the insulin resistance risk factors are there, I think it is important to do. Evaluating such an important risk factor in a systematic way, timed with the menstrual cycle, allows for early identification of women for whom this is blocking progress in weight loss and adding to the likelihood of developing diabetes and heart disease.

Moving the Body in Spite of Limitations

I have to be candid. There really are very few people who are so physically limited that they cannot exercise at all. With creativity, and guidance from physical therapists or trained exercise specialists, I have been impressed that there's exercise appropriate for almost everyone. All you have to do is look at the remarkable accomplishments of athletes in wheelchairs to know that we can find some way to exercise the body. Even when I was in a neck brace and could only walk about ten yards, the physical therapist gave me two ways of exercising aerobically to begin regaining my strength and stamina. Take a look at the picture. You don't have to sit on the *seat* to pedal a bike!

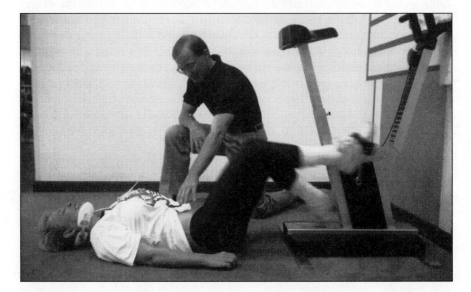

I have to admit, I made a pretty ridiculous sight, **but it worked!** The other exercise my physical therapist suggested was treading water, and I wore my neck brace in the water. Listening to music helped to stave off the boredom and keep up the pace. When I started out, I didn't have the stamina to last more than a few minutes. By the third week, I had progressed to treading water for forty-five minutes, and I had made great gains in my leg, back, and arm strength. This experience was humbling, since I had been such a strong swimmer in the past. But what a sense of accomplishment after I had built up my endurance! I continue to enjoy swimming and water exercise. I have to admit that it's easy to let my schedule demands keep me from getting in the pool as often as I know is healthy for me, but I am much better about keeping up the exercise because it helps me in so many ways. Each of us needs to find ways to increase body movement in all of our daily activities, particularly if the "exercise workouts" may be only three times a week.

I sincerely feel that if you have never exercised regularly in your life, there is *nothing* better you can do for yourself than sticking with a regular exercise program to boost your self-esteem and pride in accomplishment. Plus, you get to see the wonderful progress in your body once you start moving and keep at it. In addition to making you feel good about yourself, exercise, even simple walking, is the one wellness activity you can do that has so many profound effects on your total brain-body health and can prevent so many chronic, debilitating conditions and diseases. I have learned a great deal about the role of exercise in health through my own back surgeries and rehabilitation. I am grateful to have the strength and movement back that I have regained through exercise as a major part of each recovery process . . . even if I still miss the exhilaration of roller-blading! You may also find it worthwhile and very helpful at the beginning to hire a personal trainer to get you started and keep you on the right track until your new exercise habits are well established and you know how to do the exercises properly.

Begin now. Go for it!

Chapter 18

Osteoporosis—A Case for Preventive Medicine

Osteoporosis is a disease that may begin many years before actual menopause and can be largely prevented with proper attention to what you eat, what type of exercise you do consistently, and checking with your physician to evaluate your hormonal status. Osteoporosis occurs when bone becomes more porous, or soft, through loss of the normal bone spicules and cross-links that provide its structure and strength. In your home, this would be analogous to termites eating away at the foundation, even though the house (i.e., your body) may look fine on the outside. The problem with both termites in your house, and bone loss in your body, is that these are **silent** until there has been structural damage and areas collapse (or fracture). I find women are far more fearful of breast cancer, even though osteoporosis is much more common and can actually cause even more pain, disability, loss of independence, and early death than we see from breast cancer. Your lifetime chances of having a hip fracture are greater than your chances of breast, uterine, cervical, or ovarian cancers combined. Consider these 1999 statistics: There are 28 million women at risk, but even with our current diagnostic capability, only 4 to 5 million have been diagnosed and only about 2 to 2.5 million are being treated. These are not good numbers.

Potential consequences of osteoporosis can be devastating. We do not have any way that biotechnological medicine can "fix" the bones once the collapse and breakage process has begun. Hip fracture is not a simple thing. If we look at the number of hip fractures in this country on an annual basis, the cost to society is staggering, both in actual dollars and in individual pain and suffering. Dollar estimates run between $7 and 10 BILLION annually. Osteoporosis has an enormous adverse impact on the mobility and independence of older women and it is one of the most common reasons that older women end up having to go into a nursing home. Even more tragic is that up to 20 percent of women *die* within three months of a hip fracture due to complications. So, although you hear "just get a hip replacement" bandied about rather lightly, it is not that simple. Surgery this major requires a long and frequently painful recovery, along with hard work to regain your mobility. If you have significant bone loss, it makes some of the treatment options more limited, since hip replacements can't even be done unless there is healthy bone to support the attachment of the artificial hip device. Now you see why I am concerned that we need to help more women become aware of the preventable nature of this disease.

My goal is to help women understand, and implement, ways of preventing bone loss from starting. Then I want to help you look at ways to maintain adequate bone density so that you're not in the position of needing to be "fixed." Bone loss occurs even before menopause in women who have **risk factors** such as those shown in the chart below. Keep in mind that many of these risks can be reduced by *your* positive action and choosing healthier lifestyle practices or use of medications that are available.

RISK FACTORS FOR BONE LOSS AND OSTEOPOROSIS

- Cigarette smoking (smokers also become menopausal five to seven years sooner than nonsmokers)
- Daily and/or regular alcohol intake
- Heavy caffeine intake (coffee, tea, soft drinks, etc.)
- Poor calcium and magnesium intake (the average woman in the United States gets only about a third of the needed calcium in her diet, and less than a third of the necessary magnesium each day)
- Diet high in phosphates, which bind calcium and carry it out of the body (the biggest source for American women is *soft drinks*)
- Chronic dieting, anorexia, and/or bulimia
- Excess thyroid medication, or hyperthyroidism (such as Graves Disease)
- Prolonged use of cortisteroids, such as prednisone and others (these medications are used for asthma, arthritis, Lupus, and other disorders)
- High cortisol levels (e.g., Cushing's disease)
- Presence of endometriosis, hormone imbalances, premature menopause (whatever the cause, may be many)
- Missing menstrual periods longer than six months at any time after puberty (except when pregnant). This occurs most often in women who are too thin from chronic dieting or excessive exercise-induced suppression of the ovaries.
- Presence of other diseases such as adrenal insufficiency (Addison's Disease), chronic obstructive pulmonary diseases (e.g. emphysema), lymphoma or leukemia, malabsorption syndromes (Celiac disease, etc.), hemochromatosis, hyperparathyroidism, insulin-dependent diabetes mellitus, multiple myeloma, multiple sclerosis, pernicious anemia, rheumatoid arthritis, sarcoidosis, severe liver disease, thalessemia, thyrotoxicosis
- Regular use of aluminum-containing preparations (e.g. antacids), anticonvulsant medication (e.g., Dilantin), GnRH agonist medications (e.g., Lupron), and lithium.
- Genetic factors: ethnic group (African American women typically have denser bones than Caucasian or Asian women), family history of mother, sister, or grandmothers with osteoporosis and/or early menopause.

© Elizabeth Lee Vliet, M.D., 2000

Patsy's Story

I have been disturbed by the increasing numbers of young women who already have the beginnings of osteoporosis. In our comprehensive assessments at HER Place, we are finding that women in their late twenties and thirties have osteopenia or even osteoporosis, due to premature decline in optimal estrogen levels, poor intake of calcium, chronic dieting or excessive exercise that has stopped their normal menstruation. These young women won't even reach menopause age with a normal level of bone, and are at even greater risk of fractures later in life. It is not a correct generalization, as some authors of women's health books have stated, to say that breast cancer will get you before osteoporosis. Patsy is a good example. She is thirty-eight years old, still menstruating, and her gynecologist recently told her she was "too young" for a bone density test and would not prescribe it for her. She had many symptoms of ovarian decline and low estradiol (insomnia, fatigue, loss of sex drive, marked weight gain, PMS, depressed mood the second half of her cycle), but her doctor had not checked her actual serum hormone levels. Her other significant risk factor was her mother's severe osteoporosis. When I did my testing for her and ordered the bone density, we were shocked to find that she had already lost more than *three standard deviations* from peak bone mass of a healthy thirty-five-year-old woman at her *spine*, and more than *2 standard deviations* from peak bone mass at the *hip*. By definition, she already had osteoporosis even though she was only thirty-eight years old. Her serum estradiol level on Day 2 of her cycle was only 10 pg/ml, when it should be about 80–90 pg/ml at this cycle phase. Obviously, the bone density and hormone tests had been crucial elements in her evaluation. She and I would not have had any other way to know this information in time to do something to reverse the bone loss and help her build new bone.

1998 NATIONAL OSTEOPOROSIS FOUNDATION DIAGNOSTIC CRITERIA FOR OSTEOPOROSIS	
Category	**Bone Mineral Density (BMD) T-Score***
Normal:	Less than 1.0 standard deviation <u>below</u> young adult peak bone density
Osteopenia:	Between 1.0 and 2.0 standard deviations <u>below</u> young adult peak bone density
Osteoporosis:	2.0 or more standard deviations <u>below</u> young adult peak bone density
Severe Osteoporosis:	2.0 or more standard deviations <u>below</u> young adult peak bone density, *with* presence of fragility fractures.

NOTE: On your summary report, T-scores are reported as plus (+) numbers if bone density is <u>above</u> young adult peak bone mass, and as minus (-) numbers if bone density is <u>below</u> young adult peak bone mass.

Hormone Effects on Bone

Significant and sustained life stresses are additional factors that can cause bone loss in younger women by causing suppression of the ovaries and a decrease in ovarian hormone levels. When this happens, bone loss can be occurring *before* your periods stop. Our female hormones play a very critical role in bone growth; they deposit proper minerals into the skeleton for strength and keep the bone breakdown process from overcoming new bone formation. Estrogen helps absorb dietary calcium and magnesium from the intestinal tract and deposits these minerals into bone. Estrogen "primes" certain bone cells to respond to progesterone and stimulate new bone formation, while also helping to block the process of bone breakdown. Progesterone has a modest effect on the bone-building cells (osteoblasts) and assists in simulating new bone growth, but progesterone is a "helper" than can exert its action *only if* there is adequate estrogen present. Testosterone has a much greater bone-building effect than progesterone and it not only stimulates new bone growth to build bone density, it also enhances bone *strength*. You may not need to add hormones from an *outside* source to have enough circulating hormones to prevent bone loss. The problem is, you won't know whether you need supplemental hormones or not until you measure bone density and hormone status. It is important to keep in mind that worldwide research over the last several decades has clearly shown that there is much less bone loss in the women who are taking estrogen after menopause. There is another reason the blood level is so important for you to know. We now have additional research to show that for estradiol to prevent bone loss: there has to be consistent levels above 70–80 pg/ml (less than half the average levels of the normal menstrual cycle), which is higher than doctors have previously been taught is needed for postmenopausal women. Saliva levels don't correlate as well with the minimum threshold serum levels that are known to be protective of bone, so I don't recommend using saliva hormone tests to see if your hormone levels are adequate to prevent osteoporosis.

Women who take estrogen after menopause have been consistently found to have much greater bone density at all ages after menopause, even compared with women who exercise and consume adequate calcium. Recent studies have definitely shown that the **combination** of hormones *plus* calcium-magnesium supplements *plus* exercise has a greater bone protective effect than either calcium alone, exercise alone, or exercise and calcium without hormone therapy. In women with marked bone loss, adding testosterone, possibly with an antiresorptive medication such as Fosamax or Actonel, provides even greater benefit and can actually rebuild bone density that has been lost.

The Truth about Bone Effects of Progesterone Creams

We have talked about estrogen and testosterone effects on bone, what about progesterone effects? Although progesterone has a modest effect on the cells that build bone, this effect is more than offset by estrogen effects to prevent bone breakdown. Thus, studies have shown that if you don't have adequate levels of estradiol, you will still lose bone even if you have plenty of progesterone. Many excellent studies worldwide have failed to show a significant effect of either progesterone or progestins to prevent bone loss if given alone, without estrogen. I am seriously concerned about the current spate of misleading advertisements and health newsletters that claim progesterone skin creams *alone* are enough to protect you from bone loss. *They are not.*

There have been several recently published studies of these progesterone creams, using the gold standard of double-blind, placebo-controlled, prospective design in a variety of settings and several different countries. These studies have shown that transdermal (skin) creams containing progesterone have *no measurable effect on preserving bone density*, even though their manufacturers claim otherwise. You are gambling with your body and gambling with having silent, ongoing bone loss if you use these progesterone creams and ignore the overwhelming, well-documented studies that demonstrate estrogen's role in bone preservation. If you want to use these creams for other reasons, at least get a bone density test and measure the urine or serum markers of bone breakdown (such as N-telopeptide), to be sure you don't already have too much bone loss.

I think it is crucial that we give a more balanced picture to women concerning the roles of these ovarian hormones in maintaining bone. Many of these progesterone proponents accuse mainstream physicians of "medicalizing" menopause. This is hogwash, in my opinion. Are we "medicalizing" heart disease when we identify the biological and lifestyle causes that trigger heart attacks and then offer people various options to help prevent such a devastating problem? I don't think so. That's what medical research is all about: finding ways to help men and women stay as healthy as possible for as long as possible. I don't hear many women or men complaining about "medicalization" of heart problems. People seem to readily accept that there are both medication and lifestyle options that can be used to reduce your risk of having a premature, fatal heart attack. In my view, the same principle applies to the life transition of menopause for women. The reality is that the very medical research women have been asking for, and deserve, has overwhelmingly demonstrated the *physiological reality* of the profound brain-body consequences for women when we have many years of estrogen loss. I don't think of such research as "medicalization" but rather searching for answers to how our bodies work when they are healthy so that we can preserve that degree of health as long as possible.

Checking Your Bone Balance: Getting Tested

How do you tell if you are losing bone? There is no *more reliable* measure of bone loss than having a test of hip and spine bone mineral density. Knowing your risk factors helps, but even taking into account the best risk factor assessment, doctors can still identify only about 30 percent of the women who are actually losing bone. That means if we *just go by risk factors,* we miss *70 percent* of women with bone loss. And there really are not many observable symptoms of bone loss before a fracture occurs. The earliest change *you* can measure is a loss of height. But by the time this occurs, osteoporosis is already established and causing many small fractures in the vertebrae. With loss of bone in the vertebrae of the spine, they collapse onto each other, resulting in diminished height, increased spinal curvature, and compression of the nerve roots between each vertebra, leading to back pain. Women not on hormone therapy lose an average of two and a half inches of height over the years after menopause. **A loss of more than one quarter inch in height is considered a reliable sign of spinal bone loss.** At the time of your annual physical exam make sure that the nurse *measures* your height. Don't just tell the staff what you think or wish your height is. Always make sure the nurse tells you your height and blood pressure so you may record this in your personal health planner and make note of any changes. Most women are more concerned about their body weight, but to have a more accurate picture of your health risks, it is also important to know what is happening to your height and blood pressure.

By far the most accurate and reliable way to determine whether or not you have significant bone loss is the Dual Energy X-ray Absorptiometry (DEXA) test of both hip and spine. This test takes only a few minutes, exposes you to less radiation than you would get flying on an airplane from Los Angeles to Washington, D.C., and is considered the gold standard of bone density testing. A DEXA test is now covered by Medicare, and many states have in recent years mandated insurance companies to cover it as well. If you have any of the risk factors I have described above, or if you have lost one quarter inch or more in height, you *must* ask your doctor for a prescription to have this test done. I think we are waiting too late if we only do a bone density at menopause or afterward. I recommend that women have a DEXA test of both hip and spine bone mineral density by age thirty-five to forty, or earlier if you have many risk factors. I think it is crucial to check both hip and spine, since bone is lost at different rates from different sites in the body. Heel and finger bone density tests don't correlate very well with what is happening at the hip and spine and tend to underestimate the severity of bone loss. In addition, heel and finger fractures aren't exactly the kinds of fractures that cause women severe problems like spine and hip fractures do. DEXA is less expensive compared to CAT scans of bone density. In addition, CAT scans for bone density expose you to a far higher radiation level than needed to determine your bone density. Three companies make the DEXA equipment, and it is now more widely available at hospitals and osteoporosis centers around the country.

If bone density testing is done at a younger age, we have a window of opportunity for a premenopausal woman to help her decide what steps she must take to reduce further bone loss. It is not enough just to say we don't need to do the bone density test because all you need is to take calcium and exercise or just take hormones. You need to know the degree of loss that is there, because you may need to combine several approaches for best results. For example, if a woman has lost a great deal of bone, she may need hormones *plus* antiresorptive medications such as Fosamax, Actonel, or Miacalcin to prevent continued bone loss and increased fracture risk. Once again, the types of approaches you may need will be determined by the results of your present bone density, risk factors, your hormone levels, your personal preferences, and any side effects that may occur.

A reliable indicator of bone metabolism is the urine or new serum measure of **N-telopeptide (collagen cross-linked N-telopeptide, or NTx)**. N-telopeptide is a breakdown product of bone that is excreted in the urine. When the body is breaking down bone faster than it is making new bone, the NTx will be high (greater than 35). If you are "in balance" and the body is making new bone and breaking down old bone at about the same rates, this number will be *low,* or less than 35. The most reliable results come from using a *second morning void* urine specimen, not a random urine specimen done anytime during the day as had been thought previously. If you are taking hormone therapy to preserve bone or medications such as Fosamax, Actonel, Miacalcin or Evista, NTx levels can be used to monitor their effectiveness. You should see about a 30 percent decrease in the NTx number in about three months on medication if the antiresorptive medication and/or hormones are working properly. In addition to the urine test for NTx, there is a new NTx serum (blood) test that was recently approved by the FDA for monitoring response to bone-preserving medications. Remember the goal of medication therapy is to bring urinary NTx down to a level of 35 or less. Another urine test of bone-breakdown products that you may read about is called Pyrilinks. It is not as widely used as the NTx test and doesn't yield information that is as well correlated with future fracture risk (based on worldwide research studies) as has been found for NTx. I recommend that you request the NTx test from your physician for the most reliable information.

Women have asked me if the NTx test is enough to tell whether they have healthy bone. These two markers alone are not enough, any more than it is enough to know your financial health by simple looking at how fast you take out or put in money to your checking account. You have to also know how much the total balance of money is in your account. In this analogy, the DEXA test is like looking at your total bone "bank account," while NTx (or Pyrilinks) is like getting a snapshot of your *rate* of deposits (bone building) and withdrawals (bone breakdown). The rate of bone remodeling (formation and breakdown) is gaining more awareness as an *independent* risk factor of fracture risk, so you need this piece of information along with your actual bone mineral density determined by DEXA in order to have a complete picture of your risks and what is currently happening in your body. You need to know both if you are going to decide what you need to do to either preserve your present bone "assets," or to start agressively using strategies that will rebuild your deposits into the "bone bank" of your skeleton.

You may need to be assertive about getting a bone density test done. I have had patients tell me they asked for it and were told "you don't need it, you're too young, and you look healthy." I emphasize again: You cannot tell a woman's bone density by how she looks, any more than you can see termite damage in a house by looking only at the outside. Remember Patsy I described above, who was supposedly "too young" to need a bone density test and "looked" healthy. Even though a number of states have now mandated coverage for DEXA testing, some insurance plans still don't cover this important test for women. One approach we have found helpful for our patients is to do the less expensive NTx first, and if this number is high, along with low hormone levels, there is additional justification for you to have a bone mineral density (DEXA) test and get reimbursed by your insurance carrier. Sometimes, you may have to bite the bullet and pay out of pocket so you can have the information to guide you in your health management decisions. It is an important investment in your good health for the future.

Preventable Causes of Bone Loss

Review this inventory of "bone robbers" and work with your health professionals to make the necessary changes in diet, supplements, and medications. These are important dimensions of your health planning because each of these items is one *you* control, and each can significantly reduce your risk of later osteoporosis.

Vitamin D deficiency may be more common than had previously been recognized. A 1999 *JAMA* article, "Occult Vitamin D Deficiency in Postmenopausal US Women with Acute Hip Fracture," found that about *half* of the women hospitalized for hip fracture at Brigham and Women's Hospital in Boston between 1995 and 1998 had laboratory evidence of vitamin D deficiency with levels below 30 nmol/L. Of the 805 patients admitted to the hospital for hip replacement surgery, 262 were admitted following a hip fracture, and 543 were admitted for elective hip replacement surgery. The authors suggested that restoring vitamin D to optimal levels may reduce the risk of future fractures and may also help the healing of current hip fractures. Make sure you are getting at least 400 IU of vitamin D daily, and if you already have significant bone loss, ask your doctor to check your blood (serum) level of vitamin D to be sure your are absorbing it properly. Vitamin D deficiency is clearly a *preventable* cause of osteoporosis and future fractures.

Calcium is something we read and hear a lot about in maintaining bone, but it is also critical in mood and sleep regulating pathways, and normal muscle function. The sad part is that with as much emphasis as there has been on calcium in this country, the average calcium intake for women is still only 450 milligrams a day. The recommended amount for premenopausal women is 1000 to 1200 mg daily, and for postmenopausal women not taking estrogen, 1500 mg daily. Women have decreased their consumption of dairy products in attempts to lose weight, so their dietary calcium intake has decreased. Younger women tend to drink more diet beverages instead of milk, so they don't get adequate calcium either. At an average of 450 mg daily, we are far off the mark. Dairy products are still the richest dietary calcium sources, but there are other sources as well. Vegetables contain much less calcium per serving, and the fiber in vegetables decreases the amount of calcium absorption. If you don't eat dairy products, it really is important for you to take calcium supplements to bring your daily total up to the desired 1200–1500 mg level.

I caution you to *avoid calcium products made from oyster shell or dolomite*, since these have been found to be contaminated with toxic heavy metals such as lead, mercury, and arsenic. Calcium citrate is touted as being better absorbed, but studies have not consistently confirmed this. Since calcium citrate has *less* elemental calcium per tablet, you have to remember to take more tablets daily to get an adequate amount. Another option is Tums. Bioavailability studies of Tums (a pure calcium carbonate antacid) have shown it is readily absorbed and well-tolerated. Tums contains no aluminum, so it is safe to take daily.

It's also quite inexpensive, readily available, and easy to carry in your handbag, so there's no excuse for not taking your calcium.

You can check whether your calcium (diet and supplements) is being absorbed or not by a twenty-four-hour urine test of calcium excretion. I request this test if someone isn't responding with the degree of bone rebuilding I would expect from medications, exercise, and supplements, or if there has been greater bone loss than would be expected based on the other lab tests I have done. There are two things I look at with this test: (1) if the urinary calcium is very low, it tells me you're not absorbing calcium very well and may need additional calcium in the diet, a better estrogen level to help absorb calcium, or additional tests to find out why the calcium isn't being absorbed prop-erly; and (2) if the urinary calcium is very high, it tells me you are excreting more than you are absorbing, which typically occurs in women who are too low in their active form of estrogen, estradiol.

Magnesium. Another preventable cause of bone loss is too little **magnesium** intake each day, another mineral crucially important to bone growth and maintenance of healthy bone. The average American woman gets only about 100–200 mg a day of magnesium from her diet, and the RDA for magnesium is 400–600 mg daily. Life stress and the effects of estrogen loss cause increased need for magnesium. Drinking soft drinks daily—diet or regular—prevents absorption of magnesium and calcium since the phosphates (and phosphoric acid) in these beverages bind up magnesium and calcium and make them insoluble. The glutamate (MSG) and aspartate (Nutrasweet) added to soft drinks increase the body's need for magnesium as well. So you get a double whammy on your magnesium balance from drinking these ubiquitous beverages. Other factors that deplete our magnesium are high coffee consumption, excess catecholamine effects (e.g., from stimulant medications), and excess glucocorticoid effects (cortisone medications, and stress). People with Type-A personality have also been found to deplete magnesium stores more rapidly, likely an effect of the cortisol-stress response pathway activation.

In addition to its effect on bone, magnesium is also a critical mineral for nerve-cell conduction and muscle contraction, and it has a strong independent role in regulating blood pressure. It appears to be an important factor in preventing heart attacks, probably because it helps prevent spasms of the blood vessels throughout the body but especially in the coronary arteries. Magnesium also helps maintain normal structure and contraction strength of the heart muscle itself. In the brain, magnesium is a cofactor in the production of the important mood-regulating chemical messengers such as dopamine. It is thought to be an important mineral in helping to prevent, and possibly relieve, such mood changes as those that occur with PMS and milder forms of depression. These minerals are involved in metabolism and energy production, and they become important in weight regulation as well.

I urge my patients (and I do it myself) to take 200 to 250 mg of magnesium supplement *every morning* and 200 to 250 mg *every evening.* The calcium amount should be about twice the amount of magnesium in the morning and evening, with your remaining calcium taken in the middle of the day at lunchtime. Taking magnesium and calcium at least two times a day provides better absorption and more even levels throughout the twenty-four hours. The 2:1 ratio of calcium intake to magnesium intake is important for proper balance. I haven't been as impressed with the effectiveness of the hard tablet or caplet forms of magnesium, since these highly compressed formulations aren't absorbed very well and seem to cause more stomach irritation. I recommend either liquid forms or capsules with easily absorbed magnesium powder, such as TwinLab brand. There are now many good brands on the market, and it is important that you choose one that works for you and *use it daily.*

One very good question my patients often ask me is "How do we get enough calcium without getting constipated?" I'll almost guarantee you that if you are getting enough magnesium, which is a very effective natural laxative, you won't have to worry about constipation from your calcium! Remember, the old constipation remedy *Milk of Magnesia* is based on magnesium's ability to stimulate the intestines. Too much magnesium quickly causes diarrhea, so you have a clear indication of when to cut back on the amount. Magnesium's importance is often overlooked, and physicians often haven't paid enough attention to the importance of *optimal* magnesium intake to help treat problems such as muscle pain/spasms, fibromyalgia, PMS, headaches, high blood pressure, depressed mood, anxiety, and a host of other problems.

Manganese is another mineral often overlooked. Manganese deficiencies are associated with osteoporosis, chronic depression, chronic pain, blood sugar problems, and allergies. These multiple problems occur because manganese is involved in a number of enzyme pathways needed for the utilization of the B vitamins, vitamin E, and vitamin C, as well as the pathways of energy metabolism, glucose regulation, and immune function. Manganese is also essential to the process of forming T4 (thyroxin) by the thyroid gland, and it helps regulate pituitary function as well. Dietary deficiencies are more common today due to several factors: soils depleted of manganese, diets high in simple sugars, high-fiber diets that contain *phytates* (plant fiber substances that bind up the manganese and prevent its absorption), high intake of soda beverages that contain phosphorus and impair absorption of manganese. In addition, if you have an excess of calcium and iron supplements, this will impair manganese absorption.

Manganese is widely available in many plant foods. Examples include nuts, whole grains, raisins, spinach, carrots, broccoli, green peas, oranges, apples, tea leaves, and wheat bran. When wheat is milled to make white flour, most of the mineral is lost and is not added back in the white flours marked "enriched." The body loses about 4 mg of manganese a day, so it must be replaced in your diet or with supplements. You will probably get most of the manganese you need in a good multivitamin plus whatever you eat of the above foods. I don't think it should be necessary to take additional manganese supplements if you are taking a good multivitamin that includes manganese.

Boron is a trace mineral that is important in bone metabolism, and also helps reduce excretion of calcium and magnesium. Good dietary sources include a variety of vegetables such as green peppers and tomatoes. But, just to be sure, make certain that your multiple vitamin also contains the recommended amount of boron. As with many of these minerals, too much is not good either, so make certain that you are not taking multiple supplements that give you an excess cumulative amount.

So, don't forget your minerals! Just to review, the *most important* minerals for women experiencing hormonal problems and at risk for bone loss are **magnesium, calcium, manganese, and boron.** These minerals play crucial roles as cofactors and catalysts in building bone and regulating sleep, pain, mood, and muscle health and repair. These minerals are absolutely important to us, but you don't have to take the more expensive *colloidal* (fine particles suspended in a uniform medium) versions . . . regular capsules or tablets are readily absorbed by most people unless there is an underlying disease affecting the gastrointestinal tract. In that case, you may want to consider a liquid form.

Excess use of thyroid hormones is another preventable cause of bone loss, whether you use over-the-counter glandulars or higher-than-needed doses of prescription thyroid medication that push your TSH too low, creating a *hyper*thyroid state. Excess amounts of thyroid hormone, whether from your own body production (such as Graves disease) or from medications, cause more rapid breakdown of bone and also cause the bone that remains to be more brittle. Health practitioners, newsletters, and Internet sites that promote use of thyroid hormones just based on symptoms of low basal body temperature are creating potentially dangerous situations for midlife and menopausal woman who are also experiencing loss of their bone-building estrogen and testosterone. How does this happen?

In the first place, many of the "thyroid-only" proponents such as Drs. Broda Barnes and David Wilson have overlooked a basic fact of *women's* biology: Low body temperature and slower metabolism are *both* caused by lower levels of ovarian hormones *as well as* by low thyroid function. These men seem to have totally forgotten that the ovaries are important metabolic regulators for women. In the second place, there are now very effective and sensitive blood tests for measuring TSH, thyroid hormones, as well as tests for antibodies to the thyroid gland tissue and to your thyroid hormones. These sensitive and reliable tests had not been developed in 1978 when Dr. Barnes wrote his book and suggested tracking axillary body temperature as an indication of the need for thyroid hormone. Women who take increasing thyroid hormone trying to get their body temperature "back to normal," without checking to see what is also happening to their ovary hormones, may end up with both bone loss and heart damage from thyroid excess.

I recently saw a fifty-two-year-old woman who had a free T3 level of over 700 following the "Wilson's Syndrome" Internet protocol of increasing Cytomel doses to reach desired basal body temperature. Her free T3 level should have been only about 300 on the laboratory scale used. As result of many months of thyroid excess, she had developed high blood pressure, palpitations, significant hair loss, chronic insomnia, nervousness, anxiety symptoms, increased sweating, and her bone loss had reached the osteoporosis stage. Her TSH had been pushed down to "undetectable" levels, but at the same time, her basal body temperature was still at 97.4. No one had checked her estradiol level (or the free T3 either, for that matter), and when I did, her estradiol was less than 20 pg/ml. This is far below the estradiol level needed to preserve bone, maintain normal heart function, and restore sleep. It is also far below what the body needs in order to have a healthy basal metabolic rate and normal A.M. body temperature. You need all of these hormones checked together, with reliable measures such as blood tests, before you overdo it with just one hormone medication.

Excess adrenal hormones are another common and preventable cause of bone loss. Women who have to take daily corticosteroids to control asthma, autoimmune disorders like Lupus, or arthritis (both rheumatoid and osteo) are at especially high risk for osteoporosis. If you have one of these other illnesses and have been on steroid therapy for some time, it is imperative that you have the NTx and DEXA tests done so you can talk with your physicians about options to prevent bone breakdown and brittling due to the corticosteroids. For the same reason, it is important to avoid using "adrenal glandulars" sold in health food stores since they may also give you excess corticosteroid effect, even though they are milder than the prescription forms of these hormones. Many women are told to take the adrenal glandulars as a treatment for "chronic fatigue" on the theory that they are tired because of "adrenal insufficiency" or "adrenal exhaustion." These two terms are commonly misused by alternative medicine practitioners, and patients are given these labels without having the proper medical evaluation to determine adrenal function. Very few women that take these supplements have actually had the proper blood tests done at the right time of the day (i.e., 8 A.M. and 4 P.M.) to measure cortisol reliably and determine whether they are in fact low in these adrenal hormones. On the other hand, if you truly do have adrenal insufficiency (AI, or Addison's disease), adrenal glandulars sold over the counter are not adequate treatment. AI is a serious medical disorder and should be treated with prescription-grade medication monitored by a specialist.

Lack of exercise is another bone robber often overlooked. Many studies worldwide have clearly demonstrated the effects of weight-bearing and strength-training exercise to build and keep healthy bone. It is never too late to start exercising: Significant improvements in aerobic power, muscle endurance, and bone density have been demonstrated in women over age seventy with exercise therapy. One study evaluated women in nursing homes with an average age of eighty-one. The study participants were taught to do various exercises involving a chair; this increased their midshaft bone mineral density in the exercise group by close to 2.5 percent. Those who did not exercise continued to lose bone density. Exercise is a major component of maintaining adequate bone mineral density. Make sure that you have weight bearing and strength training exercise. It is the resistance across the joint, pulling on the bone, along with the impact of weight-bearing exercise that helps to increase the formation of bone. Studies have demonstrated that significant improvements in bone mass accrual, lean body mass, aerobic power, glucose tolerance, and mental well-being occurs among postmenopausal women who exercise regularly. Studies of the effect of exercise in humans have shown that exercise leads to higher blood concentrations of catecholamines and beta-endorphins that contribute to mood elevation. Thus, regular physical exercise may help prevent or reduce many physical and emotional symptoms that affect climacteric women. Current data further show there is also a lower incidence of cancer among women and men who exercise regularly. I have been doing individualized exercise prescriptions for my patients for close to twenty years, and these are some of the most important prescriptions I give. Remember, I said in chapter 17 that almost anyone could find a form of exercise she can do. Everyone, male and female, regardless of age, will benefit from an exercise program. Morris Notelovitz, M.D., said that "physicians need to prescribe exercise just like ERT. The physical and mental health of climacteric women can be enhanced by prescribing aerobic and muscle-strengthening exercises with, or without, hormone replacement."

Ethnic Issues: Serious Implications for African-American Women

I hear many African-American women comment that, based on race, they are not at high risk of osteoporosis and "don't need to worry about taking hormones after menopause." It turns out that this is another myth, not supported by careful review of actual statistics. More than 10 percent of African-American women age eighty or older suffer from hip fractures each year, and on average 20 percent of these women die within three months of fracture-related complications. Older African-American women have lower serum osteocalcin levels, but higher serum calcium levels when compared with older Caucasian women. Low serum levels of vitamin D occurred more frequently in older African-American women, likely a reflection of both dietary intake and darker skin pigmentation that decreases synthesis of vitamin D in the skin with exposure to sunlight. Other common risk factors for osteoporosis and increased risk of hip fracture that were identified among African-American women were thinness, previous stroke, use of aids in walking, alcohol consumption, corticosteroid use, hyperthyroidism (primary or prescribed excess medication), and diabetes. The protective effect of increased body mass appears to result primarily from weight gained since the early adult years, not from having higher body mass in early adulthood when maximum bone mass is being formed.

A multicenter study by Drs. Cauley, Ensrud, and Cummings was presented at the 1996 World Congress on Osteoporosis, showing alarming findings among elderly African-American women. In women ages seventy–seventy-nine years old, the rate of bone loss in the hip was more than *twice as fast* in African-American women compared to Caucasian women in the same age range. African-American women in the United States have a far lower rate of using hormone therapy after menopause than do Caucasian women, perhaps in part due to the incorrect belief that they are not at particularly high risk for bone loss. It appears we need to be even more aggressive in getting this information to older African-American women and helping them select appropriate treatment options to prevent such rapid bone loss.

Nonhormonal Medication Options to Preserve and Build Bone

There are alternative medication options to preserve bone for women who don't want to take estrogen or who have medical problems such as a history of breast cancer and cannot take estrogen. Next to estrogen, the *bisphosphonates* are the most effective group of *antiresorptive* medications for bone-sparing effects. **Didronel** (Etidronate) was the first one in this class that was available, and it had to be given in three-month cycles to halt bone loss. Didronel's major drawback was that it did not rebuild bone with normal strength; the new bone that was built was still more brittle and susceptible to fractures. Its use was also limited by the fact that it must be monitored carefully and can only be given for three months at one time before taking a drug-free interval of three months.

Fosamax (Alendronate) was the next bisphosphonate to be discovered by Italian researchers, and then approved by the FDA in the United States in 1995 for *treatment* of established osteoporosis in a 10 mg daily dose. It was later approved for *prevention* of osteoporosis at a 5 mg daily dose. Fosamax inhibits bone breakdown (resorption) and helps to build new bone, and stronger bone. The effects of Fosamax counteract bone loss caused by loss of estrogen. The Fracture Intervention Trial (FIT) of over two thousand postmenopausal women with a previous vertebral fracture showed that Fosamax reduced the risk of new vertebral fractures by 47 percent compared to placebo. Participants in this study were randomized to receive either placebo or alendronate 5 mg a day for two years followed by 10 mg a day for one year. Women in any group who had a dietary calcium intake of less than 1000 mg daily also received calcium supplements of 500 mg a day with vitamin D 250 IU daily. There was a 51 percent reduction in risks of hip fractures in the FIT study, and wrist fractures were also reduced by 48 percent. These are exciting and encouraging results, especially since this was a high-risk group of women who had already sustained fractures due to osteoporosis.

Studies from other countries have also shown very positive results: Australian researchers showed that women receiving 10 mg daily of Fosamax for three years *increased* their lumbar spine bone density by an average of 6.8 percent, while women on placebo had an average *decrease* in bone density at hip and spine of about 1 percent per year. The women who received Fosamax showed an average of about 6 percent increase in bone density at the hip sites as well. Being able to *increase* your bone density at a time in life when most women are *losing* bone is exciting news. In addition, the new bone formed at the hip and spine sites was normal quality and well mineralized, which means it had normal strength. This finding is a distinct improvement over the old medication Didronel.

In order to be adequately absorbed into the body so it can do its job, Fosamax *has* to be taken first thing in the morning on an empty stomach and swallowed using only water, not coffee or juice. Even taking it in the morning two hours before breakfast, only about 70 percent of the dose is absorbed. If you take Fosamax only thirty minutes before breakfast, studies have found that absorption drops to about 46 percent. If you take Fosamax with other beverages or *after* eating food, studies have shown that the amount absorbed from the stomach into the bloodstream drops way down, to less than 11 percent, which isn't enough to do your bones any good. So you must take it on an empty stomach in the morning after fasting overnight. You should also not have anything further to drink or eat for thirty to sixty minutes after you take it, and should remain standing or walking around. If you lie back down, it tends to cause burning sensations in the esophagus area, similar to reflux or heartburn. If Fosamax is taken correctly, it usually doesn't cause many side effects, and it can be taken daily rather than in the on-off cycles needed with etidronate. The chance to build strong bones for the future, I think, is worth any slight inconvenience in how you have to take it.

Actonel (risedronate) is a newer bisphosphonate medication that was initially approved by the FDA in 1998 for the treatment of Paget's Disease, and received FDA approval in April 2000 for both prevention and treatment of osteoporosis as well. Actonel has similar mode of action as Fosamax to prevent bone breakdown and build healthy bone, and has the advantage of a lower frequency of gastrointestinal side effects. Studies to date have shown impressive results with 5 mg daily dose of Actonel. As an example, a randomized, double-blind, placebo controlled clinical trial at 110 centers in North America was published in the October 13, 1999 issue of *JAMA*. In this study of 2,458 postmenopausal women, there was a fracture reduction of 65 percent observed in the first year of the study, and an overall cumulative decrease of 41 percent in new vertebral fractures over the 3-year study period. Bone mineral density increased significantly at the femoral neck (hip), at the trochanter (hip), and at the lumbar spine. The new bone formed had normal architecture and strength, an improvement over the older medication Didronel. Overall safety and side effects were similar to the placebo, an encouraging finding. Studies using Actonel in comination with hormone therapy have been done and show an even greater improvement in bone density with both therapies than with either one alone. *Actonel was also FDA-approved for the treatment of steroid-induced osteoporosis*, a serious risk of long-term corticosteroid therapy used for asthma or arthritis. Actonel was effective at improving bone density in both hip and spine in patients who had steroid-induced bone loss, so it will be a boon to the millions of women who have developed osteoporosis as a complication of many years of taking corticosteroids for other disorders.

Miacalcin (calcitonin-salmon) nasal spray is an *antiresorptive* medication that has been in use in its injectable form for over twenty years and has been available since 1991 as a well-tolerated and convenient nasal spray. It has an entirely different method of preserving bone compared to Fosamax and Actonel: Miacalcin directly suppresses the cells (osteoclasts) that break down bone. Its effectiveness in preventing bone loss and reducing risk of new vertebral fractures has been demonstrated in a variety of studies worldwide. The Prevent Recurrence of Osteoporotic Fractures (PROOF) study evaluated over 1200 postmenopausal women at 47 centers in the United States and Great Britain in a randomized, placebo-controlled trial of Miacalcin. New *vertebral* fractures were reduced by 36 percent in the group receiving 200 IU daily (1 spray) Miacalcin, but this study was not designed to test the effects on hip fractures. In addition to its benefits on preserving bone and reducing vertebral fractures, Miacalcin has another advantage over other antiresorptive medications: it has been shown to have an *analgesic effect* that reduces the back pain associated with vertebral fractures. This effect makes it quite useful for older women who may not want to start estrogen but have more severe forms of osteoporosis causing back pain. Side effects with Miacalcin have been few, primarily irritation of the nasal membranes and "runny nose" (rhinitis) caused by the chemicals in the spray itself.

Another medication recently approved by the FDA in 1999 for prevention and treatment of osteoporosis is the selective estrogen receptor modulator (SERM), raloxifene (Evista). **Evista** has estrogen-like activity (agonist) effects at bone estradiol receptors, and doesn't appear to overstimulate the lining of the uterus like tamoxifen does, but Evista *blocks* (antagonizes) estrogen activity at brain estradiol receptors and some of the vascular estradiol receptors. This is the likely mechanism by which it causes hot flashes and blood clots (deep vein thrombosis, PE or pulmonary emboli). Evista has been heavily marketed by its manufacturer for osteoporosis, but studies have found that Evista is not as effective as Fosamax for preventing bone loss or rebuilding healthy bone. Evista has only about *half* the bone-sparing effects of estrogen.

Side effects are more severe with Evista than with Fosamax or Actonel and include a marked increase in frequency of hot flashes and leg cramps. Depressed mood, memory problems, and fatigue are also problems for many women taking Evista, and appear to be due to the blocking of estrogen receptors in the brain. More serious side effects of Evista are the increased risk of blood clots, cataracts, and glaucoma. If you are considering taking an antiresorptive medication to prevent bone loss and cannot or don't want to take estrogen, I would suggest that you try Fosamax, Actonel, or Miacalcin first since these have been shown to have better bone-sparing effects than Evista. Then if you have problems with one of these, or have had breast cancer and are at higher risk of heart disease as well,

Evista may be a drug to try. Be sure that you watch for signs of serious problems like blood clots (some examples are shortness of breath, pain/swelling or tenderness in the calf area). Report any unusual changes to your physician promptly.

If You Take Premarin and Think Your Bones Are Fine—Take a Look at These Women's Stories!

So you have decided to take estrogen, and your doctor started you on the "cookbook" approach with Premarin. You coast along for several years thinking everything is just golden. Then at your annual checkup, the nurse mentions that you have lost three quarters of an inch in height! "What happened?" you say. "I thought loss of height only occurred if you were losing bone, and I can't be losing bone, I am taking estrogen." This scenario has happened all too often in my practice over the last decade. The standard dose of the horse-derived estrogen may or may not be adequate for your body to preserve bone. There needs to be some follow-up monitoring to see if it is doing the job for you. Take a look at the "numbers" from a recent patient of mine. She is fifty-six years old, and has been on Premarin 0.625 mg for six years. At her initial visit with me, her bone mineral density showed a significant loss of bone at both the hip and spine. Her hip was 2.87 standard deviations below peak bone mass, and her spine was 2.5 standard deviations below peak bone mass. According to the NOF criteria I showed you earlier in the chapter, this means she meets the definition of osteoporosis. Even though she was taking estrogen that should have improved this, her NTx was too high at sixty-five, indicating continuing rapid bone breakdown, her serum estradiol level was low at only 34 pg/ml (below the threshold for preserving bone), and her serum testosterone was low at 10 ng/dl. I see this situation commonly in women taking Premarin. Too many doctors *assume*, without checking, that Premarin gives adequate levels of estradiol to preserve bone and normalize NTx, but it often does not.

I changed this woman to a 17-beta estradiol transdermal patch, and added micronized, sustained-release testosterone 2.0 mg daily. A year later, her numbers showed marked improvement. Her estradiol level was now 105 pg/ml on the patch, her testosterone level was 40 ng/dl, and her NTx had come down to 30. More importantly, her bone mineral density (done on the same machine) showed a gain in bone mass with her hip density now only 1.75 standard deviations below peak, and her spine was now 1.5 standard deviations below peak bone mass. She now would be described as having *osteopenia* rather than osteoporosis. She also described feeling "a lot better" now that her estradiol and testosterone levels were optimal. While she couldn't feel the gain in bone, she did notice improved energy, more sexual feelings, better quality sleep, and easier time with word recall and remembering simple daily things she had been forgetting. Needless to say, she was thrilled with the improvement in bone density too!

Another young woman who had problems with the "standard" hormone therapy approaches is "Pele." Pele was only thirty-eight and had undergone a total hysterectomy and removal of her ovaries at age thirty-two. She had been on Premarin 0.625 mg daily since her surgery. She really had not been worried about bone loss but consulted me in hopes of getting her hormone therapy improved so she would feel better. She described feelings of "extreme fatigue, no libido, no energy to do things, sleepy all the time, my memory is terrible. The longer I have been on Premarin, the worse I feel. My sex drive is nonexistent, I have hot flashes, I don't feel like myself, I'm more irritable." In addition to these symptoms that were so bothersome, her laboratory measures showed some other areas for concern: cholesterol too high at 258, triglycerides elevated at 250, NTx too high at 55, and estradiol too low at 38 pg/ml. Her BMD showed an alarming degree of bone loss, particularly when you think about the fact that she is only thirty-eight years old. She was already at osteoporosis levels at both hip and spine, and understandably quite shocked to learn this. Eighteen months later, all of her lab studies and BMD had improved to the desirable levels, after changing to 17-beta estradiol using 0.1 mg Vivelle patch three times a week.

I think these two women, out of the many I have evaluated with similar findings, illustrate the importance of proper monitoring of your individual response to any hormone therapy you may be using. Don't be lulled into a false sense of security thinking you are OK on the standard doses, because no matter what name we give it—women's body chemistry, natural transition, or hormone deficiency—what cannot be ignored is that *bone loss is real*, and it accelerates rapidly as estrogen declines. If you take estrogen in any form, follow-up monitoring is essential to be certain you are getting all the benefits you seek and need.

The real tragedy is that osteoporosis is so preventable, yet 80 percent or more of peri- and postmenopausal women aren't getting the message about the importance of maintaining a normal balance of estradiol and testosterone to maintain bone. In this country, still only about 15—20 percent of the postmenopausal women who might benefit from estrogen-testosterone therapy are actually getting it. The problem is there's been so much negative information that the resulting imbalance in the press has frightened women away from options with hormones that might help them reduce their risk of bone loss and later debilitation.

In summary, *osteoporosis prevention* is like a three-legged stool that *needs all three legs* for balance and stability: (1) adequate calcium, magnesium, and other key minerals; (2) adequate weight-bearing (low to moderate impact) exercise; and (3) being hormonally complete. If any one of these "legs" is missing or wobbly, balance and stability is compromised or lost. I've had a number of women who have said, "I really prefer not to take estrogen. I'd like to monitor this and see whether or not my fitness and my diet and my calcium and all of those things are taking care of my health and my bone mineral density." That's fine. Just do it from the standpoint of knowing what your bone density is *now* by having the objective measure of the DEXA, and then recheck it in a year or two to be sure you are maintaining the desired bone density. One woman that I was following over a period of a couple of years had lost 10 percent of her bone density in spite of her very healthy lifestyle. So in giving her that information, I just said, "you might want to rethink your decision in light of this new information. Or certainly make sure you recheck the bone density in another year and if the negative trend is continuing you may want to rethink your decision about estrogen." I find that having the definitive information on bone density is the *single most important* piece of data that can help women make the important decision about adding, or not adding, hormone supplements to exercise and dietary approaches.

I still believe that with careful attention to all of the factors I have described in this chapter, we can do a lot more to help premenopausal women prevent bone loss that increases our risk of fractures in later life. For women who have already lost significant amounts of bone mass, the new treatment options offer a lot of hope for halting the progression of this debilitating illness. Ultimately, the decision about *which* approaches to use is up to each of you as individual women. I urge you to make your choices from a basis of knowledge, not fear. And don't be swept away by misleading advertising and "product pushers." Get your information from reliable sources, such as the National Osteoporosis Foundation.

And most of all: DO something. Take positive steps now to protect your bones. As Will Rogers said, ***"Even if you are on the right track, you will get run over if you just sit there!"***

Chapter 19

Patient and Physician: Imperative Agendas in Women's Health for the 21st Century

Stereotypes of Women: What Doctors Are Taught

I share this with you here because it has triggered such overwhelming confirmation of our experiences as women whenever I read it to an audience. Niki Scott's words are unfortunately as true in the year 2000 as they were when she first wrote this piece in 1982 for *The Baltimore Sun*.

WHY ARE MEN ANGRY, BUT WOMEN HYSTERICAL?

*"There is no need for hysteria," he said. Men get **angry**. Women get **hysterical**.*

*"Stop worrying," he said. Men **ask questions**. Women **worry**.*

*"Calm down," he said. Men are **adamant**. Women are **overwrought**.*

Assumptions. Expectations. Labels. They diminish us when others apply them.

We sabotage ourselves when we buy them.

Furthermore:
*Men get **annoyed**. Women get **bitchy**.*
*Men are **aggressive**. Women are **pushy**.*
*Men are **ambitious**. Women are **clawing**.*
*Men assess **their lives**. Women have **empty nest syndrome**.*
*If a man is **impotent**, it's the woman's **fault**.*
*If a woman is **frigid**, she isn't trying.*
*Men are **assertive**. Women are **uppity**.*
*Men who are assaulted are **victims**. Women who are raped **caused it**.*
*Men are **versatile**. Women are **flighty**.*
*Men **change their minds**. Women are **unpredictable**.*
*Men are **virile**. Women are **nymphomaniacs**.*

*Men have **moods**. Women have **periods**.*
*Men are **concerned**. Women are **anxious**.*
*Men analyze **people**. Women **gossip**.*
*His doctor says its **job-related stress**. Her doctor says it's **nerves**.*
*His doctor prescribes **tennis**. Her doctor prescribes **Valium**.*
*If a man is overworked, he is a **go-getter**.*
*   If a woman is overworked, she is **disorganized**.*
*Men pay attention to **detail**. Women **dither**.*
*Men **take charge**. Women **take over**.*
*Battering husbands need **help**. Battered wives **ask for it**.*
*Fathers **move away**. Mothers **desert** their children.*
*Older men are **experienced**. Older women are **over the hill**.*
*Men **react**. Women **over-react**.*
*A happily single man is **glamorous**.*
*   A happily single woman is **neurotic**.*
*Older men look **distinguished**. Older women look **dowdy**.*
*Men **communicate**. Women **talk too much**.*
This list was fun. Labels are not."

by Niki Scott, 12/5/82
The Baltimore Sun

Niki Scott has really hit the nail on the head with this powerful piece illustrating what many of us have experienced: **The same behavior is viewed and labeled differently, depending upon whether the person exhibiting it is male or female.** Unfortunately, many of these same stereotypes are operational in medical education. When you look at this entire list and all that it implies about our typical experiences as women, I think it helps clarify some reactions women encounter in many medical settings. Physicians and nurses are also products of the culture in which these stereotypes are so prevalent, and all of us to some degree carry these cultural stereotypes of women ingrained in our unconscious minds.

In addition, qualities of women are always compared against the *societal norm based on males*: male bodies, male physiology, and male behavioral patterns. If the male pattern is considered normal, then by definition women are considered "abnormal" in being *different* from males. For example, women have been labeled, in a negative sense, as "overutilizers" of health care services because we see doctors, have tests, and undergo surgeries more often than do men. This comparison assumes male bodies and male utilization patterns are "normal"; it does not take into account the obvious source of some of the differences in healthcare utilization, which is that women's bodies are physiologically more complex than men's. Women have babies and therefore *should* be expected to have more medical visits than men. It should be clear from reading this book that there is another factor why women average more doctor visits than men. Women's questions, concerns, hormonal connections, and health problems are frequently *not heard* or taken seriously, so women *continue* to seek help and try to find answers, often very *appropriately*, I might add. Many men may be *too stoic* for their own good and fail to seek medical help early in the course of an illness when consequences may not be as severe. Which gender behavioral pattern is then "normal" here: women who want to nip an illness in the bud at an early stage, or men who are stoic and wait until it's crisis time?

Women are more actively involved in all aspects of their lives and their health. I believe we are more closely attuned to our body, how it feels, what feels good for it. Through menses, pregnancy, and as ones often responsible for taking care of health problems in our immediate and extended families, we have a greater awareness and consciousness of the state of our bodies. Yet, women are still typically viewed as neurotic in their questions and focus on their health. The few studies that have been done on doctors' response to physical complaints from men and from women do indicate that physicians, especially male physicians, take those complaints from men more seriously and therefore do more extensive workups. The research indicates that in so doing, the doctors are responding to stereotypes that regard the male as typically stoic and the female as typically hypochondriacal. I have not seen any information that would indicate that female physicians are significantly *less* likely to show the same patterns, although studies have shown that women physicians are more likely to examine breasts and recommend mammograms than are male physicians.

Women not only have unique medical needs from a biological point of view, but from an emotional point of view as well. As a result of the dramatic social changes of the last thirty years, women have many more physical, emotional, and social expectations on them, and this has a significant physiological impact. Medical education and scientific research has also been based on the male norm, with the assumption that "what works for men works for women" (with the exception being reproductive function). As I have pointed out throughout this book, there simply has not been adequate recognition that the hormonal changes *normal for a women's body* have major effects on *all* organ systems in the body, not just reproductive organs. Doctors at all levels of training need to be taught how female hormones affect such functions as drug metabolism; the way alcohol is handled by females' enzymes compared to males' enzymes; the effects of estrogen and progesterone on the motility of esophagus, stomach, and bowel; how estrogen and progesterone alter insulin binding and glucose regulation and a host of other crucial dimensions affecting women's entire brain-body health.

I do not feel that this education emphasis should be limited to physicians specializing in women's health or just available to medical students and residents who are interested in women's health. I think female body physiology and hormonal influences should be taught to *all* physicians and health professionals who will provide services to women patients of any age. I think such an approach will further help to eliminate the negative stereotypes of women patients we see so much today.

Another stereotype of women that has been perpetuated in medical education is that doctors are taught to *beware* of a patient who arrives with a list of symptoms or questions because she is neurotic, a hypochondriac. Men who arrive with a list of questions are typically *not* viewed as neurotic or anxious; they are seen as *helpful and organized*. The French name for psychoneurosis is *la maladie du petit papier* ("the illness of the little paper"), referring to the lists of symptoms brought in by the typically female patients. This concept about women has been around for hundreds of years and is difficult to dispel.

It is also hard to speak up to an authority-figure physician in a white coat (male or female) if we women have been socialized to be *passive* and then are labeled "bitchy" or "difficult" when we are assertive. If we're not aware of this cultural background, our mental tapes may be telling us "it's all in my head," or "I'm making it up," or "I'm just weak," "I'm inadequate," "I'm somehow not coping." And there are certainly plenty of people around who are eager to attribute problems to midlife stress. I think it's important that we are aware of these undercurrents of unconscious self-critical images so that we don't fall into the trap of *believing the stereotype* instead of *listening to our body wisdom*.

Even when we listen to our bodies, however, it may be hard to get heard when you are in a medical office. Current managed care systems do not encourage discussion because taking time to talk to patients will decrease the volume of patients a doctor is able to see on a given day. Certainly we find that getting to the bottom of hormone-related health problems is very time-intensive. But health plan administrators typically feel that spending more time with patients increases the cost of health care. I would like to propose, however, that taking time to *listen well* might actually be *more* cost-effective. If physicians and other health professionals take a few minutes to learn more information about what the problem may be, it may help refine our thinking about what needs to be done.

In addition, patients don't get much opportunity to present a coherent description of their problems. Studies have found that physicians on average interrupt patients *within twenty seconds* of asking the first question, "What brings you in today?" That doesn't give you much time to respond, and it makes it harder for you to collect and organize your thoughts. One thing I have found as a physician is that often the *first* symptoms mentioned might not be the ones that are most troublesome for the patient. Symptoms brought up later in the interview may be more significant. In order for patients to feel free enough to talk about problems bothering them a great deal, they need to feel *listened to* in the early stages of the process. The physician and the patient must *communicate;* not just talk *at* each other, but communicate. By communicate, I mean YOU and the physician asking questions of each other, and each listening carefully to the answers so that you are each able to understand better what must be done and what options are available to best suit your needs.

Restoring Trust in Physician-Patient Relationships

Traveling to different parts of the country giving seminars and workshops on women's health has been an eye-opening, rewarding, and frequently joyful experience. It has also been painful and sad for me, as a woman and a physician, to listen to the stories of women and the breakdown of trust in their physicians because many in my profession—male and female—have simply been unwilling to *really listen* to what their patients were telling them. As a result, there is so much anger toward and distrust of physicians in general right now that we have a long way to go to rebuild a healing relationship. Unfortunately this breakdown has potentially tragic consequences when women fail to seek a physician's help for what may become life-threatening problems, and/or turn solely to the myriad alternative practitioners out there and miss out on the possible benefits of what modern Western medicine has to offer. I understand the undercurrent of frustration, dissatisfaction, and anger among women; I certainly hear it all the time. Yet women want to like and trust their doctors and are generally very loyal to their physicians, even when such loyalty may not be warranted. So where does the anger come from, and why do so many women, especially around menopause issues, now turn to nonphysician sources and therapists for help? Fundamentally what women tell me is that they are tired of not being listened to; of having their concerns discounted; of being given pills for each symptom without time to discuss side effects; of being told they "have" to take hormones and then being given the same prescription as everyone else; of having their questions trivialized or laughed off; of being told they are "neurotic," "stressed," or worse— "you just need some good sex, honey, and you'll be fine."

There is another aspect that may be underlying women's dissatisfaction with their physicians. For most women, their obstetrician-gynecologist is their primary care physician. This is the only physician many women see, and in the earlier stages of life, that may have been a good choice. As women move into midlife, however, many of them tell me they feel that their OB-GYN physician "isn't interested," or "isn't listening to what I am experiencing," or "doesn't seem to know much about menopause." Perhaps "restoring trust" in the relationship with your physician will also involve *reevaluating* exactly what type of physician is best for you **now**.

There are some important differences in the education of physicians in *surgical* fields compared to *medical* fields. OB-GYN is a surgical specialty. Most of the residency training for surgical specialties focuses on the nuances of surgical techniques, rather than the nuances of medication management that are taught in the medical fields such as internal medicine, family medicine, endocrinology, and others. OB-GYNs need to spend most of their time in training, and in continuing medical education programs, honing their surgical and obstetrical skills, so less time is spent on the nuances of hormone options. Surgeons are taught to individualize their approaches in surgery, while internists and family physicians are taught to individualize medication management. Surgeons and internal medicine/family practice physicians *think differently* about clinical problems. *Surgery* emphasizes the anatomy and *structure* of the body in health and disease, and how to *fix* body parts that are diseased, injured, or abnormal. *Medicine* emphasizes more of the physiological *function* of the body in health and disease. Medicine fields teach physicians to prescribe medications based on objective measures such as laboratory tests, adjust dose based on the individual, and monitor response with follow-up tests. Internal medicine and family practice physicians use nonsurgical approaches aimed at restoring balance and normal function for body organ systems. Both dimensions of the medicine-surgery spectrum are needed with today's complex body of medical knowledge and services; both areas have their appropriate roles for optimum patient care.

As a midlife woman, however, your needs are different from what they were when your focus was having children and needing someone skilled in delivering them and ready to perform a surgery if needed. A physician with a *surgical* background may not be the optimal choice for your *primary care* physician if what you now need is someone to manage *interrelated* medical problems that are not primarily surgical in nature. If you think about it, this would be analogous to men having their *urologist* as their primary care physician (many women laugh when I point this out, and quickly see how such a scenario would be unlikely for most men). You may decide that a different type of physician with a "medicine" background would be appropriate at this stage in your life. If you have a good primary care physician who also does pelvic exams (he or she may be a family practice or an internal medicine specialist), then you may not need to split your care with a gynecologist doing your pelvic exam and an internist checking the rest of you. Many women tell me they simply had not thought about this option. "I've always gone to my gynecologist for everything" is a phrase I hear frequently.

If your gynecologist is still doing a great deal of obstetrics, it may be difficult for this person to have the time to also keep up with the advances in the field of menopause health care. Your gynecologist may not have a broad-based background in adult women's *medicine* in order to be able to readily assimilate nonobstetrical medical advances. So, this may not be the physician for the later phases of your life. It doesn't mean there's anything bad about that, it just means there's so much knowledge today that no one person can stay up to date on everything. I specialize in preventive-climacteric medicine and women's health, with a neuroendocrine focus. I do not *also* do surgery. I would not expect a surgeon to necessarily know all that I know about hormone effects on the brain, nor do I know all that a surgeon knows about surgical techniques. You need to reflect on what your particular needs are and what type of health professional best suits those needs. You are not locked in to the physician you chose ten, fifteen, or twenty years ago to deliver your babies. You now have different needs. You may want to consider other options available to you that are better designed for your current needs.

Another way to reestablish trust and build an effective working relationship with your physician is to look for someone who is willing to work with you in a partnership approach and who values your input and questions about your health. Look for someone willing to spend the time to help you develop an individualized approach to your health needs and goals. You may have to pay extra for more time with such a physician, but isn't your health worth it? As we look at what's needed in women's health I clearly think that we must get back to the basics of the traditions and foundations from which medicine evolved. This means broadening the view of a physician's role *from* the post–World War II focus on medication and surgery, to the evolving role of a physician as a "teacher" to and partner with the patient. I use the word *patient* with a strong sense of the profound meaning of the physician/patient *helping relationship*. To me it means going back to the ancient traditions of Hippocratic medicine. The physician-patient relationship was seen as a *sacred* relationship; physicians still take the Hippocratic Oath when we receive our medical degrees, pledging to use our skills and abilities to the best of our ability to provide care to people who seek our help. The Hippocratic Oath includes a commitment to "do no harm." When I use the word *patient*, I am *not* using it as an indication of a subordinate relationship. I really see it as very much a partnership: You teach me about what you're experiencing, and I use my expertise to teach you how to improve your health. For you to get optimal health care, particularly as a woman growing older, you are going to have to be more active, involved, and knowledgeable. You are the *patient* in the sense of someone seeking help. In my opinion, *patient* does *not* mean *passive* recipient of advice or medicine; your role is *active participation* in the process of becoming more well, the process of diminishing *dis-ease* in your life, and the process of healing.

I also see *patient* as the name for the person to whom the physician has a responsibility: to listen to and take seriously. If this is not happening when you work with a physician, at some point you will need to be assertive enough to say "no more." If your needs aren't being met, look for other resources. I would encourage you to think of your health as one of the most important investments that you have; work with someone who is going to value you, listen to you, and value what you have to say about how you feel and what you are experiencing. You know that better than anyone else.

Listening to Women's Wisdom Again

I have been quite impressed over my years of medical practice with the body "*wise-ness*" of my female patients. I find that women are *far more* knowledgeable about their bodies, are more in tune with subtle as well as noticeable changes, and ask very well thought out questions about what is happening in their bodies. I find that typically women have reasoned out what might be a plausible explanation for their symptoms, and I am happily surprised to find that many of my patients are right on target with what they think is happening. Unfortunately, all too often they have been told, by both male and female physicians, that "this couldn't possibly be, hormones (or dyes or whatever) don't cause that kind of problem." Or "No, that can't be, this medicine doesn't cause those kinds of side effects."

When I had my first back problem I knew there was something terribly wrong, but I was afraid to question the pronouncement— "There's nothing wrong with you"—made by the attending neurosurgeon who was supposed to be the local expert. If I had not listened to my body, and sought another opinion, I would have ended up an incontinent handicapped woman on disability at *twenty-eight* years old. That was a crucial life lesson to learn at an early age. I have been a better physician as a result.

Pay attention to your intuition. It may save *your* life.

Ferreting Out Family History: Connections Between Your Ancestors and Your Health

I was in my early forties, preparing for a hysterectomy due to major problems with fibroids, and deciding about whether to have my ovaries out. My gynecologist told me that at my age, removal of the ovaries wasn't usually done. We talked at length about my overall health at the time, my reasons for wanting the ovaries removed, and his medical opinions about the potential advantages and drawbacks of either option. I was aware that my grandmother had developed ovarian cancer in her mid-forties, which I knew was a significant hereditary dimension. I wrote a letter to my gynecologist outlining my family history and my concerns about my own tendency to have recurring ovarian cysts, which increases risk of ovarian cancer. I just didn't want to have the continued worry in the back of my mind about developing ovarian cancer, since I knew my risk was quite a bit higher than normal. My doctor was reluctant to remove my ovaries, but he agreed it made sense after he listened to my concerns about my family history. Two years later, my mother was able to locate additional key family histories: There were two other women on my grandmother's side of the family—a sister and a niece—who had also developed ovarian cancer, with all of them having it in the *early to mid-forties*. With a shiver, I realized I was right smack in the "window of risk" based on my family genetics. I am glad I made the decision I did. The genetic oncologist who later reviewed my family data confirmed that it was fortunate I had already undergone removal of my ovaries (oophorectomy) due to my high risk of developing the disease. If I had not been proactive about my health, I may very well have been in an entirely different situation today. I did what I am suggesting you do. I made it a point to find out family history, and I used this information in making the decision that felt right for me. **Become empowered with information, explore your options, find out what you need to know to make the decision that fits you.**

As science advances, as we understand diseases better, and as we have better ways of tracking family patterns, it turns out that an astonishing number of health problems, both common and rare, have some type of hereditary, or genetic, link. Many very common disorders are now known to have a strong hereditary component: alcoholism, Alzheimer's dementia, allergies, asthma, many cancers (breast, lung, colon, ovarian, prostate, skin), depression, diabetes, heart disease, glaucoma, osteoporosis, rheumatoid arthritis. If you find that you are more susceptible to a disease because it runs in your family, you have several ways of reducing your own risk of having more serious illness:

- having earlier, or more frequent, screening tests
- having regular checkups
- eliminating nongenetic lifestyle risk factors such as smoking, alcohol, high-fat diet
- being alert to early symptoms

It really isn't all that difficult to get the information and draw a *genogram*, or family tree. Patients tell me they don't think they can find the information about people who have died. Often there is a family "historian" who knows the family traditions and problems. **It usually isn't necessary to go back many generations,** since the most important links are your parents, brothers, sisters, grand parents, aunts and uncles. A second cousin would share only about 3 percent of the same genes you do, so going this far out on the branches of the family tree really is not relevant in most situations unless you are trying to track down an inherited cancer pattern. The types of health history information you should gather include the following:

	RELATIVE	YR BORN	YR DIED
ILLNESSES (especially cancers, diabetes, stroke, heart attacks, osteoporosis, thyroid disorders, dementia, depression, alcohol abuse, autoimmune disorders, etc.)			
SURGERIES/INJURIES			
ALCOHOL/TOBACCO OR DRUG USE			
OCCUPATION			
TOXIC EXPOSURE			
AGE OF MENOPAUSE			
PROBLEMS W/MENSES OR PREGNANCIES			

© Elizabeth Lee Vliet, M.D., 1995

You simply MUST take the time to find out and write down your family medical history, before it is too late and records are lost. You need to know it, and your children and family members need to know it. You can start your own "health planner" notebook, or there are several commercial versions available in bookstores. Having the family medical information can be an important gift to yourself, to your children, and for generations still to come. You are connected to your ancestors; knowing more about *them* is a link that may have a profound effect on *your future* health.

Becoming an "Activated Patient": Getting Involved to Protect Your Health

I cannot say it strongly enough. You must become an "activated" patient in your health care. What does *activated* patient mean? This is my list:

- Become proactive about getting information, exploring options, and taking action.
- Find out your family health history; write it down and take copies with you to your medical visits.
- Know your health risks, write them down, and give a copy to your physician.
- Know your past and present "health data" (physicians call this database your "medical records"). Get copies and keep a set at home to take with you if you have an emergency or see a new physician.
- Pay attention to your "numbers" (medical results); ask for copies of your lab reports and key medical test results and keep these at home for your records and to show other physicians you may consult.
- Do your homework investigating resources for physicians and other health professionals who will best suit your needs for your health "team."
- Speak up and ask questions. Write a list of questions you want answered before each appointment with your health professionals.
- Keep track of your symptoms (charted with your menstrual cycle).
- Keep records of your over-the-counter medications and vitamin, mineral, and herbal supplements, and bring this to each medical appointment you have.

I know this kind of involvement takes time, and many of you may be saying to yourself, "I don't have time to do all of that." You are like most women, juggling multiple roles, meeting many demands and expectations in your life. "Isn't my doctor supposed to take care of all that?" Yes and no. Just as you would work with your financial planner, your tax advisor, your hairdresser, or any other person helping you, your input and your desires are crucial to a result that meets your needs. Your physician is no exception. Ideally, she or he should welcome and value your input and your questions, as well as your desire to be actively involved in the decisions about your health care options. And you have to do your homework about yourself and your health needs in order to give your physician the input needed to make suitable, intelligent recommendations for you. If your physician doesn't value your input, or the homework you do to keep track of your medical information, consider changing to one who does.

There is a lot of information out there. Most libraries have good publications on health issues. I have provided a list of resources I think are helpful and worthwhile. I do find that a lot of magazine articles either contain information that is old news or is written with more sensationalism than substance, or is slanted to promote a particular bias. Talk with your friends about health concerns, but always remember: Their cure won't necessarily be yours, their symptoms are not exactly the same as yours, and their body chemistry is not exactly the same as yours. If you are reading a research report, don't forget to check *if women were included* in the study population.

We have been so dominated by the male model of body physiology and thinking for so long that people, including health professionals, often forget to consider what is known about female physiology and the changes of the menstrual cycle that have a bearing on body functions and symptoms. You may need to remind them! Be persistent in pointing out the connections you observe. Your body wisdom, intuition, and insight are important. Some physicians are so caught up in having to be right that they have forgotten to listen to their patients . . . you may need to remind them. Sometimes physicians forget that one of the first tenets of medicine is that we should *never* say never. When you are dealing with the human body, there are all kinds of variations and almost *anything* is possible. Just because we may not be able to explain it does *not* mean that something you observe isn't real or possible. Find a physician who is willing to say, "I don't know, let's try to find out." And then *you* be willing to accept when a physician is honest enough to say "I don't know."

To be more active in their care, I encourage my patients to keep records of their physical and emotional sensations, not only when they are feeling ill, but also when they are feeling *well* so they have a baseline. I also encourage women to keep a list of health questions they want addressed at their appointments. That way their thoughts are focused, and things don't get overlooked in the discussion. In fact, I suggest that they send me this list and their symptom logs before their appointment so that I have it to read just before I see them. Physicians have been taught negative stereotypes about women patients who ask questions and who want to understand what they are experiencing. It has taken me a lot of years to undo those negative teachings about women and come to an appreciation of just how wonderful it is to have a partnership with a person who is observant about her body, shares with me her insights and thoughts about possible connections causing or aggravating her symptoms, and writes down her symptoms and questions. An involved, interested patient makes my job easier, not harder. I *like* to see lists. It shows that you care and are doing your part in our partnership. It makes the office visit more productive, is much more effective for you to get your needs met, and also is easier for me as the physician in determining what is expected.

And another important point: You may have in your life all the money, friends, family, relationships, and anything else you desire, but if you don't have your health you *cannot* fully enjoy all the rest. As someone who has *been there* in the experience of having a major health crisis and watching my good health slide rapidly into a deep, dark hole of despair, I can emphatically say that without one's health, all the other assets seem to lose a lot of value. I came to appreciate a quote I came across a few years ago: "*Your health is your greatest wealth.*"

Finding the Right Doctor for You: Questions to Ask

What are some resources to help you locate a good physician for you? Typical sources of information about doctors include friends' experiences and state and local medical societies. A doctor or nurse you know personally may have recommendations. The Yellow Pages can give you a start, and most have a section that lists those who are board certified in their specialty. An excellent resource for women in midlife is the North American Menopause Society, based in Cleveland, Ohio. Members are physicians who are interested in women's health and are attending the update conferences to learn about advances in the field. If you live in a city with a hospital-based referral resource center, these people may be able to tell you who the local health professionals interested in prevention, wellness, and midlife women's health are. You may also contact the state board of medical examiners if you have questions about whether or not a physician has ever been sanctioned for inappropriate medical practices or has had a number of malpractice suits. Don't be afraid to ask questions.

I do think that it's important to ask a potential physician or nurse practitioner what her or his interest is in preventive medicine as well as "wellness" or "complementary" approaches. What is this person's interest in women's health and has he or she been attending update medical education programs in mid-life and menopause health issues? If the answers to those questions are negative, then I would encourage you to interview someone else. It may be worth an extra consult fee to find someone whom you really feel comfortable talking with and whose medical philosophy, empathy, and competence you feel confident about. If you want to be involved in making decisions, find a health professional who is willing to work with you in a collaborative way.

The type or specialty of the physician is not as important as finding the right individual physician. My suggestion for midlife women is to locate a broad-based adult medicine generalist as the physician to oversee and coordinate your care. In such a situation, one doctor can manage the majority of your ongoing care with referral to specialists arranged when needed. Feel free to ask questions about training, interests, and payment policies. Of course price is important, but it is a little different from looking for the best price on a dress. You can always get another dress, but it is tough getting a new body.

Unfortunately the choice of health benefits for you and your family may well be determined to a great extent by your employer, their insurance company, and/or your legislators. If you get a chance to choose from several plans, be sure you do the time consuming but important task of reading all of the descriptive material. Make comparative charts, noting things like fitness and disease prevention programs, prescription plans, mental health services, physical therapy, and long-term care. The plan that has the lowest premium and co-payment may be the most expensive in the long haul if you have to cover such expenses from your own pocket. Obviously you need to read the directory of doctors and hospitals and ask questions about them. If the physician you have been assigned on your health plan doesn't seem to communicate adequately with you, speak out and request a change.

One of the first requirements of most current health insurance plans is to designate a primary care physician who will become the focal point of your health care. Not only will that doctor be the one responsible for evaluating your general state of health and treating most of your aches and pains, he or she will also be the keeper of your health information and the person who will also determine when to refer you to specialists, as well as which specialists you will see. That person will be approving prescriptions, authorizing mammograms and other screening tests, as well as ordering diagnostic tests. You need someone you trust, someone who respects and listens to you, and someone with whom you feel comfortable and with whom you are able to communicate effectively. *Select your physician carefully.* Don't be afraid to speak up. If you don't understand something, *say so.* Treat your physician with respect for her or his time and intelligence, and expect the same response in return. Do not be afraid to change doctors if you are not satisfied.

Surveys have indicated that over 90 percent of patients consider it very important for a physician to (in order of importance):

1. Be knowledgeable and competent.
2. Answer questions honestly and completely.
3. Explain medical problems in clear language.
4. Spend enough time with patients.
5. Really care about patients' health.

6. Make an effort to get patients to explain problems and symptoms completely.

It is equally important for physicians to realize that they, too, have a communication responsibility, as the above list indicates. Good communication, caring, clear communication—particularly in drawing out patients' concerns and responding to their questions to their satisfaction—go a long way toward establishing patient loyalty and compliance. Patients are more concerned with the *perceived* value of the care they pay to receive than with the dollars *per se*. Fees are not of primary importance with most patients, providing they are satisfied with the amount of time and attention they receive from the physician. A significant number of malpractice suits are triggered by poor communication, not bad results.

Women's Centers: Looking Beyond Marketing Hype

There are lots of newspaper ads promoting a new concept at many hospitals and medical practices, called women's centers. Read these ads very closely. I have seen many that are nothing more than dressed-up birthing centers with drapes, a rocking chair, and a beauty salon. Is this really any different from what we have always had? In my view, a good women's center must provide a new model of integrated health services aimed at meeting women's unique needs, not just aimed at new paint colors and a beauty shop. Is "women's health" only addressing services based on the body from breasts down and thighs up? It shouldn't be.

As an experiment, I produced a flier showing a woman's body from the neck down and had the headline question at the top: "What's wrong with this picture?" At a women's health conference for both professional and lay population, no one gave responses other than "she's overweight." I was surprised. No one noticed that the woman's *head* was missing! The functions of the brain-mind are often not considered when it comes to women's health. I mean not only hormones, but also emotions. We have many health needs for all parts of our body, which are monitored by our brain acting through our hormones. If you are looking for a women's center where you can have many dimensions of your health care *integrated*, read the fine print, and find out what programs they offer and what physicians and alternative practitioners they have on staff. Is it fluff or substance? Don't settle for window dressing or a program that is just another marketing effort. You may find it helpful to use the questionnaire in appendix III to evaluate a potential women's center to decide if it is offering services that will truly be useful and meet your needs.

Health Care Reform: Crucial Women's Issues for the Twenty-first Century

With all of the recent publicity about health care reform in the United States, and the need to improve access and control spiraling costs, I think an even more *pressing* need has been *grossly* overlooked: How do we pay better attention to the specific needs of female patients? Insurance industry profits are at an all-time high, but with their emphasis on cost containment (to maximize their profits), are we missing the boat in taking care of crucial health problems in female patients that have been ignored, overlooked, undertreated, and mistreated? I find increasing evidence that the frightening answer to this question is *yes.*

I think **HMO** or Health Maintenance Organization would be more accurately called an **HRO**—Health *Rationing* Organization. Their goal is to deny as many claims as they can to save as much money as possible to benefit their profits. Don't fool yourself into thinking otherwise. You will need to be very proactive to get the services you need. Many studies have shown that in our current climate of cost containment, *women* are more often denied important diagnostic tests. Women are more often told "you're just overworried, there's nothing wrong," "you're just under a lot of stress," "you're not at risk for anything serious," "you look healthy." I have seen this happen with everything from blood tests to treadmill stress tests (for heart disease), to bone density evaluation, and even to mammograms. There is now a significant amount of research that confirms the gender difference. When similar types of health problems affect men, men are far more likely than women to have rapid access to diagnostic tests and to get insurance reimbursement for those tests.

Mammogram coverage is a case in point. Women's health advocates finally succeeded in getting insurance reimbursement for screening mammography, and we now find that reimbursement for mammograms by Medicare has been *reduced* to coverage for a mammogram every *other* year over age fifty. You may remember my mentioning earlier that breast cancer is more common in older women. This change also comes at a time when the national guidelines for adequate cancer screening are for women to have a mammogram *every* year after age fifty. Bone density testing gives another illustration of these problems and concerns. We are beginning to have more and more data emerging to show that women actually start losing bone long *before* menopause and the end of menstrual periods. I continue to hear physicians say bone density testing isn't needed, and yet we have no better way to identify women with early bone loss. Bone loss in this stage of life is silent—it doesn't cause any symptoms to warn women that it is happening until much later, when she may notice a decrease in height. The only way women can know whether or not they have beginning bone loss is to have a specific test, usually DEXA, which measures the bone mineral content of the hip and spine. I first started doing bone density testing for perimenopause patients back in 1985. I have found it borne out just how crucial this information is for women of all ages. Medicare has finally authorized payment for bone density tests, and a number of states (Texas is one) have mandated that commercial insurance carriers pay for this test as well. But we still have states that don't require such coverage, and in a strange twist of logic, some insurance plans will pay for the *more expensive* computerized tomography (CT) bone density test that gives you unnecessary radiation exposure, but they won't reimburse for the lower cost, more useful DEXA test that exposes you to less radiation than you would get flying in an airplane across the country.

Why are we not using the information and technology that is available to help women avoid these problems? Many physicians and insurance carriers often reply that "it's too expensive" to do bone density testing in broader groups of women. The sad fact is that we could dramatically *reduce* the existing and projected health costs associated with osteoporosis, such as hip fractures, if we just evaluated women sooner, when bone loss is typically minimal and can be prevented or reversed. And this statement is based on reducing actual dollars—it doesn't even include the potential reduction in human suffering from the pain, hospitalizations, surgeries, and other costs of osteoporosis. We know that osteoporosis and its consequences and complications are one of the most devastating robbers of quality of life, independence, and longevity for older women. Women understand this logic once they know that such tests are available, and many women are willing to pay for the test, if need be, in order to have the information they need. But bone density testing remains underutilized as a tool to improve women's knowledge of their health data, particularly for younger women with premature ovarian decline or early surgical menopause. Are women once again getting the short end of the stick on health care? In my opinion, yes.

So what can you as one individual do? One of my patients from another state serves as an insurance "ombudsman" for her fellow employees, helping them understand their rights when health claims are denied. She had several good suggestions to help women obtain better insurance reimbursement. We have certainly found that many patients in our practice have often been successful with these approaches.

First of all, keep in mind that it is *common* for your first claim submission to be denied. Setting up obstacles and delays is one way the insurance carriers hold on to their money longer. Expect it, and don't give up the first time a claim comes back denied. Here are some suggested steps to follow:

1. Get all the literature on your company's health plan, check it for the specifics of their appeals process.
2. Follow the procedures exactly, and make certain that you file your appeal within the specifed time.
3. Get the name of the employee advocate in your company. It will usually be someone in human resources or the employee benefits department. There may also be a company ombudsman/woman—contact that person for help and keep a date and content log of all your conversations.
4. ˋWrite a letter to your health plan outlining the specifics of your appeal of their denial of your claim.
5. Send copies of correspondence you send to your health plan to the following people: (a) your state insurance commissioner (information such as the name and contact address for this person is available on the Internet for every state in the country), and (b) to your state legislators—this gets attention and action, and also gives your legislators ammunition to use in curbing the abuses of health insurance carriers. Patients tell us that their claims are paid rather quickly when they send their carrier a letter showing these copies being sent also!
6. Remember the words of the ombudswoman I mentioned earlier: "It can be a long, hard and demoralizing process to fight these battles, but keep in mind it is designed to be that way to keep you from getting 'their' money and to avoid paying as many claims as possible, which enhances their bottom line."

We address the issue of health care reform to benefit the people in this country who do not have insurance, and that is a worthwhile goal. But are we addressing the major overhaul that must be undertaken to provide better health care and treatment options for fully *half* the population in this country who are female? I have not yet seen much evidence that many of our leaders are even aware of this aspect of the problem, much less focusing on ways to address and correct the deficiencies in our knowledge and care of women patients. Many of the health problems that affect women do *not* fit neatly into our fragmented, specialty "boxes" based on organ systems and body parts. Women need more of an integrated, or multidisciplinary approach, that can help identify such things as endocrine changes that cause diverse symptoms, and also provide more effective treatment. So, will health care reform actually benefit women? Not unless women themselves speak up and make their voices heard as to the issues important to them. Your physicians can't do it alone. Legislators can't do it alone. The circle of empowerment is only complete when YOU are part of the circle of voices that speak out. The broader aspects of women's health need the grassroots efforts of women consumers to move the agenda forward. Together, we can make a difference for the next millennium and for generations of women to come.

Where Do We Go from Here?

Sorting fact from fiction, myth, and misinformation becomes a difficult challenge for the average consumer. I encourage you to keep in mind that all of the consumer short pieces you read in the news have to give you just that: a piece of the whole picture. You are going to have to *know yourself*, know your health history, health risks, and your values for yourself in order to make some informed, intelligent choices among the many options available to you today. One article said about hormone therapy, "it's one of the most important and difficult decisions a woman ever has to make." Women are faced with hundreds of difficult and important decisions throughout our lives. How do you make *other* decisions in your life about matters that are important to you?

Many decisions we have to make may be difficult. Most of the decisions we make have some degree of benefit to us and some degree of downside or drawback or even risk. If I take a position in Tucson, I can't live in Norfolk. If I leave Virginia, I will miss my family, close friends, and patients I have worked with for many years. I want to try the new challenges available to me in Tucson, but I can't have both. How do I decide? Think about it for you. Each choice means a road taken and a road not taken. You weigh what is meaningful, important, and beneficial against what downsides you are willing to face. There are ways to get information regarding important decisions of all kinds in our lives. Few of the really important decisions are going to be easy, and each of us has to do our homework to make them. We reevaluate other decisions and choices we have made as new information comes in or as our needs change. Media articles may have good, accurate, and helpful information, but they may also have incorrect and out-of-date information. You will have to do your homework to find out more complete answers to questions that are important to YOU to have addressed. You will also have to be assertive and diligent in seeking out a knowledgeable health professional to keep you up on new developments and to work with you in a partnership to have *your individual* health concerns addressed optimally.

The other side of that coin is to remember this admonition from

Ecclesiastes: **"If you wait for perfect conditions, you will never get anything done."** This observation is true for us today as we look at some of the issues in women's health. Women ask me, "Well, what about the studies and the fact that there's conflicting information? We don't have a definite answer and we don't have information about that." This is true. There are still many answers to be determined. The problem is that many of us early "baby boomers" are at a point *now* when we have to make important decisions about our course of action for our health. We can't wait another ten years for "definitive" answers to come in from research.

Ten years ago, when I needed to make a personal decision about using the estradiol patch, it was very unusual for a *premenopausal* woman to try estrogen. My doctor told me that, and helped me decide whether I wanted to give it a try. If I had waited for the confirming research to answer all my questions before I decided to address those needs at the time, I would likely have had reduced quality of life now, as well as progressive bone loss before I even reached menopause. My exercise and good calcium intake alone would not have made up for the decline in my body's production of the crucial estrogen. Each of us needs to make a personal decision as to whether we can afford to take more time in making a health decision or whether we need to *act now*. We will each have to make the best choice we can in light of the information available to us and our own individual values, and then stay informed as new information becomes available. And we each need to make our own decision, not just copy what our friends are doing. I foresee that with the current interest in and demand for more information tailored to women, we will have an explosion of new information over the decades ahead.

Hang on, we will *all* have to keep learning and discerning, and not just be blown like leaves in the wind with each new fad. Remember, there are no "magic bullets," and one size does *not* fit all. Consumers, both men and women, tend to want quick fixes. Our culture makes us impatient with the fine tuning and process of working over time to find solutions, then revising them as needed. Try to avoid this trap and think of this process and the time involved as an investment in your health. It is similar to investing in quality stocks for the long haul and watching them grow slowly and steadily, making minor adjustments along the way, instead of the extreme highs and lows and risks of *day trading*. As a foundation for your health investment process, seek a relationship with a health professional that will work closely with you on the journey.

Being *proactive* also means, at another level, getting involved with health advocacy organizations around the country, which are working to improve services, access, education, and research into the specific health needs of women. These organizations, some of which are listed under the resources in appendix II, are actively getting the message out to health professionals, insurance companies, legislators, researchers, and others that the specific and different health questions for women must be taken seriously and addressed. Your voice, your wisdom, your insight, and your energy are all needed in these endeavors. Tell your story, talk about your experiences, and share your ideas about how you would like to see things done differently. Get involved and speak out.

It does make a difference when women take charge in this way. All you have to do is look at what has been accomplished in this country by *one* mother who became outraged about the problem of drunk drivers when her daughter was killed by one, and you begin to see what women can accomplish when working together toward common goals that in some way will affect us all. Mothers Against Drunk Driving (MADD) as a grassroots organization did more in a short time to address the serious and potentially lethal consequences of intoxicated drivers than any other single agency or legislative group in this country. No matter what direction this organization now takes, it remains a prime example of the effect *one concerned woman,* and those working with her, can have for the broader needs in the United States. Vicki Ratner, M.D., who founded the Interstitial Cystitis Association, is another example of a woman who, after a long personal ordeal to have IC diagnosed, became an advocate for other women suffering from this unrecognized problem. AIDS and breast cancer grassroots activism by consumers have achieved remarkable results in getting research, education, and clinical services agendas met. In both cases, our increased awareness came from small groups of concerned consumers all over the country who worked together to make their voices heard. We see this support from concerned consumers become even more effective through the many Web sites that have been developed for people to share their health experiences, education, insights, and sources of help.

I have been, and plan to continue to be, a voice for change in how we educate health professionals and how we can better serve the needs of women who have been so overlooked and unheard for so long. I hope you will join me in these efforts, in whatever way fits into your life and community. You have taken a crucial first step in that change process by coming with me on the journey through the pages of this book, so don't stop now.

Margaret Mead said, **"Never doubt that a small group of concerned, committed people can make a difference; indeed, it is the only thing that ever has."** Women make a difference. YOU make a difference.

Chapter 20

Take Charge!
Creating Your Journey
to Optimal Health

Prelude

I first used a variation of this title for a talk on women's health in 1985, and it summarizes my own journey as a woman and physician, as well as the process I have described throughout this book. In the previous chapters, I have talked about the importance of caring for the physical aspects of your health: knowing your height, blood pressure, cholesterol/HDL, body composition, and hormone levels; taking time to provide your body with healthy fuel; taking time to move the body in exercise; taking time for rest and relaxation; having the appropriate preventive medicine checkups and screening tests. All of these steps are basic to health and to healthy aging. I have focused primarily on the overlooked hormonal connections in women's health because, even today, there is so little *integrated* information available for women to find answers to their questions.

People have said, "Why do you consider it so important to put the hormones so early in the process?" I think *loss* of your hormone balance, at whatever age, is like getting stuck in quicksand. You can keep working to get out, and the harder you work at it, the more you sink in the sticky muck. But if someone reaches out to you and puts a plank under your feet to give you some solid ground to gain a footing, you can begin getting out. I see the hormones as being the body's "plank" of support for all of its basic energy, growth, repair, and healing functions. Without all our hormones present in the right amounts and working properly, we just get stuck in the "quicksand" of adding more medications, more "techniques," more supplements . . . *more* of whatever is the latest trend there is to try. Yet, even with all these, you still lack the "plank" of solid support under your efforts. The use of natural forms of hormone medications helps return the body to its natural state of balance, and then the other methods all work better. So, yes, hormone balance is crucial. I do not want to suggest, however, that your physical health is the only dimension I think is important.

I have profound belief in, and respect for, the power of the mind and spirit in all aspects of health, disease, and the healing process. Indeed, these dimensions may be the most critical of all as we seek the *wellness of being* that is at the core of our human quest, instead of the cultural emphasis on *doing* and *achieving.* I know from a deep personal level and from my professional experience that healing in its fullest sense must include attention to our damaged spirit, not only our broken body. The body feels the things of our soul and spirit of which our mind is not consciously aware. Our cells know and communicate things about us that are invisible to our eyes and ears.

Even with my emphasis on the hormone connections in this book, I want you to remember this: First and foremost, my belief system emphasizes having a strong sense of faith and purpose in life as our base, then we build on this base with a wellness lifestyle, using natural options for healing, and upon that foundation add medical approaches (hormones, medications, surgery) when needed. I know firsthand how important all of these are in achieving optimal health. I want to share with you some of my thoughts on the spiritual and emotional aspects of health. And, as a dragonfly skitters over a pond, I recognize that I am just touching the surface of these dimensions. There are many beautiful and inspiring books that are available to guide you to greater depth on these subjects. I encourage you to seek out the ones that call to your heart and soul as you travel further on your journey of self-exploration and spiritual growth.

Be still . . . and listen to the unspoken messages of your body, as it calls you to pay attention to its needs and those of your battered spirit . . . you'll be guided on the steps to take toward healing and wholeness. Then let the course of your life become a beacon to others who are lost and searching.

Quiet Time: Reflection, Journaling, Meditation

Getting to know yourself takes time being with yourself.

This statement seems so obvious, and yet how often do we as women take the time to do it? We are giving to others day in and day out: We are the twenty-four-hours-a-day mother, the attentive wife, the dutiful daughter, the income-producer, the dedicated community volunteer, the caretaker of the ill, the teacher of children (at home-school-church-synagogue-daycare), the social-political activist. No matter what your particular roles, if you count them all, you will discover with amazement just how many there are.

Women are constantly "switching hats," as our multiple roles require that we dip into diverse areas of skills-insights-wisdom when new demands emerge. A man may have one primary career focus for his entire life. Women typically have several. I know you have heard these ideas and observations before. So when are you going to do something for *you?*   Janis Joplin said, not long before she died: *"Don't compromise yourself. YOU are all you've got."*

Do you really know who YOU are and what you want for yourself out of life? Have you looked within to find out? If not, when do you plan to do it? Are you going to lose yourself before you wake up and realize that you *must* take time for you? Why not take time *right now* to write down the first six things that come immediately to mind as you read this question:

If you were told you had four months to live, what do you most want to accomplish in that time? How do you want to spend those days?

Only you can see that you begin **now** to make time in your life for those meaningful activities or ways of being that you just wrote down.

Start some form of journal to give voice to this inner you. Use whatever form is helpful and useful to you: Write down your thoughts and feelings; if you don't like to write, make a collage of your feelings by gathering images and words that "speak" to you from magazines and pasting them on a piece of paper with the date; collect quotes and jot down how they affect you; use crayons and "doodles" to express your mood and feelings; write a song, poem, or story. Use your imagination. Begin now to assemble a few simple ingredients for taking care of you: solitude, time, a physical or intellectual challenge that is meaningful to you, being in nature, and taking a step outside any self-imposed limits. Combine these ingredients to make your own personal "sabbatical" to look a little deeper into your life and the aspects that you want to change, improve, and expand. Make time for play, for some undivided attention to your spontaneous, free, unrestrained inner part of you. Clarissa Pinkola Estes, Ph.D., calls this part of us the "Wild Woman," and says *"Wild Woman whispers the words and ways to us and we follow."*

> . . . . . . FIRST, WE MUST <u>LISTEN</u> TO HER WHISPERS.
> SHE is the voice within you *Screaming to be HEARD. Give her a commitment of some of your time to listen . . . . just*
> *L I S T E N . . . . listen.*
>
> From *Women Who Run wih the Wolves,*
> Clarissa Pinkola Estes, Ph.D., 1994

Food for the Soul: Feeding Women's Spirit

In the sixth century B.C. Pythagorus wrote: "The physician's task is to teach men and women the *physical and spiritual* laws of life and to live in accordance with God's purpose for them." In the ancient healing arts of all cultures, and in the tradition of the physician as "healer" or person who practices the art and science of medicine, the emphasis had traditionally been on the *whole person.* This included addressing spiritual needs as well as physical and emotional needs. Healing traditions through the centuries have also encompassed healthy lifestyle approaches in treating physical illness and emotional-spiritual pain.

Modern Western medicine has lost this connection with soul, with the spiritual dimension of human beings. As the "science" of medicine evolved, in the last hundred years or so, the care of patients has become very compartmentalized with the physical body being seen by various medical or surgical specialists, the mind needs being addressed by psychologists and psychiatrists (who usually don't do much with the medicine of the physical body), and soul-spirit pain is left for "treatment" by ministers, rabbis, or priests and placed in churches or synagogues. One "compartment" or specialty doesn't address the concerns that arise in the others. This compartmentalization is particularly prevalent in the care of women. Ultimately such partition of the mind-body and spirit leads to artificial divisions that cannot lead to true healing and wellness. I don't leave my soul or my spirituality at the doorstep when I enter the hospital or a physician's office, and I doubt that you do either.

Alexis Guirdham, Nobel prize winner, said, "*We cannot fragment our healing efforts by declaring them spiritual or medical, but recognize the total synchronizing process of healing, for the goal is wholeness and harmony.*"

I think for us as women, this statement has a particularly powerful message, since many of us live our lives in a medical model and culture that tends to fragment us into body parts and different roles. With such fragmentation and increasing high-tech (and often impersonal) approaches to *medical* care, women seeking *health care* (caring) are turning in droves to "high touch" alternative practitioners. These practitioners typically emphasize time for communication and self-empowerment, and recommend healing approaches that are promoted as more natural, more gentle, and create a better feeling of being "listened to" and "heard" in the person-to-person encounters. Many women have expressed a desire to have health care approaches that address them as a "whole" person, not just body parts.

We must take into account the role of the spiritual nature of human beings as an important dimension of healing. In using the term "spiritual" I am not referring to a person's religion. To me, one's spiritual connection with life and this universe is a personal, deeply held individual experience. It is having a sense of meaning and purpose in your life as a first step in awakening to your spiritual self. Spirituality is more than just your psychological or emotional self. It is tapping into the part of yourself that has a sense of connection to something greater than you, a source of power that transcends human limitations, whether you call that "something" God, Creator, Divine Mystery, or Great Spirit. Religion, in my view, refers to being a part of an organized group with a defined set of core beliefs. You may be deeply spiritual, yet not belong to an organized religion. I have also encountered people who are very active in their religion who are not particularly spiritual. Clearly, there are people who are both, and people who are neither. I think the unheard cries of the soul, however we may define them, are a critical dimension of the pain present in the lives of many women and men today.

I find that the more I ask patients about the role of faith in their lives, the more I hear stories of the pain from feeling a void in their spiritual lives, a sense of emptiness and meaninglessness. This has such a profound impact on one's overall health. I was taught in my formal medical training that physicians should not discuss these issues with patients. Over the years of medical practice, however, I have found that many people have been traumatized by earlier dogmatic church experiences or have not had a particular religious focus in the life experience. People like this who are in spiritual pain often have no one else with whom they can discuss their concerns. More often than not, they have been grateful that I asked about this dimension of their lives. I have had to "unlearn" my formal training and give myself permission to explore these areas of people's lives.

I find this especially true of women. Many traditional religious institutions have left women feeling invisible because of the patriarchal emphasis on God and His earthly representatives as male. I grew up attending the Presbyterian Church. I never realized how much I had been affected by not seeing women as role models in the worship services of the church until, as an adult, I went to Royster Presbyterian church in Norfolk that had a women associate pastor at the time.

For the *first* time in my life, I heard a woman minister give the sermon and watched women elders serving communion. I was truly overcome with emotion as the impact of women being part of the service hit me fully. Here I was, almost forty years old, and this was the first time in my life I had seen women in these roles. What kind of subtle, and not-so-subtle, messages have we given little girls all these years about their worth, when all they see are boys and men participating in the services and hear God always referred to as male. The soul pain with this realization was immense. I was not prepared for the impact I felt sitting in that service and listening to the Reverend Katherine Cameron present the lessons though the eyes and experiences of a woman.

Women have not always been so invisible in religions of the world. Cultures we have called "primitive" have long included the feminine qualities of the Creator as being an important dimension of balance and harmony. The ancient Chinese philosophy of Yin and Yang reflects this blend of the masculine and feminine energies and qualities. Since I moved to Tucson, I have been privileged to be able to participate in Native American prayer circles and ceremonial lodges. The depth of spiritual commitment of these people, and their deep reverence for all life in its masculine and feminine forms, has enriched me greatly. Healing the deeper spiritual wound for women is also part of health and wholeness. We physicians neglect this at our patients' peril. We must weave together all parts of the human experience in our search for health and well-being. I feel it is important to respect individual beliefs, and I believe we can do this at the same time we create healing environments that encompass the spiritual dimensions of life.

Just as our bodies and minds change, our spirit grows in new directions and we move onward in our life journey. Sometimes we look back with regret, sometimes we look back with pride; sometimes we look ahead with excitement about what lies out there, and sometimes we look ahead with fear. It seems to me much like what Ingmar Bergman must have meant in this statement: *"Old age is like climbing a mountain. You climb from ledge to ledge, the higher you get the more tired and breathless you become. But your views become more expansive."*

As we get older and wiser we have learned to cherish the considerable skills, insight, and wisdom we've accumulated adapting to all of the changes that have occurred throughout our lives. We have woven these experiences into our own unique tapestry, which we may then share with those around us. This is part of the *transcendence* of life that gives it meaning and purpose. So, no matter how busy you are, *make* time for that dimension of your life. Your very survival, at a spiritual and physical level, may depend on your listening to this inner voice that calls to you to listen. Take heed and act on her message.

As a woman at midlife and beyond, you are moving from creating *new* life to creating *your own life*. For many women, there is a sense of uncertainty as their roles change. Who am I? What do I want to accomplish? Who do I want to be? These existential questions do not have easy answers. Yet, your sense of self-worth and feeling of direction in your life is enhanced greatly by the time you set aside to explore what responses to these questions are meaningful for you. Midlife becomes a time to choose from many possibilities of thoughts, actions, feelings. We then begin to weave these into our unique pattern of responses. This weaving is our midlife creativity creating *self* anew in the womb of our soul, rather than creating a separate embryo of life and gestating it for nine months in our bodies. This is one of your most valuable assets in this phase of life. Invest it well, for its growth will nourish you for years ahead.

To create is also to *change.* As women we face many changes throughout our life journey: physical changes, role changes, emotional changes, spiritual changes. How we view *change* is a significant part of the challenge we face. Is change a *crisis* to you, or do you see change as an *opportunity*? Do you feel overwhelmed by changes in your life, or are changes exciting to you? Do you enjoy new challenges, or do you view them as threats? One woman, moving from Norfolk, Virginia, to New York City on her own, described her feelings about this major change in her life: "I feel a sense of petrified excitement!" WHAM! Her words hit me between the eyes. In those two words, *petrified excitement*, she captured the essence of the mixture of emotions that often hits us when we have significant changes in our lives.

How we view change is a big part of its impact on us. Even positive changes create a stress response in our bodies as we adapt, but the degree of impact on our body health is dramatically intensified when we perceive changes in our lives as negative ones. All of us are going through biological-psychological-social changes all the time. It's how we *perceive* these changes, what we *do* with them, and how we *use* them in our lives that makes a difference in our psychological hardiness. When we use such changes as opportunities to improve ourselves, to have an impact on others, to better the conditions around us, we create more feelings of control in our lives.

I grew up near the water in Virginia, and I loved sailing. I learned the hard way that there is no way to control the wind. I could plan a weekend sailing getaway down to the last detail, except that I had to face the inevitable: No matter how much I might want to, there is no way I can control the wind. What I had to do was *adjust the sails* to take advantage of whatever way the wind was blowing . . . and accept that sometimes it wasn't blowing at all. There were plenty of days when the wind just died, and I'd be stuck, unable to reach my destination that day. No matter how frustrated and in a dither I got, I could NOT, by force of my will, make the wind pick up. So it was a great lesson in patience, practice, and learning when to just flow with whatever is happening. Many years later, I still struggle with these same issues of learning what I can, and cannot, control in life. I may get angry and holler a lot, or cry, or withdraw. But in these moments of struggle, I also try to stop and remember, with a wry smile, those days of sailing . . . and learning to let go and adjust to the wind and its whims.

Think about this for your life. How do you view yourself? Are you kicking and screaming trying to *make* the wind blow? Or are you learning from experiences and figuring out ways to "trim the sails" to take advantage of whatever wind there is, or even just learning to kick back and flow with circumstances until the wind picks up again? Each of us, based upon how we view ourselves and how we experience our inner sense of power and control, has the ability to increase our self-confidence, self-esteem, and feelings of accomplishment in our lives. And that in turn enhances the *spirit* of the inner self, creating the individual woman who is psychologically hardy.

HARDINESS = CHALLENGE

HARDINESS = CONTROL

HARDINESS = COMMITMENT

Keep these words on your mirror or your refrigerator door, and remind yourself each day:

1. Changes are *challenges and opportunities*; they do not have to be experienced as threats unless you choose to experience them that way.
2. You have *control* in your life, no matter what the situation. You can control the choices you make, even if you cannot control the situation itself. You can control your view of the situation. Such an internal sense of control—"I have the freedom to choose my mental outlook, even in the worst adversity"—creates a strong sense of self. An internal sense of control is the *opposite of powerlessness*, the opposite of being a victim of circumstance.
3. *Commitment* is a pledge to action based on the belief that your life has meaning and purpose. Commitment is the opposite of *alienation*, the opposite of isolation and just drifting through your life. Decide what means something to you and then look for the resources around you to help you achieve it.

In thinking about all of this, remember that if you focus on *daydreaming* about the person *you would like to be,* you end up wasting the time to enjoy being the person you are *now.* Focus instead on your gifts and abilities and talents now and celebrate what is right, good, and wonderful about you as a person.

I moved to Tucson in 1992, having spent my entire life on the East Coast and very much a water-oriented person. Yet, something kept pulling me to the desert and to this land, the sky, and the mountains that protectively encircle Tucson. These mountains feel closer somehow, more *right there*, as if I could reach out and touch them. And the form is a feminine one, the rounded rocks visible down to the very earth itself, giving a sense of ruggedness and strength and permanence. These mountains are *rock*, not covered by the trees as are the mountains of the East and the Rockies. There was something primordial and powerful tugging at my spirit whenever I sat and watched the sunlight and clouds playing over the faces of the Catalina, Rincon, and Tucson mountains. I came across this poem in 1994, which for me captured this ancient connection:

Of Mountains and Women

The hearts of mountains
And the hearts of women
Are both the same. They beat to
An old rhythm, an old song.

Mountains and women
Are made from the sinew of the rock.
Mountains and women
Are home to the spirits of the earth.
Mountains and women
Embrace the mystery of life.
Mountains give patience to women.
Women give fullness to mountains.
Celebrate each mountain, each woman.
Dance for them in your dreams.

The spirit of mountains and of women
Will give courage to our children
Long after we are gone.

© Nancy Wood, *Spirit Walker*,
Doubleday/Delacort Press, 1993
Used with permission.

Each time I came to Tucson to visit over the years, I continued to hear the call of that inner voice pulling me to these mountains, even though my mind kept saying, "But you can't leave your family, friends, patients, and professional ties in Virginia. How are you going to start over *now*?"

I finally listened to the call of my soul and took the leap into the unknown and the uncertainty of a new beginning. Moving from a high rise in the city of Norfolk to a one-story stucco house in Tucson, I felt a strong sense of coming *home* to this land—this land of mountains and sky, of earth and rock; this land of incredible diversity of plants and animals that have found creative ways to adapt to the harsh desert terrain.

In the desert, I have found the connection with the earth, the mountains, and the sky, and in the quiet of the soft breeze I have reconnected with the inner voice that guides me along the path of creative change one small step at a time. And now, years later, I still feel the power of these mountains in the depths of my soul. They are my connection with the earth, and with the Creator. They bring me home, they recharge and revitalize my energy and creativity. They help me learn important lessons, like letting go of a focus on "perfection" and "completion." The way the light plays over the mountain rocks, giving different patterns every moment of every day, serves to remind me of both the permanence and of the changeability of life itself. My goal has become *experiencing* the whole process, experiencing the feelings—joys and pains—of the journey, learning to find the good that comes out of adversity as well as to celebrate the successes, and to take time to savor the moment. With each step, with each small change I make, I am becoming more *whole.*

The Physician Becomes Patient . . . Again

March 27, 1989, was a day of immense despair, pain, and hopelessness in my life. I could not recall ever feeling like I was in such a bottomless dark hole. Previously an energetic, independent, healthy woman in her early forties who had been jogging regularly three to four miles a day, I was now being discharged from Johns Hopkins after my third hospitalization and second spine surgery in three months. The two cervical spine surgeries had been only about six weeks apart, hardly enough time to recover from the first before unexpectedly being faced with a second, which was caused by a bad fall from the physical therapy table during treatment after my first neck surgery.

The last surgery had been complicated and required a fusion of two neck vertebrae using a bone chip from my hip. I was now faced with eight months in a steel two-poster neck brace from chin to chest. My neurosurgeon had just told me the *good* news that I didn't need any more surgery. The *bad* news was that the discs throughout my spine had been damaged badly in the fall and now compounded the difficulty recovering. I was able to walk only a few yards and had such little arm strength I could not even lift a full water pitcher or put on the cumbersome neck brace. The back pain was constant, debilitating, and draining, and I frequently felt exhausted in the morning, even after eight or nine hours in bed.

All of a sudden here I was, unable to do simple things for myself, feeling blind-sided by a tornado, out of control. *This* wasn't the *me* who had been in such good health and had felt so in charge of her life and career. It was definitely not a feeling I liked or wanted. I was supposed to be the one in charge, not the one on the receiving end of this bad news discussion. The neurosurgeon had told me I would need to go into a rehabilitation program for another five to six weeks to strengthen my legs, back, and arms enough that I could return to work later that spring or summer.

It was a devastating blow. I had a sinking feeling as I realized what an impact this would have on my family, my medical practice, and my patients who were counting on me. Yet, there was no choice. I either took more time out from work now for the full recovery from both surgeries, or I faced having long-term limited mobility, pain, and inability to return to work full-time. I had a sense of being outside of myself watching as I fell deeper and deeper into a seemingly endless black well of despair.

I knew enough to recognize that I desperately needed a healing environment, a place where I could get the help I needed from medical and complementary therapies, a place that could provide the mind- and bodywork I needed. I was also concerned about finding a setting where healthy food could help me start to lose the excess weight from recent months of inactivity and corticosteroid therapy. But where could I go? My fall had occurred in a hospital program in my own town; I obviously did not want to go back there. I wasn't severely injured enough to qualify for inpatient rehabilitation programs; besides I knew those programs would not have the kind of massage therapy, healthy food, and other approaches I knew I needed. Yet I couldn't really go to a health club setting in a wheelchair and a neck brace.

What to do, and how to find help? I remembered a place of healing in the Southwest desert, where I thought I could put together the program I needed. My body wisdom knew this was what I needed; yet the rest of my mental processes were so overwhelmed, I could not even think straight and deal with the enormity of the decision. I didn't have the strength or energy even to begin to think about how I could possibly get there or be able to pay for it, since I had been out of work so long.

The inner me *knew* what I needed to recover, but I hadn't yet learned to listen completely to my body wisdom. My husband, my family, my minister, and my friend–business attorney all had the clarity of thinking and insight I lacked at this point. They sorted out the issues and pointed out that I could not take care of anyone or anything else unless I first got well. They helped me make the only decision that could help me survive and begin to heal again. I simply *had* to get into a healing environment where the treatment I desperately needed could be available in one place, even if it meant going into debt and taking a long difficult journey to get there. There was simply no alternative.

But my intellect kept nagging, "wait a minute, I can't leave, I have obligations." Of course, it was apparent to everyone else that I couldn't meet those obligations anyway, even if I stayed at home. I was in such bad shape I *couldn't* work. I just could not see with the clarity they did. I finally accepted that they were right.

What a scary leap it was. I had to trust my body wisdom: I had to let go. I teetered on the edge. Then, as if at one moment, I knew I wanted to get well. I wanted to survive this ordeal and come back strong again. I had to take the leap of faith and put myself in the hands of gifted people from many fields who could help me heal. I agreed to go. I made the choice of *life*. My soul began to feel like flying again. Well, not exactly flying, I guess, when I couldn't even *walk* ten yards. But I did feel instantly lighter in spirit once I had turned the corner and made the decision my inner self knew was necessary and right for me. Mind, body, spirit: All parts of me needed help to get me back on my feet. It was time to start the journey.

Competent and compassionate people in massage therapy, hydrotherapy, physical therapy, nutrition, exercise physiology, hypnotherapy, biofeedback, acupuncture, medicine, nursing, gynecology, and endocrinology all combined their talents to help me get headed back in the right direction and regain my strength and vitality. The healing presence of nature and her beauty, the sunshine, the mountains, the desert air and soft breezes all soothed my body and my weary psyche. My soul was being revived. I felt close to my Creator, grateful to be alive and to have loving people in my life to give my courage a boost. I felt and experienced the recuperative power of combining the best of Western medicine with all that complementary modalities can offer in the healing process. It was a truly transformational experience in my life. I now know that it was a crucial part of my process and preparation to continue my role as a physician, healer, and teacher of other health professionals. A decade later, the year 2000 brought the need for yet another back surgery, but I felt a sense of calm and confidence in dealing with that setback because of all I had gained in wisdom and knowledge of healing approaches from the earlier devastating events. I even see beautiful symbolism in the way the physical body changes and problems parallel the emotional and spiritual lessons.

When you see me today, remember these experiences in my life, and know that I, too, have much in common with those of you who have suffered pain in your lives. I am much like Rainer Marie Rilke, who said of himself in *Letters to A Young Poet:*

Do not believe that he who seeks to comfort you lives untroubled among the simple and quiet words that sometimes do you good. His life has much difficulty and sadness and remains far behind yours. Were it otherwise he would never have been able to find these words [of comfort and healing].

Rilke is saying that his wounds of pain and sadness had awakened his imagination, his creativity, and his care of people. Likewise, had I not been a patient in so many surgeries, and in such physical pain and despair many times in my life, I would not have been able to have such an empathy for what my patients are describing. Sages down through the ages have referred to this as "the wounded healer." Only by passing through the struggles of anxiety, fear, hopelessness, and even the "dark night of the soul," can we find a path leading to faith and trust. I know this feeling well. Historian Roy Nichols also described this process when he wrote about the impact on soul and mind, as well as body, as he dealt with his own terminal illness:

The most beautiful people I have known are those who have known defeat, known suffering, known struggle, known loss and have found their way out of the depths. These people have an appreciation, a sensitivity, and an understanding of life that fills them with compassion, gentleness and a deep loving concern. Beautiful people do not just happen.

In times of crisis in your life, I am sure that each of you has felt a sense of clarity about what "ought" to be done. Finding the courage and strength to carry out what "ought" to be done is another matter. Many times we are afraid to accept that insight because of all the "what ifs" that might happen, or the gamble that we might be taking on a bad choice. Oftentimes we are so confused or disoriented by the darkness of the "hole" we have been sucked into, the hole in which we see ourselves trapped or forced, that we need someone to shine a light in the hole for us to see things more clearly and be able to find a way out. Each of us has these "lights" in our lives, but many times we forget to use them, or to ask people close to us to share *their* light with us to guide the way.

You have the power to be a major influence on the course of your life. Albert Einstein, who had difficulty even getting passing grades in school, said: *"Great spirits have always encountered violent opposition from mediocre minds."* Don't let negative, mediocre minds, even your own, get in the way of what you want to be and accomplish. Be the "great spirit" that you can be, and take charge of your life and well-being. The moment of YOUR power and strength is NOW.

LISTEN to what lies within you. Take a step NOW to *claim* your life for what is important and meaningful to YOU.

Benediction

It has been an awe-filled journey with these women who cross my doorstep in search of answers, in search of ways to rekindle hope. I don't take these responsibilities lightly. And because I don't take these issues lightly, and because I see the devastation in women's lives that can come from misinformation and mistreatment, I find myself at times overcome with anger and immense sadness at what women have been told, at the gross misinformation in the press and books by those who seek only to be a "guru" and sell the most books, or tapes, or vitamins, or wild yam creams, or herbs, or saliva tests or "designer" estrogens . . . or whatever the latest gimmick may be. The appalling morass of myth, hype, misinformation, and distortion, along with the fear tactics frequently used in advertising, creates untold damage and suffering for the women who are seeking help to feel better. Damage is also done by those who fear to venture out of the narrow tunnel vision of their specialty, or who make pronouncements based on their medical training from twenty-five years ago. I don't have an easy answer for you, but I do encourage you to rely on your own wisdom and common sense, and on medical professionals you feel care about you and whose knowledge you can trust, and who are willing to admit when they don't know something.

The following diagram shows how I visualize this process of putting it all together to create a circle of wholeness and integration of the body chemistry/nutritional balance, the body hormonal balance, the body mechanical balance, the psychological balance, and the spiritual balance.

DR. VLIET'S MODEL OF OPTIMAL HEALTH

MEANING IN LIFE
SOUL-SPIRIT
Desire to live,
Desire to get better,
Sense of purpose

SHARING WITH OTHERS
Gives meaning to pain,
Positive benefits of altruism,
Gain new insights, coping skills

EATING WELL—BODY FUEL
Healthy food, vitamins, and
minerals provide chemicals for
body to use to heal and grow,
and benefit from

HORMONES
Provide balance for normal energy,
sleep, brain function, and increase
in pain-relieving chemicals (beta-
endorphins, serotonin, etc.)
Then, you can better use
and benefit from

MEDICATIONS
AND/OR SURGERY
Individually tailored to
relieve residual symptoms

BODYWORK, STRESS RELIEF
TECHNIQUES, HABIT CHANGES,
EXERCISE
These combine to decrease
need for Rx meds or surgery.
If such are needed, they can
be better tailored to relieve
residual symptoms

© Elizabeth Lee Vliet, M.D., 2000

Keep in mind as you design your health plan: Balance is the key. Your body is exquisitely sensitive and precious. It is a beautiful tapestry that needs the proper balance of all its many "threads" to fulfill its mission optimally. That balance will be achieved in different ways, and with different techniques, for different individuals, using the tools of modern medicine coupled with the tools of complementary medicine therapeutics. Each one of us is an individual with different needs. The key is to blend the therapeutic approaches into the blend that is right for you. I know that it is possible to find a way out of the *hormonal haze* with careful attention to healthy food; optimal hormonal balance; exercise; optimal vitamin and mineral supplementation; body therapies; other medications as appropriate; as well as practicing positive mental attitudes, meditation, and prayer. You will be able to find pleasure again, to regain your health, zest, and vitality. New treatment options blossom every year, offering a lot of hope and help. I hope this book has given you new ideas and insights to add to others you have gained in your search.

If we in the healing arts are honest with ourselves and our patients, we must admit that we, too, have doubts and fears and pain like you . . . but when you come to see us for our help, it is our responsibility to focus on your needs, not our own. It is not really appropriate to share our problems with those who are coming to seek help for themselves. So if we seem on the surface to "have it all," or "have it all together," that's not likely to be the complete picture.

As you reflect on your own journey to find health and wellness of being, the decision about which approaches to use is ultimately up to you. I urge you to make your choices from a basis of knowledge, not fear, and when fear does occur, face it head on. Most important: Just **do** something positive to take charge of your journey to finding vitality and meaning in your life. Remember, there are no single answers and one right approach. Start with the options that feel right to you, trust your intuition, and get moving.

Three critical elements are necessary:

- a positive, healing relationship with your health professionals,
- the blend of therapies needed for you as an individual, and
- the active involvement of your own capacity for developing internal self-healing awareness and abilities.

Tap into the power of your mind in taking an active role in your journey to health. Spend time in solitude, or being in nature, or taking a step outside the limits of your own culture. Combine these ingredients to make your own personal sabbatical to look a little deeper into your life and the aspects that you want to change, improve, and expand. When we combine our internal healing power with the appropriate external therapies available to us, the integration enhances our ability to achieve the best state of health we can. It's a different way of looking at things: Someone who has no disease or illness or an easy transition in menopause may still be *unwell*; another person who practices the integration of internal and external healing options may be much more *well* even in the face of significant health problems. If we CHOOSE to use it, engaging our minds to activate the healing ability within us is the most powerful medicine that exists for all of us.

My emphasis throughout my career and in this book has been on creating a health partnership between you and your physicians, to assist you to feel in control of your choices and options. Without YOU having an active commitment to and involvement in YOUR own health care, the healing process breaks down. YOU are the most crucial member of any health care team. My desire is to help you learn the information and skills to take responsibility for your own well-being, and then help you find the necessary resources to reach your goals. I hope this book has given you ideas, new insights, and options to better understand the wonderful miracle of your body and the means to help you achieve your best level of health, wherever you are on life's journey.

The guiding principal for my life and work has been dominated by Ralph Waldo Emerson's thought: *"Do not go where the path may lead, Go instead where there is no path and leave a trail."* Blaze *your* trail into pleasure and zest for the years ahead.

To each of you reading this, I wish for you this Gaelic blessing:

> Deep peace
> Of the running wave to you,
> Deep peace
> Of the quiet earth to you,
> Deep peace
> Of the flowing air to you,
> Deep peace
> Of the shining star to you.

And as I finish my soul's call of writing this book, the words of a Navaho prayer come to mind, as a guide for the trail that lies ahead:

> Happily may I walk.
> May it be beautiful before me.
> May it be beautiful behind me.
> May it be beautiful below me.
> May it be beautiful all around me.
> In beauty it is finished.

> *Mi takuye oyasin*
> All my relations.

LISTEN to what lies within you; make the most of the beautiful and unique person you are. Take a step NOW to *claim* your life for what is important and meaningful to YOU.

SCREAM if you need to.

BE HEARD! Your health, indeed your very soul's survival, depends on it.

It's never too late to be who we might have been.

—GEORGE ELIOT

Appendix I

Glossary of Terms

This is a glossary of some medical terms I have used in my book. If you are going to take charge of your health, it will help for you to become informed about what these terms mean, so you will understand terms used by your physician to explain what is happening to your body.

ABLATION: To remove, as in *endometrial* ablation—a surgical technique to remove as much as possible of the uterine lining (endometrium) to prevent heavy bleeding and reduce the risk of endometrial cancer.

ADRENAL GLANDS: Two small glands situated on top of the kidneys, which secrete steroid hormones (cortisol, aldosterone, DHEA) and the stress hormones epinephrine and norepinephrine (sometimes grouped together in common usage and called *adrenaline*).

AFFECT (AFFECTIVE): A term used to mean "mood" or range of emotional expression. Affective refers to emotional content or to disorders of mood.

AIDS: Acquired Immune Deficiency Syndrome, a sexually transmitted viral disease with a long incubation period; leads to a severe chronic illness that is usually fatal.

ALOPECIA: Loss of hair that is excessive and abnormal. There are many medical, dietary, and lifestyle causes. Anorexia, bulimia, and decline in ovarian and thyroid hormones are common causes in women.

AMENORRHEA: The absence of menstrual bleeding in a woman who has not gone through menopause; may be due to prolonged stress, thyroid disorders, excessive exercise, eating disorders, premature ovarian failure, and other causes.

AMINO ACIDS: Chemical molecules found in foods that serve as the "building blocks" for the body to make its proteins. **Essential amino acids** are those that the body cannot synthesize and that must be included in the food we eat. Dietary protein containing all of the essential amino acids is "complete protein" and can be obtained from animal/dairy products and also by combining at one meal any three of the following: nuts, grains, seeds, or legumes.

ANABOLIC: A term meaning "to build up," as in the *anabolic* phase of metabolism, a process of using nutrients to build larger molecules that are used by the body for growth, repair, and healing. See also **Catabolic** and **Metabolism.**

ANABOLIC STEROIDS: Hormones that stimulate the growth of bone and muscle (lean body mass) and have male ("virilizing") effects on body chemistry and shape.

ANDROGENS: A group of hormones that produces masculine effects on the body. This group of hormones is produced by both the adrenal glands and the gonads (testes in males and ovaries in females). Androgens are produced in much smaller amounts in women compared to men. Androgens decrease with aging in both men and women, but after menopause in women the levels of androgens in women are higher relative to the amount of estrogen that remains. This change in balance of androgens to estrogen produces the characteristic body changes (waist area fat, hair growth on face and chin, etc.) seen in older women.

ANDROGENIC: An adjective used to describe substances (natural or synthetic) that produce masculine changes in the body, stimulating: male pattern hair growth (or loss), oily skin, acne, deepening of the voice, increased appetite, increased muscle mass, increased bone mass, and increased total cholesterol with lower HDL.

ANDROSTENEDIONE: An androgenic hormone produced by the ovaries, testes, and adrenal glands; excess levels in women (such as in PCOS) lead to unwanted facial hair, acne, infertility, body-fat gain around the middle of the body, oily skin, and other masculinizing effects.

ANGINA: Pain in the arm, neck, or chest caused by lack of blood supply (ischemia) to the heart.

ANTIBODIES: Protein substances produced by the body (or transferred from a mother to infant during pregnancy) that react with foreign substances called antigens as part of our immune process. Antibodies are made to foreign tissue such as grafts, bacteria, and viruses; antibodies may also be produced against our own body organs (thyroid, ovary, etc.) in the autoimmune disorders.

ANTIGEN: A substance that triggers the formation of antibodies to stimulate an immune reaction; may be introduced from external sources (bacteria, viruses, etc.) or formed within the body.

ANTIOXIDANT: Substances such as vitamins A, C, and E, beta-carotene, and selenium, which protect the cellular structures from oxidative damage caused by free radicals.

ATHEROSCLEROSIS: artery-clogging deposits formed by cholesterol, fibrin, and "sticky" platelets; a major cause of heart attacks, strokes, angina, and other cardiovascular diseases.

ATROPHY: Wasting or thinning of tissues or organs.

BALLOON THERAPY: See **Uterine balloon therapy.**

BENIGN: Noncancerous or nonmalignant.

BIOAVAILABLE: A substance, often carried in the bloodstream, that is unattached to carrier proteins and therefore able to bind to special receptor sites on cells throughout the body. The amount of a compound or hormone that is "bioavailable" is also called "active" or "free fraction."

BIOFLAVINOIDS: Substances found in plants along with vitamin C that exert a beneficial effect upon the walls of the blood and lymphatic vessels.

BIO-IDENTICAL: A molecule that is exactly the same makeup and configuration as those made by the body. Hormones that are bio-identical may be made in the laboratory from building blocks found in plants, but end up with the same chemical structure as the hormones made by body organs such as the thyroid and ovary. Bio-identical hormones are often called "natural" hormones, but "natural" may also refer to a biological source (such as the horse) that produces molecules different from those made by the human body. Bio-identical is a more correct term than "natural" when referring to the types made by the human body and pharmaceuticals that are designed to duplicate ones made by the body.

BISPHOSPHONATES: A group of medications that prevent excess bone breakdown and stimulate the formation of healthy new bone. Examples are Fosamax, Actonel.

BODY MASS INDEX (BMI): A scientific way of determining body composition. It is calculated according to the formula BMI = weight (kilogram) /height squared (meters). The normal BMI for women ranges from 20 to 25 kg/m2 and many hormonal and menstrual problems can be overcome by keeping weight in the normal range.

BONE RESORPTION: The normal process of bone breakdown or "remodeling" that occurs throughout our lives to allow healthy strong bone to replace older, brittle bone. Resorption can lead to osteoporosis if the bone-building process slows down too much and breakdown (or "withdrawal") of bone exceeds bone formation.

BOUND HORMONE: Hormone that is circulating in the bloodstream connected to a carrier protein (such as sex-hormone-binding globulin, SHBG, or corticosteroid-binding globulin, CBG), and therefore is not "free" to be biologically active at cell receptor sites. (See **Free hormone.**)

BREAKTHROUGH BLEEDING (BTB): Irregular vaginal bleeding or spotting occurring in women when they are taking oral contraceptives or postmenopausal hormone therapy.

CALCITONIN (Thyrocalcitonin): A hormone produced in the thyroid gland that regulates calcium balance in the body.

CALCIUM: A crucial mineral involved in maintaining normal bone strength/density, and normal nerve and muscle function.

CANCER: A malignant growth/tumor with rapid multiplication of abnormal cells that may spread to and invade distant body parts.

CARDIOVASCULAR DISEASE (CVD): Disease of the heart, arteries, veins, and capillaries, which make up the circulatory system.

CATABOLIC: A term meaning "to break down," as in the *catabolic* phase of metabolism, a process of breaking nutrients into smaller molecules that are either utilized by the body for growth and repair, or excreted through the skin, lungs, kidneys, and bowels. See also *Anabolic* and *Metabolism.*

CAT SCAN: A computerized X ray of consecutive sections of the body, which is used to look for tumors, masses, and other abnormal structural changes inside the body.

CELL: The basic unit of structure of all animals and plants that carries out the physical functions of life processes, either by itself or working together with other cells making up organs.

CELLULITE: Fatty deposits resulting in a dimply or lumpy appearance of the skin. It is gradually lost with proper fluid intake, exercise, and overall weight loss.

CERVIX: The opening of the uterus that projects into the vagina. It is also called the mouth of the womb. Some women report that the penis thrusting against the cervix during intercourse leads to greater sexual stimulation and more intense orgasm, which may be a reason to leave the cervix if a woman needs to have the uterus removed.

CHLAMYDIA: A sexually transmitted bacteria that is a common cause of pelvic infection and infertility.

CHLOASMA: Brownish pigmentation of the face that can occur in pregnancy (may also be caused by some types of hormonal imbalance and progestin-dominant birth control pills).

CHOLESTEROL: An important body molecule that is the precursor for the body to make sex hormones, adrenal hormones, and other molecules. It is found in the blood in three forms: (1) High Density Lipoprotein (HDL), which *protects* against plaque formation in the arteries (atherosclerosis); (2) Low Density Lipoprotein (LDL), which *promotes* plaque formation (atherosclerosis); and (3) Very Low Density Lipoprotein (VLDL), also a plaque promoter. Cholesterol is produced in the liver even when dietary intake is lowered, and it is found in all animal fats and oils (butter, milk, meat, cheese, etc).

CIRCADIAN RHYTHM: The regular, rthymic pattern of changes in biological activity and function that occurs over the course of a day. Examples of circadian rhythms are our sleep-wake cycle and the daily cyclic variation in cortisol and melatonin secretion.

CLIMACTERIC: The span of years in a woman's life when hormone levels are gradually decreasing, leading to changes in body shape and function ultimately ending in the last menstrual period.

CLITORIS: The female equivalent (embryologically) of the penis. It is a small bulb found at the top of the vulva, just below the pubic bone, and is covered by a hood of tissue. It contains erectile tissue and nerve endings that are very sensitive to stimulation and enhance a woman's sexual arousal and orgasm. Clitoral nerve endings become less sensitive at menopause with declining hormone levels.

CLOTTING FACTORS: Substances carried in the bloodstream that promote coagulation (the process of clotting), such as prothrombin, thrombin, thromboplastin, calcium in ionic form, and fibrinogen. Clotting can be retarded by cold, smooth surfaces, and other substances. Clotting is hastened by warming or by providing a rough surface (such as plaque inside arteries). Medications may be given to promote or decrease clotting.

CLUSTER HEADACHE: A severe and intense headache, more common in males, which lasts several hours and may recur frequently over a six-to eight-week period.

COMBINED ORAL CONTRACEPTIVE PILL (OC): A contraceptive pill containing both female sex hormones, estrogen and a synthetic progestin. To contrast the *combined* OC, there are also progestin-only contraceptives (Micronor is an oral tablet; Norplant and Depo-Provera are long-acting implants/injectables).

COMPLEX CARBOHYDRATES: Carbohydrates are macronutrients that provide a quick energy source. Complex carbohydrates refers to those found occurring naturally "complexed" with fiber, minerals, and other nutrients (such as whole grains, fruits, vegetables). They are more slowly absorbed and utilized than processed or refined carbohydrates (sweets, pasta, white bread).

CONCEPTION: The fertilization of the female egg by the spermatozoa (sperm).

CONJUGATED ESTROGENS: A mixture of estrogens, chemically different from those made in the human female ovary, that may come from animals (Premarin, horse) or plants (Cenestin).

CONSENT FORM: A legal document that you are required to sign, thereby giving your consent before undergoing a surgical operation or before taking some medications.

CONTRAINDICATION: A medical condition that makes it inadvisable to use a certain medication, for example, the presence of breast cancer would usually contraindicate taking estrogen; cigarette smoking is a contraindication for using the oral birth control pill.

CORPUS LUTEUM: The yellow, progesterone-producing sac that is formed within the ovary from the remains of the follicle after it has released its egg at ovulation.

CORTICOSTEROID: (also glucocorticoid) Any of a number of steroid hormones produced by the cortex of the adrenal gland. Cortisol is an example.

CORTISOL: An adrenal cortical hormone (glucocorticoid), usually referred to as our body's "stress" hormone because it prepares the body to respond to emergencies or stresses. It is closely related to cortisone in physiological effects.

CORTISONE: A steroid compound made naturally by the adrenal glands and also produced synthetically in laboratories for use as a drug. It has a powerful anti-inflammatory effect but may produce many adverse side effects with high levels over long periods of time.

CREATININE: The end product of creatine metabolism; found in muscle tissue, blood, and urine. High levels may indicate excess muscle breakdown, for example, or advanced stages of kidney disease.

CUSHING'S SYNDROME (DISEASE): A group of symptoms and signs such as moon-shaped face, buffalo hump, and high blood pressure caused by excessive amounts of cortisone either produced by the adrenal gland or taken as medication.

CYSTIC ACNE: A skin disorder manifesting as blocked pores and pimples, many of which are blind cysts containing pus. It is a severe form of acne.

DAIDZEIN: Isoflavone compound (also called phytoestrogen) found in soy and other plants that has weak estrogenic effects.

DEXA (Dual Energy X-ray Absorptiometry). A highly reliable means of measuring bone mineral density using very small amounts of radiation. Recommended for women with multiple risk factors for osteopenia/osteoporosis, or women who want a baseline measure before beginning menopause.

DHEA: Dehydroepiandrosterone. One of the androgens ("male" hormones) produced in the adrenal glands and ovary in women. Excess levels cause facial hair, scalp hair loss, oily skin, and acne among other changes.

DISOGENIN: A steroid compound found in wild yam and other plants that is used by pharmaceutical companies as a "building block" or precursor molecule to make bioidentical forms of human hormones such as progesterone and 17-beta estradiol. Disogenin in extracts of wild yam (found in skin creams) cannot be converted by the human body to progesterone or estradiol because we lack the necessary enzymes to do this.

DIURETIC: A substance, whether synthetic or natural, that stimulates the kidneys to excrete salt (sodium chloride) and water, thereby relieving fluid retention.

DIURNAL: Variation by time of day. For example, hormones in the body often are higher at one time of day and lower at another in a predictable pattern. Diseases may alter the normal diurnal pattern. An example: melatonin is normally highest at night (promotes sleep) and lowest in the bright sunlight of daytime. Melatonin that doesn't shut off properly in the daytime is considered a cause of seasonal affective disorder syndrome ("winter depression" or SAD).

DOPAMINE: A mood-elevating chemical messenger produced in the brain and body; it is also important in preventing Parkinson's disease, and as an inhibitory neurotransmitter preventing inappropriate milk secretion by the breast.

DOWN-REGULATION: A process in the brain and body in which the number (or function) of cell receptors is decreased. May occur as a natural process or due to medication effects.

ECTOPIC PREGNANCY: A pregnancy implanted in an abnormal position, usually inside a fallopian tube; may cause severe pain, hemorrhage, and infection if it ruptures into the pelvis.

ENDOCRINE GLANDS: Glands that manufacture and secrete hormones.

ENDOCRINOLOGIST: A medical specialist in diseases of the endocrine glands and their hormones; Endocrinology is the study and treatment of disorders of the glands and the hormones they secrete.

ENDOMETRIAL ABLATION: A surgical technique to remove as much as possible of the uterine lining (endometrium) to prevent heavy bleeding and reduce the risk of endometrial cancer.

ENDOMETRIAL HYPERPLASIA: Abnormal degree of thickening of the lining of the uterus, usually due to excess estrogen effect with insufficient progesterone or progestin effect. If left uncontrolled, may lead over time to the development of endometrial cancer.

ENDOMETRIAL LINING (ENDOMETRIUM): The lining of the uterus. This tissue grows under the influence of estrogen (*proliferative* endometrium), and thickens under the influence of progesterone each month (*secretory* endometrium) in the menstrual cycle. The fall in progesterone (or a progestin, such as Provera, Aygestin and others), triggers the secretory endometrium to "slough" and then be shed from the uterus in the monthly bleeding.

ENDOMETRIOSIS: The presence of small islands (implants) of endometrium lying outside of the uterus, scattered about the abdomen and pelvic cavities and many times stuck on the outside of the intestine and bladder. Endometrium tissue is normally found only *inside* the uterus, and menstrual blood is released to the *outside* of the body via the vagina. When these implants bleed at the time of menses, they cause such severe pain because the blood is *released into* the abdomen and pelvis and acts as a significant irritant to other organs.

ENDORPHINS (ENKEPHALINS): Natural pain-relieving and mood-elevating compounds (peptides) produced in the brain, spinal cord, and body to produce a morphine-like analgesia.

ENTEROHEPATIC CIRCULATION: Blood flow from the gastrointestinal tract to the liver, which prolongs the action of compounds such as estrogen and other hormones by allowing them to "recirculate" rather than being excreted in the stool.

ENZYMES: Proteins produced by living cells that assist body functions by acting as catalysts in specific biochemical reactions. Enzyme catalysts are not themselves consumed in the reactions.

EPINEPHRINE (ADRENALINE): A chemical messenger made by the adrenal gland that prepares the body to handle emergencies, called the fight-or-flight response. Epinephrine is also made in the laboratory to be used as a drug to treat severe allergic reactions, asthma, severe bleeding, and certain types of heart rhythm problems.

EQUINE ESTROGENS, EQUILIN: Estrogens derived from **pregnant mares'** urine and used to make the animal-derived estrogen, Premarin. These estrogens are chemically different from the ones made by the human ovary. They have some effects that are similar to human estrogens, and some effects that are quite different from human estrogens. See chapters 5, 13, and 15 for detailed explanations.

ESSENTIAL FATTY ACIDS: Fatty acids necessary for cellular metabolism that cannot be made by the body but must be supplied in the diet. Good sources are fish oil, oils from nuts and seeds, and evening primrose oil.

ESTROGEN: The group of three sex hormones produced by the gonads (ovary in women, testes in men), and by the adrenal gland. In women, the higher amounts of these sex hormones are responsible for the female characteristics of breasts, feminine curves, menstruation, pregnancy.
  • **ESTRONE (E1):** One of the human estrogens made by the ovary, adrenal gland, and body fat before menopause. It is the one found in higher amounts after menopause because it is still made by body fat and to a lesser extent, the adrenal glands. Estrone serves as a "storage" form of estrogen for the ovary to make the more active estradiol before menopause. High estrone levels are more associated with breast and uterine cancers, a good reason to maintain a healthy percentage of body fat and weight.

- **ESTRADIOL (E2, 17-beta estradiol):** The primary estrogen produced by the ovary before menopause. It is the biologically active estrogen at the estrogen receptors and the most potent of all the natural human estrogens. Estradiol is involved in over 400 functions in a woman's body and is the form of estrogen that is lost at menopause when the ovary follicles are depleted.
- **ESTRIOL (E3):** The weakest of the primary human estrogens, it is produced in large amounts during pregnancy. It is barely detectable in the *nonpregnant* female body, so women do not normally have estriol present to a measurable degree on a continuous basis, and it has not been shown to have bone-, heart-, or brain-preserving effects.
- **ESTRADIOL VALERATE:** A more potent, synthetic estrogen, chemically different from the 17-beta estradiol produced by the ovary; used for menopausal hormone therapy in Europe for many years, but not used very often in the United States.
- **ETHINYL ESTRADIOL:** A more potent synthetic estrogen used in birth control pills where the higher potency is needed (with the synthetic progestins) to adequately suppress the ovaries and provide reliable contraception. Not generally used in the United States for menopausal hormone therapy.

EVENING PRIMROSE OIL: The oil extracted from the evening primrose plant. It is a good source of the omega-6 fatty acids, in particular the essential fatty acid know as gamma linolenic acid (GLA).

FALLOPIAN TUBES: The tubes that carry the egg (ovum) from the ovary to the uterus. Fertilization of the egg occurs in the outer part of the fallopian tube.

FEEDBACK: The process by which products made in a series of reactions provide messages back to the beginning of the process to control further reactions. Feedback may be electrical, chemical or mechanical, or thermal. Example of a thermal "feedback" is the thermostat that controls your furnace. Chemical feedback occurs with hormone levels reach a critical level and feed back to the brain that no more is needed for awhile.

FEMALE SEX HORMONES: The two sex hormones produced by the female ovary and placenta during pregnancy, estrogen (see above for types) and progesterone.

FERTILIZATION: The union of the female egg (ovum) with the male sperm (spermatozoa), which occurs in the fallopian tube.

FETUS: A developing human from the end of the eighth week of pregnancy until birth.

FIBROCYSTIC: Development of dense, lumpy, ropy (fibrous) changes in tissue. About 60–70 percent of healthy women will have "fibrocystic" changes in their breasts, and this does not indicate a disease process. Similar changes may occur in muscle tissue in chronic pain syndromes.

FIBROIDS (FIBROMAS): Noncancerous growths of the uterus consisting of muscle and fibrous tissue. The medical term is leiomyoma, or sometimes just "myomas." The presence of fibroids tends to cause heavy, painful bleeding and cramps. At times they cause back pain, referred pain to the hip, or bladder pain and pressure with incontinence, depending on where the fibroids are found in the uterus.

FIRST-PASS METABOLISM: Breakdown of chemicals, medications, hormones, et cetera, by the liver as a first-step after being absorbed into the bloodstream from the gastrointestinal tract. First-pass metabolism can eliminate as much as 70 percent or more of an oral dose of a medication or hormone. This step is omitted when medications and hormones are absorbed directly into the bloodstream from the skin (patch or cream) or muscle (injection).

FOLLICLE STIMULATING HORMONE (FSH): A hormone secreted by the pituitary gland that reaches the ovaries via the blood circulation and stimulates the growth of ovarian follicles to form the egg that is released at ovulation. FSH above 10–15 when the brain senses a decline in ovarian hormones, and levels of FSH greater than 20 are defined as menopausal. FSH also functions in men to stimulate the sperm-producing cells in the testes; high FSH levels in men indicate low levels of testosterone, sometimes called "andropause."

FOLLICULAR (PHASE): The first half of the ovarian hormone cycle leading up to the release of the egg at ovulation. Estrogen (estradiol) is the dominant hormone for this part of the cycle, and there is very little progesterone present.

FREE HORMONE: Hormone that is circulating in the bloodstream not connected to a carrier protein, and therefore "free" to be biologically active at cell receptor sites. See also **Bound hormone.**

FREE RADICAL: "Scavenger" molecules that attack and damage body cells and tissues because they are so highly reactive. Antioxidant compounds in the body, such as vitamin E and C, bind up these free radicals and help prevent damage to cells.

FRIGID (SEXUAL): A negative term applied to women who are considered by their partner to be sexually unresponsive and disinterested. Hormonal, medical, and relationship factors may cause loss of sexual desire and responsiveness, and all of these should be properly evaluated to determine the cause of sexual difficulties.

GALACTORRHEA: The presence of milk or milky fluid in the breasts when not breastfeeding. It is usually a symptom of elevated prolactin, which may be caused by some medications (such as antidepressants) or by benign hormone-producing tumors (adenomas) of the pituitary gland.

GAMMA AMINOBUTYRIC ACID (GABA): An inhibitory neurotransmitter in the brain and nerves throughout the body; activation of this neurotransmitter produces a calming or antianxiety effect.

GAMMA LINOLENIC ACID (GLA): An omega-6 essential fatty acid that is used to synthesize prostaglandins. It has an anti-inflammatory effect in the body. Good sources: breastmilk, evening primrose oil, borage plant oil, and black currant seed oil.

GENISTEIN: Isoflavone compound (also called phytoestrogen) found in soy and other plants that has weak estrogenlike effects. In some concentrations it acts to block estrogen receptors, while in other concentrations it may stimulate the estrogen receptors in certain tissues.

GLANDS: Body organs or tissues, generally soft and fleshy in consistency, that manufacture and secrete or excrete hormones, chemicals that exert their effects on target organs elsewhere in the body.

GLUCOCORTICOID: A group of hormones produced in the adrenal cortex that are primarily active in protecting against stress and in regulating protein and carbohydrate metabolism. These compounds (such as cortisone) tend to increase blood glucose, liver glycogen, and suppress the immune response and inflammatory response. Levels that are too high over time cause bone loss.

GYNECOLOGY: Surgical specialty of medicine that provides surgical and medicinal treatments for problems related to women's reproductive organs.

HALF-LIFE: A measurement of how long it takes for half of a substance to be lost or removed; for example, drug half-life refers to how long it takes for the concentration of a drug or hormone to be decreased by one-half due to metabolic breakdown or excretion. It is usually estimated that it takes five half-lives for a substance to be completely gone from the body.

HDL: See **Cholesterol.**

HIRSUTISM: A condition of excessive facial and body hair (excluding hair on the scalp) and often in women is due to excess of androgens.

HORMONE RECEPTOR SITE: A "binding" or "docking" site in or on cells for hormones to connect in order to exert their actions. The hormone and its receptor create what is called a "receptor complex" that sends signals to the cell to carry out various functions.

HORMONE REPLACEMENT THERAPY (HRT): Technically, the administration of any hormonal preparations (natural or synthetic) to replace the loss of natural hormones produced by various glands (thyroid, ovary, testes, pancreas, adrenal, pituitary, etc.). HRT in *common* usage now refers to administration of female hormones (estrogen and progestin) after menopause.

HORMONES: Chemicals produced by various glands that are then transported around the body to exert their multiple metabolic effects.

HOT FLASH (FLUSH): Episode of vasodilation in skin of head, neck, and chest, accompanied by sensation of suffocation, sweating, feeling suddenly hot or cold. Occurs commonly during menopause due to falling hormone levels that trigger changes in the brain heat regulatory center.

HYPERTHYROIDISM: A condition caused by excessive hormone secretion of the thyroid glands that will increase the basal metabolic rate, increase heart rate and blood pressure, disrupt sleep, and may cause marked weight loss.

HYPOTHALAMUS: The "master conductor" or "control center" situated at the base of the brain regulates body temperature, thirst, appetite, sex drive, and all other hormonal glands. It releases hormones that travel directly to the pituitary gland and stimulate the release of pituitary hormones, which govern the other endocrine glands.

HYPOTHYROIDISM: A slowing of overall body metabolism due to deficiency of the thyroid hormone production or function. There are many diverse symptoms, but common ones include obesity, dry skin and hair, low blood pressure, slow pulse, sluggishness of all functions, constipation, depressed mood, muscle aches/weakness, hair loss, low energy, goiter.

HYSTERECTOMY: Surgical removal (abdominal or vaginal) of the uterus only. In common usage, women may say "hysterectomy" when both the uterus and ovaries have been removed or when just the uterus has been removed. The medical term for removal of the uterus and ovaries together is *hysterectomy with bilateral salpingo-oophorectomy (BSO).*

IMMUNE SYSTEM: The defense and surveillance system of the body that protects against infection by microorganisms and invasion by foreign tissues and substances. The immune system is made up of specialized blood cells (lymphocytes, B-cells, T-cells, etc.), blood proteins (antibodies), the spleen, thymus gland, lymph nodes, bone marrow. Immune function is impaired with a variety of endocrine imbalances, such as menopause and thyroid disorders.

IMPLANT: A device that is surgically implanted into a part of the body for cosmetic or therapeutic purposes. Hormone-containing implants are sometimes used for contraception or for menopausal hormone replacement therapy.

INFLAMMATION: A condition characterized by swelling, redness, heat, and pain in any tissue as a result of trauma, irritation, infection, or imbalances in immune function.

INSULIN: A hormone secreted by beta cells of the pancreas that is essential for the proper metabolism of blood sugar (glucose), for maintenance of proper blood sugar level, and for promoting storage of fat. Insulin medication is used to control high blood sugar in diabetes.

ISOFLAVONE: Chemical compounds found in a variety of plants (soy, red clover, etc.) that are weakly estrogenic in their effects and are often called phytoestrogens (*phyto* meaning "derived from plants"). Common isoflavones that are being studied for their health effects are genistein, daidzein, biochanin, and formononetin.

IUD: Intrauterine device, an object inserted into the uterus, typically used for contraception, but may also be a means of delivering hormones (e.g., Progestasert progestin delivery sytem).

LAPAROSCOPE: A long, thin telescopic instrument utilizing a fiberoptic lighting system, which is inserted through a small incision in the abdominal wall. It functions like a hollow flashlight enabling the surgeon to view internal organs and insert operating instruments through its hollow tube.

LAPAROSCOPY: Surgical techniques used in gynecology, general surgery, orthopedic surgery and others that are performed through the laparoscope in order to use smaller incisions and still visualize areas inside the body. In many cases, laparoscopic surgery means shorter recovery time.

LDL: See **Cholesterol.**

LIBIDO: Level of sexual desire, sexual energy, or drive.

LUTEAL (PHASE): The progesterone-dominant second half of the menstrual cycle, from ovulation until menses begin. The primary hormone of this phase is progesterone. It is also the time of the cycle when PMS occurs.

LUTEINIZING HORMONE (LH): A hormone produced by the pituitary gland that triggers ovulation and the egg release to become the corpus luteum. In men, LH stimulates production of testosterone by the testes, and LH levels will rise in men with low testosterone.

MALE HORMONE: A hormone that promotes masculine characteristics in the body such as facial and body hair, acne, deepening of the voice, increased muscle mass, and increased libido.

MALIGNANT: Cancer, cancerous.

MANIC DEPRESSION (BIPOLAR DISORDER): A biological disorder of brain function that produces episodes of euphoria, delusions, and abnormally increased energy, alternating at variable intervals with severe depressions.

MELATONIN: A hormone produced by the pineal gland in the brain; it is involved in regulating the sleep-wake cycle; levels rise during darkness and fall at daylight. Excess melatonin levels that fail to shut off during the day have been thought to cause seasonal affective disorder (SAD).

MENOPAUSE: The cessation of menstruation. The last period. May be natural (due to depletion of the ovarian follicles) or due to surgical removal of the uterus (without or with removal of ovaries). When the ovaries are gone or have lost their follicles, the body loses the hormones estradiol, progesterone, testosterone, and much of the DHEA. The period of time leading up the menopause, when hormone production by the ovaries is decreasing, is called the climacteric.

MENSTRUAL CLOCK: A specialized part of the hypothalamus regulating the cyclical timing of the phases of the menstrual cycle.

MENSTRUATION: Monthly bleeding from the vagina in women from puberty until menopause, caused by shedding of the lining of the womb (uterus) if there is no fertilization of an egg.

METABOLIC HORMONES: Hormones that are involved in regulating cellular energy processes, synthesis of body proteins, and other functions involved in tissue growth and repair.

METABOLIC RATE: The rate at which the body converts chemical energy in foods into heat (thermal) and movement (kinetic) energy. Metabolic rate is governed by hormones from the thyroid, ovary, testes, adrenal glands, and pancreas.

METABOLISM: Chemical processes, regulated by hormones, utilizing the raw materials of food nutrients, oxygen, minerals, vitamins along with enzymes to produce energy for body functions such as growth, repair, healing. See also **Anabolic, Catabolic metabolism.**

METABOLITE: Any product of metabolism. Some metabolites are active and needed for other functions, and some metabolites may be toxic and need to be excreted. An example of a toxic metabolite is ammonia from the breakdown of protein; an active metabolite of progesterone has anxiety-relieving properties when it binds to the brain's GABA receptor.

MICROGRAM: One-millionth part of a gram. One thousandth of a milligram. The abbreviation on prescriptions is mcg.

MILLIGRAM: One-thousandth of a gram. The abbreviation on prescriptions is mg. See also **Picogram, Nanogram.**

MILLILITER: One-thousandth of a liter, or about 1 cc. The abbreviation on prescriptions is ml.

MINERALOCORTICOID: Hormones produced by the adrenal gland that primarily function to regulate electrolytes (sodium, potassium, chloride) and water balance in the body. An example is aldosterone.

MOLECULE: A chemical compound made up of different arrangements and types of atoms; a molecule is the smallest unit into which a substance may be divided without loss of its unique characteristics.

MYOMECTOMY: Surgical removal of fibroids (myomas) but leaving the uterus and cervix intact. This procedure preserves fertility, but frequently may become a more complicated surgery with greater blood loss than hysterectomy. Complications and risk of damage may be similar to hysterectomy. Careful evaluation by an experienced surgeon is important to determine whether a woman is a good candidate for myomectomy.

NANOGRAM: One-billionth of a gram, abbreviated as ng.

"NATURAL" HORMONE: Bio-identical hormones are often called "natural" hormones, but "natural" may also refer to a biological source (such as the horse) that produces molecules different from those made by the human body. *Bio-identical* is a more correct term than natural when referring to the types made by the human body and pharmaceuticals that are designed to duplicate ones made by the body. Hormones that are bio-identical may be made in the laboratory from building blocks found in plants, but end up with the same chemical structure as the hormones made by body organs such as the thyroid and ovary.

NEURON: A nerve cell, the structure and functional unit of the nervous system. Neurons function in initiation and conduction of electrical and chemical "nerve" impulses.

NEUROTRANSMITTERS: Chemicals that transmit messages from nerve cell to nerve cell in the brain, and between the brain and the tissues and organs of the body. Common ones referred to throughout this book are serotonin, dopamine, acetylcholine, GABA, norepinephrine.

NONANDROGENIC: Not causing masculine hormone effects in the body.

NOREPINEPHRINE (NORADRENALINE): A hormone produced by the adrenal gland and certain areas of the brain that helps the body prepare for and cope with stress. It also has a mood-elevating effect, but levels that are too high may cause feelings of anxiety, raise blood pressure, and cause insomnia. Epinephrine (adrenaline) is another "stress hormone" produced by the adrenal gland with similar effects in some tissues and opposite effects in others.

NUCLEUS: The vital body inside cells that contains the genetic material (DNA) and is responsible for regulation of essential functions for cell growth, protein synthesis, metabolism, reproduction, and transmission of characteristics of a cell.

OOPHORECTOMY (OVARIECTOMY): Surgical removal of the ovaries.

ORAL: Indicating something is to be taken by mouth.

ORGASM: The physical and emotional release of sexual arousal tension; also called *climax*.

OSTEOBLAST: Cells that function to build new bone. These cells are stimulated by estradiol, testosterone, and, to a lesser extent, progesterone.

OSTEOCLAST: Cells that are responsible for resorption (breaking down) of old, brittle bone. Their action is regulated primarily by estradiol and testosterone to a lesser extent.

OSTEOPENIA: Loss of bone density that is not yet severe enough to be considered osteoporosis. Osteopenia will progress to osteoporosis if active measures are not taken to maintain bone (such as calcium, magnesium, exercise, and hormone therapy).

OSTEOPOROSIS: Loss of bone density (mass) due to loss of bone minerals and reduction of the normal bony architecture that provides strength to the skeleton. Causes bones to become porous, brittle, and more easily broken.

OVA (OVUM): An ovarian follicle that has been released to become the egg (ova) at ovulation. An ova that is fertilized with sperm becomes an embryo that develops into a fetus.

OVARIAN BLOOD SUPPLY: The blood carried to the ovaries via the ovarian arteries, which branch off from the uterine blood vessels. The ovarian arteries run alongside the fallopian tubes and may be injured or damaged with surgical procedures on the tubes (such as tubal ligation or hysterectomy, even if the ovaries are not removed).

OVARIES: The female sex glands (gonads) located on each side of the uterus, which produce eggs and the female sex hormones (estrogen and progesterone), along with small amounts of testosterone.

OVULATION: The release of the egg from the ovary occurring around mid-cycle.

OVULATION PAIN: "Mittelschmerz" pain occurring at ovulation, which may be sharp and severe and last from a few minutes up to twelve hours.

PANCREAS: A gland situated behind the stomach that produces pancreatic juice (contains digestive enzymes such as lipase and amylase) and also the hormones insulin and glucagon, which function to regulate blood sugar and carbohydrate metabolism.

PARASYMPATHETIC NERVOUS SYSTEM: The part of the autonomic nervous system that regulates body relaxation and functions of growth and repair such as digestion. Its primary chemical messenger or neurotransmitter is acetylcholine.

PARATHYROID GLANDS: Located close to the thyroid gland, one of several small endocrine glands that secretes a hormone, parathormone, that regulates calcium-phosphorus metabolism.

PARENTERAL: A method of delivering substances (such as medications) directly to the bloodstream, bypassing the digestive system and liver metabolism. Parenteral routes include: vaginal and rectal suppositories/tablets, sublingual tablets/capsules, transdermal (skin patch), subcutaneous (implant), intramuscular (IM), and intravenous (IV) injections.

PEAK LEVEL: The highest level of a hormone or medication that is reached after taking a dose or being produced by the body. ("Trough" level is the lowest point reached after a medication or hormone is taken or produced by the body.)

PELVIC INFLAMMATORY DISEASE (PID): Inflammation of the pelvic organs, particularly the uterus and fallopian tubes, caused by infectious microorganisms, typically occurring from sexually transmitted bacteria, fungi, and viruses.

PERIMENOPAUSE: Time frame of several years prior to menopause when menstrual periods start to be skipped and continuing through menopause to the first few years just after periods stop. It has a variable age of onset and symptoms commonly include insomnia, mood changes, bone loss, cholesterol changes, disrupted sleep, hot flashes, and other phenomena. See also **premenopause.**

PESSARY: An oval object designed to be inserted into the vagina for support of a prolapsed uterus or bladder; may also be used to deliver medications or hormones to vaginal tissue.

PHARMACOKINETICS/ DYNAMICS: Study of drug absorption, delivery to tissues of the body, metabolism, and excretion.

PHYSIOLOGICAL: Normal body processes and functions.

PHYTOESTROGENS: Plant-derived (phyto) chemical molecules that may attach to the body's estrogen receptors and trigger certain estrogenlike actions; some of these compounds have estrogen-blocking actions (antagonists) that may or may not be desirable. These occur naturally in several hundred different types of plants, including soy, clover, and a variety of grains.

PICOGRAM: One-trillionth of a gram, abbreviated pg.

PITUITARY GLAND: A mushroom-shaped gland connected by a vascular stalk to the base of the brain. The pituitary gland manufactures hormones (FSH, LH, TSH, ACTH, and others) that in turn control other hormonal glands such as the thyroid, adrenals, ovaries, and breasts.

PLACENTA: The hormonal organ designed to provide for the nourishment of the fetus and the elimination of its waste products. It produces a number of hormones, such as progesterone and estriol, that have roles in sustaining pregnancy and adapting the mother's body to adjust to the increased physiological demands of pregnancy. It is formed in the uterus by the union of uterine mucous membrane with membranes of the fetus.

PLAQUE: A deposit of platelets, fibrin, calcium, cholesterol, and other fatty substances that build up in arteries and cause clogging that leads to reduced blood flow and may cause angina, heart attacks, or strokes. The whole process of plaque buildup and artery damage is referred to as atherosclerosis.

PLASMA: The liquid part of blood and the lymph (minus the red and white blood cells) that contains proteins, clotting factors, and other chemicals such as glucose, hormones, et cetera.

PMS: See **Premenstrual Syndrome.**

POLYCYSTIC OVARY SYNDROME (PCOS): A hereditary disorder of the ovaries in which the usual female hormonal balance is altered, and there are excessive levels of insulin and male hormones accompanied by changes in body shape and irregular menstruation. It may also be triggered by stress or weight gain. In PCOS the ovaries have multiple small follicles or "cysts," which can be seen on an ultrasound scan of the pelvis. Other common features: truncal obesity, acne, glucose intolerance and insulin resistance, hypertension, infertility, and changes in mood related to the hormonal imbalances.

POSTMENOPAUSE: The years following the end of menstruation and decline in production of ovarian female hormones (menopause).

POSTNATAL, POSTPARTUM: The time period after childbirth.

PRECURSOR: A substance (building block) that is used to make another compound, hormone or medication. For example, cholesterol molecules are used as the building blocks for the body to make other steroid hormones, such as progesterone.

PREMATURE MENOPAUSE: Cessation of menses and decline of ovarian hormone production occurring before the age of forty-two.

PRE-MENOPAUSAL: The time leading up to menopause characterized by hormonal changes and irregular menstrual flow. It may begin as much as ten years before actual menopause, but more commonly occurs about four to five years before menopause (see also perimenopause).

PREMENSTRUAL SYNDROME (PMS): A collection of variable symptoms such as mood disturbance, headaches, abdominal bloating, et cetera, recurring on a cyclical basis in the week or two before menstrual bleeding. See also **Perimenopause.**

PROGESTERONE: A steroid hormone produced by the corpus luteum (formed from the egg released at ovulation in the ovary) or placenta during pregnancy. Small amounts are also made by the adrenal glands. Responsible for secretory changes in uterine endometrium in second half of menstrual cycle to prepare the uterus to receive and nourish a fertilized egg. Progesterone also has many metabolic functions designed help a mother's body change in ways that will support a pregnancy (progestation hormone = progesterone).

PROGESTIN: A group of hormones that have progesterone-like effects on the uterus and body; progesterone is correctly included in this larger class of hormones, but common usage usually means that "progestin" refers to synthetic compounds that are made in the laboratory and are chemically different from the natural ovary compound progesterone.

PROGESTIN-ONLY PILL ("mini-pill"): A contraceptive pill containing only a progestin such as norethindrone (Micronor and others). Unless it is given with estrogen to balance the unwanted side effects, the progestin-only pills are not recommended for midlife women due to the potential for adverse effects on cholesterol, glucose control and body weight. Progestin-only pills, implants, or injections are not recommended for women with a history of depression, diabetes, headaches, hypertension, or weight gain as progestins aggravate all of these problems unless estrogen is also given.

PROGESTOGENS: Natural or synthetic substances that have effects similar to the natural female hormone progesterone. Synthetic progestogens (called progestins) are commonly used in birth control pills and HRT to regulate menstrual bleeding. Examples are medroxyprogesterone acetate (Provera, Cycrin), norethindrone (Aygestin, Micronor), norethisterone, norgestrel, et cetera.

PROLACTIN: A hormone secreted by the pituitary gland that stimulates milk production in the breasts. At times other than nursing, high levels of prolactin may cause headaches, weight gain, depression, and breast discharge (galactorrhea).

PROSTAGLANDINS: Chemicals manufactured throughout the body that exert a hormonelike effect and influence muscular (including the uterus) contraction, circulation, and inflammation. Release of prostaglandins in the uterus at the time of menstruation is a cause of menstrual cramps.

PROSTATE GLAND: This gland is located just below the bladder in men and secretes fluid into the ejaculate of semen during male orgasm.

PSYCHOSIS: A severe biochemical disorder of brain function characterized by delusions, hallucinations, and abnormalities in thinking and reasoning. It may be due to many causes: schizophrenia, major depression, manic-depressive disorder, alcohol intoxication, severe endocrine illness (e.g., hyper- and hypothyroidism), drug abuse (cocaine), and medication toxicity (such as atropine, digitalis, lidocaine, stimulants, and many others).

PSYCHOSOMATIC: Physical symptoms that are triggered by psychological and emotional causes and not due primarily to physical disease. This term is often misused when applied to women, as in "the cause isn't known so it must be psychosomatic, or stress-related."

PSYCHOTHERAPY: The process of using systematic "talking" approaches to treat stress-related problems, emotional issues, and disturbances in self-image. Many different methods may be used, depending upon the training of the therapist.

PSYCHOTROPIC DRUGS: Drugs that act primarily on the brain to produce effects on mood, thinking, sleep, and other functions. Examples are sedatives, tranquilizers (antianxiety agents), antidepressants, antipsychotics, analgesic and anesthetic agents.

PUERPERIUM: The period of time after childbirth required to return the reproductive organs to their prepregnant size and condition. This takes six to eight weeks.

RECEPTOR: See **Hormone receptor site.**

RECEPTOR ANTAGONIST (BLOCKER): A compound, hormone, or medication that binds at a cell's receptor site but blocks the normal action of that receptor system. Examples are beta-blockers, which block the normal action of the beta adrenergic receptors; tamoxifen, which blocks the estrogen receptors of the breast and brain even though it will activate the estrogen receptors in the uterine lining (endometrium).

RECTAL: Pertaining to the rectum.

SEBACEOUS GLANDS: The tiny oil-producing glands in the skin. If they overproduce oil and/or become obstructed, pimples or acne will result.

SERMS: An abbreviation for a class of medications called Selective Estrogen Receptor Modulators. These drugs have both agonist (activating) and antagonist (blocking) actions at the body's estrogen receptors, depending on the particular organ. Examples are tamoxifen and raloxifen; both drugs *block* breast estrogen receptors and *stimulate* estrogen receptors elsewhere (such as bone). Because they block important actions of estrogen, they are not a pure replacement for all of estrogen's actions in the body. Side effects of both medicines include hot flashes, formation of blood clots, pulmonary emboli, cataracts, and increased risk of uterine cancer (tamoxifen).

SEROTONIN (5-HT): A potent brain chemical that regulates sleep, mood, libido, appetite, pain, and repetitive thoughts and actions. Serotonin's chemical name is 5-hydroxytryptophan and it is made by the brain and body from dietary sources of the amino acid tryptophan (milk, turkey, whole grains, et cetera.).

SERUM: The fluid portion of the blood after coagulation has removed the cells, fibrin, and fibrinogen.

SEX-HORMONE-BINDING GLOBULIN: A carrier protein in the bloodstream (made in the liver) that binds or carries estrogen, testosterone, progesterone to provide a reservoir of hormones ready for release into the free fraction to become the active form.

SEX HORMONES: The male and female hormones produced from cholesterol by the testicles, ovaries, adrenal glands, and body fat: testosterone, estrogens, progesterone, androgens.

STEROID DRUGS AND HORMONES: The group of chemical substances that has a chemical structure consisting of multiple rings of carbon atoms. Cortisone (the drug), estrogen, progesterone, and testosterone (sex hormones).

STRESS (URINARY) INCONTINENCE: Loss of urine due to pressure on weakened bladder structures and supporting ligaments; this weakness occurs as a result of estrogen loss and damage during childbirth. Increased pressure on the bladder may come from coughing, sneezing, laughing, straining to lift objects, or prolonged standing.

STROKE: Brain damage resulting from diminished blood supply and oxygen (ischemia) to the brain; usually occurs as a result of a clot blocking the arteries.

SUBLINGUAL: Something (medication, hormones, allergy drops, etc.) given underneath the tongue to be absorbed into the bloodstream.

SUSTAINED (TIMED) RELEASE: A process in which a medication is prepared or formulated in such a way as to deliver small amounts over a longer period of time.

SYMPATHETIC NERVOUS SYSTEM: The part of the autonomic nervous system that prepares the body for stress through effects of the stress hormones it releases (e.g., by increasing oxygen to the tissues; increasing heart rate, blood pressure, and glucose release; etc.). Its primary chemical messengers (neurotransmitters) are norepinephrine and epinephrine.

SYMPTOMS: Any physical or emotional change in the body that is perceived as distressing or painful. "Symptom" usually means a change that makes a person feel unwell. "Phenomena" is a word used to describe changes that don't necessarily cause distress.

SYNDROME: A group of symptoms and objective signs that typically occur together and serve to characterize a disease or disorder.

SYNERGISTIC: Substances interacting in ways that produce an effect *greater than* just adding the effects of the combined substances.

SYNTHETIC: Made by synthesis; can be identical to a natural compound found in the body, or may be synthesized to be chemically different and have different properties. Synthetic simply means "made by synthesis," it **does not** mean "artificial" (although common useage often implies "artificial" when the term *synthetic* is used to apply to a hormone).

TESTES: The male gonads; two reproductive glands located in the scrotum, which produce the male reproductive cells or spermatozoa and the male hormone testosterone.

TESTOSTERONE: The major male sex hormone produced in the testes and also in smaller amounts by the female ovary; plays a major role in men and women for sexual arousal, maintaining bone and muscle mass, and psychological well-being.

THYMUS: A gland located at the base of the neck that is important in development of immune response in newborns, with lesser activity as we get older. The cortex of the gland is composed of dense lymphoid tissue that produces the T-cells of the immune system.

THYROID GLAND: The endocrine gland situated in front of the larynx that produces the major hormones of metabolism; thyroxine (T4) and tri-iodothyronine (T3); also produces calcitonin, which regulates calcium balance.

THYROID STIMULATING HORMONE (TSH): The hormone produced by the brain that regulates the production and release of thyroid hormones from the thyroid gland. TSH levels are **low** in *hyper*thyroidism, and **high** in *hypo*thyroidism.

TRANSDERMAL: Absorbed through the skin into the bloodstream from a cream or patch or injection; this form of delivery bypasses the liver's "first-pass" metabolism.

TRIGLYCERIDES (TG): One of the blood fats that the body can use to make cholesterol; elevated TG (from diet, alcohol intake, lack of exercise, and some drugs) is a significant and *independent* risk factor for heart disease in women and also increases the risk of diabetes. Consists of one glycerol and three fatty acids.

TRYPTOPHAN: An amino acid found in foods that is the major precursor (building block) for the body and brain to make serotonin (5-hydroxytryptophan, 5-HT).

TUBAL LIGATION (BTL): The surgical procedure to cut or tie the fallopian tubes and prevent eggs released from the ovary from reaching the uterus. BTL is used as a method of contraception, considered permanent because it is difficult and expensive to reverse, with low probability of success. Some women notice worsening PMS and other symptoms of imbalance or decrease in ovarian hormones after tubal ligation, and this is thought to be due to changes in ovarian blood flow from the procedure.

TUMOR: An abnormal growth; may be cancerous or benign. An example is a uterine fibroid, a benign abnormal growth in the uterus. See **Fibroid.**

ULTRASOUND SCAN: A method of using very high frequency sound waves to visualize internal organs, blood vessels, and the fetus in pregnancy. The sound waves used are more than 20,000 hertz, and above the level that humans can hear. Ultrasound images do not involve using radiation sources, so there is no exposure to radiation during the procedure.

UP-REGULATION: The process of increasing the number or function of cellular receptors.

URETHRA: A muscular tube that carries urine from the bladder to the outside of the body. Inflammation of this tube is called urethritis, and causes painful burning sensations on urination.

UTERUS: The womb or female reproductive organ that carries and nourishes a growing fetus; made up of an inner layer (see **Endometrium**) and a thick muscular layer that undergoes rhythmic contractions during labor and delivery, during menstruation, and during orgasm (although not all women feel this).

UROLOGIST: A surgeon who specializes in diseases of the kidneys, urinary tract, and bladder.

VAGINA: The birth canal or genital passage leading from the uterus to the outside of the body at the vulva; it is muscular and elastic, expanding to accommodate the penis during intercourse, or to accommodate a baby during delivery.

VAGINAL DIAPHRAGM: A soft rubber cap that fits snugly over the cervix and is used for contraception.

VAGINAL RING: A small, soft plastic or Silastic device containing hormones or other medication for direct topical delivery to the vagina and urinary system. An example is Estring, containing 17-beta estradiol, used to treat vaginal dryness.

VASOACTIVE HORMONE or DRUGS: Drugs or substances acting on the blood vessels to cause either dilatation (e.g., estradiol, nitroglycerine) or constriction (e.g., nicotine) of the arteries.

VASOMOTOR: A term that refers to the way that nerve cells connect at the smooth muscle wall of arteries and govern the opening (vasodilation) and closing (vasoconstriction) of blood vessels to control blood flow.

VIRILIZATION: The development of masculine physical characteristics due to presence of male hormones. Virilization may occur in women if the androgen hormones are too high.

VULVA: Female external genitalia. Also known as the lips of the vaginal opening.

WILD (MEXICAN) YAM: A root vegetable that grows in many areas and contains precursor compounds that can be extracted and used in the laboratory as building blocks to make the hormones estradiol, testosterone, and progesterone. Extracts of wild yam cannot be converted by the human body to the human forms of active hormones, since we do not have the enzymes to carry out these chemical reactions.

RESOURCES

I. Sources for Natural Hormones

Belmar Pharmacy, Charles Hakala, R.Ph., Lakewood, CO (Denver area)
Phone 800-525-9473   Fax 303-763-9712

Charles has been a pioneer in compounding prescriptions for patients with challenging medical problems such as chemical sensitivities, multiple allergies to dyes/binders, in addition to his outstanding reputation in the field of compounding natural, bio-identical hormone preparations for thyroid, ovary, and adrenal hormones. He uses micronized natural forms of estradiol, testosterone, progesterone, and DHEA derived from soybeans and wild yams, and will make prescriptions in whatever form is needed for best results. Although I don't recommend estriol and estrone as desirable forms of hormone therapy, Charles does make these compounded prescriptions for those women who wish to use these types of estrogen. Belmar pharmacists will make up prescriptions using lactose-free hypoallergenic formulations with no dyes; they also make vaginal creams that are hypoallergenic and omit some of the common irritants found in most commercial products.

For those of you with thyroid problems, it may be helpful to know that I have been working with the addition of T3 to Synthroid (T4) since about 1985. Since commercial preparations containing T3 were fixed dose combinations that did not allow the "fine-tuning" that many people need, I turned to Charles many years ago to help me with hypothyroid patients who needed a reliable, sustained-release form of T3 when they could not tolerate the short-acting Cytomel. After seeing my patients do so well, Charles's formulation is the one I personally use and trust. Charles is also knowledgeable about important differences between the more reliable *serum* methods of hormone testing versus methods such as saliva and urine that commonly give misleading results. He will discuss these issues with both consumers and physicians.

Spence Pharmacy, Daryl Spence, R.Ph., Ft. Worth, TX (Dallas metroplex)
Phone 800-209-7364   Fax 817-625-8103

Daryl Spence is a dedicated and reliable compounding pharmacist who has created innovative topical pain relief medications, in addition to his work with bio-identical, natural micronized hormones such as estradiol, testosterone, progesterone, DHEA. Although I don't recommend estriol and estrone as desirable forms of hormone therapy, Daryl does make these compounded prescriptions for those women who wish to use these types of estrogen. In trying to find testosterone options for women, Daryl and I have collaborated on forms that will provide sustained effects over the day, and I am pleased with the success of his formulations for my patients. Daryl's sustained-release testosterone capsule formulation is the one I have personally found works the best for my own testosterone replacement, since I no longer have ovaries to make it. Spence Pharmacy will also make up prescriptions using lactose-free hypoallergenic formulations with no dyes, and no preservatives that are potentially irritating or may aggravate allergies.

General Comments

Both Belmar and Spence Pharmacies are *full-service pharmacies* with ability to fill all of your prescription needs, not just compounded prescriptions. Both pharmacies also work with many major health insurance plans. In addition, I have found that both of these pharmacies often have better prices on common commercial prescriptions (such as estradiol patches) than my patients find at the big chain drugstores. I encourage you to do a little price-shopping to decide where you want your prescriptions filled before you automatically assume the big chain drugstores are cheaper.

There are many pharmacies around the country that are now providing compounding services. There are several important reasons I have continued to collaborate primarily with Belmar and Spence pharmacies on prescriptions for my patients. First, both of these pharmacists have many years' experience in the art and science of compounding and are not just starting these services in the wake of the revived interest now. Second, each compounding pharmacist has his or her own formula for making the various forms of prescription hormones, and each formulation will vary in how it is metabolized in the body. Therefore, each formulation will act somewhat differently in a given person and adds yet another variable to the equation of trying to solve the problem when a person has side effects. It is difficult enough clinically to sort out individual differences in metabolism and response when I know the pharmacology of a given preparation. If the preparation also varies, it can become almost impossible to sort out the Gordian knot of factors that could alter a person's response. That's why I prefer to work with brand name products instead of generics, and to limit my prescriptions to just a few compounding pharmacists whose preparations I can rely upon.

Third, I have seen a disturbing trend in recent years as some compounding pharmacies have begun to move into the area of advising patients on dosing of hormones, which violates the laws governing pharmacy practice. I have treated too many patients who have been significantly overdosed on hormones when getting their information from pharmacists making the dose changes, and I have chosen to put my prescriptions at pharmacies where the pharmacists do not engage in this practice.

Disclaimer: *I have no financial interest in any of these pharmacies or their products.* I provide this information as a service to you and your physician because reliable information on these topics has been difficult for the average consumer to obtain. Compounded and "natural" hormones are not new, in spite of all the recent marketing of such products. Many of these options have been around for forty years or more. I have been a longstanding advocate for the use of bio-identical, "natural" human forms of hormone preparations, and I have seen over many years of my practice the marked positive difference that occurs when women change from the animal-derived, conjugated estrogens and synthetic forms of progestins.

Comments about FDA-Approval

Women often ask, "Are these compounded hormones FDA-approved?" The answer is no, because the individual compounded prescriptions are not manufactured and distributed for sale in quantities that would require FDA-approval. At reputable compounding pharmacies, the ingredients used are *pharmaceutical-grade* (U.S.P.) bases that are then made up into tablets or creams or suppositories to your individual needs. Individual pharmacists operate within their training and state licenses when they prepare (compound) individual prescriptions based on your own physician's decision about dose and type of medication best for you. Pharmacists are not, however, licensed to determine the *dose* that is correct for you; that function is by law the task of the physician. The two pharmacies above are resources I have depended upon to provide individual prescriptions for my patients and family; we have been pleased with the results. These pharmacists are skilled, knowledgeable, and committed to providing quality service to you and your physician. I have found them to be ethical and responsible in working *with* the physician. Neither of these pharmacy owners allows their staff to go outside the bounds of pharmacy licensing and make dose changes on their own. I am increasingly concerned at the degree to which some pharmacists are now practicing medicine by adjusting women's hormone doses based on questionable test methods, such as saliva and urine hormone levels, without having access to other laboratory measures that need to be included in decision making about appropriate hormone dose and route.

Although many types of medications used to be compounded individually, it is no longer advantageous to do so with the current quality of manufactured products widely available. Much of the current use of individual compounding is for patients with allergies, marked sensitivities to dyes and binders in commercial preparations, patients who need smaller doses, and in particular, women who want to take natural, bio-identical human forms of hormones that aren't yet available in commercial products at regular drugstores. Natural ovarian hormones have been in widespread use in Europe, Australia, Canada, Japan and other countries for many years, generally with better clinical response and fewer side effects than the synthetic progestins, conjugated equine estrogens, and synthetic methyltestosterone compounds used in the United States. When these natural, or bio-identical, forms of hormones are not available commercially at the chain drugstores, the compounding pharmacies can make up ones similar to those available in Europe and other countries.

For estrogen, however, there are several *brands* of the natural human form, 17-beta estradiol, available in the United States that are FDA approved and made by commercial pharmaceutical companies: **Estrace** tablets and vaginal cream, **Alora**, **VivelleDOT**, **Climara** and **Estraderm** transdermal (skin) patches. All of these products contain the same natural, bio-identical form of 17-beta estradiol that our ovaries made before menopause. These products are made with the precursor, or building block, molecules that come from soybeans. The primary difference in the various patches is the type of adhesive (which may affect frequency of skin rash and how well it stays on your body) and the duration of effect from the patch. We work with whatever brand a woman likes best. There are also now available several generic versions of 17-beta estradiol tablets now that **Estrace** has gone off patent. Unfortunately, I have found that the quality varies widely from one generic manufacturer to another, so I don't usually recommend the generic estradiol tablets. I have had many patients who had marked relapse of their symptoms when switched to a generic form of estradiol.

In addition to the commercial estradiol products, there are now two new FDA-approved commercial products for natural progesterone: **Prometrium** tablets and **Crinone** vaginal gel. You no longer have to turn to compounded natural progesterone products that are often not covered by insurance plans. Both Prometrium and Crinone are available through regular drugstores and are usually covered by most health plans that provide prescription plans. Both of these commercial products are made from yam and soybean precursors and are micronized for optimal absorption. They both work well for endometrial protection, so the choice of which product for your use depends on such aspects as personal preference and side effects, which will vary depending on whether progesterone is taken orally or is absorbed vaginally and therefore bypasses the liver "first-pass" metabolism.

We do not have a major pharmaceutical company in the United States that has yet developed natural micronized testosterone preparation approved by the FDA for widespread consumer use. A testosterone patch for women is in development by several companies, but it is not yet on the market in the United States. The testosterone patches for men are quite good, but the dose is too high for women to use. It is my hope that as we understand more about the important differences between the native human forms for hormones and the synthetic or animal-derived ones, the women of this country will have better options widely available. Until that time, you may ask your physician to work with reputable pharmacists to compound the natural testosterone to suit your needs.

Update on Saliva Hormone Tests

Initially, I thought saliva tests had some promise for ease of use and convenience, and I prescribed these tests for my patients through both Aeron Labs and Diagnos-Techs. I had to stop using the saliva tests several years ago because they simply were not reliable and did not correlate with women's descriptions of their symptoms. The saliva tests also did not correlate with the blood serum tests, yet the serum tests were the ones that fit closely with what the women themselves described regarding symptoms. I tried to figure out these discrepancies and I repeatedly asked both companies to provide me any data they had correlating serum and saliva results in the same patient. I never received this information from either company selling saliva test kits.

Another problem is that saliva results provide only *part* of the picture we need in order to determine optimal hormone dose, since they only measure the *free* hormone, rather than the combination of total and free hormone available for the body to use. The most useful clinical information to guide you and your physician in determining the optimal hormone dose comes from looking at the total hormone available, as well as other laboratory parameters that provide an indirect measure of hormone effect. When needed, the *free* fraction of a given hormone can also be done with serum, and is a more reliable measure than the amount that is "excreted" into saliva. Just think about all the kinds of variables that affect your saliva production: Everything from what medicines you take, whether you use antihistamines, whether you chew gum, whether you are stressed, and a host of others. Then you will understand why measuring hormones excreted into saliva isn't the best way to go when you are trying to decide a complex matter like what hormones to take and how much to use. Your blood system is much more stable over time, and the components in the blood are more finely regulated by the body's balancing (homeostasis) mechanisms. Plus, keep in mind that the hormones are constantly moving back and forth from free to bound state as they interact with cellular receptors, so knowing the level of the total hormone available becomes quite important in deciding what you may need.

As I researched the saliva tests further, I found that colleagues in reproductive endocrinology (fertility specialists) had also encountered difficulty with the wide variance in saliva tests and with the lack of correlation with other hormone measures used to determine hormone balance for fertility. The international menopause studies use serum hormone levels, and the serum hormone tests are considered the gold standard hormone assay in international research. Over the years since I first wrote *Screaming to Be Heard,* I have treated too many women who got into significant difficulty when relying just on saliva tests, and I no longer recommend this test or pharmacies and practitioners that promote these test kits. If you are going to invest the time and money to get hormone levels checked, I encourage you to use the serum tests that are the most reliable methods at this time.

When you have your hormone levels done, be certain that you have them drawn at the appropriate time of your menstrual cycle (if you still have one), or at appropriate intervals from your last hormone dose or patch change. In chapters 4, 5, 6, and 15, I have provided target ranges for serum hormone levels that I have found in my practice over the years correlate well with when women feel their best and their symptoms have improved or resolved. Once you have reviewed the information on ranges that are desirable for optimal well-being, your own physician can order these tests and then use the information to guide you on dose adjustments for your hormone prescriptions.

II: Resources —Books, Clinical Centers, and National Organizations

There has been an explosion of information in women's health since the first edition of *Screaming to Be Heard* was published. It is impossible to list all of the good resources here, and I encourage you to first turn to the Web sites and publications of the national not-for-profit organizations dedicated to providing reliable educational resources for women. A few key ones are listed in the material that follows. As you try to evaluate the plethora of women's health books now available, remember to retain a healthy skepticism for books by authors who are also trying to sell you products such as nutritional supplements, hormone creams and various types of test kits. Many of these books have a primary focus of selling the author's products and are not always the most up-to-date or accurate on the scientific information. Keep in mind the analogy I used earlier about buying a car from a used car salesman, and ask yourself the question: "Do I unquestioningly accept the pitch from the salesman, or do I want an independent opinion from someone who has nothing to gain financially?"

For each of the following books, I have provided my comments about strengths, weaknesses, content overview or other aspects I think may be relevant for you to consider in selecting ones to read. These are my best opinions from my own extensive reading of both the scientific literature and many consumer books, and from our patients' feedback as to which resources are both practical and helpful. I have listed reading materials that, in my professional opinion, are both useful and reliable in the medical information presented. I have updated some of the suggested readings below, but I also decided to keep in the list some of the more meaningful classics that I included in the first edition of *Screaming to Be Heard*. Further reading suggestions are listed chapter by chapter, and in some cases, I have also included Web site information.

CHAPTER 1: SCREAMING TO BE HEARD: LISTENING TO WOMEN'S VOICES
1. <u>Woman As Healer.</u> Jeanne Achterberg, Ph.D., Shambhala, Boston, 1991, paperback. Dr. Achterberg examines the role of women and their pivotal roles in healing traditions in ancient cultures, as well as the loss of the feminine influences in the Western medical traditions. A profoundly moving and inspiring book that helps us understand women's vital contributions and influence in the past, and sheds more light on the problems in the world today, medicine in particular. I was deeply moved as I journeyed through the pages of this book!
2. <u>Medicine Women, Curanderas, and Women Doctors.</u> Bobette Perrone, H. Henrietta Stockel, and Victoria Krueger, University of Oklahoma Press, Norman, OK, 1993, revised edition. Presents ten Southwestern female healers from three cultures (Native American, Hispanic, and Western) and provides an in-depth analysis of alternative healing methods along with remarkable insights about the profound impact of the psyche/soul on physical illness. Inspirational reading about our rich history as women healers.
3. <u>BACKLASH—The Undeclared War Against American Women.</u> Susan Faludi, Anchor Books/Doubleday, New York, 1992. Ms. Faludi makes a compelling case that whenever women make progress in their efforts for equality, an antifeminist backlash strikes on all fronts—in the media, politics, fashion, and the workplace. Many of these issues are even more prevalent today than when the author first wrote this book, so I encourage you to read it.
4. <u>Women & Self-Esteem-Understanding and Improving the Way We Think and Feel About Ourselves.</u> Linda Tschirhart Sanford and Mary Ellen Donovan, Penguin Books, New York, 1992. An excellent overview of issues affecting women, still relevant today. Helps women understand cultural sources of low self-esteem and provides practical approaches for building an enhanced self-esteem; a valuable resource.
5. "Still Killing Us Softly" 1995 Update: Advertising's Impact on Women. Cambridge Documentary Films, Inc. 617-354-3677. Resource for rental or

purchase of Dr. Jean Kilbourne's films *Killing Us Softly* and *STILL Killing Us Softly* as well as other important documentary films on significant topics of interest to women and their families. Although these films were made several years ago, the issues they raise are still quite current, and Dr. Kilbourne has a wonderful presentation style that I found provocative *and* entertaining. I highly recommend these films and encourage readers to rent them for showing/discussion to community and school groups. Time has gone on, but the images in the ads have tended to get worse, not better. You need to be aware of how the images affect you. We need consumer activism to help solve these issues.

CHAPTER 2: HORMONES: A GUIDE TO YOUR BODY CYCLES
1.   **Woman's Body: A Manual For Life.** Dr. Miriam Stoppard, Dorling Kindersley, London and New York, 1994. Compiled by a team of health experts from many fields, this book covers physical and emotional concerns of women throughout the life span and is illustrated with hundreds of color charts, graphs, and photos. It is one of the most comprehensive and practical women's health books I have found.
2.   **The Good News About Women's Hormones.** Geoffrey Redmond, M.D., Warner Books, New York, 1995. This book was not available at the time I first wrote *Screaming to Be Heard* in 1994 or I would have included it in the references for my first edition since his book is an excellent resource. There are many parallels in the work Dr. Redmond has done to identify and treat women's hormone problems and the hormone connections I have been addressing in my own work. Dr. Redmond has been President of the Foundation for Developmental Endocrinology and has also edited medical texts on hormone disorders. This book is written for consumers, is easily understandable, and has excellent sections on androgenic disorders (excess hair growth, acne, and other problems) and alopecia (hair loss) as well as the many other hormone problems he discusses. He gives a balanced view of benefits and risks of hormone treatments, and a logical approach to helping women decide about hormone use and how to get reliable lab tests.
3.   **Listening to Your Hormones.** Gillian Ford, Prima Publishing Co., Rocklin, CA, 1997. Gill is a health educator, not a physician, but she has spent many years reviewing medical articles on hormone issues as a result of her own hormonal problems that she describes in her book. Gill worked with me for about a year in our Texas center, and I valued the contributions she made to educate women about these problems even though I don't agree with all of her approaches and opinions. In addition, some of the physicians she cites have questionable theories not supported by the current medical literature, so you need to be cautious about accepting without question all of the opinions presented. One of the strengths of this book is the bibliography of over 200 references for those who would like to be able to locate original medical articles.

CHAPTER 3: HORMONES AND THE BRAIN
1.   **"New Perspectives on the Relationship of Hormone Changes to Affective Disorders in the Perimenopause."** Elizabeth Lee Vliet, M.D., and Virginia Lee Hutcheson Davis, M.S., Clinical Issues in Mid-Life Women's Health (NAACOG), vol. 2, no. 4, October/December 1991, pp. 453–471. An eighteen-page detailed review of over thirty years of world-wide neuroendocrine

research on hormone effects on brain and mood. Includes list of references of classic papers in the field of neuroendocrine research. Available from medical libraries, or you may order a copy by sending a check for $10.00 to *HER Place*, P.O. Box 64507, Tucson, AZ 85728.

2.   The Thyroid Solution. Ridha Arem, M.D., The Ballantine Publishing Group, a division of Random House, Inc., New York, 1999. An excellent reference book on thyroid disorders, written by an endocrinologist with solid credentials and clinical experience. Dr. Arem validates what I have seen in my practice for my entire career: Many women in particular have subclinical forms of thyroid disorders that affect mood, fertility, weight and a host of other problems. In addition, Dr. Arem goes into more depth on the value of adding T3 to a thyroid medication regimen, as I have espoused and used for many years as well. I do not think Dr. Arem's information on estrogen therapy is either comprehensive or up-to-date, and I am very concerned about his emphasis on the use of Premarin and Provera based on the issues I have described in *Screaming to Be Heard*. I do, however, think his information on thyroid is outstanding.

3.   Living Well with Hypothyroidism. Mary Shomon, Wholecare/Avon Books, New York, New York, 2000. An excellent, practical guide to improving the quality of your life and health if you suffer from hypothyroidism. Mary is a lay person who has suffered from a thyroid disorder, and she has done extensive research on the subject to bring the latest information to her readers. She also has a thyroid newsletter (*Sticking Out Our Necks*), and Web site (www.thyroid-info.com) that you will also find full of useful tips and the latest scientific studies.

CHAPTER 4: HORMONES OF PREGNANCY AND STRESS: PROGESTERONE AND CORTISOL

1.   Why Zebras Don't Get Ulcers. Robert M. Sapolsky, W.H. Freeman & Co., New York, NY, 1998. Excellent and humorous review of the adverse effects over time due to high cortisol levels from stress. If you ever wondered just how "stress" affects your entire body, this is a terrific and well-written book.

2.   There is not space to provide all of the medical references for the progesterone material, but some readers might want to locate this classic paper for further reading: "Progesterone suppression of the Plasma Growth Hormone Response," Bhatia SK, Moore D, and Kalkhoff RK, J. Clin Endocrinol Metab 35: 364-369; 1972.

3.   I have not included any of the current consumer books on progesterone as a resource since these all contain serious errors and incorrect medical information about the roles of estrogen and progesterone, with most of them emphasizing incorrectly negatives about estrogen and failing to give balanced view of the drawbacks of progesterone. Most of the authors are promoting or selling progesterone creams as *the* answer to all of women's hormone problems. If you are interested in more detailed material on the roles of progesterone, I refer you to the medical studies described in my book.

CHAPTER 5: THE BIG QUESTION: HAS ANYBODY SEEN MY ESTROGEN?

1.   Menopause and Midlife Health. Morris Notelovitz, M.D., and Diana Tonnessen, St. Martin's Press, New York, 1994. Written by a pioneer in osteoporosis and menopause, this book presents accurate and up-to-date information about managing your health, including the role of healthy lifestyle habits.

Discusses hormone therapies, pros and cons of gynecological procedures, issues about breast cancer and other concerns of importance to women.

2. **Menopause.** Miriam Stoppard, M.D., Dorling Kindslerly Publishing, London and New York, 1994. A beautifully illustrated book that addresses the total woman during this important transition and the years beyond. Color charts and graphs make it easier to understand difficult medical concepts and help women manage their menopause in optimal ways.

3. **The Silent Passage: Menopause.** Gail Sheehy, Pocket Books (paperback), New York, 1998. The best-selling book that brought the M word out of the closet and into mainstream. Although it originally came out in hardcover in 1991, it is still a good one to provide an overview of what to expect and to read other women's experiences.

CHAPTER 6: TESTOSTERONE AND DHEA:
THE FORGOTTEN WOMEN'S HORMONES

1. **The Magic of Sex. The Book That Really Tells Men About Women and Women About Men.** Miriam Stoppard, M.D., Dorling Kindersley, Inc., New York, 1992. Men and women approach love and sex with different expectations; they respond to physical love in different ways; and even when their responses are similar, they often happen at different times and are brought about by different stimuli. With beautiful photographs, *The Magic of Sex* covers this subject from both the man's and the woman's point of view. I think this is THE best, most comprehensive and beautifully written book on sex I have found, and I highly recommend it.

2 **The Art of Sexual Ecstacy: The Path of Sacred Sexuality for Western Lovers.** Margo Anand, Jeremy P. Tarcher, Inc., Los Angeles, CA, 1991. A comprehensive and clearly written work on contemporary Tantric and Taoist practices adapted and made understandable to Western readers. Helpful for those who wish to explore ways to intensify their sexual experiences.

3. **Becoming Orgasmic; A Sexual and Personal Growth Program for Women.** Julia Heiman, Ph.D., and J. Lopiccolo. Ph.D., Simon and Schuster, New York, 1988. If you have any inhibitions about sex or want to enhance the pleasure you get from sex, the program presented will help you feel comfortable with yourself and your ideas about sex.

4. **Dancing With Myself: Sensuous Exercises for Body, Mind and Spirit.** K. dePeyer, Nucleus Publications, Willow Springs, MO, 1991. Intuitive approach to physical fitness that embraces mind, body, and spirit; suggest exercises that enhance body/sensual awareness.

CHAPTER 7: THE PERSNICKETY P'S: PMS, PCOS, PREMATURE
MENOPAUSE, PERIMENOPAUSE, AND POSTPARTUM DEPRESSION

1. **Menopause.** Miriam Stoppard, M.D., Dorling Kindersley Publishing, London and New York, 1994. A beautifully illustrated book that addresses the total woman during this important transition and the years beyond. Color charts and graphs make it easier to understand difficult medical concepts and help women manage their menopause in optimal ways.

2. **PCOS: The Hidden Epidemic.** Samuel S. Thatcher, M.D., Ph.D. Perspectives Press, Indianapolis, IN, 2000. Dr. Thatcher is a renown expert in reproductive endocrinology and brings to this book many years of clinical experience as one

of the early advocates for increased understanding of this complex and serious metabolic disorder. The book gives an overview of what PCOS is, our current understanding of causes, and information on helpful treatments based on research findings. This is an excellent resource, recommended by the Polycystic Ovarian Syndrome Association. The order line for Perspective Press is 317-872-3055, 8:00 A.M. to 4:00 P.M. Indiana time, Monday through Thursday, or through their Web site at www.perspectivespress.com.

3.   **PolyCystic Ovarian Syndrome Association, Inc.** An excellent resource for educational materials, support groups, web discussions of PCOS. The organization also hosts an outstanding annual conference on PCOS, with presentations from many of the leading experts in the field. Check out their Web site at www.pcosupport.com, or call 630-585-3690. Mail address is P.O. Box 7007, Rosemont, IL 60018

4.   **The Premature Menopause Book.** Kathryn Petras, Avon Books, Inc., New York, 1999. This is a good book written by a lay person sharing her own story about struggling with premature menopause. This book provides an abundance of resources and other helpful consumer information including Web sites and support groups for women finding themselves in menopause at an early age.

5.   **Women's Moods: What Every Woman Must Know About Hormones, the Brain, and Emotional Health.** Deborah Sichel, M.D., William Morrow and Co., New York, 1999. This book extends what I have written in 1991 and 1994, as well as in *Screaming to Be Heard,* about the crucial hormone effects on mood syndromes in women. Dr. Sichel has included additional material on postpartum mood syndromes that many readers will find helpful. Although her emphasis is more on the serotonin connections than on the ovarian hormones, the book does provide validation for women experiencing these bewildering mood shifts.

CHAPTER 8: IS IT CHRONIC FATIGUE, "YEAST," OR PERIMENOPAUSE?

1.   **From Fatigued to Fantastic!** Jacob Teitelbaum, M.D., Avery Publishing Group, Garden City, New York, 1996. A good overview of chronic fatigue causes and suggestions for evaluation and treatment options for CFS to pursue with your physicians. The hormonal recommendations for women are a weakness of this book, and I don't recommend following the ovarian hormone protocols he suggests, since this is not reflective of the current international research information in the menopause field. He puts more emphasis on use of androgens prior to appropriate restoration of estrogen balance for women, which commonly leads to more side effects of androgen-excess. He is also recommending use of "tri-est" that contains too little estradiol to provide the protective effects on bone, brain, and heart and other vital estrogen target tissues. I do think this book provides very helpful suggestions for chronic fatigue treatment approaches, as well as crucial validation for the sufferers of this disorder.

2.   **Betrayal by the Brain: The Neurologic Basis of Chronic Fatigue Syndrome, Fibromyalgia Syndrome, and Other Neural Network Disorders.** Jay A. Goldstein, Haworth Press, Binghamton, NY, 1996. An in-depth discussion of neurological connections in these syndromes, with some attention to hormone systems such as the adrenal and pituitary. This book, however, has very little material on women's hormones and their role in these disorders as I have described in my book.

3. <u>Chronic Fatigue and Tiredness: A Self-Help Program</u>. Susan M. Lark, M.D., Westchester Publishing Co., Los Altos, CA, 1993. A more in-depth exploration of the role of nutrition, vitamins, minerals, and herbs in the treatment of chronic fatigue. This book has many helpful and practical suggestions for enhancing energy level and well-being but doesn't address any of the ovarian hormone issues in fatigue syndromes.

4. <u>Doctor, Why Am I So Tired?</u> Richard N. Podell, M.D., FACP, Pharos Books, New York, 1987. Although this book may now be difficult to find, it addresses unrecognized medical causes of fatigue as well as suggestions for nutritional and other mind-body approaches to help improve your energy and well-being. Dr. Podell also includes helpful approaches to discuss symptoms and problems with your physician.

5. <u>The Yeast Connection.</u> W. Crook, M.D., Professional Books, Jackson, TN, 1986. Written by a leading proponent of the candida theory, this book gives an overview of the ideas developed by Orian Truss and W. Crook. It has not been well accepted by most allergists because of the lack of adequate studies to verify the "yeast connection." Dr. Crook has also written another book, *The Yeast Connection and the Woman,* but I do not recommend this one since his medical information on women's hormones is not accurate, complete or up-to-date, and he is often incorrect on *which* hormones have what functions in a woman's body. I include my comments on these books here because so many women have been told they have this syndrome without ever having the proper reliable tests of their ovarian hormones. I recommend a careful evaluation of your ovarian and thyroid hormones (and other medical conditions) as outlined in my book before you accept the diagnosis of "chronic candidiasis" and spend a great deal of money on unproven treatments. In spite of its limitations, Dr. Crook does have helpful dietary and lifestyle suggestions.

6. **"Position Paper on the Candida Yeast Theory."** American Academy of Allergy and Immunology, 611 E. Wells St., Milwaukee, WI 53202. Provides a detailed evaluation (from an objective, albeit somewhat skeptical, point of view) on the scientific evidence pertaining to the yeast theory. A good balance for the above books that attribute every symptom a woman experiences to "yeast overgrowth."

7. **National CEBV Syndrome Association.** P.O. Box 230108, Portland, OR 97223. Support group organization for people diagnosed with Epstein-Barr syndrome. Write to them for information and suggested reading list.

CHAPTER 9: ESTROGEN AND MEMORY: THE WORDS ESCAPE ME
In the first edition of *Screaming to Be Heard.* I wrote that I had not seen consumer books that focused on the hormonal connections in memory function. Since that time, a consumer book was published that brings together the scientific literature on menopause and memory and other issues affecting the mind: <u>Menopause and the Mind,</u> by Claire Warga, Ph.D., Simon & Schuster, New York, 1999. Although not the first (as she claims) to identify these "cognitive" connections with hormone change at menopause, the author has summarized over thirty years of research in the field of hormone effects on the brain and mental functioning. This book is based on the extensive research over the last 25 years by such pioneers as Dr. Barbara Sherwin of Canada and other experts world wide. It extends material I wrote about in 1991 and 1994 on these sub-

jects and the author has provided references to the extensive medical literature about hormone effects on the brain.

CHAPTER 10: MIGRAINES AND HORMONAL HEADACHES
Organizations: The following organizations provide educational materials and referral lists of headache specialists and you may find them helpful: **National Headache Foundation,** 1-888-NHF-5552, www.headaches.org; **American Council for Headache Education,** 800-255-ACHE.
The following books do not address much information on the hormone connections that trigger migraines as I have described in *Screaming to Be Heard,* but the authors provide other helpful background information on causes and treatments of a variety of headache syndromes.
1. **Help for Headaches.** Joel Saper, M.D., Warner Books, New York, 1987.
2. **Headache Relief for Women**. Alan Rapoport, M.D., and Fred Sheftell, M.D., Little Brown and Co., New York, 1996.
3. **The Headache Book**. Seymour Solomon, M.D., and Steven Fraccaro, Consumers Union, Mount Vernon, NY, 1991.
4. **Overcoming Migraine**: **A Comprehensive Guide to Treatment and Prevention by a Survivor.** Betsy Wyckoff, Station Hill Press, Tarrytown, NY, 1998. May be ordered through *Amazon.com.* A very helpful book, and more useful than many since the author has herself struggled with the migraine problem for many years.

Headache Centers. I have listed the following programs because the physician directors have more experience in addressing the hormonal issues many programs overlook. There are also many medical centers with pain clinics that treat headache problems, as well as pain programs affiliated with university medical centers that have headache specialists. Either of the national organizations above can provide additional referral resources in your area, but make sure they pay attention to the hormone connections and will evaluate those as part of a comprehensive treatment program.

Stephen D. Silberstein, M.D., Chief of Neurology and Co-Director, The Comprehensive Headache Center at The Germantown Hospital and Medical Center, Philadelphia, PA

Joel Saper, M.D., The Michigan Neurological Institute, Ann Arbor, Michigan

Elizabeth Lee Vliet, M.D. HER Place Tucson, Arizona, and Dallas area, Texas. These two programs designed by Dr. Vliet are tailored to women and include complete hormonal measurement to check this overlooked trigger of migraines. Both provide comprehensive hormonal evaluations and multidisciplinary recommendations including alternative therapies (such as acupuncture, myofascial release, neuromuscular therapy, massage therapy, dietary changes, biofeedback, hypnotherapy, water therapies, chiropractic, osteopathic manipulation, and others) along with traditional medical options. Women's previous medical test results are reviewed to be certain that disorders more common in women have not been overlooked.

You may download information forms from the ℋℰℛ 𝒫𝓁𝒶𝒸ℯ Web site at www.herplace.com, or contact the staff in either office for guidance on the process to arrange consultation:

1. ℋℰℛ 𝒫𝓁𝒶𝒸ℯ: **Health, Enhancement and Renewal for Women, Inc.** For information package, mail request to P.O. Box 64507, Tucson, AZ 85728, or call 520-797-9131, fax 520-797-2948.

2. ℋℰℛ 𝒫𝓁𝒶𝒸ℯ: **Health, Enhancement and Renewal for Women, Inc.**, 2700 Tibbets Drive, Suite #100, Bedford (Dallas area, near DFW airport), TX 76022, 817-355-8008, Fax 817-355-8010

CHAPTER 11: FIBROMYALGIA, ACHES AND PAIN: THE ESTROGEN FACTOR
Unfortunately, very few programs in the country at this time are addressing women's hormone levels as part of a comprehensive pain evaluation and treatment program even though there are many excellent, accredited, pain treatment centers across the country. The national organization of pain specialists, <u>The American Academy of Pain Management,</u> reviews credentials of specialists in pain management from many different professional backgrounds (physicians, nurse practitioners, psychologists, acupuncturists, physical therapists, etc.), provides a referral resource to help identify pain programs and specialists around the country, and also provides information on upcoming conferences, books, and other resources. You may contact them at 209-533-9744, 13947 Mono Way, Suite A, Sonora, CA 95370, or their Web site at <u>www.aapainmanage.org</u>. Another resource is the **Fibromyalgia Network,** 1-800-853-2929, P.O. Box 31750, Tucson AZ 85751. This organization publishes a very good newsletter that gives an overview of current research on fibromyalgia, helpful pointers for people with this problem, and news of upcoming conferences. Web site: www.fmnetnews.com.

<u>Centers that include detailed assessment of women's hormones as contributing factors in chronic pain syndromes:</u>
ℋℰℛ 𝒫𝓁𝒶𝒸ℯ, Tucson, Arizona and Dallas-Ft. Worth, Texas, designed by **Elizabeth Lee Vliet, M.D.** These two programs are tailored to women and include complete hormonal measurement to check this overlooked cause of fibromyalgia and other chronic pain conditions. Both provide comprehensive medical/hormonal evaluation, with recommendations for multidisciplinary therapy approaches including alternative therapies (such as acupuncture, myofascial release, neuromuscular therapy, massage therapy, dietary changes, biofeedback, hypnotherapy, water therapies, chiropractic, osteopathic/craniosacral manipulation, sound therapy, and others) along with traditional medical options. Women's previous medical test results are reviewed to avoid duplication of testing, and to be certain that disorders more common in women have not been overlooked. **You may download information forms from the Web site at www.herplace.com.**

1. ℋℰℛ 𝒫𝓁𝒶𝒸ℯ: **Health, Enhancement and Renewal for Women, Inc.,** for information package, mail inquiries to P.O. Box 64507, Tucson, AZ 85728, or call 520-797-9131, Fax: 520-797-2948 .

2. ℋℰℛ 𝒫𝓁𝒶𝒸ℯ: **Health, Enhancement and Renewal for Women, Inc.,** 2700 Tibbets Drive, Suite #100, Bedford (Dallas area, near DFW airport), TX 76022, 817-355-8008, Fax 817-355-8010.

CHAPTER 12: INTERSTITIAL CYSTITIS, VULVODYNIA, AND LEAKY BLADDERS

1. **Alliance for Aging Research.** 2021 K Street, N.W., Suite 305, Washington, D.C. 20006, 202-293-2856
2. **Interstitial Cystitis Association.** (Vicki Ratner, M.D., Founder), P.O. Box 1553, Madison Square Station, New York, NY 10159
3. **The Bladder Health Council, American Foundation for Urologic Disease.** 1120 N. Charles Street, Baltimore, MD 21201, 1-800-242-2383.
4. **National Association for Continence.** PO Box 8310, Spartenburg, SC 29305, 1-800-252-3337 or 864-579-7900, Web site: www.nafc.org
5. **HIP, Help for Incontinent People.** P.O. Box 544, Union, SC 29379, 1-800-BLADDER
6. **The Simon Foundation for Continence.** P.O. Box 835, Wilmette, IL 60091, 1-800-23-SIMON (patients) 708-864-3913 (health professionals)
7. **Women Leaders in Urology:**
   Tamara G. Bavendam, M.D., Center for Pelvic Floor Disorders, Medical College of Pennsylvania, 3300 Henry Avenue, Philadelphia, PA 19129, 215-842-7007
   Kristene E. Whitmore, M.D., Director, The Incontinence Center Clinical Associate Professor of Urology, University of Pennsylvania, Philadelphia, PA
8. The Urinary Incontinence Sourcebook. Diane Kaschak Newman, R.N.C., M.S.N., C.R.N.P., F.A.A.N., Lowell House, Chicago, IL, 1997.

CHAPTER 13: ESTROGEN AND YOUR HEART: NOT JUST A MENOPAUSE PROBLEM

1. The Female Heart: The Truth About Women and Coronary Artery Disease. Marianne Legato, M.D., and Carol Colman, Harper Collins Publishers, New York, 1996.
2. Nutrition, Hypertension & Cardiovascular Disease. Smith R., Lyncean Press, Beavertown, Oregon, 1989. Although this was published in 1989, it is clearly written, and provides understandable explanations of hypertension and cardiovascular disease, emphasizing risk factors you can control and ways to prevent development of disease.
3. No Ifs, Ands or Butts: A Smoker's Guide to Kicking the Habit. Julie Waltz, Northwest Learning Associates, Tucson, AZ, 1989. Quite simply, one of the best and most practical guides for helping "kick the tobacco habit." Full of helpful tips and very human stories of dealing with change at all levels.
4. Syndrome X: The Complete Nutritional Program to Prevent and Reverse Insulin Resistance. Jack Challen, Dr. Burton Berkson, and Melissa Diane Smith. John Wiley and Sons, New York, NY, 2000. An excellent resource for understanding the role that elevated insulin plays in causing heart disease, hypertension, elevated triglycerides, abnormal cholesterol patterns, and diabetes. Gives helpful information on nutritional approaches to correct these problems and reduce later risk of diabetes and cardiovascular disorders.
5. American Medical Women's Association (AMWA) Continuing Education Workshop: **Coronary Heart Disease in Women** (CME credit for physicians, educational materials for consumers). Contact AMWA at 703-838-0500.

CHAPTER 14: BREAST CANCER: CONTROVERSIES
AND RISKS YOU AREN'T TOLD, OPTIONS TO EXPLORE
1. **Breast Cancer: If It Runs in Your Family, How to Reduce Your Risk.**
Mary Dan Eades, M.D., Bantam Books, New York, NY, 1991. An excellent
review of the known risk factors for breast cancer (even if it doesn't run in your
family), and more in-depth discussions than I had space for in my book. It is
thorough, very readable, and gives sound practical approaches for changes in
your lifestyle. I highly recommend it for all women.
2. **Dr. Susan Love's Breast Book.** Susan Love, M.D., with Karen Lindsey,
Perseus Press, Cambridge, MA, 1995. A comprehensive book on total breast
health for women of all ages. Very detailed and well researched. I highly recommend this book. Sadly, I *cannot* recommend *Dr. Love's Hormone Book*
because I have found it to be seriously flawed in its medical content, and not
accurate in presenting many women's health risk beyond breast cancer (osteoporosis and heart disease in particular). Dr. Love also does not address the crucial differences between types of estrogen and progestins or progesterone as I
have done in *Screaming to Be Heard*. In my opinion, these are serious deficiencies in her book. In addition, Dr. Love has an anti-hormone message that
is not warranted by our current science or in keeping with many women's needs
as well as positive experiences with HRT.
3. **Breast and Cervical Cancer Education Project.** A program offered by the
American Medical Women's Association (AMWA) as a continuing education
workshop for physicians and other health professionals. For information about
obtaining a speaker or for a list of consumer educational materials, contact
AMWA at 703-838-0500.
4. T. L. Bush, and M.K. Whiteman, **"Hormone replacement therapy and risk
of breast cancer"** (editorial). *JAMA* 1999, 281, pp.2140-2142.

CHAPTER 15: HORMONE THERAPY: FACTS AND FALLACIES
1. North American Menopause Society. Check their Web site at
www.nams.org for information on hormone therapy, a list of health professionals specializing in menopause around the country, consumer educational
materials and other helpful resources.
2. **Menopause and Midlife Health.** Morris Notelovitz, M.D., and Diana
Tonnessen, St. Martin's Press, New York, 1994. Written by a pioneer in osteoporosis and menopause, this book presents accurate and up-to-date information about managing your health, including the role of healthy lifestyle habits.
Discusses hormone therapies, pros and cons of gynecological procedures, issues
about breast cancer and other concerns of importance to women.

CHAPTER 16: COMPLEMENTARY MEDICINE:
MAKING "HOLISTIC" MEDICINE WHOLE
1. **Pharmacist's Letter/Prescriber's Letter Natural Medicines Comprehensive
Database.** J. M. Jellin, F. Batz, and K. Hitchens, Therapeutic Research Faculty,
Stockton, CA, 1999. This group publishes a newsletter and a comprehensive
reference book of detailed information on vitamins, herbs, and natural medicine supplements. Their reference book has been prepared by pharmacists who
have reviewed the medical studies from around the world and then compiled
summaries of uses, side effects, and symptoms of overdose for thousands of

supplements. It is one of the most comprehensive, reliable, scientifically-based compilations of information on natural medicines that I have found anywhere. It is not supported by advertising, is objective and medically sound. For more information on how to subscribe to their newsletter or purchase a copy of the reference book, call 209-472-2244 or visit their Web site: www.naturaldatabase.com.

2.   **Mind/Body Medicine: How To Use Your Mind For Better Health**. Consumer Reports Books, Consumers Union of the U.S., Inc., New York, 1993. A well-researched book written by the leading authorities from the nation's top medical centers. Full of practical suggestions and descriptions of what works and how to find resources in your area.

3.   **The Wellness Book: The Comprehensive Guide to Maintaining Health and Treating Stress-Related Illness**. Herbert Benson, M.D., and Eileen M. Stuart, R.N., M.S., Birch Lane Press, New York, 1993. Competent overall look at wellness with practical how-to information.

CHAPTER 17: FAT TO FIT: HEALTHY LIFESTYLE
CHANGES FOR ALL AGES

1.   **Cooking Low Carb.** Brenda Laughlin and Kelly Nason, Two N's Publishing, P.O. Box 35, Littleton, MA 01460, 1999. Order from www.cestbon.com. A practical and easy-to-follow cookbook written especially for sufferers of PCOS, but useful for anyone with problems managing waistline weight gain.

2.   **CPSI/Nutrition Action Health Letter**, 1875 Connecticut Avenue, N.W., Suite 300, Washington, D.C. 20009. Web site www.cspinet.org/nah. A hard-hitting, scientifically-based newsletter that exposes frauds and fads in all the nutrition-supplement hype abounding today. An excellent resource to get reliable information since it is NOT supported by advertising.

3.   **40-30-30 Fat Burning Nutrition.** Joyce and Gene Daoust, Wharton Publishing, Del Mar, CA, 1996. An excellent, easy-to-read, practical and easy-to-follow meal plan that helps you reduce the fat-storing insulin excesses caused by our current high-carbohydrate, low-fat diets. The Daosts have done a terrific job of providing healthy meal plans for both vegetarians and non-vegetarians, and they have also provided a list of prepared foods that fit well into the 40-30-30 balance. Our patients have really found this book helpful, and they have lots of lost pounds to back them up!

4.   **Mastering The Zone.** Barry Sears and Mary Goodbody, Harper Collins, New York, 1996. I think this is an excellent meal plan, and addresses important points about the role of excess insulin in causing a number of serious health problems that become more common in women during the years of transition to menopause and beyond. I have recommended it to our patients since 1996, but the feedback from patients has been that it is difficult to read, comprehend, and follow as a meal plan. For that reason, I have turned to the simpler, more "user-friendly" book by the Daousts. Dr. Sears has recently published a new book, *The Soy Zone,* which I have also reviewed and do not recommend as positively as his original "Zone" meal plan. In his new emphasis on soy, he does not take into account the latest science showing competitive inhibition of ovarian hormone production in premenopausal women by high dietary intake of soy protein or soy supplements. Nor does he address the

potential for a high soy diet to markedly interfere with thyroid function, particularly a common problem in women. For these reasons, if you have any symptoms suggestive of either ovarian hormone imbalance or thyroid disorders, I suggest if you want to follow the "Zone" meal plan, stay with the original book and recipes rather than the "soy zone."

5.   Syndrome X: The Complete Nutritional Program to Prevent and Reverse Insulin Resistance. Jack Challen, Dr. Burton Berkson, and Melissa Diane Smith. John Wiley and Sons, New York, NY, 2000. An excellent resource for understanding the role that elevated insulin plays in causing heart disease, hypertension, elevated triglycerides, abnormal cholesterol patterns and diabetes. Gives helpful information on nutritional approaches to correct these problems and reduce later risk of diabetes and cardiovascular disorders.

6.   The Callaway Diet: Successful Permanent Weight Control for Starvers, Stuffers, and Skippers. Wayne Callaway, M.D., Bantum Books, New York, 1990. An older book (and possibly hard to find), but still an excellent resource to explain the effects on the body from chronic diets, how to reduce the problem of insulin resistance and how to break out of the trap of "skipping and stuffing." Dr. Callaway has extensive experience in obesity treatment and provides medically sound overall information.

7.   The Bodywise Woman: Reliable Information About Physical Activity and Health. Written by the staff and researchers of the Melpomene Institute for Women's Health Research, Prentice Hall Press, New York, 1990. Well-researched and specific to the needs of women of all ages. Write to this organization for updates of their consumer materials.

8.   The Protein Power Plan. Michael R. and Mary Dan Eades, M.D., Bantam Books, New York, NY, 1996. Similar to the above meal plans in providing background understanding of the ways to reduce excess insulin through your meal plan schedule and food choices. Although it is a bit expensive, their complete package of materials (sold as a set with videotape, audiotapes, workbook guide, professional references, et cetera) provides a wealth of practical tips for success as well as medical references for you to discuss with your own physician before starting this meal plan.

9.   "Long-term effects of oral estradiol and dydrogesterone on carbohydrate metabolism in postmenopausal women." U.J. Gaspard, O.J. Wery, A.J. Scheen, et al, Climacteric: The Journal of the International Menopause Society, vol. 2, no2, June 1999, pp. 93-100.

CHAPTER 18: OSTEOPOROSIS—
A CASE FOR PREVENTIVE MEDICINE

1.   National Osteoporosis Foundation (NOF), 2100 M Street N.W., Suite 602, Washington, D.C. 20037, 1-800-223-2226, Web site: www.nof.org. An excellent source of cutting edge information about osteoporosis prevention and treatment. Join NOF and become an advocate in your community. I highly recommend their educational materials.

2.   Strong Women Stay Young. Miriam E. Nelson, Ph.D., Bantam-Doubleday-Dell, New York, NY, (paperback) 1998. An excellent book outlining the benefits of both aerobic and strength-training for women to preserve and build healthy bone and muscle. I highly recommend it.

CHAPTER 19: PATIENT AND PHYSICIAN: IMPERATIVE AGENDAS IN WOMEN'S HEALTH FOR THE TWENTY-FIRST CENTURY

1. <u>The Complete Guide to Women's Health: Revised Edition.</u> Bruce D. Shephard, M.D., F.A.C.O.G., and Carroll A. Shephard, R.N., Ph.D., Plume, 1997, paperback. This is an excellent reference book to have in your library. Available from Amazon.com.

2. <u>Take Charge of Your Hospital Stay.</u> Karen Keating McCann, Perseus Books, Cambridge, MA, 1994. A must-read before you go in for tests, out-patient surgeries or other procedures or you find that you have to be hospitalized for anything. It may be difficult to find in bookstores, but is available on Amazon.com.

CHAPTER 20: WEAVING YOUR TAPESTRY OF HEALTH AND WHOLENESS

The following books are ones I have used often in my women's growth groups and seminars because I feel they offer a great deal of clarity about our lives as women, how we have reached the place we are now and the opportunities to discover the fullest dimensions of ourselves as women for the times ahead. In my opinion, these remain classics and I have kept this list for the revised edition to encourage you to explore them.

1. <u>Women Who Run with the Wolves.</u> Clarissa Pinkola Estes, Ph.D., Ballantine Books Div. of Random House, Inc. 1997. A powerful and moving book about recovering the creative, spontaneous, passionate soul force within each individual woman that is too often masked by societal roles and expectations. I found this a moving and inspiring book and still turn to it often.I agree with the description by Jean Shinoda Bolen, M.D., "Full of wonderful, passionate, poetic, and psychologically potent words and images that will inspire, instruct and empower women to be true to their own nature and thus in touch with sources of creativity, humor and strength."

3. <u>The Crone: Woman of Age, Wisdom and Power.</u> Barbara G. Walker, Harper, San Francisco, 1988. Many women have a negative image of a "crone." Barbara Walker's book clarifies the derivation of *crone* as being from "crown," representing "wise woman" after menopause. This book chronicles the historical roots of devaluation, repression, and denial of the wisdom of older women, and offers a wealth of insights into ways women may develop the kind of constructive healing power that will benefit themselves as well as present and future generations. I highly recommend it.

4. <u>The Heroine's Journey: Woman's Quest for Wholeness.</u> Maureen Murdoch, Shambhala Publications, Inc., Boston and London, 1990. A meaningful exploration of feminine psyche and female psychological development, and a guide to help women find the spiritually alive feminine self who will be actively engaged in personal and cultural empowerment. If you are just beginning your inner quest, this book has many suggestions for helping you explore your feelings and gain appreciation of your full self.

5. <u>The Road Less Traveled.</u> M. Scott Peck, M.D. Simon and Schuster, New York, 1977, and Buccaneer Books, 1995. The power and enduring quality of this book is indicated by it being on the N.Y Times best-seller list for *over ten years*. It is one of the most meaningful books I have read; I continue to find new levels of thought-provoking ideas each time I go back to it. It is truly a classic, and I highly recommend that you read it.

6. **Healing Words. The Power of Prayer and the Practice of Medicine**, Larry Dossey, MD, Harper, San Francisco, 1993. A meaningful book about the ways that modern medicine has overlooked the crucial role of prayer in healing, and how to help you re-connect with your spiritual needs as you face life's challenges. I have read most of Dr. Dossey's books and have found they are inspiring and encouraging of the steps we need to take to make medicine and healing more focused on the whole person.

7. **Sacred Journey.** An inspirational journal of readings, prayers and reflections on life written by contributors of all faiths and published by the interfaith organization, A Fellowship in Prayer, Inc. 291 Witherspoon St., Princeton, NJ 08542. This little journal is a wealth of short, inspiring readings that will help facilitate your daily meditation and spiritual awareness.

III. Newsletters

Nutrition Action published by the Center for Science in the Public Interest, Washington, D.C. **Web site: www.cspinet.org/nah**. An excellent, progressive newletter which is NOT supported by advertising. It is hard-hitting and unbiased by commercial influences. Contains practical advice on reading food labels, selecting healthy options and avoiding hidden sources of fat, salt, and sugar and other useful pointers.

The Harvard Women's Health Watch Newsletter. In my opinion, of all the many women's health newsletters that have brought out since the first edition of my book, this is by far the best in terms of quality and depth of information. It is published monthly by Harvard Health Publications, 10 Shattuck Street, Suite 612, Boston, MA 02115. The authors provide timely, well-researched information on many topics of interest to women of all ages, and the content is provided in enough depth to make it useful to guide your discussions with your own health professionals. I subscribed to a number of other women's health newsletters for at least a year or so with each one so that I could evaluate their material over time. After this detailed review, I am not recommending any other women's health newsletters because in my professional opinion, they are either (1) pushing supplements and other products, (2) have unreliable medical information, (3) have too much "fluff" without enough depth to their content to be overly useful, or (4) they push a narrow point-of-view without sufficient balance to be objective.

What's Wrong?
Quiz Yourself Before You
See the Doctor

Self Test: Do You Have PMS?

PMS, premenstrual syndrome, is characterized by a wide variety of emotional and physical symptoms that appear regularly before a woman's period (sometimes as long as two weeks before menstruation), end with the onset of menses, and are followed by a *symptom-free phase* EACH cycle. The following questions are aimed at helping you identify whether or not you suffer from a cluster of PMS symptoms. Please answer each question as accurately as possible. **At about the same time each month, prior to the beginning of your menstrual period:**

1. Do you experience any of the following mood changes?
    a. anxiety ___YES ___NO
    b. irritability ___YES ___NO
    c. feeling nervous and tense ___YES ___NO
    d. mood swings ___YES ___NO
    e. crying spells ___YES ___NO
    f. depressed mood ___YES ___NO

2. Do you experience any of the following changes in your behavior?
    a. impulsivity ___YES ___NO
    b. anger outbursts ___YES ___NO
    c. becoming withdrawn ___YES ___NO
    d. lethargy ___YES ___NO
    e. fatigue ___YES ___NO
    f. craving for sweets, chocolate ___YES ___NO
    g. craving for carbohydrates, alcohol ___YES ___NO
    h. craving for salty foods ___YES ___NO

3. Do you experience any of the following symptoms related to the central nervous system?
    a. forgetfulness ___YES ___NO
    b. indecision ___YES ___NO
    c. difficulty concentrating ___YES ___NO

d. memory problem	___YES	___NO
e. lack of coordination	___YES	___NO
f. restless sleep	___YES	___NO
g. altered sex drive	___YES	___NO
h. marked appetite changes	___YES	___NO

4. Do you experience any of the following physical symptoms?

a. weight gain	___YES	___NO
b. breast tenderness	___YES	___NO
c. bloating	___YES	___NO
d. swelling of hands and feet	___YES	___NO
e. constipation	___YES	___NO
f. headaches	___YES	___NO
g. heart palpitations	___YES	___NO
h. dizziness	___YES	___NO
i. low back pain or joint pain	___YES	___NO
j. crawly, itchy, dry skin	___YES	___NO
k. dry eyes	___YES	___NO
l. hair loss or thinning	___YES	___NO

Discussion of Results

If you answered YES to more than *five* of the above questions, and you feel that the symptoms regularly affect your daily functioning, you may have PMS. I suggest you consider the following steps:

- Seek a comprehensive medical/psychological evaluation from physicians who are knowledgeable about PMS and who will do appropriate lab tests also.
- It is important to get your hormone levels reliably tested, at the proper time of your cycle, as I have outlined in my book. Blood Serum tests will give you a more complete and reliable picture than will saliva or urine tests.
- Seek the guidance of trained professionals to help you make lifestyle and dietary changes that will help reduce PMS symptoms.

PMS affects women of all backgrounds, races, ages, and nationalities. About four out of every ten women have moderately severe premenstrual symptoms. Five to 10 percent of women with PMS have symptoms severe enough to disrupt their personal and professional lives. PMS symptoms are not caused by psychological or mental problems, but stress may make the PMS symptoms worse. There is no one established theory as to what causes PMS; it is generally considered to be a biochemical disorder involving the interaction of many hormonal systems.

PMS is a problem that has *many* approaches to help reduce your discomfort. Ideally these approaches should be combined in an integrated program suited to your individual needs. Options to help you feel better include diet changes, stress management, vitamins, herbs, acupuncture, and a variety of medications for severe symptoms. Hormonal therapies may be beneficial for some of you. Don't just sit there and feel terrible. Take charge of your health and seek the help that is available!

PMS Self-Check by Elizabeth Lee Vliet, M.D., 1984 revised 1990, 1995, 1999

Self Test: Are You Beginning or in Menopause?

Current Medications/Hormones_____

| Hysterectomy: | ___No | ___Yes | (Date:_____) |
| Ovaries Removed: | ___No | ___Yes | |

Directions: Circle number that best describes *degree* of symptom intensity you have experienced over the past month(s):

	No	**Mild**	**Moderate**	**Severe**
	0	**1**	**2**	**3**

1. Hot flushes, perspiration, and/or chilly sensations

    0   1   2   3

2. Sensations of numbness and/or tingling of the skin

    0   1   2   3

3. Insomnia or restless, fragmented sleep

    0   1   2   3

4. Irritability, feeling anxious or apprehensive

    0   1   2   3

5. Feeling of depression and unhappiness and/or being miserable without any obvious reason

    0   1   2   3

6. Sensations of dizziness or swimming in the head

    0   1   2   3

7. Feeling of weariness of mind and body associated with desire for rest; disinclination to make further efforts

    0   1   2   3

8. Pain of any kind affecting joints or muscles

    0   1   2   3

9. Headaches of any kind (tension, migraine, etc.)

    0   1   2   3

10. Quickening or acceleration of heartbeat or a fluttering/pounding heartbeat in a sitting or resting position

    0   1   2   3

11. Sensation of ants or other insects creeping over the skin ("crawly skin")

    0   1   2   3

Directions: Circle number that best describes *degree* of symptom intensity you have experienced over the past month(s):

Never	Infrequently	Sometimes	Most of the Time	Always
0	1	2	3	4

12. Vaginal burning or itching

    0   1   2   3   4

13. Painful urination or increased frequency of urination

    0   1   2   3   4

14. Leaking of urine when coughing, laughing, sneezing, or on hard work

    0   1   2   3   4

15. Leaking of urine when walking, running, climbing steps, or on light work

    0   1   2   3   4

16. Leaking of urine, regardless of activity, even when in a lying position?

    0   1   2   3   4

Scoring and Discussion

To calculate your total score:

    Question 1: **Multiply** the number corresponding to your response **by 4** and write the resulting number on the line   ————

    Questions 2–4: **Multiply** the number corresponding to each answer **by 2** and then **total the points**, write the total points on the line   ————

    Questions 5–16: **Add** together all of the numbers corresponding to your response for each question, and write the total points on the line   ————

                                       Total from Above: ————

If your total score is **between 7 and 15**, you *may* be in the early phases of the menopause transition, or (if taking hormones) your HRT regimen may not yet be optimal for you.

If your score is **between 16 and 30**, you clearly have menopausal symptoms, and I think you would benefit from having hormone levels checked (ovary and thyroid) along with your usual medical checkup. There are many lifestyle changes, herbs, vitamins and/or hormones that may be helpful to you and should be discussed with your primary physician or an experienced and knowledgeable menopause specialist.

If your score is **greater than 30,** you have marked to severe menopausal *symptoms, which also suggest the presence of other risk factors such as bone loss and cholesterol changes.* You would be wise to have a *comprehensive midlife women's health evaluation* to determine the best options to improve your immediate well-being as well as to reduce the risks of later diseases such as osteoporosis and heart disease. You may want to have this done by your present physician, or consider one of the centers around the country where the comprehensive evaluations, tailored to midlife women, are provided.

Reference: Kupperman Menopausal Index; modifications by Elizabeth Lee Vliet, M.D., 1992

Self Test: Cancer Risk Questionnaire for Women

Name_____ Date of Birth_____ Age:_____

YES NO GENERAL HEALTH
___ ___ I have had cancer
___ ___ There is a history of cancer in my immediate family
___ ___ I am 15 or more pounds overweight
___ ___ I eat a diet high in meats/dairy products and fat content
___ ___ I eat fewer than 5 servings of fruit and vegetables per day
___ ___ I use chewing tobacco or snuff, or smoke cigarettes
___ ___ I have not had a complete physical in at least five years
___ ___ I drink alcohol regularly
___ ___ I have not been to a dentist in over three years

YES NO BREAST CANCER
___ ___ I have had breast cancer
___ ___ Someone in my family has had breast cancer
       Who? _____ **(Risk increases if person with cancer is mother or sister)**
___ ___ I am over 50 years of age
___ ___ I have had surgery for "lumps" in the breast
___ ___ I have had a female cancer (ovary or womb/uterus)
___ ___ I gave birth to my first child after age 35
___ ___ I am 35 or older and have not been pregnant to full term (9 months)

YES NO ENDOMETRIAL CANCER
___ ___ My mother and/or sister(s) have had endometrial or breast cancer
___ ___ I have had breast or ovarian cancer
___ ___ I am over 50 years of age
___ ___ I am more than 20 percent over the recommended body weight for my height
___ ___ I have never had a full-term (9 months) pregnancy
___ ___ I have high blood pressure
___ ___ I have a uterus and have taken estrogen **alone** (without progestin or progesterone) for a long period of time (more than two years)

YES NO OVARIAN CANCER
___ ___ I have a family history of ovarian cancer
___ ___ I am over age 50
___ ___ I have had either breast or endometrial cancer
___ ___ I have never had a full-term pregnancy
___ ___ I have a history of infertility and/or menstrual irregularities, cycles with no ovulation
___ ___ I have a history of recurring ovarian cysts
___ ___ I am or have been a cigarette smoker
___ ___ I have taken fertility drugs such as Clomid and/or Pergonal
___ ___ I regularly use(d) talcum powder in underwear and/or on sanitary pads

YES	NO	COLON CANCER
___	___	I have had colon cancer
___	___	A family member has had colon cancer
		Who? _____
___	___	I have had polyp(s) in the colon
___	___	I have had Crohn's disease or ulcerative colitis
___	___	I have had a recent change from my usual bowel movements
___	___	I have noticed blood in my bowel movements
___	___	I am over 50 years of age
___	___	I eat a diet high in meat, fat and/or grilled foods
___	___	I eat very few fruits, vegetables and whole grains

YES	NO	LUNG CANCER
___	___	I smoke cigarettes
___	___	I have smoked cigarettes How long?_____ When quit?_____
		(If you stopped smoking more than 15 years ago, risk decreases almost to the normal expected risk based on your present age.)
___	___	I am over 40 years of age
___	___	I am exposed regularly to other people's cigarette smoking
___	___	At work, I am exposed to arsenic, asbestos, chromates, nickel, organic solvents, uranium, or petroleum products
___	___	Someone in my family has had lung cancer. (**Risk is higher if parent or sibling has lung cancer, especially if person is a nonsmoker.**)

YES	NO	SKIN CANCER
___	___	I have light-colored hair, eyes, or complexion
___	___	I have a large number of moles or moles that are large or irregular in shape or color
___	___	I frequently work or play in the sun
___	___	I rarely use sunscreen or sunblock when I am out in the sun
___	___	I was sunburned (blistered) several times before age 20
___	___	My skin is frequently exposed to chemicals or radioactive materials (arsenic, coal, petroleum, uranium, radioisotopes)
___	___	I have a family history of skin cancer
___	___	I have been to tanning salons

Discussion of Results

The more YES answers you have, the higher your cancer risk. If the YES answers are clustered in a particular type of cancer, you should take this self-test information to your physician and discuss what preventive screening is desirable for you to have and how frequently such screening evaluations should be done. Even if you do not appear to have a high risk of a particular cancer, I would encourage you to copy this information for your physician to have as part of your medical record. Then you and your physician should reassess your risks whenever you have your annual checkup.

Adapted from "SPOT: Cancer Risk Questionnaire," a joint program developed and funded by the University of Texas, M.D. Anderson Cancer Center, and the Texas Academy of Family Physicians. Copyright UTMDACC 1993. Material added by Elizabeth Lee Vliet, M.D., © 1994.

Self Test: Are You at Risk for Serious Bone Loss and Osteoporosis?

Osteoporosis is called a "silent enemy" because you may not find out you have it until significant irreversible damage has occurred. Even if you do not have any clear symptoms, use this test to evaluate your risk level according to factors that have been scientifically identified through extensive medical research.

Directions: Answer each question, then write down the number of risk points shown for each answer, and total your score.

I. Risk Factors that Can't Be Controlled

____	Do you have a family history of osteoporosis?	No (0 points)	Yes (4 points)
____	Are you White, northern European, or Asian?	No (0 points)	Yes (3 points)
____	Do you have a fair complexion?	No (0 points)	Yes (2 points)
____	Do you have a small-boned frame?	No (0 points)	Yes (4 points)
____	Are you over 40 years of age?	No (0 points)	Yes (2 points)
____	Are you over 70 years of age?	No (0 points)	Yes (4 points)
____	Have you had both your ovaries removed (and are NOT taking replacement hormones)?	No (0 points)	Yes (4 points)
____	Have you breast fed at least one child?	No (0 points)	Yes (1 point)
____	Are you allergic to milk or other dairy products?	No (0 points)	Yes (3 points)
____	Have you not had children?	No (0 points)	Yes (2 points)
____	Did youy menopause occur around age 45?	No (0 points)	Yes (3 points)
____	Have you lost more than ½ inch in height?	No (0 points)	Yes (4 points)

I. ____   **Subtotal for risk factors that can't be controlled**

II. Risk Factors that Can Be Controlled

____	Do you smoke cigarettes?	No (0 points)	Yes (4 points)
____	Do you drink alcoholic beverages?	No (0 points)	Yes _____

Yes: 1–2 ounces a day (2 points)
3 or more ounces per day (4 points)

___ Do you avoid milk and other dairy products?	No (0 points)	Yes (3 points)
___ Do you exercise?	Regular exercise (0 points) Little or none (3 points)	
___ Are you a person who exercises a great deal, with irregular or no menstruation?	No (0 points)	Yes (4 points)
___ Is your diet high in animal protein such as meats?	No (0 points)	Yes (2 points)
___ Do you add salt to foods at the table?	No (0 points)	Yes (3 points)
___ Are you a vegetarian, or have a diet heavily weighted toward vegetables?	No (0 points)	Yes (2 points)
___ Do you have an eating disorder, or consume too little nutritious food?	No (0 points)	Yes (4 points)
___ Do you have high amounts of fiber in your diet?	No (0 points)	Yes (4 points)
___ Do you have 3 or more cups of coffee a day—or an equivalent amount of caffeine from other sources, such as cola-type beverages?	No (0 points)	Yes (2 points)

II. ___ Subtotal for risk factors that can be controlled

III. Risk Factors that You Might Be Able to Control

___ Do you have a low percentage of body fat (less than 18% of total body weight)?	No (0 points)	Yes (4 points)
___ Have you ever used anticonvulsants (medications designed to prevent convulsions or fits)?	No (0 points)	Yes (2 points)
___ Have you had hyperparathyroidism (an excessive secretion of the parathyroid glands that causes loss of calcium from the bones, formation of cysts in the bones, and kidney stones)?	No (0 points)	Yes (3 points)
___ Have you ever used steroid (cortisone) drugs?	No (0 points)	Yes (4 points)

_____ Have you had biliary cirrhosis   **No** (0 points)   **Yes** (3 points)
       (an inflammatory disease of
       the bile system connecting the
       liver and the intestines)?

_____ Have you had an overactive thyroid   **No** (0 points)   **Yes** (4 points)
       gland with symptoms such as fast
       pulse and heart rate, loss of weight,
       "hyped up" metabolism?

_____ Have you had stomach or small-   **No** (0 points)   **Yes** (4 points)
       bowel disease?

III. _____ Subtotal for risk factors that you might be able to control

To evaluate your level of risk, add ALL subtotals: _____

Your **total point level (from I, II, and III subtotals)** determines your risk category:

0–8 Low Risk Category: As you grow older, your risk will increase. So take steps now to minimize threats to your bones by paying close attention to good nutrition, exercise, and the other controllable risk factors.

9–16 Moderate Risk Category: Pay close attention to changeable risk factors. Ask your doctor about drugs that may be causing bone loss. If you're past menopause, discuss estrogen replacement therapy or antiresorptive medication if you aren't already on one of these.

17–25 and Above: High and Very High Risk Categories: Take steps immediately to counteract bone loss. With your doctor, formulate a personal bone-protection program. You may want your doctor to measure the density of your bones to evaluate their present condition and to serve as baseline to be sure the bone loss is not getting worse.

From: *Preventing Osteoporosis*, by Kenneth Cooper, M.D., M.P.H., © 1989, Bantam Books. Used with permission.

Self Test: Do You Have a Sleep Disorder?

1. Do you have an irregular or abnormal sleep-wake schedule? ___YES   ___NO

2. Do you have a problem falling asleep at night ___YES   ___NO

3. Do you regularly wake up several times during the night? ___YES   ___NO

4. Do you regularly wake up too early, unable to go back to sleep? ___YES   ___NO

5. Do you have difficulty getting up and functioning effectively the first thing in the morning? ___YES   ___NO

6. Do you frequently feel overly sleepy or drowsy in the daytime? ___YES   ___NO

7. Do you regularly have discomfort or pain disturbing your sleep? ___YES   ___NO

8. Do you snore loudly on a fairly regular basis? ___YES   ___NO

9. Do you have any abnormal breathing during sleep? ___YES   ___NO

10. Do you have abnormal movements, jerkiness of the legs, or excessive restlessness during your sleep? ___YES   ___NO

11. Do you need medication to help you sleep at night? ___YES   ___NO

12. Do you need stimulants or medication for daytime alertness? ___YES   ___NO

13. Does your bed partner or anybody else who has observed your sleep say that you snore too much, are too restless, have jerky movements, or ever stop breathing briefly during sleep? ___YES   ___NO

14. Do you experience an unusual degree of fatigue or lethargy during the day? ___YES   ___NO

15. Do you notice that you no longer seem to dream normally, or have abnormally vivid or frightening dreams? ___YES   ___NO

Scoring and Discussion

If you have *two* or more YES answers, you should discuss these problems with your physician. Ask the question, "Could I have a sleep disorder that needs to be checked further?" I encourage you to *avoid just taking sleeping pills,* thinking that is treating the problem. Sleeping pills lose their effectiveness after about two weeks, and most are addictive when taken for longer than seven to ten days. These medications can actually be dangerous if you have sleep apnea, since these medications may further depress breathing.

For women in midlife, restless sleep with several awakenings may be one of the earliest indicators of declining estrogen. This is even more likely if the waking episodes are also accompanied by "fluttering" or racing heartbeat, sweating, feeling too hot and/or suddenly chilled. If the cause of the sleep disturbance is an endocrine change, it won't help to just take sleeping pills.

If you answered yes to *any* of the questions 8 through 12, you should be evaluated for sleep apnea, myoclonus, "restless legs syndrome," and narcolepsy. Sleep apnea, if unrecognized and untreated, can cause sexual dysfunction, major depression, high blood pressure, chronic fatigue, problems with memory and concentration during the day, and potentially a heart attack.

It is important to have sleep problems such as these checked properly by a physician knowledgeable about sleep disorders. If your physician dismisses your concerns, seek a consultation with a sleep specialist.

Sleep Disorders Questionnaire by Elizabeth Lee Vliet, M.D., © 1988, revised 2000

Self Test: Do You Have Fibromyalgia?

Fibromyalgia is such an elusive medical problem that it is difficult to design a questionnaire that would be specific for this pain syndrome. I have provided these questions as a guide for you to evaluate what you are experiencing. If you answer YES to **more than 3 questions**, I suggest you review the chapter on fibromyalgia, write the resource organizations in the appendix for more information, and consult with your physician or a pain-management specialist in your area. The more you know about this pain syndrome, the better you will be able to put together effective approaches to reduce pain and feel better overall.

1. I have trouble sleeping on a regular basis due to pain.   ____YES ___NO

2. I notice the pain on a constant, almost daily basis.   ____YES ___NO

3. I experience pain in multiple areas of my body: neck, shoulders, back, hips, joints, head, etc.   ____YES ___NO

4. My pain is not usually relieved by aspirin, Tylenol, or over-the-counter antiinflammatory (pain) medications.   ____YES ___NO

5. I have reduced or eliminated activities that I used to enjoy due to limitations caused by my pain.   ____YES ___NO

6. I no longer enjoy sexual activity due to constant pain.   ____YES ___NO

7. I experience a worsening of my pain in cold, damp weather.   ____YES ___NO

8. I have experienced a decrease in my ability to work at home or in my outside-the-home job due to pain.   ____YES ___NO

9. I have been depressed or irritable and tenset o a degree that is unlike my usual self because of the pain.   ____YES ___NO

10. I experience numbness, burning or cold sensations in my muscles and/or my arms and legs.   ____YES ___NO

11. I have generalized stiffness and soreness, often worse in the mornings.   ____YES ___NO

12. I have a lot of tender places where muscles come together around my joints, shoulders, back, and neck.   ____YES ___NO

13. My memory and concentration are getting worse due to the pain.   ____YES ___NO

14. My pain is so difficult for me to live with, I have had thoughts of taking my life. (If this answer is YES, **you must get professional help NOW.**)   ____YES ___NO

© *Elizabeth Lee Vliet M.D., 1994, revised 2000*

Self Test: Are You at Risk for Heart Disease?

These questions address some of the common genetic, lifestyle, and medical factors that increase risk of *atherosclerosis*, or disease of the heart and blood vessels. If you are a *postmenopausal* woman, you will want to know what your estradiol level is in addition to cholesterol and other measures of risk. The items shown here do not all have the same degree of importance in determining your heart disease risk. They are ones that you should be taking into account as you make healthy lifestyle changes. Your physician can discuss the relative importance, or weighting, given to each of these risk factors, based on your individual health profile as a whole.

The items shown in bold are ones that should be checked by your physician. If you do not know the answers to the statements shown in bold, I urge you to *find out*. This is information you should keep in your personal health file to help you keep track of how you measure up on heart disease risk.

Directions: Answer YES or NO to the following questions:

No one in my family has heart problems, high blood pressure, stroke(s), diabetes, or is overweight.   ____YES ___NO

My body weight is in the normal range for my age, height, and sex.   ____YES ___NO

My waist-to-hip ratio is <u>less</u> than 0.85 (divide waist measurement by hip measurement, with hips measured 7 inches below the waist).   ____YES ___NO

I walk briskly or do other aerobic exercise three or more times a week.   ____YES ___NO

I never used or have stopped using cigarettes and tobacco products.   ____YES ___NO

I drink alcohol occasionally or only one drink a day.   ____YES ___NO

I manage stress in my life effectively.   ____YES ___NO

I have eliminated or reduced my intake of meat, butter, cheese, lunch meat, and salty and fatty snack foods.   ____YES ___NO

I take regular vacations and weekend breaks.   ____YES ___NO

I feel pretty calm most of the time, able to relax after work.   ____YES ___NO

I take a low dose of aspirin every other day (low dose is one-quarter to one full tablet of regular-strength aspirin, 325 mg/tablet)   ____YES ___NO

My total cholesterol is 200 or less. ____YES ___NO

My HDL-cholesterol is 50 or higher. ____YES ___NO

My blood triglycerides are in the normal range. ____YES ___NO

My blood pressure is in the normal range for my age. ____YES ___NO

My fasting blood glucose is in the normal range. ____YES ___NO

My estradiol levels are in the normal premenopausal range. ____YES ___NO

(If you are postmenopausal) I take estrogen therapy daily. ____YES ___NO

My fasting insulin is in the normal range ____YES ___NO

My levels of ferritin and homocysteine are in the normal range. ____YES ___NO

My level of hsCRP is in the normal range (see chapter 13). ____YES ___NO

Scoring and Discussion

The more **NO responses** you have, the *higher* **your risk** of heart disease. You will notice that *all* of the risk factors above, *except* for your family history, are ones that YOU CONTROL by CHOICES you make each day and by how effectively you work with your physician as an active partner in your health care. Think about this: If YOU don't take care of your heart, who will? Review chapters 13, 15, 19, and 20 for more help on heart disease and how to decrease your risks.

Women's Heart Disease Risk Checklist by Elizabeth Lee Vliet, M.D., © 1987, revised 1995, 2000

Self Test: What's Your Stress Index?

How do you cope with the stress in your life? There are numerous ways, and some are more effective than others. In addition, some coping approaches you might turn to can actually be as *harmful* as the stress they were intended to alleviate. This scale is a self-assessment *educational* tool, not a *diagnostic* one. Its purpose is to inform you of healthy ways in which you can effectively cope with the stress in your life. Using a point system, this self test is designed to give you some indication of how important or desirable specific coping strategies are.

Directions: Simply answer the questions, score each one as directed. Then total your points and see how you did. Do you see some ways to improve your score?

_____ 1. Give yourself 10 if you feel that you have a supportive family member near you.

_____ 2. Give yourself 10 points if you actively pursue a hobby.

_____ 3. Give yourself 10 if you belong to some social or activity group that meets once a month (other than your family).

_____ 4. Give yourself 15 points if you are within five pounds of your "ideal" body weight for your height and bone structure.

_____ 5. Give yourself 15 points if you practice some form of "deep relaxation" at least three times a week (such exercises include meditation, imagery, Yoga, etc.).

_____ 6. Give yourself 15 points *for each time* you exercise thirty minutes or longer during the course of an average week.

_____ 7. Give yourself 5 points for each nutritionally balanced and wholesome meal you consume during the course of an average day.

_____ 8. Give yourself 5 points if you do something that you enjoy and that is "just for you" during the course of an average week.

_____ 9. Give yourself 10 points if you have some place in your home that you can go to relax and/or be by yourself.

_____ 10. Give yourself 10 points if you practice time management techniques in your daily life.

_____ 11. Subtract 10 points for each pack of cigarettes you smoke during the course of an average day.

_____ 12. Subtract 5 points for each evening during the course of an average week that take any form of medication or chemical substance (including alcohol) to help you sleep.

_____ 13. Subtract 10 points for each day during the course of an average week that you consume any form of medication or chemical substance (including alcohol) to reduce your anxiety or just calm you down.

_____ 14. Subtract five points for each evening during the course of an average week that you bring work home (work that was meant to be done at your workplace).

_____ 15. Subtract five points for each day during the course of an average week that you overeat or binge to cope with feelings (anxiety, anger, depression, etc.).

_____ NOW CALCULATE YOUR TOTAL SCORE

A maximum score would be 115 points.

This stress assessment test was created by Dr. George S. Everly, Jr.,
University of Maryland. Available from U.S. Gov. Department of Health Education.

Discussion and Reflection

If your score was *less than 30,* I encourage you to seek a professional in stress management, counseling, or psychotherapy to help you improve your stress-coping skills, behaviors, and attitudes, which will lead to improved" psychological hardiness" and a better sense of wellness in your life.

If your score was *between 30 and 50,* it's time to take a serious look at your lifestyle and think about the choices you are making that cause stress to mount up and have a negative effect on your health. Time to wake up and practice some new (or unused) stress-coping skills.

If your score was *over 50,* you probably have adequate coping strategies for the common sources of stress. Keep in mind, the higher your score the greater your ability to cope with stress in an effective and healthy manner. The higher your score, the better your "resilience" when major stresses hit!

You may have been surprised with your results. Maybe you thought you cope pretty well with stress but got a lower score than you expected. Maybe you found you were doing pretty well but would like to improve. Whatever the case, each of us can find ways to bring more joy, playfulness, and spontaneity into our lives to reduce tension and overload. Create fun rewards for yourself as you carry out adding new coping skills.

REFLECTION

Another important dimension of "stress management" is to feel good about the way you live your life, that your life has meaning and purpose, and that you are reaching those goals that are important to you. You may find it helpful now to jot down your thoughts, feelings, and reactions to these "reflection" questions.

Self-Reflection and Exploration

1. Describe an experience in which you had the feeling of being totally alive. How long ago was this? When are you going to schedule time for such an experience again?

2. What makes you feel life is really worth living?

3. Make a list of at least five things you like about yourself and another five things you feel you do very well. Put these lists in a place where you will see them daily.

4. List at least five things in your life that you are happy with and do not want to change. Put this list where you will see it daily, and *add* at least one item a month!

5. What ways have you found to maintain these positives in your life?

6. What are the five most pressing things in your life that you are *not* happy with and would like to change?

7. Which of these are within *your control* to change and which are *not* within your control? Begin a list of ways to change the things within your control.

8. What are some ways to help you accept the things that are not within your control? Do you need an objective outside person (e.g., therapist) to help you with this accepting?

9. List at least five ways you contribute positively to the lives of others?

10. List at least five things you can do for your own well-being without the assistance of anyone else. Pick one of these when you are tempted to overeat or drink alcohol.

11. Make a list of your five to ten most important aspirations. What do you have yet to learn to do? Is it time to take a class or tackle learning something toward an aspiration?

12. What are some self-destrucive or self-defeaing behaviors you want to stop? List several ways to "neutralize" or eliminate obstacles to your success that are created by your old behaviors.

13. What are several things that you tell yourself you "should/ought" to do that you really *do not want to do?* List several ways you may **begin now** to elliminate these "should" and "ought tos" and be gentler on yourself.

14. List five positive changes that have occurred in your life since menopause. Focus on adding one to the list each month.

Reflection Self Inventory: by Elizabeth Lee Vliet, ©1989, revised 1995, 2000

Self Test: How's My Sexuality?

Most women I talk with say they are embarrassed to initiate discussion of their questions about sexuality. I think it will help if you take time by yourself to consider these questions, write down your responses, and then make a list of the specific questions you would like to ask your doctor or a therapist. There are no right or wrong answers to these questions. I have written them in hopes it will help you reflect honestly about areas you may wish to improve, or possible health issues that should be addressed with a professional you trust.

1. *Am I satisfied with the frequency of my sexual activity?* Has it declined in recent months or years? If so, what ideas do I have about causes? Suggestions for reflection: Think about your body (are you satisfied with how you look and feel?), your partner, your lifestyle (do you drink too much alcohol, use drugs or medications, smoke tobacco?), your stresses (are you overworked and too tired to relax and enjoy sex?), and other pissible causes.

2. *Am I as interested in sexual activity as I have been in the past? Is my partner healthy and interested in sex? Do either my partner or I have any difficulty performing sexually?*

3. *Have I noticed a change or decline in my level of sexual desire?*

4. *Am I experiencing any pain or discomfort (burning, itching, etc.) with sexual intercourse?*

5. *Have I been having decreased vaginal lubrication and feeling too dry to enjoy sexual activity?*

6. *Does it take longer or is it harder to achieve an orgasm, making me feel like it's just too much effort to try?*

7. *Am I experiencing any painful muscle (e.g., uterus) contractions with intercourse or with orgasm that inhibiting my interest or desire?*

8. *Am I angry or upset with my partner and not communicating these feelings?*

9. *Are there other relationship problems (including my relationship with MYSELF) affecting my sexual activity and enjoyment?*

10. *What would I like to see changed or improved in my sexual activity and relationship with myself and others?*

"How's My Sexuality?" by Elizabeth Lee Vliet, M.D., © 1982, revised 1992, 1995

Self Test: Do You Have a Problem with Alcohol ?

The AUDIT, or Alcohol Use Disorders Identification Test, was designed to help physicians and patients better identify people who have problem drinking patterns and encourage treatment interventions *before* the addictive illness of alcoholism develops. I have included the self-assessment part of the AUDIT here so that you can answer these questions in a private setting. In our culture, women who are problem drinkers or alcoholics are more adversely stigmatized than are men; as a result, women are usually too ashamed to bring this up to their physicians. Even when they do talk with their physicians about drinking problems, women are commonly *not* referred for appropriate substance-abuse treatment as early in the disease as are men. Consequently, women are more seriously ill and have experienced more destructive consequences of alcohol abuse before they get help.

Be honest with yourself when you answer these questions. If you are not, you hurt primarily yourself and those who love you. **I *urge you to get professional help* if you have a score of 4 or more on this self test.**

AUDIT Self-Assessment: The following questions are about the past year.

1. How often do you have a drink containing alcohol?   <u>POINTS</u>

    _____Never   (0)
    _____Monthly or less   (1)
    _____2 to 4 times a month   (2)
    _____2 to 3 times a week   (3)
    _____4 or more times a week   (4)

2. How many drinks containing alcohol do you have on a typical day when you are drinking?

    _____None   (0)
    _____1 or 2   (1)
    _____3 or 4   (2)
    _____5 or 6   (3)
    _____7 or 9   (4)
    _____10 or more   (5)

3. How often do you have six or more drinks on one occasion?

    _____Never   (0)
    _____Less than monthly   (1)
    _____Monthly   (1)
    _____Weekly   (3)
    _____Daily or almost daily   (4)

4. How often during the past year have you found that you were unable to stop drinking once you had started?

    _____Never   (0)
    _____Less than monthly   (1)
    _____Monthly   (2)
    _____Weekly   (3)
    _____Daily or almost daily   (4)

5. How often during the past year have you failed to do what was normally expected from you because of drinking?

    _____Never   (0)
    _____Less than monthly   (1)
    _____Monthly   (2)
    _____Weekly   (3)
    _____Daily or almost daily   (4)

6. How often during the past year have you needed a first drink in the morning to get yourself going after a heavy drinking session?

    _____Never   (0)
    _____Less than monthly   (1)
    _____Monthly   (2)
    _____Weekly   (3)
    _____Daily or almost daily   (4)

7. How often during the past year have you had a feeling of guilt or remorse after drinking?

    _____Never   (0)
    _____Less than monthly   (1)
    _____Monthly   (2)
    _____Weekly   (3)
    _____Daily or almost daily   (4)

8. How often during the past year have you been unable to remember what happened the night before because you had been drinking?

    _____Never   (0)
    _____Less than monthly   (1)
    _____Monthly   (2)
    _____Weekly   (3)
    _____Daily or almost daily   (4)

9. Have you or someone else been injured as the result of your drinking?

    _____No   (0)
    _____Yes, but not in the last year   (2)
    _____Yes, during the last year   (4)

10. Has a relative, friend, a doctor, or other health worker expressed concern about your drinking or suggested you cut down?

    _____No   (0)
    _____Yes, but not in the last year   (2)
    _____Yes, during the last year   (4)

11. Have you ever experienced blackouts, "D.T.s," or loss of consciousness from drinking too much?

    _____No   (0)
    _____Yes, but not in the last year   (2)
    _____Yes, once during the last year   (4)
    _____Yes, more than once in the last year   (8)

Reference: Schmidt, et.al.

Self Test: Do You Have a Major Depression

Directions: Answer each question below according to the following key:

	None of the time	Some of the time	Good part of the time	Almost always
1. I feel downhearted, blue, and sad.				X
2. Morning is when I feel the best.			X	
3. I have crying spells or feel like it.				X
4. I have trouble sleeping through the night.		X		
5. I eat as much as I used to.	X			X
6. I enjoy looking at, talking to, and being with interesting women and men.				X
7. I notice that I am losing weight.	X			
8. I have trouble with constipation.	X			
9. My heart beats faster than usual.				
10. I get tired for no reason.				
11. My mind is as clear as it used to be.				
12. I find it easy to do the things I used to do.				
13. I am restless and can't keep still.				
14. I feel hopeful about the future.				
15. I am more irritable than usual.				
16. I find it more difficult to make decisions.				
17. I feel that I am useful and needed.				

18. My life is pretty full.				
19. I feel that others would be better off if I were dead.				
20. I still enjoy the things I used to.				

Make sure you answer every question. You cannot accurately score this quiz according to the formula below unless there is a response to each question!

Scoring and Discussion

Questions **2, 5, 6, 11, 12, 14, 16, 17, 18, 20**: Score according to the following key:

None or a little of the time = 4 points
Some of the time   = 3 points
Good part of the time   = 2 points
Almost always   = 1 point

Questions **1, 3, 4, 7, 8, 9, 10, 13, 15, 19**: Score according to the following key:

None or a little of the time = 1 point
Some of the time   = 2 points
Good part of the time   = 3 points
Almost always   = 4 points

After you have given the proper points to each of your responses, add all of these numbers to get your total raw score. To convert your raw score to the Depression Index score, use the following formula:

$$\text{INDEX} = \frac{\text{Raw score total points}}{\text{Max score of 80 points}} \times 100$$

Once you have calculated your index score, you can then interpret it based on the following ranges:

Index Score Less than 50:   normal range
Index Score of 50–59:   presence of minimal to mild depression
Index Score of 60–69:   presence of moderate to marked depression
Index Score of 70 and above: presence of severe to extreme depression

Depression is a very treatable problem—don't ignore it! If your score is over 55, I encourage you to consult with your personal physician or a psychiatrist to see that you have a more in-depth evaluation for possible medical factors affecting your mood and well-being and to also evalutate the possibility of a major depression, which could respond well to medications and supportive therapy

© W. W. K. Zung, "A Self-Rating Depression Scale," *Arch.Gen.Psychiatry*, 1965, 12:63–70. Zung Depression Scale also copyrighted 1974, 1989.

Self Test: Do You Have an Anxiety Disorder?

Directions: Answer the following questions according to the following key:

a. **None or a little of the time**
b. **Some of the time**
c. **A good part of the time**
d. **Almost always**

1. I feel more nervous and anxious than usual. _____
2. I feel afraid for no reason at all. _____
3. I get upset easily or feel panicky. _____
4. I feel like I'm falling apart and going to pieces. _____
5. I feel that everything is all right and nothing bad will happen. _____
6. My arms and legs shake and tremble. _____
7. I am bothered by headaches, neck and back pains. _____
8. I feel weak and get tired easily. _____
9. I feel calm and can sit still easily. _____
10. I can feel my heart beating fast. _____
11. I am bothered by dizzy spells. _____
12. I have fainting spells or feel faint. _____
13. I can breath in and out easily. _____
14. I get feelings of numbness and tingling in my fingers and toes. _____
15. I am bothered by stomachaches or indigestion. _____
16. I have to empty my bladder often. _____
17. My hands are usually dry and warm. _____
18. My face gets hot and blushes. _____
19. I fall asleep easily and get a good night's rest. _____
20. I have nightmares. _____

Make sure you answer every question. You cannot accurately score this quiz according to the formula below unless there is a response to each question!

Scoring and Discussion

Questions **5, 9, 13, 17, 19**: Score according to the following key:

a. None or a little of the time   = 4 points
b. Some of the time   = 3 points
c. Good part of the time   = 2 points
d. Almost always   = 1 point

Questions **1, 2, 3, 4, 6, 7, 8, 10, 11, 12, 14, 15, 16, 18, 20**: Score according to the following key:

a. None or a little of the time   = 1 point
b. Some of the time   = 2 points
c. Good part of the time   = 3 points
d. Almost always   = 4 points

Reference: W. W. K. Zung: "Self-Rating Anxiety Scale," © 1974

After you have given the proper points to each of your responses, add all of these numbers to get your total raw score. To convert your raw score to the Anxiety Index score, use the following formula:

$$\text{INDEX} = \frac{\text{Raw score total points}}{\text{Max score of 80 points}} \times 100$$

Once you have calculated your index score, you can then interpret it based on the following ranges:

Index Score Less than 45:   normal range
Index Score of 46–59:   presence of minimal to moderate anxiety
Index Score of 60–74:   presence of marked to severe anxiety
Index Score of 74 and above: presence of extreme anxiety

Anxiety disorders are very treatable—don't ignore it!. If your score is over 55, I encourage you to consult with your personal physician or a psychiatrist to have a more in-depth evaluation for possible medical factors causing your anxiety symptoms and negatively affecting your well-being. Don't forget that hormonal problems such as perimenopause, postparum ovarian decline, or throid imbalance can also cause significant anxiety symptoms that may mimic a primary anxiety disorder. It is also important to evaluate the possibility of panic disorder or a significant generalized anxiety disorder, which could respond well to medications and supportive therapy. Many types of alternative or complementary therapies are very useful in alleviating anxiety disorders. Among the ones I have recommended for my patients are those in the list that follows. You may find others to be helpful as well. I do think it is crucial to your health to have a good medical checkup, before assuming that your problems are "just" due to anxiety. There are over a **hundred different medical disorders** that can cause identical symptoms and may need specific and different treatments. Make sure your physician and your other therapists are working together to help you with the anxiety problems

Complementary Therapies Helpful for Anxiety

- acupuncture
- biofeedback
- hypnotherapy
- visualization and guided imagery exercises
- therapeutic massage for deep muscle relaxation
- jacuzzi herbal baths (using calming herbs)
- dietary changes and proper vitamin balance
- brisk walking
- aerobic exercise (to relieve buildup of excess adrenaline)
- eliminating alcohol, caffeine, and over-the-counter decongestants and sinus medications

Self Test: Do You Have an Eating Disorder?

This quiz is not diagnostic for the presence of an eating disorder. It can serve to alert you to problem areas that need to be changed or improved, and it will also alert you to the possibility that you may have an eating disorder. Both anorexia and bulimia may have serious medical complications, so it is important to have a professional evaluation if you suspect you may have an eating disorder. Anorexia nervosa is often called the starvation disease and it is far more common in women than men, particularly adolescents and college-age women. It is potentially fatal if not treated in a comprehensive approach by experienced medical and psychiatric professionals. Bulimia is often called the binge-purge disease and is also seen in the same age group as anorexia, with a similar prevalence in women. It may be cyclically aggravated by the menstrual cycle hormonal effects on appetite regulation mechanisms.

Directions: Answer each question YES or NO, then total the number of YES answers and the number of NO responses.

Are you presently at the optimal body weight for your height?	____YES	___NO
Do you feel overcome with fear of becoming fat?	____YES	___NO
Do you feel totally preoccupied with weight and thinness?	____YES	___NO
Do you feel fat most of the time?	____YES	___NO
Do you avoid letting people close to you see you without any clothes?	____YES	___NO
Do family and friends tell you that you are too thin or underweight, even though *you* feel *fat?*	____YES	___NO
Have you regularly restricted the amount of food you eat daily?	____YES	___NO
Do you tend to fuss around the kitchen, fixing food for others and not eating it?	____YES	___NO
Do you take laxatives or diuretics on a regular basis?	____YES	___NO
Have you ever taken laxatives and diuretics to lose weight?	____YES	___NO
Have your menstrual periods gotten *lighter, less frequent, or have they stopped completely?* (not due to hysterectomy or birth control pill use)	____YES	___NO
Has your body and scalp hair become thin and fine, or are you losing a lot of hair?	____YES	___NO
Do you exercise frantically, trying to burn off	____YES	___NO

calories and keep your weight down?

Have family and friends told you that you appear ____YES ___NO
to eat a large quantity of food, but you don't
gain weight?

Do you fast (not eat) for long periods of time? ____YES ___NO

Have you become *secretive* about eating, the food ____YES ___NO
you buy, and other food-related activities?

Have you made yourself vomit after large meals to ____YES ___NO
keep from gaining weight?

Have you frequently had weight fluctuations ____YES ___NO
greater than 10 pounds due to alternating binges
and fasts?

Do you frequently binge on high-calorie, easily ____YES ___NO
consumed foods like ice cream, cookies, fast food,
snacks, etc.?

Do you frequently end such eating episodes due to ____YES ___NO
falling asleep, to abdominal pain, or self-induced
vomiting?

Scoring and Discussion

The more YES answers you have, the more serious the eating disturbance. A score of 2 to 3 YES answers suggests that you have abnormal eating behaviors, which may lead to a serious eating disorder. You would benefit from seeking professional help to make healthy changes in your eating habits.

A score of 4 or more YES answers suggests that you have an existing eating disorder, which may already have created significant hazards to your health, such as bone loss and menstrual disruption. It is very important that you seek professional help **now** from an experienced eating disorders specialist. You should also talk honestly with your physician about your eating problems and ask to have a complete medical evaluation to determine what medical problems may be present or likely to happen. Eating disorders can be lethal. They are treatable, and help is available. Choose to *use* it!

Eating Disorders Questionnaire by Elizabeth Lee Vliet, M.D., 1988, revised 2000

Self Test: Do You Have OCD? Obsessions and Compulsions Checklist

	Current	Past
Aggressive Obsessions		
Fear might harm others	—	—
Fear might harm self	—	—
Violent or horrific images	—	—
Fear of doing something embarrassing	—	—
Fear will act on other impulses (e.g. rob bank, shoplift, cheat cashier)	—	—
Fear will be responsible for things going wrong (e.g., company will go bankrupt because of actions of self)	—	—
Fear something terrible will happen (e.g., fire, burglary, death or illness of relative/friend, miscellaneous superstitions)	—	—
Other:_____	—	—
Contamination Obsessions		
Concerns or disgust with bodily waste or secretions (e.g., urine, feces, saliva)	—	—
Concern with dirt or germs	—	—
Excessive concern with environmental contaminants (e.g., asbestos, radiation, toxic wastes)(e.g., asbestos,	—	—
Excessive concern with household items (e.g., cleansers, solvents, pets)	—	—
Concerned will get ill	—	—
Concerned will get others ill (Aggressive)	—	—
Other_____	—	—
Sexual Obsessions		
Forbidden or perverse sexual thoughts, images, or impulses	—	—
Content involves children	—	—
Content involves animals	—	—
Content involves incest	—	—
Content involves homosexuality	—	—
Sexual behavior toward others (Aggressive)	—	—
Other _____	—	—
Hoarding/Collecting Obsessions	—	—
Religious Obsessions	—	—
Obsession with Need for Symmetry, Exactness, or Order	—	—
Miscellaneous Obsessions		
Need to know or remember	—	—
Fear of saying certain things	—	—
Fear of not saying things just right	—	—
Intrusive (neutral) images	—	—
Intrusive nonsense sounds, words, or music	—	—
Lucky/unlucky numbers	—	—
Colors with special significance	—	—

<u>Ordering/Arranging Compulsions</u>   ___   ___

<u>Counting Compulsions</u>   ___   ___

<u>Somatic (Physical) Obsessions/Compulsions</u>   ___   ___

<u>Cleaning/Washing Compulsions</u>
Excessive or ritualized handwashing   ___   ___
Excessive or ritualized showering, bathing, toothbrushing,
    or grooming   ___   ___
Involves cleaning of household items or other inanimate
    objects   ___   ___
Other measures to remove contact with contaminants   ___   ___

<u>Checking Compulsions</u>
Checking doors, locks, stove, appliances, emergency brake
on car, etc.   ___   ___
Checking that did not/will not harm others   ___   ___
Checking that did not/will not harm self   ___   ___
Checking that nothing terrible will happen   ___   ___
Checking for contaminants   ___   ___

<u>Miscellaneous Compulsions</u>
Mental rituals (other than checking/counting)   ___   ___
Need to tell, ask, or confess   ___   ___
Need to touch   ___   ___
Measure to prevent: harm to self   ___   ___
     (Not checking)   harm to others   ___   ___
     terrible consequences   ___   ___
     other_____   ___   ___

Obsessive compulsive disorder is another type of biological illness, thought to be due to dysfunction in the serotonin-regulating mechanisms in the brain, which is manifested by intrusive unwanted thoughts (obsessions) and actions (compulsions). In its milder forms, it may not be noticed or may be seen as simply odd behavior. In its severe forms, it can be debilitating and may interfere with one's ability to live a normal life because the sufferer is so preoccupied with carrying out the actions that he or she is unable to carry on normal activities. It is much more common than previously thought and is no longer considered to be due primarily to unconscious *psychological conflicts*. This illness is now treated, usually very successfully, with the new serotonin-augmenting medications such as Prozac, Paxil, Luvox, or Celexa. Behavior therapy is also used as a component of treatment. Milder forms of obsessional thinking may also occur as symptoms of endocrine imbalance affecting the brain chemical messengers that regulate our thought processes. Examples include declining estradiol in postpartum or perimenopause, hyperthyroidism, and others.

If you have checked several of the items on this list and are troubled by OCD symptoms, I encourage you to consult with a hormone specialist to rule out endocrine problems, and then consult a psychiatrist knowledgeable with the newer treatment options. You may want to call the national OCD Foundation for a list of specialists in your area.

Reference: Yale OCD Checklist

Take Charge! Dr. Vliet's Guide to Periodic Personal Health Screenings

There are many different resources and recommended frequencies for health risk screenings. These are the recommendations that I feel are important for women and that will provide the best possibility of identifying disease in early and more treatable stages.

1. **Start your personal medical records notebook.** Keep an up-to-date list of diseases present in your family, copies of all your laboratory tests, mammograms, Pap reports, and other important health information.

2. **Self-exams:**
Breast - monthly, just after menses
Skin - a nurse practitioner colleague calls this "Your Mole Patrol," giving yourself a good look to see if any moles or skin "bumps" exhibit changes in size, shape, or color over time. **Frequency:** every six months from adolescence through age 35, monthly along with your breast exam after age 35. Report any suspicious changes to your physician or nurse practitioner.

3. **Physical Examination by your physician:**
Height and weight : annually
Blood pressure: Every year ages 14 to 40 ; two or more times per year after age 40 ; Two or more times a year **before age 40 if you**
 • have elevated or borderline blood pressure
 • take oral contraceptives
 • have had a hysterectomy (with or without ovaries removed)
 • have a history of heart disease
 • smoke cigarettes or use other tobacco products
 • are more than 10 percent overweight
 • have chronic diseases that require periodic blood pressure screening
 • take corticosteroids
 • have kidney disease.
 • have thyroid disease
 • drink alcohol on a daily basis

Breast: Every 1 to 3 years, ages 16 to 39; *annually after age 40.*

Pelvic exam: Every 1 to 2 years beginning when you become sexually active. *Every year after age 40 ; every 3 three years if you had a complete hysterectomy (removal of uterus, cervix and ovaries) for non-cancerous reasons (ACOG guidelines).*

Pap smear: Begin when you become sexually active. Ages 18 to 39, every 1 to 3 years after two negative results. *Every year after age 40 ; every 3 three years if you had a complete hysterectomy (removal of uterus, cervix and ovaries) for non-cancerous reasons (ACOG guidelines).*

Endometrial (uterine) tissue biopsy: American College of Obstetrics and Gynecology recommends an *annual* biopsy in women who are intolerant to progestin or progesterone and are taking estrogen alone. American Cancer Society recommends *one screening test* for the following situations (frequency of additional tests based on physician recommendations):

- if you have anovulatory cycles
- if you have a history of infertility
- if you have abnormal uterine bleeding
- if you are postmenopausal and is considering estrogen replacement therapy (ERT)
- if you develop bleeding a year or more after menopause and are not on any hormone therapy
- if you are taking tamoxifen

Rectal exam for occult blood (digital): Once a year after age 40.

Proctosigmoidoscopy or colonoscopy: for polyps, tumors, bleeding, etc. Every 3 to 4 years after age 50; annually if at high risk for cancer.

4. Laboratory/Screening Tests

Bone density measurement: I recommend this be done for a baseline by age 40, *or earlier* if multiple risk factors for bone loss are present. Waiting until after menopause is too late in my opinion. I recommend Dual Energy X Ray Absorptiometry (DEXA) as the safest and most useful procedure. DEXA uses far less radiation and is much less expensive than CT scans. Heel and wrist scans are not as reliable as DEXA scans of hip and spine: the former are often normal even when significant bone loss is present in the hip or spine.

Mammogram, alone or with breast ultrasound: Baseline exam at age 35 if no family history of breast cancer.
If there is a **positive family history** of breast cancer in mother or sister(s), the baseline should be done **before age 35.**
Normal risk: every 1 to 2 years from age 40 to 50.
High risk (positive family history): annually from age 35 onward.
Normal risk: Every year after age 50.

Electrocardiogram: Baseline at age 40, then every 3 to 5 years. There is controversy about the value of screening exercise (treadmill) "stress" EKG in women. I recommend that this be done if you are beginning a new exercise program and are overweight or have existing medical problems. Such testing may also be recommended by your physician if you develop chest pain or shortness of breath with mild exertion.

Chest X ray: Annually if you are a smoker or have a significant family history of lung cancer. Every 3 to 5 years if symptoms warrant.

Cholesterol testing (must be done fasting for reliable results, and must include HDL cholesterol to be useful in assessing risk of heart disease. Women also need to include fasting triglycerides with the fasting cholesterol profile):
Every 5 years, beginning in early teen years. Twice or more per year if the following situations exist:
- extreme changes in weight
- marked changes in level of activity have occurred
- if you have been ill or begin new medications that may affect cholesterol
- if you become menopausal (after surgery or naturally) and do not take estrogen; once a year if taking estrogen
- if you have high blood pressure or diabetes mellitus
- if you suspect or have been diagnosed with a thyroid disorder
- if you had previously been found to have high cholesterol or triglycerides

- if you smoke cigarettes or use other tobacco products
- if you drink more than 2 glasses of wine (or equivalent) daily
- if you take corticosteroids over a long period of time
- life changes or other chronic diseases that affect cholesterol

Fasting blood glucose (sugar): Every 3 to 5 years after age 20, if within normal limits. **Annually after age 35 if you are at high risk of diabetes based on:**
- family history of diabetes
- overweight
- have gained more than 20 pounds in the last year
- have gained weight around the middle of your body
- experience new onset sweet cravings, increased thirst, increased urination

Thyroid: Baseline test at age 35, unless indicated earlier. Then every 2 years. **Should include TSH for women and thyroid antibodies since these are more sensitive indicators of subtle (subclinical) thyroid disorders.**

Ovarian Hormones: Baseline estradiol, progesterone, testosterone, DHEA, in your 20s or 30s when you are feeling really well. Be sure that you have the blood serum tests done to give a picture of both total and free hormones. Urine and saliva tests do not give as complete a picture of the hormone reserve that is available for action in the body. Do at the mid-luteal phase and early follicular phase of your menstrual cycle as discussed earlier in my book. Then recheck these levels if/when you develop symptoms, or after a tubal ligation, after hysterectomy, or when you change your hormone Rx. Having your healthy baseline gives you a target range to aim for with any later hormone replacement. Checking levels after starting hormone therapy helps you be certain that you are above the currently accepted thresholds for preserving bone, brain, heart and other benefits of estradiol.

CA 125 : A cancer antigen that may be elevated in both ovarian cancer and several benign conditions such as endometriosis, fibroids, ovarian cysts and early pregnancy. Although not diagnostic for ovarian cancer, it is the best early warning test we have at this time and I think it is important to have done if you have a familiy history of ovarian cancer, or if you have vague abdominal symptoms (gas, bloating, distension, change in bowel movements, pain, etc.) that are not responding to other measures.

Ferritin : A measure of iron stores, associated with fatigue syndromes if too low *or* too high. Iron overload, or *hemachromatosis*, is a potentially serious disorder that may lead to increased risk of heart attack, liver damage and other problems. I recommend including this in your annual check-up, along with the complete blood counts.

Hemoglobin and hematocrit: Every 3-5 years, unless anemic (then annually until stabilized).

Sexually Transmitted diseases: Annually or more often if high risk based on having multiple sexual partners **or if you have failed to use a condom**

Tuberculosis: Annually if in health care profession. If high risk, as indicated.

Personal Prevention Guidelines by Elizabeth Lee Vliet, MD ©1994, revised 2000

Check List: Questions to Ask Your Women's Health Center

Many facilities are now calling themselves "women's health centers," but the resources and types of staff available vary considerably. Some are just traditional medical practices repackaged under a new name designed to attract women. Evaluate *your* center by asking the following questions. Is the women's health center you are visiting the real thing? It probably is if the answer to most of these questions is YES.

1. Is the first step a careful and thorough assessment of you as a total person, rather than just treating the presenting symptom? Are hormonal factors checked?

2. Is the initial visit at least 45 minutes, with subsequent visits at least 20 minutes?

3. Are the physicians interested and do they listen to YOUR ideas about your health?

4. Are the physicians willing to take time to talk with you about your concerns and to answer your questions about your health?

5. Does the care you receive emphasize **prevention** of health problems in addition to the treatment of acute problems?

6. Does the center utilize a range of health care providers including such professionals as nutritionists, exercise physiologists, massage therapists, chiropractors, and others?

7. Is there an emphasis on noninvasive treatments (such as lifestyle changes) first, rather than just giving medications for symptoms?

8. Do the physicians offer a choice of treatment options and explain the pros and cons (or the benefits and risks) of each, rather than using only the medication approach?

9. Does the center offer evaluation of your emotional well-being as well as your physical problems?

10. Does the center offer counseling and psychotherapy with psychiatric physicians who are able to treat the mind *and* the body together?

11. Does the center have or urge patients to use a medical library that includes non-technical resources for the layperson? Does your physician give you references to read further about your health concerns?

12. Are there free or low-cost educational programs and self-help support groups available on site?

13. Does the staff make you feel comfortable, secure, and confident that they care about you as a woman and treat you as an individual?

14. Does the staff take your concerns seriously, and do you feel they listen?

15. Does the center make an effort to solicit your feedback and ideas about how to improve services?

The more YES answers you have, the more likely you will find that this women's center is able to meet your individual health needs and provide you with additional resources beyond those provided on site at the center.

Check List by Elizabeth Lee Vliet, MD ©1984, revised 2000

Index

For <u>Individual Medical Consultations</u>:

1. We have a centralized appointment scheduling process for our consultations, and this is managed from the Texas office, whether your consult occurs in either Tucson or Texas. Please contact the Patient Services Coordinator in Texas at *HER Place: Health, Enhancement and Renewal for Women, Inc.* To receive an **information package,** you may **mail request** to 2700 Tibbets Drive, Suite #100, Bedford TX 76022 (Dallas area, near DFW airport), **or call** 817-355-8008, Fax 817-355-8010.

2. Our Web site at <u>www.herplace.com</u>. You may download and print the information forms and personal history forms that are used to schedule an appointment in either location. Then contact the Texas office as shown above.

To arrange SPEAKING ENGAGEMENTS, SEMINARS, WORKSHOPS, or a PRECEPTORSHIP FOR HEALTH PROFESSIONALS, please contact:

Kathryn A. Kresnik
Vice President, Director of Operations
HER Place
Phone: *972-564-5089,* FAX 972-564-1786
Email: <u>kkrez@aol.com</u> or <u>www.herplace.com</u>
Regular mail: P.O. Box 64507, Tucson, AZ 85728

Arizona office information: *HER Place:*
Health, Enhancement and Renewal for Women, Inc.
Mailing address: P.O. Box *64507,* Tucson, AZ 85728
Or call *520-797-9131,* fax 520-797-2948.